Cambridge History of Medicine

EDITORS: CHARLES WEBSTER AND CHARLES ROSENBERG

Health, race and German politics
between national unification and
Nazism, 1870–1945

OTHER BOOKS IN THIS SERIES

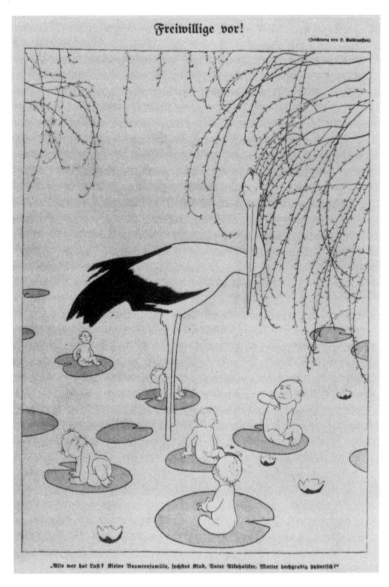

„Also wer hat Lust? Kleine Beamtenfamilie, sechstes Kind, Vater Alkoholiker, Mutter hochgradig hysterisch!"

'Volunteers to the fore' by Olaf Gulbransson, from *Simplicissimus*, vol. 18 no. 31 (1913).
'Who wishes to join the family of a minor official as the sixth child? The father is an alcoholic
and the mother suffers from high-grade hysteria.'

Health, race and German politics between national unification and Nazism, 1870–1945

PAUL WEINDLING
University of Oxford, Wellcome Unit for the History of Medicine

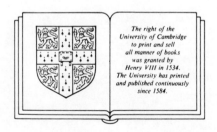

The right of the
University of Cambridge
to print and sell
all manner of books
was granted by
Henry VIII in 1534.
The University has printed
and published continuously
since 1584.

CAMBRIDGE UNIVERSITY PRESS

CAMBRIDGE

NEW YORK   NEW ROCHELLE   MELBOURNE   SYDNEY

Published by the Press Syndicate of the University of Cambridge
The Pitt Building, Trumpington Street, Cambridge CB2 1RP
32 East 57th Street, New York, NY 10022, USA
10 Stamford Road, Oakleigh, Melbourne 3166, Australia

First published 1989

Printed in Great Britain by The University Press, Cambridge

British Library cataloguing in publication data

Weindling, Paul
Health, race and German politics between national
unification and Nazism, 1870–1945.
1.Germany. Health service. Policies of government
1870–1945
I.Title
362.1'0943

Library of Congress cataloguing in publication data

ISBN 0 521 36381 0

CONTENTS

ILLUSTRATIONS AND TABLES

ILLUSTRATIONS

TABLES

PREFACE

During the writing of this book, public interest in the politics and funding of health has steadily increased. The same is true for the record of the German medical profession under Nazism. Although my study was originally conceived as a more modest account of state public health administration between 1900 and 1933, it became impossible to ignore broader questions of the interaction with professional organizations and concerned public groups. Today's debates on the costs of services resonate with echoes from a past age when the German welfare state, often referred to as pioneering, began its rapid but ramshackle pattern of growth. Ironically, it achieved its most complete and coherent development in the midst of terror and mass killing. The state and the people were brought into ever closer contact, as the rise of eugenics led to the invasion of the home and control over personal behaviour.

There have been many reasons why the completion of this book has surprised no one more than its author. The following list of thanks is no perfunctory courtesy but testifies to a combination of great personal kindness and generous support on the part of others. My first expression of thanks is owed to Charles Webster. For the past ten years I have been fortunate to be a member of the Wellcome Unit for the History of Medicine, University of Oxford, and under his direction, the Unit has been a continuously lively and challenging place to develop new approaches to the social history of health care. I also owe especial thanks to Margaret Pelling, who has been immensely supportive in all aspects of research and writing. I have benefited from contacts with German researchers that go far beyond the strictly academic, for I have received much generous help and hospitality when visiting archives. A seminal event was a conference on the social history of medicine held in 1981 at the Centre for Inter-Disciplinary Research, Bielefeld, and organized by Alfons Labisch (Kassel) and Reinhard Spree (Konstanz), both of whom have published highly innovative studies on health and social change. Many of the papers presented to the first and subsequent meetings have been published as substantial monographs, and I am all too aware that this book comes at the end of a long line of pioneering academic initiatives. I have also enjoyed fruitful relations with Florian

Tennstedt (Kassel), who not only sent me his fundamental publications on the German welfare state but also encouraged me with advice and source materials. Similar encouragement and help has been received from Stephan Leibfried, Dietrich Milles and Rainer Müller of the University of Bremen. Georg Lilienthal (Mainz) has provided a link between social history and the history of medicine. I consulted an important collection of printed sources at the Medizinhistorisches Institut (Mainz), when under the directorship of Gunter Mann, who has initiated a series of dissertations on *Biologismus*, and has published a number of valuable articles on themes dealt with in this book. The Institut für Geschichte und Theorie der Medizin, Münster, allowed me generous access to their library. Manfred Stürzbecher, the historian of public health in Berlin, has been a valued source of advice. I have had lively discussions with Peter Weingart and his group of researchers at Bielefeld, and with Sheila Weiss (Potsdam, New York) who have parallel projects on the history of eugenics. I have exchanged ideas with medical historians in the German Democratic Republic in connection with the major project on medicine under fascism, directed by Achim Thom (Leipzig). British colleagues who have provided crucial help are Richard Evans (Norwich), Elizabeth Harvey (Salford), Jon Harwood (Manchester), and Jeremy Noakes (Exeter), and I also wish to thank Volker Berghahn (Brown University). Gunnar Broberg (Uppsala) and Ann Harrington (Harvard) kindly sent copies of archival material, and during the final stages of writing I was sent a manuscript on German genetics by Adela Baer (Oregon).

The families of leading figures in this study have generously shared their memories, and provided documentation, often in considerable quantities. I wish to thank Hermann Blaschko (Oxford), Iring Fetscher (Frankfurt-on-Main), Widukind Lenz (Münster), Kurt Nemitz (Bremen), Wilfrid Ploetz (Herrsching), Otto Spatz (Munich), and Edith Zerbin-Rüdin (Munich). Professor Lenz commented at length on a draft of my manuscript. I am also indebted to archivists and librarians at institutions mentioned in the list of archives.

As regards financial support, I wish to thank the Wellcome Trust for funding my posts as Research Assistant and Research Officer at the Wellcome Unit. The research expenses associated with foreign travel have been largely financed by the Deutscher Akademischer Austauschdienst, the Economic and Social Research Council/Deutsche Forschungsgemeinschaft scheme for visiting social scientists, the British Council exchange scheme with the German Democratic Republic, the Royal Society, and the Rockefeller Archive Center.

Perhaps it is appropriate to dedicate a book that makes much of family allegiances and the birth rate to Julia Taplin and Silvia.

ABBREVIATIONS

ARGB	Archiv für Rassen- und Gesellschaftsbiologie
BA	Bundesarchiv
BAK	Bundesarchiv Koblenz
DMW	Deutsche Medizinische Wochenschrift
GSTA	Geheimes Staatsarchiv
HSTA	Hauptstaatsarchiv
MMW	Münchener Medizinische Wochenschrift
MPG	Max Planck Gesellschaft
RAC	Rockefeller Archive Center
STA	Staatsarchiv
VGB	Veröffentlichungen aus dem Gebiet der Medizinalverwaltung
ZSTA M	Zentrales Staatsarchiv Dienststelle Merseburg
ZSTA P	Zentrales Staatsarchiv Dienststelle Potsdam

Introduction
Science and social cohesion

The rise of science during the nineteenth century was associated with liberal values of education, intellectual freedom and humanitarianism. These values were incorporated into medicine, as it developed as a scientifically based profession with the humanitarian task of the relief of suffering. The health of the individual and family were regarded as the basis of personal well-being and prosperity, and of a civilized and productive society. A progressive and educated society was to be sustained by free trade, manufacturing and technical progress. Advances in science and medicine were synonymous with social progress.

In addition to their instrumental roles in improving health and harnessing the powers of nature, science and medicine served to define the social status of intellectual elites. Scientifically educated experts acquired a directing role as prescribers of social policies and personal lifestyle. The scientific creeds of Social Darwinism and eugenics offered general models for constructing an ordered and developing society. As such, science and medicine provided an alternative to party politics, by forming a basis for collectivist social policies to remedy social ills. Whereas the state was reluctant to intervene in industry and commerce in order to limit the ill-effects of industrialization, eugenicists planned intervention in family life and sexuality. The concept of a fit and healthy social organism provided a means for realizing renewed stability, social integration and national power. The achievements of German unification were considered to be threatened by the fragmentation of economic competition, class conflict, the rise of industrial technologies, concentrations of the poor in factories and insanitary tenement blocks, and declining family size. Health was not only an ideology of national integration at a time of rapid social change, but it also could ensure national unity through a uniform life style in everyday life. Scientific medicine thus defined an elite profession which would take a leading role in consolidating national unification.

Party politics in Imperial Germany was exceptionally narrow because of the restrictive franchise and a distinctive disdain of party political machinations. During the 1870s liberal convictions were on the wane among university academics who became sceptical of party politics as divisive and partisan and as lacking in an impartial concern for the national interest. The liberal political inputs into the sciences weakened, and science itself became regarded as the basis for authoritative pronouncements on social ills. To understand processes of decision-making in the sphere of social reforms, one has to look beyond the political parties to interest groups, administrators and elite groups of notables or *Honoratioren* in Imperial Germany. These joined the emergent professions in participating in health and welfare organizations as part of a broad movement of social imperialism entailing domestic social reform. There was intense public involvement in welfare organizations, and their official functions were extended to give considerable scope to professional experts and administrators. Public health reformers had only a rudimentary sense of accountability to the public, as they developed an institutional infrastructure in associations and the state for the provision of welfare. Control of sickness insurances, municipal welfare and voluntary organizations was recognised as of strategic political importance. The political values underlying social institutions were transformed by the rise of authoritarian and collectivist forms of social organization.

Science and medicine were shaped by the politics of social status and the economics of class relations. This study is concerned with how German bourgeois values, which nurtured and inspired science and medicine, became associated with collectivist plans for social reform. As science enlarged areas of social activity, it became subject to conflicting socialist and nationalist strategies of development. Underlying party political differences were diverse conceptions of a collectivist welfare state reliant on technocratic administration and professional expertise of a scientifically educated medical profession. Doctors became imbued with a sense of social responsibility to promote the nation's health and to ensure the survival of the nation as a competitive world power. Eugenicists argued that doctors should treat patients in the interests of society and future generations. The sense of responsibility of the doctor to sick individuals weakened as awareness dawned of the economic costs of poverty and disease. Although German science and medicine lost their position of world leadership during the twentieth century, scientific social planning was to re-build the German economy and the health of the population after the catastrophic defeat of 1918. Medical sciences became caught up in authoritarian politics and posed threats to personal liberties and autonomy. Ultimately a racial concept of health was central to National Socialism. The illiberal creeds of racism and National Socialism became paradigmatic for the abuse and misapplication of science and medicine.

Popular ideology and technocratic expertise

The nineteenth century was rich in alternative types of science and medicine, associated with conflicting social interests. Public opinion included many varieties of scientistic and socio-biological beliefs. There was the vision of science as a democratic and open type of knowledge. Popular science lectures went with ideas of self-education and self-help, and with socialist expectations of co-operation and unity. Some of the most widely disseminated forms of science were part of a broader movement for secular materialism. There were holistic alternatives to mechanistic theories that emphasized how nature was greater than any fragmentary analysis in rational and experimental terms of academic science. There was the potential for science as a form of democratic ideology; mass education would purge societies of ignorance, privilege and superstition. But as science became the domain of privileged professionals, it became ever more inaccessible to the average citizen; science and democracy could be conceptualized as antitheses. Doctors believed that the collective well-being of society meant that they could experiment on, treat and segregate the sick and the deviant without individual consent. Self-help and radical ideas of the individual's right to health weakened as medical and welfare institutions proliferated and the medical profession consolidated its power and status. The common spheres of public discourse became enclosed by expert groups.

Science was polarized between elitist and populist models. As a popular ideology, science used the means of mass communication that it had helped to invent. Printing – becoming both cheaper and technically more sophisticated – created the possibility of a mass market for scientific literature with strikingly illustrated encyclopaedias, popular magazines and textbooks. Diagrams became vibrant visual images when transferred to wall charts, dioramas, slides, and models such as the spectacular Visible Man at hygiene exhibitions. Societies and lecture halls for every branch of the natural world from astronomy to zoology, and commercial and public associations for aquaria, museums and zoos provided education and entertainment. Newspapers and journals helped to keep the public informed of intellectual breakthroughs so that science and medicine were part of a common cultural context. Railways and postal services sustained networks of communication facilitating scientific congresses and informal networks of correspondence, and the telegraph and newspapers communicated news of sensational discoveries like X-rays and of bacterial causes of diseases. Mass universal education from primary schools to public lectures for workers broadened access to knowledge. Advances in technology created possibilities for the mass production of high quality and reasonably priced instruments such as microscopes and telescopes. In addition to dissemination of the facts of science came the public expectation that this knowledge would be culturally and materially enriching, as well as providing a respectable leisure or professional pursuit. Such associations symbolized a popular commitment to liberal and secular culture based on natural laws and forces. During the mid nineteenth century there was a potential for science and medicine to be open, participatory and democratically organized.

Contrasting to science as a popular ideology was science as the expert knowledge of a technocratic elite. Knowledge as power motivated the appropriating of science to the domain of expert groups. Indeed, the very concept of the professional 'scientist' was a nineteenth-century invention, that pointed to the separation of the natural sciences from broader cultural movements. Scientific education and discoveries were accompanied by hopes of enhanced social status in the form of academic degrees, titles, medals and offices, as well as career opportunities and wealth. Statistical, historical, and anthropological data were collected on every aspect of society and nature. Although the natural sciences retained a commitment to the philosophical generalities of *Wissenschaft*, there was a tendency to reduce social and moral problems to scientific terms. Such an approach opened the possibility for scientific solutions to social problems. This was attractive to a state concerned with defusing socialist analysis of poverty, sickness and crime as the result of economic inequalities. Scientific solutions to social ills avoided public consultation, participation and accountability. The state fostered the development of pure research institutions in such areas as bacteriology. This had implications for health which became divided between strategies of self-help and popular learning (symbolized by the 'hygiene eye' of the entrepreneur August Lingner), and medical expertise. Technocratic science can be contrasted to science as a popular ideology supporting the democratic values of an open society.

While 'the age of the natural sciences' was to be based on liberal values of freedom of speech and publication, tolerance, and a free and thriving economy, there was no unanimity on the type of science to be deployed. Although the cultural and social values attached to science were associated with middle–class demands for German unification, there was a clash of interests. University teachers and students had taken a lead in the agitation for a united Germany. Traditions of academic freedoms were equated with liberal social freedoms and with culture as a form of national assertion. Yet there was division of opinion over whether science and culture should be the basis of an alternative set of reforming values, or primarily should augment national power. Universities and the sciences stood at the cross roads where the social interests of the educated middle classes and the state intersected. As university institutions were state funded and professors were appointed by the state, German academic life reflected the changing relations of the educated middle class, the *Bildungsbürgertum*, to the state. It was in the interests of both the middle class and the state to provide professional education for those who would be recruited into the ranks of officials, and into liberal professions such as medicine and law. Yet the value attached to learning went beyond either utility or scholarship. The vast effort devoted to science was envisaged as realizing higher ethical and social qualities. Scientific achievement would build Germany into a *Kulturstaat*, enshrining liberal values, and gaining international respect as the cultural leader of the civilized world.

The need to provide health and welfare for large urban populations was satisfied in a variety of ways. The state supported medical research as a basis for effective therapies. Municipal, state and insurance authorities financed expansion of hospitals and welfare institutions. These were to be staffed by scientifically educated professionals. The 'scientizing' of health was a product of industrialization and population growth with the need to prevent wastage of valuable resources of labour. Public health served to discipline and restrain the industrial workforce. There was a system of medical police with powers to quarantine, disinfect and, in the case of certain contagious diseases and mental illnesses, to detain in custody in hospital. Beyond its policing function, medicine was an agent of informal processes of socialization. The production of a healthy lifestyle, sanctified by scientific laws, was the outcome of subtle and informal processes of education, emulation, fashion and economic consumption. Processed foods, mass-produced clothing, contraceptives and such leisure activities as sports or walking reflected consumer demand for health promoting products and leisure activities. Bourgeois status was expressed not only in terms of economic and political power, but also in an orderly, self-disciplined and sober lifestyle that achieved widespread acceptability. Health was a means of attaining a cohesive and integrated society during the upheavals of industrialization. Yet whether scientific medicine or nature therapies and other popular anti-scientific ideologies held the keys to health was controversial. In such a conflict-ridden situation, the state initially tried to preserve a role as impartial umpire, but as it succumbed to the influence of professional experts, it adopted interventionist policies.

Eugenics and national health

Eugenics offers insight into the process of extending the dominance of a professionally controlled and biologically based form of health care. Eugenicists were prepared to do battle with rival strategies for reforming lifestyle and democratic socialization of medical services. They clashed with lay nature therapists and sexual reformers, and were critical of the socialist-dominated sickness insurances. Eugenicists demanded a reform of state authorities with powers being conceded to the medical profession. There were internal conflicts within the medical profession and among biologists over the role of biological heredity in determining health. The politics of health care can be gauged by the establishing of state, municipal and insurance authorities, and welfare associations, and by the influence within these of cliques of eugenic enthusiasts. Medical advance was to provide a de-politicized surrogate for civic rights and welfare reforms.

German eugenics raises the issue of how the noble vision of the civilized *Kulturstaat* took on authoritarian forms. Welfare policies undermined individual rights and reinforced state and professional power, creating an authoritarian social structure. The right of the individual to health was an important demand of the 1848 revolutions. Radical medical reformers instigated a campaign for a national ministry of health headed by a doctor. These democratic and professional demands were consistent as long as doctors were to be democratically accountable to workers' associations. But as science became more technical and the professions more organized, a contradiction developed in liberalism. Liberal schemes for universal education conflicted with the campaigns of liberal professions for freedoms from state controls and sovereign rights within their occupational sphere.

The public became reliant on the services of the medical profession, as medical scientists became an exclusive and privileged status group. While some perceived that a contradiction had emerged between the professional and the public interest, the professions claimed that they had authority to override individual rights in the interest of society and of future generations. Biology took a major role in the genesis of a distinctive form of racial ideology, and in establishing the threats of genetic defects to the health of the 'social organism'. There was loss of individual rights in the field of family affairs, health care and reproduction. The sick, the handicapped and the mentally disturbed were subjected to professional and state controls, which could result in compulsory institutionalization, sterilization or medical killing such as 'euthanasia'. Medicine was transformed from a free profession, as it was proclaimed by the German Confederation in 1868, to the doctor carrying out duties of state officials in the interests not of the individual patient but of society and of future generations. The medical profession demanded that it be granted a state-enforced medical monopoly of health care. Doctors became part of a growing state apparatus for registering the population and for eradicating undesirable diseases and racial characteristics. Scientific and medical advances were accompanied by the rise of authoritarian social values.

The social bases of German biology, its patronage by the state and popularity among a broad social spectrum, must be regarded as crucial elements in the transformation of German biology and medicine. Eugenics thus raises the issue of the middle-class response to national unification, to the rapid industrialization, population growth and urbanization in Imperial Germany, and to the First World War and its catastrophic aftermath. The 1860s and 1870s saw a wide dissemination of biological values, penetrating many features of scientific and middle-class culture of the *Bildungsbürgertum*. The development of the *Bildungsbürgertum* into the professional sector of the middle class with the growth of responsibilities of doctors, welfare workers and psychologists provided the circumstances for the transformation of general biological values into an organized eugenics movement. There was assimilation of hereditarian biology into medical techniques with the expectation of social control of the deviant and the biological reproduction of the social order in ways favourable to professional middle-class interests.

Eugenics, as a product of middle-class values and as associated with public health, poses historical questions which transcend the limitations of the conventional history of German racism. Hitherto the history of eugenics has been neglected because it has been seen as a product of ultra-nationalist racial (or *völkisch*) movements. According to this interpretation, the new anti-semitic rhetoric of the purity of blood and race which gathered force from the 1880s was realized inevitably in the Nazi genocide. But although there were connections between racial hygiene and anti-semitism, the situation was complex, and eugenics did not necessarily point the way towards Nazi racism. There were those of other political persuasions, liberal and socialist, who looked to biology and medicine as the means to engineer social improvements. It was not without good reason that one of the first attempts to explore the history of eugenics, organized by SS medical officials in the German heartland of Thuringia, concentrated on the issue of eugenics and socialism. My interpretation stresses that eugenics was authoritarian in that it offered the state and professions unlimited powers to eradicate disease and improve the health of future generations. But it was neither a product of the theory of a superior Aryan race, and nor was it inherently Nazi. The synthesis between Nazism and eugenics was a process of adaptation and appropriation on both sides.

Eugenics was closely linked to the attempt to move beyond party politics as divisive and partial, and to use science and medicine to obtain real improvements in social conditions. This presented a novel role for the professional expert. Most eugenicists were doctors, frustrated at the lack of career prospects in the overfull universities and in the overcrowded medical profession. They sought to colonize new areas for medicine, such as sexuality, mental illness, and deviant social behaviour. What had been private or moral spheres were subjugated to an hereditarian social pathology. Scientific solutions to such social problems as crime, vagrancy and poverty appealed to state authorities concerned with neutralizing social and political tensions. Yet inherent within eugenics were tensions between a modern science-based professional technocracy and racial ideology; while eugenics legitimated strategies of professional imperialism and of social control, it had a broader appeal to a populist movement of racial nationalism.

The scientificity and the professionalism of German eugenics endow it with similarities to eugenic movements in other countries. There was a widespread concern with racial degeneration in those countries undergoing comparable social processes of industrialization, declining birth rates and the emergence of professional elites. Lombroso's criminology and French hereditarian psychiatry provided two influential models for eugenic social engineering. In Britain, France and Germany there was a scientific and public debate on degeneration as produced by industrialization. There was a considerable time lag between Galton's proposing the term 'eugenics' in 1881 and the founding of the Eugenics Education Society in 1907 or the Racial Hygiene Society in Berlin in 1905. A liberal and secular cultural movement preceded the organization of special leagues and societies. Scientists such as Galton and Huxley in Britain, and Haeckel and Virchow in Germany, propagated scientistic values as surrogates for Christianity. Discussions of the social implications of Darwinism had penetrated many aspects of middle-class culture and welfare provisions before the founding of the Racial Hygiene Society. The experience of industrialization and of demographic change meant that issues such as the declining birth rate, the hereditary consequences of chronic diseases, and the problem of the degenerate residuum in the population could be seen as of widespread international relevance. Negative eugenic measures, such as steriliza-tion, were imitated in many countries. This was facilitated by hereditarian principles becoming standard in medicine and the social sciences.

The tendency in assessing the German path to social modernity has been to concentrate on the most extreme features differentiating Germany from the rest of the 'civilized world'. Anti-semitism, hostility to liberal democratic values, nationalism and the distinctive course of socio-political development have been identified as causes of how Germany came to threaten world stability and civilized values. It has been more comforting to heap the guilt for racism onto extremes that are remote from bourgeois liberalism than to investigate authoritarian elements in liberal science, professions and perceptions of social issues endemic in modern society, such as poverty, disease and crime. While it cannot be denied that anti-semitism and Aryan racism were forces in the eugenics movement, eugenics represented far more than these. Indeed, there were factions seeking to purge eugenics of 'unscientific' racialism. At one level this study is meant to provide an analysis of the changing intellectual and social composition of eugenics. It is also necessary to assess the influence of eugenic and racial theories, in order to specify at what point in time and to what extent eugenic and racist beliefs permeated diverse social sectors. Extensive use of archives of key individuals, scientific institutions and of state administrations has been made in order to assess the influence of eugenics, and to investigate the interaction of popular culture, medical and scientific expertise and professional organizations with the state apparatus of bureaucrats. Permeating these institutions and social strata were political and national ideologies. Eugenics illustrates social stratification and regional differences within the social and administrative structure of Germany. This interpretative approach will serve to isolate those features of German society and ideologies of social cohesion both distinctive from and comparable with other societies.

The transformation of utopia

The issues of science as the expression of the social interests of the educated middle classes, the rise of professionalism and the shift to authoritarian social values, result in the following scenario. The birth of German national unity in 1870 was accompanied by more profound economic and social change than the Prussian architects of national unity expected. Rapid industrial expansion and a surge in population growth meant that a range of political structures and values were resented as restrictive. The 1880s saw the repression of socialism, a peak in the numbers of emigrants, and dissident, middle-class groups disappointed by the lack of professional opportunities and by cultural and moral restrictions. Interventionist and repressive state social policies coincided with demands for overseas colonies and political campaigns against socialists and against the Jews as an alien race. The criticism of industrialization as divorcing humanity from nature was widespread. Public concern over industrial living and working conditions gave rise to innovative schemes of welfare legislation and social insurance from the 1880s. A vociferous lobby argued that society would be healthiest if the laws of biological evolution were allowed to function freely. Controversies erupted over human and animal experiments. Those who shrank from applying natural selection to society proposed 'humane' social mechanisms to improve the conditions of the population through fertility control.

Plans for utopian breeding settlements were formulated in the 1880s and 90s. These colonies were a reaction to the political and cultural repression, and harsh living conditions during German industrialization. During the 1890s the emphasis shifted to nationalist concerns with domestic social reform. Guidelines for a reformed life style were drawn up in accordance with the laws of biology and hygiene. These were variously termed *Volkshygiene, Rassenhygiene,* or *Sozialhygiene,* and were designed to prevent a supposed racial degeneration. Struggling young professionals sought the patronage of leading experts in biology, hygiene, and ethnology, and launched a movement for racial hygiene after the turn of the century. Moral decadence, chronic diseases like tuberculosis, venereal diseases and alcoholism, crime and deviant social behaviour – which included merely having two children or less – were diagnosed as symptoms of hereditary degeneration.

From the 1890s until the 1930s the movement for biological purity gathered strength. In Imperial Germany the eugenic movement was an elitist association, and sought to be a biologically regenerated type of aristocracy. Attempts were made to organize elite elements in other countries into an International Society for Racial Hygiene. The First World War marked a turning point in the transition from eugenics as cultural elitism to state social planning. During the war eugenic schemes to improve the quality of the race were considered by state officials concerned with the falling birth rate and with high military casualties. Defeat brought a profound transition in social values. Biology was looked to for providing guidelines for national reconstruction and for reinvigorating the German family and people. Eugenic concepts like that of an inherited constitution were accepted in medicine, biology, sociology and social work. There was a rapid expansion of custodial and therapeutic institutions such as mental hospitals designed to detain the large proportion of the population considered biologically inferior.

The economic crisis of 1929 brought support for the view that the costly state welfare apparatus could not be maintained. Negative eugenic measures such as sterilization gained support in a more authoritarian political climate. By 1932 sterilization legislation was prepared, and accepted by a wide range of Catholic, Jewish and socialist eugenicists. The Nazi takeover marked a fundamental change in the course of German eugenics. There was great emphasis on racial factors, and bureaucratic mechanisms were constructed for the implementation of public health policies on a racial basis. The concern with the economic burdens of the racially degenerate intensified; the category of the degenerate was enlarged to include 'races' such as Jews, gypsies, and slavs, social 'problem' groups such as criminals or the feeble minded, homosexuals, and women as the weaker sex. Biology justified the subordination and mass killing of the greater proportion of the population. Compulsory sterilization and 'euthanasia' of congenitally disabled children and mental patients were instituted. Yet racial hygiene in the Third Reich was far from a monolithic and unified body of ideology and policies. There were many conflicts between competing and diverse groups of racial hygienists in a power structure designed to proliferate competing hierarchies. Far from inevitable, the transition from sterilization to expansive 'euthanasia' measures provoked considerable dissension, and radical changes of principle. Nordic ideologies, medically oriented racial hygienists, and factions in the NSDAP (Nationalsozialistische Deutsche Arbeiterpartei) and SS (Schutz-Staffel) were in constant conflict.

During the Third Reich a heroic history of the racial hygiene movement was constructed. The movement was said to have paved the way for Nazism, owing to the appearance of schemes for improving the German race during the 1880s. Its founding fathers could claim prescience for having articulated and organized racial hygiene in such a way that it could be readily applied in the new order. Yet this history was a fabrication. Those who have assumed that eugenics was an offshoot of Aryan ideologies for racial purity and of anti-semitism have considered only the ultra-conservative fringe and have failed to understand the course, intention and scope of German eugenics. While there were links with *völkisch* racism and extreme nationalist groupings, eugenics has a history better understood from the perspectives of public health, social policy, and of the bio-medical sciences. Professional and bureaucratic groups disengaged from party politics as they sought a scientific basis for administration and for an ideology of social cohesion. As German academics prided themselves on their a-political objectivity, but also on their national commitments, eugenics was well suited to be an ideology of social integration. German biology and medicine assumed social tasks of national reconstruction.

This account of German eugenics has broader aims of providing insight into perceptions of major social changes: the declining birth rate, urban and rural social conditions, and debates on national identity. Eugenicists were confident that they could root out and exterminate the causes of mental and physical degeneracy, and transform daily life into a hygienic utopia of large, prosperous and patriotic families of sound 'eugenic' quality. This sense of power was accompanied by secularization of attitudes to life and confidence that biological processes could be fully brought under human control. Social cohesion was reinforced by biologistic ideologies of health, of a progressing social organism and of society as a 'human economy' for the reproduction of the population rather than profit. These developments resulted from changes in the fortunes of the academically educated, professional middle class, the *Bildungsbürgertum*, in their attitudes to an increasingly assertive working class. The medical profession's quest for social power was pursued through the channels of eugenics.

I

Social Darwinism

The vigour of German science and medicine derived from the emerging industrial economy. From the 1870s Germans were in the grips of processes of industrialization, population growth and urban expansion that were among the most rapid in Europe. Although German industry boomed, its development wavered between staggeringly high growth rates in some years and recession in 1878, 1891 and 1901.[1] Rapid expansion of iron and coal production was followed by the development of science-based industries for chemicals and electrical engineering. From the 1880s manufacture of dye-stuffs and pharmaceuticals began to take off. Industrial products such as Krupp steel, such aniline dyes as Bismarck Brown, or Siemens' telegraph, symbolized modern Germany. Agriculture, by way of contrast, stagnated and had to be artificially protected by high tariffs – itself an erosion of liberal economic principles.[2] The cataclysmic pace and contradictions of social change resulted in immense disparities between incomes, life expectancy, the growing labour market and employment opportunities. There were great differences in prosperity, working conditions and life style between regions, occupations and classes. The expanding cities lacked an adequate infrastructure of housing, education, sanitation and medical care. In addition to the purely economic costs of wages and machines, industrialization involved human and political costs, with sickness and poverty on an unprecedented scale.

German population growth outstripped the nation's productive capacity. By the 1860s there was a crisis of overpopulation with a 60 per cent growth since 1815. In the ten years from 1864 until 1873 one million emigrated. Germany became a nation of migrants, with the increase of seasonal labour, wholesale migration to cities and overseas emigration. Between 1871 and 1911 the population rose from 41 million to 65.3 million. The population was static or declining in rural areas,

---

[1] H. Rosenberg, 'Political and Social Consequences of the Great Depression of 1873–96 in Central Europe', in J.J. Sheehan (ed.), *Imperial Germany* (New York, 1976), pp. 39–60.
[2] V. Berghahn, *Modern Germany* (Cambridge, 1982), pp. 1–15.

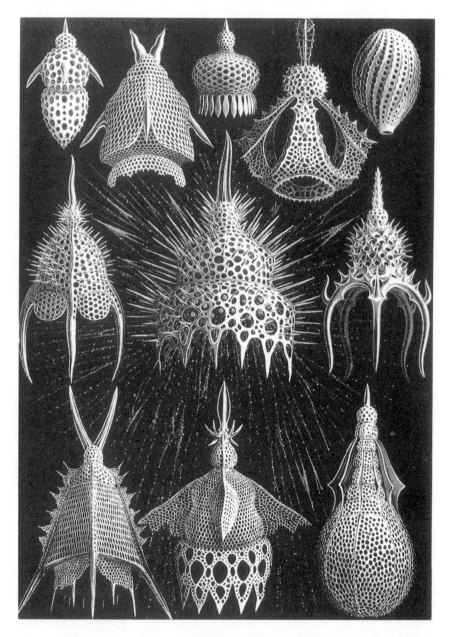

1 Ernst Haeckel, *Cyrtoidea* (or *Actinozoa*), from *Kunst-Formen der Natur*, Leipzig and Vienna 1899. Haeckel's vibrant images of marine organisms captivated the imagination of naturalist authors and artists. Wilhelm Boelsche's three-volume study of *Love Life in Nature* is an example of the popularization of Haeckel's monist biology.

whereas the population of the large cities with populations of over one million grew in size by sixfold.[3] In 1907 only half of the 60 million Germans still lived in their birth place. The effect of such mobility was to create great contrasts between those regions and localities retaining traditional characteristics, and the centres of population where the social fabric was bursting at its seams. These tensions heightened a sense of rootlessness, which was compensated for by national patriotism and an idealizing of biological values. From the 1890s attention was focused on solving the problems of large urban centres where industrial and population growth were concentrated.

The condition of the population was a cause for concern. Mortality reached an all time high in the early 1870s with 28.7 deaths per 1,000 inhabitants in 1872–73. Infants suffered the highest rates of mortality due to adverse social conditions, and the infant death rate remained high until the twentieth century. Despite the decline in adult mortality, there were a number of indicators of worsening social conditions. During the 1870s the rapidly expanding cities had far higher rates of mortality than small towns or rural areas. Major causes of mortality were diseases associated with poverty and industrial working conditions – the two most significant causes being tuberculosis and respiratory diseases. These diseases had a high (though unquantifiable) incidence, especially in overcrowded urban tenements. Officials and white collar workers were, in terms of health, highly privileged. The infant mortality rate in the families of unskilled industrial workers was twice as high as in the families of officials.[4] The norms for industrial workers were working days of between ten and twelve hours, for six days a week in often hazardous conditions involving contact with noisy and dangerous machinery, poisonous fumes, and dusty, toxic substances. Families lived in one or two rooms in dank tenement blocks, and generally took in overnight lodgers. The lack of drainage, sanitation and planning laws became evident, not least because the bourgeoisie felt threatened by epidemics.[5] The problems of industrial society were evident in the staggeringly high incidence of chronic degenerative diseases like VD, TB and alcoholism. Despite the continuing political dominance of the East Elbian Junkers, urban problems encroached on the political arena. Berlin was not only the centre of government but a rapidly expanding industrial city: it meant that leading administrators and notables could not fail to be struck by how the growth of the urban proletariat was accompanied by social misery and political radicalism. 'The social question' preoccupied a range of political parties as well as the ruling elite. Whether Germany should be an 'agricultural state' or an 'industrial state' was debated. The inexorable rates of population growth prompted the question as to whether Germany should alleviate mass poverty and become a 'social welfare state'. How the anxieties over the nation's industrial future permeated the ideas and aspirations of middle-class professionals in the expanding centres of population is of

[3] P. Marschalck, *Bevölkerungsgeschichte Deutschlands im 19. und 20. Jahrhundert* (Frankfurt-on-Main, 1984). [4] R. Spree, *Soziale Ungleichheit vor Krankheit und Tod* (Göttingen, 1981), p. 56.
[5] Spree, *Soziale Ungleichheit*, pp. 30–49.

special interest as medical experts documented and offered solutions to the social problems of poverty and disease.

The demise of liberalism

The decade between 1866 and 1877 is often characterised as a 'liberal era'. This was also a period when liberals divided between National and Progressive Parties, a political split which resulted from parliamentary disagreements over proposals of Bismarck for a financial indemnity for the victorious Prussian army of 1866. The principle of 'unity versus freedom' exposed the contradiction in liberalism between the yearning for a strong and vigorous nation and the quest for enlarging individual autonomy. Whatever the political fluctuations of the two wings of liberalism, as a social movement liberalism had an impressive effect during the 1860s and 70s.[6] Liberalism set the tone of middle-class and official attitudes. The oppressive burdens of state regulations of commerce, education and population movements – with restrictions on marriage and mobility – were steadily eased. In its administrative procedures, political constitution and commercial regulations, Germany acquired many liberal institutions that shaped the basic ground rules of the Imperial state. Municipalities took pride in the principle of autonomous self-administration. Professions such as medicine campaigned for the removal of the burden of state controls on practitioners. In 1868 medicine was proclaimed a 'free trade', open to all to practice. In addition to academically educated doctors, anyone could trade in healing or cures without legal penalties against quackery.[7] The only restrictions concerned general penalties against fraud and physical assault, and the legal protection of the title *Arzt*.[8] Leaders of the profession such as Rudolf Virchow were convinced that scientific excellence guaranteed the future of the profession.

From about 1878 there was a sharp change of mood. A political crisis arose due to Otto von Bismarck breaking his alliance with the liberal parties; he switched economic allegiances from free trade and a non-interventionist state to protectionism in order to shore up the Junker agrarian elite. The reassertion of conservative authority was rooted in an economic crisis. But the changes in values were so profound as to require explanation at a deeper level. The crisis shattered the faith of many Germans in liberal freedoms. Bismarck implemented the draconian laws banning the recently united SPD (Sozialdemokratische Partei Deutschlands) in 1878. Attempts were made by the Association for Social Policy[9] to use social scientific analysis as a surrogate means for attaining social reform, so providing an academic alternative to both liberalism and socialism. The commercial and

---

[6] J.J. Sheehan, *German Liberalism in the Nineteenth Century* (London, 1982), pp. 123–40.
[7] *Kurpfuscherei.*
[8] I have generally used 'doctor' as a translation for *Arzt*, although the title *Doktor* could apply to someone with a doctorate in any discipline. The less common English term 'physician' excludes surgeons and therefore also has misleading connotations.   [9] *Verein für Sozialpolitik.*

academic status groups in the middle class were becoming more cohesive, as the newly enriched sectors of society accounted for an increasing proportion of students. This precipitated a crisis in that the universities were producing a surplus of qualified graduates. Reactions to these developments were varied, but intense. Strategies of political mass mobilization for national ends were initiated, bringing with them the appearance of anti-semitism and popular imperialism, and the repression of socialism. The advent of racial and political anti-semitism in the 1880s indicates the public mood; the movement for overseas colonies was supported by a popular imperialist crusade. Among those profoundly influenced by the emergence of racism and social imperialism was a group of schoolboys, who were to provide the germ of the eugenic movement.

Historians have pursued the themes of political mobilization either in terms of the major political parties, and their performance in national and local elections, or in 'imperialist' or 'radical nationalist' associations. The crisis of industrialization affected not only the party political system, but also shaped in less demonstrative but perhaps ultimately more enduring terms the social structures of the emergent professions, and welfare associations and institutions. Scientistic ideologies of the nation as an organically cohesive social organism show the limits of party politics in a social system that relied on expertise and welfare mechanisms to solve social problems. The professional and welfare organizations were intensely political in that conflicts in social values were apparent in the aims of directing elites and in the organizing of popular participation. Frequent disagreements over the structure and aims of hygiene organizations reflected national political divisions. There was awareness that the industrial social order required controlling institutions that had to be set up on a collectivist model. Doctrinaire individualism was exposed as inadequate to solve social problems. This was especially clear in the sphere of public health where sanitation, water supply, and control of infections all required supervisory state or municipal sanitary and medical officials and institutions. The Hamburg cholera epidemic of 1891–92 dealt a death blow to government on the model of oligarchic and non-interventionist liberalism.[10] The problem of welfare reforms was apparent to revisionist socialists, who felt that revolutionary Marxism was inappropriate, given the opportunities provided by participating in the expanding system of sickness insurances and municipal welfare. Expertise and social organization required a collectivist philosophy that was supplied by social biology.

Biological expertise

Industrialization transformed the medical sciences and institutions. There were fundamental scientific breakthroughs, which in the short-term were controversial and inconclusive, but which in the long-term subordinated conceptions of life to

[10] R.J. Evans, *Death in Hamburg* (Oxford, 1987).

medicine and biology. The years of the late 1870s and early 80s saw biological discoveries of laws of health and reproduction. In the mid 1870s Darwinian biologists discovered the process of fertilization as the fusion of the egg and sperm as two cells. Observations and experimental manipulation of the cell nucleus and chromosomes led to the belief that heredity and evolution could be somehow controlled at reproduction through selective breeding or improving conditions surrounding conception and pregnancy. The sensational discovery of bacteria as causes of such infections as anthrax (in 1876) and TB (in 1882) led to the germ theory of disease: a specific bacillus was postulated as the cause of a specific disease, by showing that a disease could be reproduced experimentally. Such discoveries were part of a series of breakthroughs in scientific medicine. Others included diagnostic innovations and the discovery of antiseptics. While the actual effect of such discoveries on health was limited, they enhanced the prestige of the medical profession both with the public and with state officials. Medical discoveries ushered in interventionist health and social policies as diagnostic and therapeutic institutions proliferated.

Coinciding with these scientific developments were innovative 'social technologies' of integration.[11] Drawing together ideas of health as a means of social and economic integration, and appropriating a radical and self-help tradition of independent sickness funds, Bismarck instituted sickness insurance in 1883. This was part of a package of legislation which also included invalidity benefits, accident insurance (in 1885) and pensions (in 1887). These had limited impact in the short-term but over the next decades set a pattern of state-regulated social welfare. Hitherto, there had been coercive Poor Law regulations, segregating the visibly destitute such as the vagabonds and beggars. Poor Law welfare entailed a loss of political rights, and detention in workhouses. Classification, custody and control applied only to a small strata of the impoverished. Demographic and industrial expansion made the connection between poverty and disease a question of broader political importance, and special concern was voiced over the health of industrial wage earners. Whereas the activities of friendly societies and sickness funds had been largely unregulated, compulsory insurance was a mechanism that regulated social relations in the expanding industries.[12] The state legislated for insurance on the basis of compulsory contributions by employers and workers. In 1885 there were 4,294,000 insured workers compared with 13,566,000 in 1913, a rise from 9 per cent to 20 per cent of the population.[13] Attention shifted from the destitute to more prosperous workers. Sickness insurance was restricted to selected groups of workers – who happened to be those deemed especially prone to socialism. Insurance spread more rapidly in the largest cities such as Berlin. Benefits were only for the insured individual – so excluding dependant wives and children – and were at low levels and of short duration. Widespread diseases such as VD were excluded

[11] G. Göckenjan, *Gesundheit und Staat machen* (Frankfurt-on-Main, 1985).
[12] U. Frevert, *Krankheit als politisches Problem 1770–1880* (Göttingen, 1984).
[13] Spree, *Soziale Ungleichheit*, p. 102.

(because the sickness was attributed to immorality), as well as benefits at childbirth. As the insurance system was extended, it provided mechanisms of socialization and integration. From the 1890s categories of insured workers and the scope of insurance benefits steadily increased. Medical science took part in the socializing of the industrial populace, as many workers visited a scientifically educated doctor for the first time. Hunger and exhaustion were to be 'treated' with hospital stays and medicines. A few renegade insurances experimented with allowing payment for nature therapists, but they were subjected to bitter attack by the medical profession as subsidizing 'quackery'. The most innovative insurances offered medical care to family dependants, subsidized TB sanatoria and health education. The effect was to erode the traditions of lay care and self-help in medicine.[14]

There was a rush to study medicine in order to profit from the opportunities of insurance-financed practice. A catastrophic overproduction of doctors resulted. In 1876 there were 13,728 doctors in the Reich; by 1900, there were 27,374 doctors.[15] These doctors were concentrated in towns and cities. In the longer term, sickness insurance was fundamental to the establishment of corporate social structures. The Bismarckian law laid down strict parameters regarding the operation of the system, but it was not as such a state system. The sickness insurances were autonomous bodies governed jointly by employers and insured workers on the liberal principle of 'self-administration'.[16] They drew workers into developing reformist strategies. When the SPD was legalized in 1890, many socialists found a career in the administration of the insurances. Although insurances could not reduce the risks to existence entailed by industrial work, they at least provided rudimentary care for the sick and the invalids. Insurance statistics were frequently cited by socialists as evidence for the crippling effects of industrial work. They reinforced workers' sense of solidarity. When sanatoria were provided, socialists formed groups for politicizing patients. Medical insurance and institutions were regarded as means of health education, and for the inculcating of an orderly and healthy lifestyle. Socialist doctors retrospectively welcomed the insurance laws as creating a means of socializing the old, sick and invalid in a way equivalent to mass schooling.[17]

The insurance system was the making of the medical profession. During the liberal decades of the 1860s and 1870s, medical associations were founded which were mainly of a scientific character. Leaders of the profession, such as the National Liberal Eduard Graf, campaigned from 1884 for representative organizations to offset the influence of the insurances. A law of 1887 required that medical chambers representing doctors be established by doctors in each province. These official bodies known as *Ärztekammer*[18] enabled the profession to articulate economic and socio-political demands. Doctors began to campaign for self-regulation as they

[14] F. Tennstedt, *Vom Proleten zum Industriearbeiter. Arbeiterbewegung und Sozialpolitik in Deutschland 1800 bis 1914* (Cologne, 1983).   [15] Spree, *Soziale Ungleichheit*, p. 99.   [16] *Krankenkassen*.
[17] Frevert, *Krankheit*, pp. 314–32; Tennstedt, *Vom Proleten*, pp. 462–4.
[18] There is no English equivalent; based on analogy to 'chambers of commerce', I have used 'medical chambers' or 'chambers of doctors'.

resented the economic controls by which sickness insurances were able to dictate fees and select practitioners. The *Ärztekammer* extended their competence to general questions of public health and hygiene, and after 1900 were consulted by the state on such matters as midwifery reform and the declining birth rate. The counter-movement to defend the economic interests of the medical profession became institutionalized in 1900 in an association known as the Hartmannbund. This league for the defence of the economic interests of the medical profession demanded certain 'freedoms', which in effect were monopolistic powers. Doctors resorted to the tactics of the labour movement in instigating strikes, blacklists and propaganda in protest against the control of the sickness insurances. It was a step towards the establishment of a monopoly of health by a scientifically educated profession.[19]

Doctors benefited from an expanded market for medical services opened up by sickness insurance. As insurance became available to ever widening categories of workers, so the market broadened for the services of medical practitioners. Doctors gained authority with the powers of certification for medical benefits and sick pay. Accident insurance claims required that safety standards be established and policed. Cleanliness was 'scientized': there were medical authorities for the disinfection of homes, railway facilities and factories, for analyzing air pollution in terms of constituent dust particles and fumes, and for calculating levels of toxicity.[20] As medical science assumed prominence in economic life, doctors became arbiters of social relations. It is in this context of social crisis, economic needs and the reinforcing of bourgeois values that the importance of health should be understood. On the one hand, medicine was to sustain the labour force at a time when the excess labour supply was diminishing owing to the rapid upswing in production. On the other, health was seen as a way of guaranteeing orderly behaviour. Hygienic standards were to be imposed as a way of reforming lifestyle. Public health offered a subtle means of social integration by civilizing the *Volk*.[21] The doctor took on a leadership role as Führer to guide the nation to an industrious, clean and healthy lifestyle.

While the people had long been prepared to expend substantial amounts of meagre incomes on doctors and medicines, sickness insurance brought a wider clientele to the doctor's surgery. Consultation and medical knowledge underwent a process of rationalization. The rational procedures of science were deployed in the laying bare of the sinews and nerves of human existence in terms of medical facts. The doctor was confronted not by sick persons but by specific diseases and cellular malfunctions. Sickness insurance practice accelerated the rapidity and frequency of

---

[19] C. Huerkamp, *Der Aufstieg der Ärzte* (Göttingen, 1985), pp. 216–40.

[20] D. Milles and R. Müller, 'Die relative Schädlichkeit industrieller Produktion. Zur Geschichte des Grenzwert Konzepts in der Gewerbehygiene', *Umweltrechtliche Studien* (Düsseldorf, 1986), I, pp. 227–262.

[21] This interpretation has been developed by Alfons Labisch, 'Doctors, Workers and the Scientific Cosmology of the Industrial World: The Social Construction of the "Homo Hygienicus"', *Journal of Contemporary History*, vol. 20 (1985), 599–615.

consultations. The basis of medicine shifted from home visits to doctors' surgeries and hospitals. As practitioners resorted to inventions like X-rays or electrotherapy, medicine for the masses became more technological. A division of labour resulting in new medical specialisms benefited the profession as further extending the market for care. It was in the economic interests of a struggling young physician to see patients frequently, even if fees were moderate.[22] The greater the scientificity of medicine, the greater became the expectations of the control of diseases, and the more consolidated became the medical profession. The more science advanced, the more de-humanized it tended to become, as personal and social elements were gradually refined out of the medical *Weltanschauung*. In keeping with the mechanization of society, the body was conceptualized in terms of division of labour, machinery and production. Cells were compared to small workshops, and organs to factories. Yet between 1860 and 1890 mechanistic concepts gave way to a stress on the distinct organicist and vitalist features of life. Biology became a means for subordinating historical, economic and political processes to the laws of evolution. Social problems could be treated as diseases in a malfunctioning social organism. The more such biological categories were extended to hitherto moral, social and religious spheres, as in the explanation of mind and sexuality, the greater became the possibilities of control of a wide range of social and psychological spheres. There was a rapid proliferation of medical institutions such as psychiatric and general municipal hospitals and sanatoria. In 1876 there were 140,900 hospital beds in the Reich, and by 1900 there were 370,000. In one year (1898–99), 1,650,000 sick and infirm cases were treated.[23] As the medical categories invaded the terrain of social categories, the greater became the potential for creating a society corresponding to a total institution.

During the 1880s there was a critical reaction to the repressive norms of Imperial Germany when utopian theorists planned alternative models for a rational and scientifically based society. Eugenics was initially limited to certain dissident young doctors and intellectuals, but it can nonetheless be understood as a response to the crisis of industrialization as experienced by urban bourgeois elites. There was disenchantment with the conventional political alternatives of conservatism, doctrinaire liberalism or even revolutionary socialism. Bismarck's authoritarianism and the alarming consequences of industrialization in terms of poverty, disease and homelessness inspired the sense of the need to provide collectivist (but not socialist) solutions to social problems. Politics could be replaced by scientific planning and administration. Organicist welfare schemes and eugenics were responses to the need to create social institutions to ensure the integration of the urban and industrial population. The close association of eugenics with 'social hygiene' shows how it was instrumental in bringing to light and offering solutions

---

[22] P.J. Weindling, 'Medical Practice in Imperial Berlin: The Casebook of Alfred Grotjahn', *Bulletin of the History of Medicine*, vol. 61 (1987), 391–440.

[23] Spree, *Soziale Ungleichheit*, p. 101; A. Guttstadt, *Krankenhaus – Lexicon für das Deutsche Reich* (Berlin, 1900), pp. iv–v.

for the social problems that were perceived as manifest in such chronic diseases as TB, VD and alcoholism. Instead of conceptualizing these in either moral or political terms, eugenicists applied the categories of hereditary biology, which could be extended to everyday life. Eugenics represented a process of substitution of biological values where hitherto the categories of political economy and civil society had predominated. In this sense, eugenics was a form of 'technocratic anti-politics'.[24]

The dynamic of professionalization

The improvement of individual and public health provided an ideological basis for welding the great regional disparities of urban and agrarian Germany into national unity. Health expressed liberal convictions of science, self-help and social reform, and was an index as to whether rising productivity actually benefited the people. Health as an ideology combined the promotion of national and economic efficiency with individual benefits. Political unification in 1870 involved not only the development of national institutions of government and political organizations, but also the growth of national markets in terms of labour, capital finance and consumer goods. Science and culture were major expressions of unification as expressed by the ideal of the nation as a *Kulturstaat*. One further constituent of the social basis for national unity was the development of a uniformly healthy lifestyle. This was the product of a growing market for scientific medicine, an increasingly cohesive medical profession and the rise of state concern with health and population growth. These concerns represented an attempt to overcome regional and class differentials in health. Standardization of lifestyle was facilitated by the spread of sickness insurance, particularly in industrial regions and large cities. The crusade for a healthier lifestyle was not only the making of a cohesive medical profession, but was also regarded as a matter of national importance.[25]

The medical profession sought to control conditions of medical practice in order to dictate what constituted good health. As sickness insurances began to press for preventive medicine and social reforms, the medical profession stiffened its resistance to what it regarded as the insurances' insipient socialism. The profession demanded a free market for medical care with patients having a 'free choice of doctor'. This liberal rhetoric concealed the striving for a monopoly by the profession over health care. The liberal ground rules of Imperial Germany meant that a 'welfare state' emerged to only a very limited extent. Health and welfare were administered by constituent states which had only limited concerns of policing public order by controlling epidemic, infectious diseases. Medicine remained a free trade; only the title *approbierter Arzt* (qualified doctor) was

---

[24] H. Luebbe, *Politische Philosophie in Deutschland* (Munich, 1974), pp. 161–5. The concept of 'anti-politics' arose in the context of Sombart's critique of Naumann in 1907; see R. vom Bruch, *Wissenschaft, Politik und öffentliche Meinung* (Husum, 1980), p. 187.

[25] For this process see Spree, *Soziale Ungleichheit*, pp. 138–63.

restricted by law to those who passed the state medical exams. The sickness insurances were autonomous institutions under dual employer-worker control. The state had certain sickness insurance funds at its disposal to encourage and direct welfare initiatives such as hospital building. Until 1900 the state preferred informal methods of co-ordinating welfare by laying down legislative guidelines and encouraging voluntary philanthropic associations.

The medical profession fought an aggressive campaign against lay practitioners. This conflict exemplifies the transition from popular self-help and lay medical practice, which were tolerated by the scientific elite of the profession during the 1860s and 70s, to a militant movement for a medical monopoly over all aspects of health by 1900. During the early nineteenth century the absolutist states had erected elaborate hierarchies of medical policing agencies and officials: these ranged from elite university-educated physicians to a broad base of such practitioners as midwives and barber surgeons. Although the official system was finely gradated, there flourished alongside a buoyant and highly varied mass of lay practitioners that fulfilled popular demands for health care. In theory medical practice was to be regulated by state licensing authorities, but in practice the official regulations were generally flouted. The medical profession by the 1880s conducted its own policing activities against its popular rivals. It stigmatized 'quackery' as a major public health hazard. Quacks were accused of carrying out abortions, and incompetent treatment of VD and of other infectious diseases. Moreover, lay therapists were charged with being crooks and swindlers. The medical profession turned from scientific elitism, reinforced by state medical qualifications, to an aggressive campaign for a controlling monopoly on health.

Popular healers resorted to professional defence mechanisms. They formed associations and lobbied the authorities. Earlier in the century (particularly during the 1830s and 40s), diverse lay health associations as for homoeopathy or hydrotherapy were formed. There were many regional and status group variants; lay homoeopathy was, for example, vigorous in the small towns of Württemberg. In 1872 homoeopathic practitioners founded the Central Association for Nature Therapy. The Association was based in Saxony which, as highly industrialized, remained a lively centre for alternative medicine.[26] A further stage of unification was attained in 1888 when this association banded together with nature therapists to form the German League of Associations for Health Care and Therapy without Drugs.[27] It had 14,000 members in the 1890s and its membership reached a peak of 885 local associations and 148,000 members in 1913. It provided welfare benefits, holiday colonies and 'air baths'.[28] Nature therapists were staunch defenders of the

[26] E. Wolf, '". . . nichts weiter als eben einen unmittelbaren persönlichen Nutzen . . .". Zur Entstehung und Ausbreitung der homöopatischen Laienbewegung", *Jahrbuch des Instituts für Geschichte der Medizin der Robert Bosch Stiftung*, vol. 4 (1985), 61–97.

[27] *Hundert Jahre Deutsche Naturheilvereine* (Berlin, 1935); *Zur Geschichte der Naturheilbewegung* (Berlin, 1934).

[28] G. Stollberg, 'Die Naturheilvereine im Deutschen Kaiserreich', *Archiv für Sozialgeschichte* (1988).

right of the laity to choose alternatives to the officially sanctioned 'school medicine'. The variety of practitioners was inexhaustible. Some were aggressively anti-scientific; others used terms like 'biological' and 'biochemical' in a naturalistic sense opposed to orthodox medical science. A wide variety of popular beliefs were synthesized with science such as magnetotherapy, phrenology and chiromancy. Entrepreneurial pioneers of therapies, such as Vincenz Priessnitz, Sebastian Kneipp and Friedrich Eduard Bilz, gave an air of authority to such associations. Air, water and light were essential elements in the efforts to reform lifestyle.

The nature therapists were active in defence of their position. The medical profession competed with nature therapists to form alliances with conservatives, liberals and socialists. The future socialist *Kultusminister*, Konrad Haenisch, defended nature therapists in the Prussian House of Representatives. Although the leadership of the SDP was much in favour of conventional medical science, the lobby supporting nature therapists meant that the SPD could never achieve unanimity of health policy. Nature therapy had its devotees on the right, and even among the medical profession, an example being Bismarck's physician Ernst Schweninger. *Völkisch* renegades such as Paul Förster (Nietzsche's brother-in-law and a critic of vivisection experiments) were activists in the nature therapy movement.[29] In 1897 the German *Magnetiseurs* petitioned the Reichstag in their defence. In 1903 the furore was so great that the Reich Chancellor ordered an inquiry on the prevalence of quackery. Homoeopathic doctors urged that they be granted special dispensing privileges.[30] In 1904, the physician Carl Alexander, established a Medical League to Oppose Quackery with widespread support among doctors. The Prussian Medical Department provided small financial subsidies. The sympathy of the medically qualified officials outraged legal officials of the Ministry of Justice, who pointed out that the state had no right to side with the doctors and use such terms of abuse as 'quack'. Justice officials insisted that the only defence against quackery was the law of assault. As long as it was not possible to demonstrate that body, life or property had been violated, no action could be taken against lay therapists.[31].

The Medical League to Oppose Quackery fought a vicious public propaganda battle. It had a widely distributed journal, *Der Gesundheitslehrer*, and flooded the nation with anti-quackery propaganda, such as publicity stamps, posters and pamphlets. Their symbol was a knight slaying the alien beast of quackery and evil. There was venomous hostility to those insurances (for example, in Saxony) which upheld their right to pay for members' treatment by nature therapists.[32] Anti-quackery meetings and exhibitions, such as that held in Dresden in 1908, drew a vigorous response from nature therapists, whose counter-propaganda defended their cause with messianic fervour. When the Dresden Hygiene Exhibition of 1911

---

[29] Stollberg has made an analysis of the participation of workers and the middle classes in nature therapy associations.   [30] ZSTA M Rep 76 VIII B Nr 1320 Die Homoeopathie 1897–1926.
[31] ZSTA M Rep 76 VIII B Nr 1342.
[32] STA Dresden Ministerium des Inneren Nr 10209/21.

excluded nature therapy, a petition of 300,000 signatories showed the extent of popular support. The profession fought against the spread of such popular self-help manuals of medicine as those by M. Platen (*Das neue Heilverfahren*) and Bilz (*Die neue Heilmethode*), which had circulation figures that reached the million mark. It was clear that the number of lay therapists was rising as fast as the demand for doctors' services. Nature therapists became a cohesive and organized lobby in order to defend their interests. Their associations pressed their case with vigour. In 1903 the nature therapists organized a mass petition to defend their position.[33] Some institutes gave training in nature therapy, but on the whole the irregular practitioners were so varied that they defied the demand for unified standards of practice. Often masseurs and magnetopaths were carrying out types of inexpensive therapy for the poor. A few were therapists who were much in demand with the rich and influential.

There were special interest groups who felt vulnerable to the encroachment of physicians. Intermediate groups with apprenticeship qualifications, such as the dentists or *Zahntechniker*, were outraged by the professions' claims for control over dentistry, as well as by the increase in unqualified dentists. From the 1880s the Association of German *Zahnkünstler* fought against quackery, while itself being attacked by the medically qualified specialists.[34] There were rival claims of dentists, general physicians and specialized *Zahnärzte* with medical qualifications. The latter established a special association to fight the dentists, because of their apprenticeship rather than academic qualifications. Dentists, they said, consisted of 70 per cent barbers, 5 per cent locksmiths, mechanics and goldsmiths, 7 per cent lower types of barber surgeon and 18 per cent of other trades such as tailors, waiters and washerwomen.[35] A survey carried out by the state in 1907 indicated that the Reich contained 2,198 dental surgeons and 4,264 dentists, mostly in towns. The medically dominated Prussian Scientific Advisory Committee recommended the suppression of dentists.[36]

The state authorities began to consult the profession on issues concerning health. A turning point came in 1897. The Reich Minister of the Interior was concerned that hypnosis could be harmful if demonstrated at public performances. Hypnosis was condemned as a dangerous form of lay therapy. A special report was commissioned in 1902 on medical uses of hypnosis and mass suggestion in relation to VD and TB. The Prussian state sought the opinion of *Ärztekammer* and scientific specialists.[37] Following a suggestion by the psychiatrist August Forel, medical chambers urged that the state ban public exhibitions of hypnosis, magnetism and suggestion, but that its use for medical research be supported. Hypnosis was used by a wide range of lay healers for such complaints as hysteria, epilepsy, alcoholism, and

[33] STA Dresden Ministerium des Inneren Nr 15232. [34] GSTA Rep 84a Nr 10991.
[35] Pamphlet of the *Deutsche zahnärztliche Gesellschaft zur Bekämpfung des Kurpfuschertums*.
[36] GSTA Dahlem Rep 84a Nr 1240 Kurpfuscherei.
[37] GSTA Rep 84a 10992 Hypnose und Suggestion 1897–1931; ZSTA M Rep 76 VIII B Nr 1324 Die Anwendung des Hypnotismus und des Magnetismus zu Heilzwecken 1881–1927.

VD.[38] These were the very areas of chronic and psychiatric disease with which eugenicists were concerned. Medical officers joined with police authorities to keep lay practitioners under surveillance. The medical chambers were keen to advise the state on issues of science and public order, and from this time there was a growing sense of mutual interest between state authorities and the medical profession.

The tension arising from a scientific elite attempting to gain control over health care had a deep impact on the general public and on state authorities. The public was concerned that it was liable to be a subject for scientific experiments. By 1906 the Prussian *Kultusministerium* was considering bringing in a special law to control quacks, and the Reich Chancellor, Bethmann Hollweg, endorsed this in 1908. The law proposed registration with the police and obliged the practitioner to keep a register of the date and course of treatment, the diagnosis, number of visits, therapy and payment. There would be prohibition on treatment at a distance (*Fernbehandlung*), the treatment of VD and sexual weakness, the improving of sexual potency, the prevention or termination of pregnancy and the use of hypnosis or suggestion. These categories show the influence of venereologists and psychiatrists in shaping the law. Judicial officials had severe misgivings on the basis of constitutional issues and with regard to effective controls. They pointed out that police intervention was ineffective. At a time when birth control methods and devices were becoming popular among the public, the medical profession came into conflict with what amounted to a social movement to limit family size. There was popular recognition that birth control could improve individual health and prosperity, and allow women fuller participation in social life. Birth control was one of the most effective forms of lay self-help in maintaining personal health.

The issue of 'quackery' illustrates the highly charged atmosphere of conflict over what constituted the basis of a healthy society. The conflict had broad implications and a direct impact on the controversy surrounding the declining birth rate, with quacks accused of carrying out abortions and of peddling contraceptives. There were demands that advertisements should be subject to strict control. Medical officers were outraged that lay practitioners were holding public lectures on sex, selling such devices as vaginal douches and distributing neo–Malthusian birth control propaganda. By 1909 these lectures had been banned by towns such as Stuttgart, Karlsruhe and Munich, and there was deep concern among the police and health officials in Dresden and Berlin.[39] The lay therapists were joined by groups opposed to vaccination, serum therapy and salvarsan (the anti-syphilis drug). The lay movement for sexual reform was to reach a climax in the abortion law repeal agitation of the early 1930s.

There were popular campaigns for dietary reform, sporting facilities and a natural and healthy lifestyle. Health and nature constituted a politicized terrain

[38] ZSTA M Rep 76 VIII B Nr 1325 die Sammlung der Berichte auf den Runderlass vom 5 April 1902 betr. die Anwendung der Hypnose.
[39] STA Dresden MdI Nr 15233 Ausübung der Heilkunde.

over which lay and professional groups competed for influence. For its part, the medical profession strengthened its resolve to fight the incipient socialism represented by sickness insurance funds, and agitated against malpractice by 'quacks'. The result was a highly militant profession, incessantly lobbying state and police authorities and keen to extend the scope and responsibilities of scientific medicine. Eugenics represented an attempt to synthesize elements of both embattled parties on the basis of biology and experimental science. Eugenics incorporated the *Lebensreformer's* values of physical fitness and air, sun and light as preconditions for national health and racial purity. The eugenicists attempted to win support among both the medical profession and clients of scientific medicine, as well as among those idealizing the virtues of a reformed lifestyle. The publicity given to issues such as alcoholism and TB prevention was a means for eugenic measures against chronic degenerative diseases to reach a broad public. Popular participation in health associations matched those of nationalist associations since health was part of the movement for social imperialism. While the Navy League could muster virtually one million affiliations by 1914, welfare and health organizations attained similarly high levels of popular mobilization.[40] Organizations for TB and alcohol prevention were deeply patriotic and emphasized the social benefits of an orderly and decent lifestyle. The eugenicists attempted to resolve the clash between socialism and conservatism on the basis of scientific expertise. They sought to infiltrate and restructure the medical profession. But eugenicists were divided over whether individual therapy should be replaced by collectivist social reforms or by populist revival of a primitive racial vigour. Eugenics was a response by dissident bourgeois groups to the social conflicts generated by industrializing Germany.

DARWINISM AND LIBERALISM

Darwinism reinforced the importance of health as an ideology of national integration. Evolutionary biology offered 'objective' criteria for evaluating fitness, welfare and the struggle for survival in urban and commercial life. Darwinism had a popular appeal, and at the same time offered a means of scientizing and extending the scope of medicine. There was a transition in Darwinism from being a liberal and secular ideology of social reform during the 1860s to reinforcing monopolistic professional interests during the social imperialism of the 1890s. The popularity of Darwinism meant that the public was responsive to scientific medicine and to organicist portrayals of the nation as a social organism. German Darwinists combined scientific research with such distinctive cultural concerns as historical development and organic unity. These ideological, institutional and scientific issues were a precondition for the dissemination of racial hygiene.

---

[40] Compare the figures of Stollberg with those of G. Eley in *Reshaping the German Right. Radical Nationalism and Political Change after Bismarck* (New Haven and London, 1986), p. 366.

Scientific impacts

The widespread public and academic debate on Darwinism from the 1860s gave it the character of a liberalizing movement for social reform. Evolutionary biology was 'a Whitworth gun in the armoury of liberalism' with the expectation that education and science would secure secularization of social institutions, the removal of aristocratic privilege, and establish government on a rational and scientific basis. At the same time, biology was the foundation of professional education in medicine. The superiority of German medicine derived from the application of experimental science and biology. As there were few specific drugs and only a limited medical capacity for cure, biology offered superior insights into the diagnosis and classification of disease by such means as the science of cellular pathology. Cell theory and embryology contributed to the understanding of the inflammation of tissues and the formation of tumours. The doctor was compared with a cellular defender of the organism from invasive micro-organisms. Darwinism had dual functions of being both a popular and professional ideology. As a popular ideology it stood for a progressive and integrated *Kulturstaat* at a time of traumatic political and social change. Biology, as a unified science of life, not only provided the basis for professional expertise, but it also inspired an ideology for the social role of the medical profession.

The amalgam of biological theories of social change known since the 1890s as 'Social Darwinism' poses complex problems of interpretation. Historians have portrayed Social Darwinism as an offshoot of a persistent 'Germanic ideology' of nationalist culture, racist impulses and militarism.[41] However, it has been argued that there was an intermediate ideology common to bourgeois elites in Britain and Germany. Comparison between bourgeois ideologies has rejected both 'Manchester liberalism' and 'German cultural pessimism' as caricatures of a common bourgeois faith in technological efficiency and mechanization.[42] While the shift away from assumed national stereotypes is welcome, the distinctive quality of German intellectual life associated with developing institutional structures as in higher education or the professions is underrated. Contrasts between German and British Social Darwinism provide a means of comparing liberal bourgeois ideologies and political aspects of social structure. A distinctive climate of liberal organicism was established as scientists contributed to academic and popular periodicals, gave public lectures, and encouraged the popular fashions for national history and anthropology. While an exhaustive account of their proseletyzing activities lies beyond the scope of this book, it is worthwhile explaining the different ways in which the sciences linked family life, careers and commercial activity with German liberal patriotism.

Darwinism contributed to academic expansion at such German universities as

[41] G.L. Mosse, *The Crisis of German Ideology* (New York, 1964).
[42] D. Blackbourne and G. Eley, *The Peculiarities of German History* (Oxford, 1984).

Jena; in contrast, British universities were slow to expand their intake of students, to develop research facilities and to offer professional training. German visitors to England, such as the zoologist Anton Dohrn, were puzzled that the greatest intellects, such as Darwin, John Stuart Mill and Charles Lyell, were *Privatgelehrte* (private scholars) rather than professors.[43] Huxley's London chair and research interests were analogous to those of a German professor like Haeckel. Yet he was exceptional when compared with Darwin, who settled for the lifestyle of a country gentleman, or with the self-supporting collector and co-discoverer of natural selection, Alfred Russel Wallace, or with the entrepreneurial author, Herbert Spencer. Huxley perceived the risks of autonomous groups of experts and joined with Spencer and Wallace in objecting to the idea of state-funded science as undemocratic.[44] Distinctive social, institutional and intellectual factors shaped the attitudes of German Darwinists to the state and to a range of national questions. The superior technical quality of the German biological synthesis of Darwinism with cell biology and embryology should also be taken into account. From debates over vitalist and mechanist interpretations of evolution, there emerged an organicist consensus by the 1890s. Darwin's most original contribution to evolutionary theory, that of natural selection, was often lost from sight. During the 1890s some scientists reformulated natural selection not as competition between organisms but as selection from an immutable germplasm. Others rejected ideas of selection as a relic of a redundant liberal individualism. Darwinism thus meant a general conviction of the truth of evolution, and could include such diverse mechanisms as 'Lamarckian' adaptation and psychic factors such as 'will' and learning powers. German biologists drew on distinctive organicist philosophical and historical concepts in analyzing developmental processes. These biological ideas were distinct from other traditions of racial thought including that of Aryan racial purity.

Political implications

The changes in Darwinism resulted from broader political and social developments. The rapid dissemination of biological theories of social change coincided with the rise and disintegration of liberalism between 1860 and 1914 in the context of rapid industrialization in an authoritarian social structure. The 1860s saw the rise of liberal parties as a national political force throughout Europe; in Germany the *Fortschrittspartei*[45] was founded in 1861. Leaders of the *Fortschrittspartei*, most notably the pathologist Virchow, drew on biological concepts to support their ideology of progress. Initially, Darwinism was closely connected to advocacy of laissez-faire and self-improvement and the lifting of restrictive controls by archaic states. By the 1890s Darwinism reflected the shift away from individualism to

[43] T. Heuss, *Anton Dohrn* (Stuttgart and Tübingen, 1948), pp. 85–90.
[44] T. Heyck, *The Transformation of Intellectual Life in Victorian England* (London, 1982).
[45] Progress Party.

corporate ideologies, emphasizing organic unity as opposed to class struggle and the fitness of national populations. There were attempts to make Darwinism the basis of national politics in order to secure a basis of support greater than the constituency of any single party. Social imperialism and national efficiency inspired the conservative Friedrich Alfred Krupp and the liberal Friedrich Naumann to use Darwinism to justify national coalitions supporting social welfare reforms. There was growing concern in the state over the degeneration of the population as a result of industrialization. Social Darwinism gave legitimacy to a variety of interests in an 'expanding industrial society, and cannot be identified as an exclusively right-wing racist ideology. It enabled the formulation of concepts of a unified and developing society which were part of transformation of liberal and left-wing thought.

The social basis of German biology lay in the universities and among families anxious to gain academic status; its ideological basis lay in a distinctive organicist tradition and the agitation for national unification. These factors suggest that underlying the apparent similarities of concern with social progress shared by British and German Darwinists during the 1860s and 1870s were fundamentally different social structures and cultural traditions. German Darwinists developed historicist and organicist themes, employing the Goethean term 'morphology' and the Pietist concept of *Organismus*, and priding themselves on a radical scientific tradition stretching back to Paracelsus as a popular healer and to the Reformation tradition of nature mysticism. Whereas the German Darwinists idealized the state in their science, there was a greater commitment to liberal political economy and utilitarian doctrines among the British. The vigour of German politics was matched by local and national scientific and medical societies. Accounts of popular politics overlook other related processes such as professionalization that enhanced the authority and power of bourgeois groups. National unification channelled bourgeois energies into administration, the professions, philanthropy, education and the sciences. These activities were regarded as of 'national' and 'social' significance, and as contributing to strengthening the cohesion and unity of German society. The natural sciences and medicine were buoyed up by expectations of social and economic progress, suggesting that science was a modernizing and reforming force. Darwinism was part of the process of adaptation to urban and industrial social forms. The popularity of Darwinism indicated that a social transformation was taking place outside the scope of state power. Darwinism as embedded in science, art and social thought was a public, cultural movement. Only at the turn of the century did biological social thought penetrate state institutions as the state turned to professional groups like public health officials for guidance on social problems.

The social bases of Darwinism

Britain and Germany saw the rise of voluntary associations for education, philanthropy and entertainment. Science encompassed all these functions, and scientific societies were a forum for progressive-minded intellectuals. Lively debates erupted on evolution, materialism and vitalism in both Germany and Britain. The *Gesellschaft Deutscher Naturforscher und Aerzte*[46], which was a sister organization of the British Association for the Advancement of Science, acted as a national public forum for scientific debate to which academics and other middle-class intellectuals flocked. It was at the meeting of 1863 that the zoologist, Ernst Haeckel, raised Darwinism as an issue of development and progress.[47] National scientific organizations enabled scientists and other members of the middle class to share common cultural interests to develop sub-disciplines and raise petitions for state support and funding. Yet these large-scale scientific assemblies should not obscure how scientific programmes were generated by small, closely-knit groupings, and were financed by personal wealth, private patrons or publishers. These networks were often informal and held together by such ties as family, politics or philanthropy. Darwinism, eugenics and social hygiene were generated by groups motivated by such convictions as national unification or abstinence from alcohol, or by alienation from repressive bourgeois morality. The cultural specificity of their values raises questions of how distinctive were the German forms of association. While universities were state institutions, academics were well integrated into municipal life, and associated in societies with civic dignitaries. At societies such as the Scientific Society of Jena, Darwinism and liberal politics would be discussed by professors, and bourgeois professionals and industrialists.[48] Major commercial centres such as Frankfurt did not have a university, but made up for this through civic museums like the Senckenberg Society, which was administered by amateurs. Newspapers such as the *Augsburger Nachrichten*, and bourgeois 'family journals' such as *Über Land und Meer* and *Die Gartenlaube* from 1853, published liberal interpretations of animal societies. The popular writer on animals, Alfred Brehm, exemplifies how it was possible to finance expeditions and natural history from the 1850s by publications, working for zoos and aquaria, and the patronage of notables such as Crown Prince Rudolf. Brehm was inspired by the democrat Emil Adolf Rossmässler, a veteran of the 1848 Frankfurt assembly.[49] Scientific materialism and radical polemics were popularized by such journals as *Die Natur*, *Das Jahrhundert* and, from 1877, the Darwinian *Kosmos*.[50] These periodicals disseminated such liberal types of science as the progressivist concepts of hygiene and the organicist writings of liberal politicians such as Hermann Schulze-Delitzsch.

Darwinism enhanced the reputation, popularity and prosperity of university academics. In the 1860s patriotic students clamoured for lectures on Darwinism at Jena. Professors found that nationalist metaphors were popular with the ever-expanding numbers of medical and science students. Professors coloured science

---

[46] Society of German Doctors and Naturalists.   [47] *Entwicklung und Fortschritt.*
[48] *Die medizinisch-naturwissenschaftliche Gesellschaft zu Jena.*
[49] S. Schmitz, *Tiervater Brehm* (Frankfurt-on-Main, 1986), pp. 101–2.
[50] *Kosmos. Zeitschrift für eine einheitliche Weltanschauung auf Grund der Entwicklungslehre in Verbindung mit Charles Darwin und Ernst Haeckel*, ed. O. Caspari, G. Jäger and E. Krause (Leipzig, April 1877), I.

and medicine with nationalist metaphors of organization, integration and hierarchical control. As students paid fees to attend lectures, the better lecturers were rewarded by fatter incomes. This was an incentive to make lectures relevant with the use of topical social analogies. Universities competed in the appointment of professors, so an offer of a chair at another university would be a valuable bargaining counter with a state for a greater salary. Behind the rising academic productivity resulting in voluminous publications, there was the financial incentive of payment per *Bogen*. Publishers paid handsomely for monographs, textbooks and popularizations. Whole firms grew up that profited from the expanding market for academic and professional publications. This is exemplified by the success of Gustav Fischer in Jena, the publisher of much Darwinian biology[51] and by that of the Lehmann Verlag in Munich which published medical periodicals and textbooks.[52] There were lucrative possibilities in popularizing science. Books on expeditions to exotic parts of the world, on evolution and reproductive biology, on the wonders of technology or on health care were eagerly read. Darwinism was a means of improving scientific reputations, and creating lucrative opportunities to extend science into the public sphere.[53] Because state control over the universities limited the extent to which radical theories could be developed, public platforms were erected to popularize science as a form of progressive, secular culture. Nationalism went hand in hand with a naturalistic world view. The public mind linked the unity of mankind and the animal world, with the politics of national unification. The nation was the culmination of the evolution of life from simple to complex organisms, and science offered insight into the laws of social progress.

The motivating ideologies of association differed in Britain and Germany. In 1858 the liberal advocate of co-operatives, Schulze-Delitzsch, rejected the term *Association* as alien in its nationalist tone, favouring instead the German term *Genossenschaft*.[54] Liberals were attempting to promote an alliance of the educated and propertied bourgeoisie with the *Handwerker*[55] during the 1860s.[56] Civil society was defined by means of a distinctive organicist vocabulary. Liberal terms such as *Constitution* and *Gesamtperson* were used to establish the concept of society as a distinct and higher form of life.[57] Mechanistic ideas permeated social discourse only to a limited degree since they denied the very essence of the social. Virchow's concept of the 'cell-state'[58] and Haeckel's deployment of concepts of society as a

[51] F. Lütge, *Das Verlagshaus Gustav Fischer in Jena* (Jena, 1928).

[52] G.D. Stark, *Entrepreneurs of Ideology. Neoconservative Publishers in Germany, 1890–1933* (Chapel Hill, 1981).

[53] C. Hünemörder and I. Scheele, 'Das Berufsbild des Biologen im Zweiten Deutschen Kaiserreich – Anspruch und Wirklichkeit', in G. Mann and R. Winau (eds.), *Medizin, Naturwissenschaft und Technik und das Zweite Deutschen Kaiserreich* (Göttingen, 1977), pp. 119–51.

[54] W. Conze, 'Möglichkeiten und Grenzen der liberalen Arbeiterbewegung in Deutschland. Das Beispiel Schulze-Delitzschs', in H.J. Varain (ed.), *Interessenverbände in Deutschland* (Cologne, 1973), pp. 85–102, 95.   [55] craftsmen.   [56] Sheehan, *Liberalism*, pp. 90–4.

[57] L. Gall, 'Liberalismus und "Bürgerliche Gesellschaft": Zu Charakter und Entwicklung der Liberalen Bewegung in Deutschland', *Historische Zeitschrift*, vol. 220 (1975), 324–56.

[58] *Zellenstaat*.

Gesamtperson illustrate how biology incorporated organicist terminology. There was a concern to establish elemental categories such as the cell, the individual or the family in a way that would not lead to atomistic disintegration but would reinforce organic unity. It was a vision of society in which the talented intellectuals were to be rewarded with privilege and influence. The underlying sentiments were corporatist (in the sense that society was a federation of privileged corporations) rather than democratic, and geared to a vision of small-scale productive units as the basis of society. The 1860s marked a high point of when national spokesmen, drawn from the class of the *Gebildeten*,[59] sought to work with organizations such as the *Verein deutscher Handwerker*. This limited the spread of laissez-faire liberalism, and resulted in a preference for stabilizing co-operation and corporations.[60] Positivist science conferred prestige and authority, enabling academics to project their opinions in the general interest of 'the nation'.

Corporate ideology fused the family, the emergent professions and the sense of privileged identity of those with educational qualifications. These elemental structures of social life shaped science and medicine as means of securing income, status and influence. Science integrated the economic, intellectual and social aspirations of bourgeois – or aspiring bourgeois – families. The German obsession with university education was distinctive. Pressure from the lower middle class resulted in the mid-century university enrollment boom.[61] Culture had an important role in giving cohesion to the bourgeois family, and by extension the nation was idealized as a *Kulturstaat*. The German bourgeoisie pressed for liberalization and modernization of universities. While universities were state administered, study required substantial investment by the student's family. The importance of such financial support from families, the role of university academics in civic associations and their informal economic and political ties to urban communities have been underrated. Science was a form of family investment to secure social status. That civil servants were university trained, and the fact that officials responsible for universities were drawn from the ranks of professors indicates a symbiosis between the *Bildungsbürgertum* and the state.[62] There was an overall rise in university matriculations, which between 1870 and 1906 were twice as large as the rate of population growth.[63] Universities took a growing share of a GNP which was itself dramatically rising. The percentage of state funding of higher education and science increased by 465 per cent between 1873 and 1914. Prussia spent 2.5 million marks between 1850 and 1859, amounting to 0.15 marks per head of population; between 1900 and 1909, expenditure rose to 50.1 million marks, amounting to 1.22 marks per head of population.[64] Palatial institutes were built to accommodate the burgeoning numbers of students and researchers.

Following national unification, the popularity and importance of biology rose.

---

[59] educated bourgeois. [60] Sheehan, *Liberalism*, pp. 77–107.

[61] H. Kaelble, *Historical Research on Social Mobility* (London, 1981), pp. 64–7.

[62] W. Conze and J. Kocka (eds.), *Bildungsbürgertum im 19. Jahrhundert* (Stuttgart, 1985).

[63] C.E. McClelland, *State, Society and University in Germany 1700–1914* (Cambridge, 1980), p. 249.

[64] F.R. Pfetsch, *Zur Entwicklung der Wissenschaftspolitik in Deutschland, 1750–1914* (Berlin, 1974).

The numbers studying biological subjects greatly increased, partly because of their importance for expanding professions such as medicine, and partly because of intrinsic fascination with the laws of evolution. Between 1882 and 1907 the Prussian *Ministerialdirektor* in the *Kultusministerium*, Friedrich Althoff, established eighty-six medical institutes, laboratories and clinics.[65] While research drew on evolutionary biology, this did not attain official recognition because of suspicions that Darwinism led to materialism and political radicalism. The subject remained divided between the disciplines of botany, zoology, anatomy, physiology and hygiene. Classical, legal and historical studies still enjoyed greater prestige, but the subject had an attractive modern air and was linked to the growth of medical studies, and to such economic fields as agriculture, forestry, fisheries and pharmaceutical manufacturing. The idea of biology as a unified discipline that included everything from botany to social science gained in popularity, despite its lack of an institutional base.

Family status

Families were concerned to sustain inherited economic interests which for their part were necessary to support secondary and university education. Investment in a scientific career could improve social status from that of *Kaufmann* to *Akademiker*, as well as promise a viable income and social influence. Marriage reinforced the cohesion of scientific elites. Many a budding scientist married a professor's daughter. Examples of two leading biologists indicate the prevalence of kinship strengthening the cohesion of the intelligentsia. Although Haeckel, the son of a civil servant, first married his cousin, he had a second marriage to the daughter of Emil Huschke, a professor of anatomy. Virchow, the son of a merchant, cemented his ties with the Berlin medical profession by marrying the daughter of a leading gynaecologist, and his career owed much to family connections through a high-ranking military uncle. Virchow's son, Hans, became an anatomist, and his daughter married the biologist, Carl Rabl. Darwinism was used to establish professional dynasties. The Darwinist brothers, Oscar and Richard Hertwig, were sons of a manufacturer; they became students of Haeckel (paternalistically referred to as his *Goldsöhne*), and Oscar's son and daughter became geneticists. More broadly, between 1870 and 1914 professors of medicine at Berlin tended to be the sons of other doctors or professors.[66] Examples were Virchow's son, or Rudolf Fick, the son of a physiologist, Adolf Fick, who formed part of a nationally minded academic dynasty.[67] Professional education and early steps in a career required support by the family.

Cultural pursuits within the family, efforts to sustain inherited family economic interests, and professionalization channelled intellectual and social concerns into

---

[65] McClelland, *State, Society and University*, pp. 281–3.
[66] P.J. Weindling, 'Theories of the Cell State in Imperial Germany', in C. Webster (ed.), *Biology, Medicine and Society 1840–1940* (Cambridge, 1981), pp. 99–155.

science. The limitations of school education in science meant that science was a force integrating economic, intellectual and political interests in families and civic life beyond the official culture of the class room and church. This can be illustrated by the career of the zoologist, Ludwig Plate, who became Haeckel's successor at Jena, supported the Pan-German League and anti-semitism, and founded the Racial Hygiene Society. He was the son of a Bremen school teacher and his early interests in natural history were fostered by a godparent, by the city's collections for natural history and ethnology, and by the Bremen Scientific Society which was established in 1868. His godparent, a Senate scholarship, and additional support by a Senator financed his zoological studies under Haeckel in Jena. Throughout his career Plate combined the commercial and public spheres with science as at the Museum for Marine Studies in Berlin and at the Phyletic Museum in Jena.[68] Biologists were concerned with the rise and decline of ability and the problems arising from primogeniture of aristocratic titles and of property. The widespread concern with heredity from the 1870s reflected a bourgeois concern with whether ability was acquired through education or inherited. Darwinism expanded teaching and research opportunities in the universities, and a biologically based social hygiene boosted the medical profession's claim for expertise over social questions.[69] In contrast to the elitism of Berlin professors, the founders of the Racial Hygiene Society in Berlin in 1905 were recruited from outside exclusive academic circles:

Name	Father's Occupation
Nordenholz	Commerce
Plate	Teacher
Ploetz	Commerce
Rüdin	Commerce/Teacher
Thurnwald	Manager

Eugenics defended the status of vulnerable middle-class academics by offering biological rationales for the privileged position of intellectual and professional elites.

Scientists were entrepreneurial in expanding their research facilities and in seeking sources of additional income. The expansion of hygiene as an academic discipline illustrates this. The first professor of hygiene, Max Pettenkofer, not only believed that economic progress was conducive to health, but he also invested in Justus Liebig's discovery of a beef extract. During the 1890s bacteriologists such as Robert Koch and Emil Behring were shrewd in negotiations with such chemical manufacturers as Hoechst. Successive Berlin professors of hygiene had economic interests, such as Max Rubner in nutritional products, and Martin Hahn used his family's manufacturing interests in seamless piping to good effect in studies of

[67] 'Die Familie Fick', *ARGB*, vol. 14 (1922), 159–75.
[68] W. Lührs, *Bremische Biographie 1912–1962* (Bremen, 1969).
[69] P.J. Weindling, *Darwinism and Social Darwinism in Imperial Germany* (Stuttgart, 1989).

sewers and heating.[70] Medical professors could earn additional income in private practice. Laboratory researchers could be called on to adjudicate in law cases and to provide analyses for commercial and state purposes; if they were prepared to sponsor a product by endorsing its scientific and medical value then chances for its market success improved. Manufacturers of foodstuffs, pharmaceutical products or articles for personal hygiene cultivated contacts with the academic establishment. This reached a high point when the Odol manufacturer, August Lingner, used his marketing expertise to publicize scientific discoveries in hygiene.

Biology and hygiene became more and more technical disciplines, reliant on aniline dyes and precision optics for the observation of cells, chromosomes, or bacteria. Technical skills reinforced the authority of experts when they came to pronounce on national issues. After 1900 biology became dominated by a group of researchers from socially well-connected families. Theodor Boveri, an eminent cytologist, employed his brother, the engineer and partner in the Brown-Boveri engineering works, to intercede in negotiations over the Kaiser Wilhelm Institute for Biology in 1911. Although the Institute was staffed by scientists with heterogeneous social backgrounds – such as Richard Goldschmidt (whose father owned a confectionary business), Hans Spemann (the son of a publisher), Max Hartmann (the son of an official) and Carl Correns (the son of a historical painter) – the ethos of the Kaiser Wilhelm Gesellschaft was to fuse commerce with national culture. In medicine there were similar connections between the established elite and commerce. For example, the pathologist, David von Hansemann, came from a Bavarian banking family, and the immunologist, August von Wassermann came from a Jewish banking family. These social connections enabled scientific ideas to have a social impact. Wassermann inspired the industrialist, Walther Rathenau, to develop a symbiotic theory of society as composed of interdependent living entities.[71] The Krupp dynasty supported biological research and neurobiology as well as launching a competition on social evolution in 1900. Bankers and industrialists provided crucial support for medicine and biology. For their part, scientists tempered industrial expansion with pleas for welfare and cultural cohesion.

If a family was poor or socially marginal as with Jewish physicians, family and political ties provided alternative channels of advance. Radical intellectuals frequented the 'red salon' of the mathematician, Leo Arons (dismissed from the university in 1899 for membership of the SPD). The Arons family was a clan of wealthy bankers and academics, who could support the socialist convictions of their less well-off scions. The fourteen children of Marcus Mosse, a liberal-minded medical officer, became another such clan of commercial tycoons and academic leading lights.[72] Socialist doctors such as Ignaz Zadek (the brother-in-law of the

[70] P.J. Weindling, *From Bacteriology to Social Hygiene: the Papers of Martin Hahn* (Oxford, 1985).   [71] H. Pogge von Strandmann, *Walther Rathenau* (Oxford, 1985), p. 109.
[72] W.E. Mosse, 'Rudolf Mosse and the House of Mosse 1807–1920', *Leo Baeck Institute Yearbook*, vol. 4 (1959), 237–59.

revisionist politician Eduard Bernstein) formed influential groups campaigning for extension of social medicine. Bernstein was friends with a group of young radical Jewish doctors, who included Hermann Lisso, Alfred Blaschko, Paul Christeller and Mieczyslaw Epstein. These migrated from eastern towns like Danzig and Posen to Berlin as an intellectual centre. In 1877 Zadek, Blaschko and Lisso organized a secret socialist society in the University's anatomical dissecting rooms. Eduard Bernstein's cousins included the physiologist Julius Bernstein whose son Felix was the mathematician and serologist. Another frequenter of Arons' red salon was the leading theoretician of social hygiene, Alfred Grotjahn, who was the son of a provincial doctor. But it became difficult to penetrate the bastions of academia, and he joined forces with other marginalized doctors to campaign for social hygiene. While many of the radical socialist physicians were academically inclined, very few found a career in medical research.[73] They sought alternative outlets in private clinics or public health services, and they transposed biology to the broader realm of the social organism.

As long as there was growing public prosperity and expansion of university facilities, it seemed that the newly educated scientific elite could enter science or other science-based professions and be assured of an income and career. But this educational expansion, that worked to the advantage of those beginning careers during the 1870s and early 1880s, could not sustain the later generations of graduates. Rising numbers of graduates coincided with a renewed industrial depression in the late 1870s. Prospects deteriorated for academic careers in the universities and professions.[74] A divide opened between the elite professors and the growing 'academic proletariat' of lecturers who were unsalaried and unrepresented on faculties and without much hope of a permanent appointment. Professors in such traditional disciplines as anatomy and pathology resisted specialization as devaluing the general status of science. Moreover, they saw the 'mass university' with expanding student numbers as debasing the quality of research and teaching. They were uneasy with the prospect of the university as a 'teaching factory'. In contrast, advocates of new disciplines – like genetics or paediatrics – or of intellectual currents – like neo-vitalism or political anthropology – found themselves without career prospects.[75] The young eugenicists were to be troubled by the problem of establishing racial hygiene as an intellectual discipline, and then securing financial support for research and for career-posts. There arose a sense of alienation from the social establishement. Such disgruntled academics turned to a range of socially critical ideologies, and prophetic philosophies were in vogue. They venerated cultural ideologists who raised issues beyond the confines

---

[73] F. Tennstedt, 'Arbeiterbewegung und Familiengeschichte bei Eduard Bernstein und Ignaz Zadek', *IWK*, vol. 18 (1982), 451–81.
[74] F. Eulenburg, *Der 'akademische Nachwuchs'. Eine Untersuchung über die Lage und die Aufgaben der Extraordinarien und Privatdozenten* (Berlin and Leipzig, 1908).
[75] A. Busch, 'The Vicissitudes of the *Privatdozent*: Breakdown and Adaptation in the Recruitment of German University Teachers', *Minerva*, vol. 9 (1962), 319–41.

of academic science. Cults arose around the figures of Friedrich Nietzsche, Haeckel and the *Lebensphilosoph*, Rudolf Eucken, who were venerated as offering the basis for a critique of social conventions. Contempt arose for the narrow specialization of academic study as irrelevant to the broader problems of life and society.[76]

The educated bourgeoisie rallied to an organicist ideology of mutual dependence. Such organicism was a basis for social imperialism, for mobilization of public opinion on national issues, and for integrating the state with the diverse social interests, institutions and expectations arising from rapid industrialization. Reforming associations, municipalities, industrial, professional and agrarian interest groups could all be linked by organicist social theory to each other and to the state. Organicism could overcome the contradictions of liberal society: as between professions and popular self-help, or between defence of property and the rise of democracy. Theories of social evolution proved that individual interests were linked to higher ethical and social ideals in the corporate body politic. Family wealth and status was to be sustained by professional careers, and the ideal of a fit and healthy family life was to be realized through medical advance and through social reform.

DARWINIAN DEMAGOGUES

Public associations and pressure groups provided fertile ground for the spread of organicist ideas of social unity. As German scientists took a world lead in biology and medicine in the 1880s, they gave the credit for their achievements not to industry that created the wealth that financed the universities, but to the newly united nation-state. Nationalist ideology permeated biology with terms such as 'the cell state' and 'organic integration'; discussions of the mechanisms of evolutionary adaptation were related to the founding of Reich institutions. The rise of socialism meant that liberal leaders no longer could assume that there was an identity of interests between liberal reformers and artisans. Instead, academics resisted the use of Darwinism by socialists, while pontificating on national issues as objective academic experts. Professors applied evolutionary theory to a range of issues such as the Catholic Church, education, socialism, German armament, colonial policy, feminism and the Polish problem, and gave their opinions the authority of science by using biological analogies. But state authorities took scant regard of such outpourings. The state alloted a functional role to the universities. Officially, university academics had the limited tasks of educating students for professions such as medicine, law and teaching, and of conducting research in their academic specialism. Professors acted as ideologists, spokesmen for professions and the educated bourgeoisie, setting the pattern for dictatorship over social affairs.[77]

---

[76] J. Most, 'Die Stellung der Gelehrten zur Socialdemokratie', *Die Zukunft*, vol. 1 no. 4 (15 November 1877), pp. 97–106.

[77] A. Kirchhoff, *Die akademische Frau. Gutachten hervorragender Universitätslehrer, Frauenlehrer und Schriftssteller* (Berlin, 1897); Kirchhoff, *Deutsche Universitätslehrer über die Flottenvorlage* (Berlin, 1900).

Underlying this was the situation that bourgeois family and professionalizing interests came to be expressed through state-controlled university traditions in Germany, at a time when the British bourgeoisie preferred autonomous channels. Differential rates of industrialization, the preoccupation with unification and removal of restrictions on the freedom of commerce and ideas, and contrasting intellectual traditions and scientific organization combined to create a distinctive intellectual climate in Germany.

The demise of radicalism

The rise of bourgeois professionalism and of scientific institutions took the radical ideological sting out of biology. A reversal of liberal reformist values occurred in biology. The rapid growth of interest in biology among academics and the general public owed its origins to the liberal movement for enlarging economic opportunities and removing the relics of aristocratic privilege and clerical superstition. The writings by such as Alexander von Humboldt, whose *Kosmos* was published between 1845 and 1862, generated the expectation that biology was internationalist, popular and respectful of other races and cultures. Such scientific cosmologies inspired the imagination of the educated public for the realization of a humane and unified nation. The radicalism of the mechanistic biology of the 1840s gave way to a more authoritarian type of biology emphasizing hierarchy and integration. This can be seen in the ideas of biologists such as Vogt, Virchow and Haeckel. During the 1848 revolutions, physicians such as Virchow campaigned for social medicine based on 'a science of man'. All aspects of public and private life, including therapy and politics, were subject to natural laws. Scientists were high priests of nature able to determine guidelines for a humane society.[78] The materialist doctors, Carl Vogt and Ludwig Büchner, agitated for a scientific explanation of human evolution. It was hoped that science could give insight into the origins and development of living organisms and reveal the laws of their organization. Such laws ought also to explain the physical evolution of humanity, human psychology and social organization. Materialists looked to physics and chemistry for the laws of the spontaneous generation of new forms of life. Only later would biologists turn to continuous historical sequences of evolution.[79]

In 1855 two brilliant statements of materialism attacked the vestiges of theism in science. Büchner's *Force and Matter*[80] received a stormy response because of its use of the latest scientific discoveries to support mechanistic materialism. He argued that as a result of education in naturally based laws 'a new race will gradually be evolved, whose faculties and organization will be of a higher type'. Racial characteristics were the result of the natural environment; he cited Galton's geographical observations to support this.[81] Vogt was a marine zoologist whose

---

[78] R. Virchow, *Vier Reden über Leben und Kranksein* (Berlin, 1862).
[79] O. Temkin, 'The Idea of Descent in Post-Romantic German Biology: 1848–1858', in B. Glass, O. Temkin and W.L. Straus (eds.), *Forerunners of Darwin 1745–1859* (Baltimore, 1968), pp. 323–56.
[80] *Kraft und Stoff.*   [81] L. Büchner, *Force and Matter* (London and Leipzig, 1884), pp. 464, 490.

views were radicalized by friendship with the revolutionaries Michael Bakunin and Alexandre Herzen in Paris from 1845–48. Vogt took a leading role in the 1848 revolution. Although 'Herr Vogt' earned the scorn of Karl Marx, he established a pattern for a socially radical type of science. His 'Zoological Letters' portrayed 'animal states' and denounced the middle class, religion and all forms of government; the state was a primitive relic of animal life that ought to be transcended by mankind. Individual freedom required the abolition of government, as well as necessitating sex education. Vogt was attacked by vitalist and conservatively inclined scientists for scientific heresies and for denouncing Prussian militarism. Vogt's scientific anarchism could be interpreted as standing for a radical liberalism. Büchner also espoused the self-help creed of the radical liberal, Schulze-Delitzsch during the 1850s.[82]

This polarity between materialism and the vitalism of more conservative zoologists such as Johannes Müller was overcome by an intermediate historicist and organicist philosophy. That Müller brandished his sword to defend his systematic zoological collections from the revolutionary mob in Berlin during 1848 indicated that organicist ideas had to be reformulated before they could be turned to reformist ends by such Müller students as Virchow and Haeckel. Biological reformism was pioneered by liberal and radical spirits, who used the discovery of the cell to establish continuous historical processes of development. The radical physician, Robert Remak (a staunch upholder of his Polish-Jewish identities), discovered cell division in 1851. Virchow confirmed (and virtually appropriated) the theory that all cells grow from pre-existing cells, and developed its potential for pathology.[83] The 1860s saw a culmination of this reorientation with the fusion of liberalism, cell biology and Darwinism. In 1861 – the year that Virchow was active in founding the German liberal party – a 'constitutional reform' in the laws or *Staatsgrundgesetz* of the cell was proclaimed by Max Schultze, a secular and liberal-minded Bonn anatomist. Rather than cells being a membrane surrounding a structureless substance, he argued that this 'protoplasm' was the basis of cellular organization. In 1861 Virchow introduced the concept of an aggregate of cells as citizens forming a 'cell state'. The idea of spontaneous generation was replaced by the theory of the historical continuity of cells. The fusion of Darwinism and cell biology was to be the achievement of Haeckel, who was encouraged in this by Schultze and Virchow. In 1863 Haeckel proclaimed Darwinism as raising the issues of 'development and progress' at the Society of German Naturalists and Doctors. Haeckel ignited a fiery public and academic debate on Darwinism.[84]

Cell biology marked the way forward into a multiplicity of fields. As the basic organic unit in all plants and animals (including man) knowledge of the cell could be used to good effect in such areas as reproductive biology, neurology and brain

[82] F. Gregory, *Scientific Materialism in Nineteenth Century Germany* (Dordrecht, 1977).
[83] B. Kisch, 'Forgotten Leaders in Modern Medicine: Valentin, Gruby, Remak and Auerbach', *Transactions of the American Philosophical Society*, vol. 44 (1954), 141–317.
[84] P. Corsi and P.J. Weindling, 'Darwinism in Germany, France and Italy', in D. Kohn (ed.), *Images of Darwin* (Princeton, 1985), pp. 683–729.

anatomy. The cell became the basis of medicine with the study of cellular defence mechanisms against infections, arising from the minute bacteria, and of disease processes. The cell acquired significance as the germ of psychological and social life. Cells as individuals were studied as endowed with primal characteristics of hunger and sensibility, and were compared to labourers. Virchow's concept of the 'cell-state' opened the way to analyzing organisms as multi-cellular composites. Biology resounded with social analogies, drawn from an expanding and industrializing society: scientists spoke of cellular 'production', 'learning', 'cultures', 'colonies', 'migration', and 'division of labour'.[85] Virchow compared the cell to an individual citizen, and he was opposed to hierarchical concepts of controlling substances or regions. Liberal biology was a constituent part of organic social theory. Virchow combined rigorous laboratory research with social concepts in his pioneering of cellular pathology. Other liberals echoed these views. Karl Twesten in the 1860s popularized Comtist ideas of the state as an organic part of human society. He drew on biological anthropology and physiology. Mechanical inventions were conceptualized in organicist terms. For example, the liberal, Werner Siemens introduced the idea of the telegraph integrating society like the nervous system in biological organisms. Writers on technology used a theory of machines as *Organapparaten*, with a basis in animal physiology. Later generations of scientists would move away from such individualistic liberalism and stress the importance of organic processes requiring cellular interaction and interdependence.

Despite the stimulus of liberalism, cell biology pointed in authoritarian and professional directions. Virchow attempted to use science as an authoritative basis for professional and political activity. He proclaimed in 1860: 'the freer the society or the state is, the more science is supported'. A contradiction emerged between freedom and unity. Although there were concessions to liberal demands in education and commerce, the authoritarian nature of Bismarck's government meant that Virchow became a leading opponent. But despite the rhetoric of freedom, Virchow's outlook was meritocratic rather than democratic. He demanded privileged status for the educated at a time when access to higher education was limited by constraints of class and gender. Science-based politics was itself highly privileged, and aspirations for cosmopolitan science gave way to ideas of a German national science. In 1865 Virchow celebrated the 'liberation' of German from French medicine, and boasted of German cultural superiority.[86] He resisted both the idea of a democratically accountable medical profession and state plans for expanding numbers of university chairs. Virchow's professional politics were elitist.[87] Science was a basis for authoritative pronouncement on social conditions.

---

[85] G. Mann, 'Medizinisch-biologische Ideen und Modelle in der Gesellschaftslehre des 19. Jahrhunderts', *Medizinhistorisches Journal*, vol. 4 (1969), 1–23; Weindling, 'Theories of the Cell State in Imperial Germany', pp. 99–155.

[86] E. Ackerknecht, *Rudolf Virchow, Doctor, Statesman and Anthropologist* (Madison, 1953), p. 151.

[87] N. Andernach, *Der Einfluss der Parteien auf das Hochschulwesen in Preussen 1848–1918* (Göttingen, 1972), p. 54.

Monist unity

Between 1860 and 1900 the crusaders for biological reform became less hostile towards the aristocratic and clerical ethos of the ruling elite. The political implications of mobilizing public support for rational, civilized and progressive biological values changed from the radical liberalism of Virchow to expectations of co-ordination and integration. Industrialization meant that the educated elite feared that science and culture would be debased by socialist materialism. At the same time, many biologists and doctors withdrew from active participation in party politics, and instead preferred to act as professional experts on issues of social reform and public health. Biology was to provide objective solutions to social problems. That Darwinism was both a scientific and a social movement boosted the authority of scientific experts. By the twentieth century biologists came to stress the values of hierarchy, order and historical traditions.

Darwinism offered a means of expanding career opportunities in research and teaching. Ideologically, evolutionary theory was well suited to the competitive and decentralized university system.[88] Universities were seen as organisms competing for students, funds and the best brains. A number of universities enhanced their reputation with Darwinian professors. How this came about is exemplified by rapid growth of the University of Jena. Generations of patriotic and scientifically gifted students flocked to Jena, which gained the reputation as a 'citadel of Darwinism'. Reconstruction of the history of life was a mammoth research programme that could justify new institutes, collections and equipment. The 1860s and 1870s were decades of opportunity when gifted young researchers rapidly acquired chairs. The state administrator, Moritz Seebeck, appointed a cluster of Darwinians in the 1860s. The state authorities were prepared to match the growth of student numbers with research facilities. Among the academics who made their mark at Jena were Eduard Strasburger, the botanist, Carl Gegenbaur, Oscar Hertwig and Gustav Schwalbe in anatomy; and Thierry William Preyer, the physiologist. All were keen Darwinists.[89] At the same time the university benefited from public and industrial support, such as that from the Zeiss Foundation, managed by the left liberal physicist Ernst Abbe, and from other commercial sources.

Haeckel exercised a charismatic influence. He led bands of students on walks in the Thuringian hills, where on the summits they sensed 'the spirit of freedom'. Politics and Darwinism were constant sources of discussion. Major discoveries were made in the heady atmosphere of patriotism and belief in evolution as a naturalistic religion. When Haeckel accompanied research students on marine biological expeditions, they spent their evenings discussing Darwinism and

---

[88] J. Ben-David and A. Zloczower, 'Universities and Academic Systems in Modern Societies', *European Journal of Sociology*, vol. 3 (1962), 45–84.

[89] G. Uschmann, *Geschichte der Zoologie und der zoologischen Anstalten in Jena 1779–1919* (Jena, 1959).

politics. Haeckel was a leading actor in the social transformation of Darwinism. He popularized biology as the basis for a monistic world view, and projected biology as a naturally based system of ethics and social organization. He shifted in political sympathies from liberal radicalism to a politically more quiescent and hierarchical nationalism. His monistic creed inspired biologists to participate in a scientistic public movement. In addition to advocating biological nationalism, Haeckel made important scientific contributions. German Darwinism was characterized by rapid advances in cell biology and embryology. The intensity of biological research was due to the conviction that every original fact – each discovery of a species of microscopic plankton or observation on the contortions of embryos – was a nail in the coffin of Christianity as an archaic superstition.

Haeckel's synthesis of evolution and cell biology reinforced his position as an ideologist of social evolution. He assumed the task of demonstrating the evolutionary implications of cell theory, and applying historicist ideas of human progress and economic theories to biology. He developed the concept of an animal economy in such a way that it could be reapplied in a biological form to social problems. On a marine biological expedition to Italy in 1859, he became enraptured with the beauty of the minute 'social' *Radiolaria*, which were united into 'colonies' by networks of protoplasm. Coinciding with his reading of Darwin, and with nationalist enthusiasm aroused by the Risorgimento, these *Radiolaria* prompted Haeckel's speculations on the first-formed organisms as composed of plasma. Encouraged by Virchow's principle of continuous cell division, Haeckel developed a powerful synthesis of cell theory and Darwinism. He deduced that all organisms were organized plasmatic bodies, and were historically derived from a single ancestor. He set himself the task of historical explanation of the laws of formation of evermore complex species. The key to the problem was provided by study of the early stages of embryological development: the embryo recapitulated the evolutionary sequence passing through the forms of extinct or as yet undiscovered 'lower' organisms. The development of the embryo passed through a sequence of primitive organs – for example, a combined organ for reproduction and digestion – and extinct types of organisms such as the *Gastraea*. Embryology was historical in its approach, and could be extended to mankind and the evolution of societies.

When Haeckel suffered the death of his first wife in 1864, it triggered off the sense of a scientific mission. He became aware of a hardening of character. He felt that a life of sensuous contemplation of the beauties of nature must give way to a life of the intellect in the service of science and mankind. In 1866 he published a major polemic on behalf of Darwinism, the *Generelle Morphologie*. Haeckel made evolution stand for progressive philosophical and nationalist viewpoints .Darwinism had symbolic value, representing a constellation of evolutionary theories including cell theory, historical recapitulation of lower forms, direct adaptation by an organism to its environment and the cultural traditions of Goethe's morphology. Huxley warned Haeckel in 1867 that 'one public war dance against all sorts of humbug and imposture is enough'.[90] After reading Spencer in 1870 (the year of national unification), Haeckel concluded that 'higher', more complex organisms required integrative powers. Haeckel saw in his scientific studies the proof of the unity of man and nature, a natural ethics and an evolutionary cosmology. All these were within the grasp of the German nation as among the highest evolved of social organisms. This gave organicism relevance to the development of social and educational institutions. Biology was not a separate science but, Haeckel said, an extension of history and archaeology. Nature thus reinforced rather than replaced theories of historical progress culminating in national unity.

Darwinism came at a crucial moment for German biologists. Darwin's work offered the basis for a history of development from 'lower' to 'higher' organisms. That Darwin did not use these hierarchical terms did not deter those scientists who employed nature to reveal laws of organization and reproduction. The conflict can be seen in the widening rift between Virchow and Haeckel. Haeckel was alarmed by Bismarck's blood-and-iron politics for unifying Germany by Prussian military conquests. Haeckel pleaded with Virchow that the *Fortschrittspartei* should oppose Prussian expansionism as not in the interests of German patriotism. He warned that Southern German liberalism was in jeopardy and suggested that Virchow ally himself with the radical doctor Johann Jacoby and other radical democrats against Bismarckian Caesarism.[91] Haeckel was disillusioned that Virchow did not use his influence to lead a secularizing and patriotic popular movement to achieve unity.

There was a growing disenchantment with liberal individualism during the 1870s. The split found expression in a clash between Virchow's egalitarian concept of the cell state and Haeckel's hierarchical nationalism. There were parallel shifts in other disciplines such as jurisprudence: Otto von Gierke's legal theories developed the concept of a social organism as opposed to utilitarian individualism. There were very different sets of values in Britain and Germany. Whereas in Britain Darwinism was an off-shoot from political economy, in Germany historicist concerns were pre-eminent. Although Spencer and Haeckel share concepts such as 'the social organism', their overall aims differ. Spencer was well known for his hostility to the state, and for his advocacy of individualism, as expressed in his phrase 'survival of the fittest'. Haeckel was impressed by Spencer's concept of 'organic integration' – the more an organism is differentiated, the more centralizing control is necessary. Haeckel used this theory after 1870 to formulate a hierarchical concept of the social organism. But in contrast to Spencer, he emphasized the need for central state direction, just as 'higher' organisms require a more developed brain. German biologists thus transformed Darwinism, placing it on an organicist and hierarchical basis.

[90] G. Uschmann and I. Jahn, 'Der Briefwechsel zwischen Thomas Henry Huxley und Ernst Haeckel', *Wissenschaftliche Zeitschrift der Friedrich-Schiller-Universität Jena. Mathematisch-naturwissenschaftliche Reihe*, vol. 9 (1959–60), 13.

[91] P. Klemm, *Der Ketzer von Jena* (Jena, 1966), pp. 104–6.

Haeckel maintained hostility to Prussian Junkers as repressive and authoritarian. Unification did not satisfy his expectations that Germany should develop as a progressive, civilized and educated society. Bismarck's anti-Catholic crusade, christened the '*Kulturkampf*' by Virchow, was a hopeful sign, but Haeckel soon fell foul of fellow biologists and the political establishment. He applauded the *Kulturkampf* in his popular account on human origins, the *Anthropogenie*. Soon after unification, however, restrictions were imposed on the teaching of biology in schools. In 1876 a school teacher, Hermann Müller, was censored for having taught the evolutionary popularization by Carus Sterne, stating the chemical origins of life from carbon. Haeckel reacted with a campaign for reinstating the teaching of biology in schools, leading a series of ferocious debates at the *Naturforscher Versammlungen* in 1877, 1882 and 1886. At the height of the campaign, in February and March 1878, he toured Germany and Austria holding popular lectures on the cell soul and the monistic unity of man and nature.[92] In 1879 a debate on the teaching of Darwinism in schools in the Prussian House of Representatives resulted in the banning of the teaching of evolution in schools. In 1882 an education order excluded natural history teaching from higher classes in schools.[93] The authorities suspected biology of subversive materialism and as aiding the spread of socialism. Biology was a casualty of the anti-socialist laws.

These political tensions over the teaching of biology coincided with socialist electoral successes in the Reichstag elections of January 1877. A savage debate flared up between Haeckel and Virchow over whether Darwinism was a proven law, suitable for teaching in schools, or whether it was only a hypothesis. They examined the social implications of teaching Darwinism. Whereas Virchow was a critic of Bismarck, and remained individualistic and anti-hierarchical in his politics and science, Haeckel glorified the German Reich as highly evolved. He argued that evolutionary theory should be the basis of education in the newly united nation. Indeed, he went further and suggested that study of cellular organisms proved the existence of a natural religion based on duty, division of labour and the subordination of egoism to the social whole. Unicellular organisms like the *Radiolaria* showed that the single cell was the basic unit of mental life, and could be termed a *Seelenzelle*. Protoplasm was composed of molecules, termed by Haeckel 'plastids'; hence the lowest psychological unit was a *Plastidulseele*, which arose from the unity of inorganic substances. The evolution of social instincts made it possible for the sense of duty to arise in higher organisms. Each citizen was a cell in the social organism. At the same time Haeckel took a stand against socialist materialism. Darwinism stood for order, differentiation and specialization in contrast to egalitarian socialism.[94]

[92] G. Uschmann, *Ernst Haeckel. Eine Biographie in Briefen* (Leipzig, 1983), p. 155.
[93] I. Scheele, *Von Lüben bis Schmeil* (Berlin, 1981), pp. 101–6.
[94] E. Haeckel, 'Die heutige Entwickelungslehre im Verhältnis zur Gesamtwissenschaft', *Amtlicher Bericht der 50. Versammlung Deutscher Naturforscher und Aerzte in München vom 17. bis 22. September 1877*, (Munich, 1877), 14–22; Haeckel, *Freie Wissenschaft und freie Lehre* (Stuttgart, 1878).

Virchow ridiculed such an attempt to construct a Darwinian cosmology as based on hypothesis rather than fact. Only positive knowledge was suitable for teaching in schools. If evolutionary theory was made the basis of social and ethical principles, then this would lead to dangerous speculations. The theory of a 'plastidul soul' was a possibility, but it could not be proved. Virchow believed that such dangerous half-knowledge was based on false scientific premises and opened the way to socialism.[95] Virchow's views found sympathy with many academics who preferred empirical laboratory-based research in the proliferating university institutes and clinics.

In the 1870s biology entered an experimental phase from which Haeckel recoiled. Experimental methods intervened in the normal processes of growth and reproduction in order to establish causal factors in development. Experiments on changing the constitution of egg cells and spermatozoa, and in producing malformed embryos supported the conviction that the human constitution could be altered or at least that pathological traits could be bred out. Regulation and heredity were the major concerns of experimental biology. Both Haeckel and Virchow were casualties of experimental biology, as representing a shift away from historical approaches and as more professional and career-oriented, and embedded in medical and research institutions. Virchow became perceived as dogmatically egalitarian, and Haeckel clung to his evolutionary causal chains of supposed phylogenies according to which scientists could locate the causal forces within the cell and metabolism of organisms. This can be seen in debates on localization of brain functions. Virchow maintained a localistic and non-hierarchical theory of the nervous system. This was refuted in 1870 when the physiologists, Eduard Hitzig and Gustav Fritsch, experimentally demonstrated cerebral localization and the fact that the brain cortex directed the motions of different body parts. Hitzig conducted high voltage electro-therapeutic experiments on patients while a military doctor in 1867. Experiments on dogs established that electrical stimulation of the cortex led to distinct motor responses. Fritsch, a strongly nationalistic Darwinist and racial anthropologist, compared the motor centre to a government minister. Any movement after removal of the centre was similar to the continuation of bureaucratic activity while the minister was on holiday. Experimental biology revealed the mechanisms of order, control and hierarchy.[96] Haeckel similarly emphasized how the organs formed from tissues were like state departments and institutions: rule by central government was comparable to the power of the brain as nerve centre.[97]

A generation of physiologists and histologists localized mental processes,

[95] R. Virchow, 'Die Freiheit der Wissenschaft im modernen Staat', *Amtlicher Bericht der 50. Versammlung Deutscher Naturforscher und Aerzte in München* (1877), 65–77.

[96] P.J. Pauly, 'The Political Structure of the Brain: Cerebral Localization in Bismarckian Germany', *International Journal of Neuroscience*, vol. 21 (1983), 145–50.

[97] E. Haeckel, *Zellseelen und Seelenzellen. Vortrag gehalten am 22. März 1878 in der 'Concordia' zu Wien* (Leipzig, 1920).

reducing them to the categories of neurology. This justified control and authority of the intellectual elite in society; in the expanding medical sphere, doctors were achieving total control over proliferating numbers of clinics and sanatoria. Doctors led public agitation for the founding of modern mental hospitals, as they were convinced that brain research could result in cures for mental diseases. Hitzig was appointed as director of a modern mental hospital in Zürich, the Burghölzli. Yet he was so authoritarian that after a few years he was forced to resign from his post. (The Burghölzli was to have a crucial role in the genesis of eugenics.) Those seeking to promote national integration and social reform could draw on corporatist biology. Doctors and other converts to biological values promoted concepts of individual and national health as in campaigns against alcohol, or for school health education.

Professionalism meant a retreat from the overt political activism of Virchow or the anticlerical campaigning of Haeckel. Darwinian monism continued to provide critical perspectives. After his dispute with Virchow, he wrote to his friend, the poet Hermann Allmers, of the need to continue 'propaganda' for the evolutionary world view.[98] Haeckel despised the piety and compromises with the churches of successive Prussian ministers. When judged from his biological vantage point, it appeared that government, education and justice remained in a state of barbarism. Even the liberalizing policies of the 'new course' of the social reformers during the early 1890s were too tame for Haeckel, who insisted on the separation of church and schooling.[99] It was only when Bismarck had been dismissed that Haeckel proclaimed him 'doctor of phylogeny', and recognized his historical achievement of national unification. The debate on school biology of 1892 prompted a fiery statement of his philosophy of monism which expressed the unity between science and the spirit.[100] The campaign for nature to be the basis of education reached a climax at the turn of the century. Haeckel demanded a reduction in classical studies, and the instatement of biology, physics, chemistry and anthropology as part of the culture of every educated citizen; at the same time there should be physical education and country excursions. He scored a major popular success when the author Emil Strauss prompted him to restate his views. The resulting publication of *Die Welträthsel* (The Riddles of the Universe) in 1899 showed how mechanistic features of evolutionary theory gave way for Haeckel to a mystic idealism. This pantheistic nature philosophy was expressed in vibrant language, giving the work immense popular appeal. The *Welträthsel* had very few specifically Darwinian features, and fitted in with a mood of scientific and popular sympathy with vitalism and organicism.[101] While scientists were dismissive of the lack of originality, the *Welträthsel*, as with all Haeckel's works, was informative about human reproduc-

---

[98] Uschmann, *Ernst Haeckel*, p. 118.

[99] E. Haeckel, 'Die Weltanschauung des Neuen Kursus', quoted by Uschmann, *Ernst Haeckel*, p. 169.

[100] E. Haeckel, *Der Monismus als Band zwischen Religion und Wissenschaft* (Bonn, 1892); E. Krause, *Ernst Haeckel*, (Leipzig, 1983), pp. 103–5.

[101] P.J. Weindling, 'Ernst Haeckel and the Secularization of Nature', in J. Moore (ed.), *History, Humanity and Evolution* (Cambridge, in press); E. Haeckel, *Die Welträthsel* (Bonn, 1899).

tion and embryology. Such readily available popularizations of biology provided useful facts about sexuality, presented in lucid and sensuous language.

The campaign for biological values after 1900 continued with popular editions of *The Riddles of the Universe* and *The Wonder of Life* (1904), and the Jena Prize for an essay on the application of biological laws to society.[102] This biological evangelism culminated with an adulatory reception at the International Congress of Free-Thinkers in Rome in 1904 and in the establishment of the Monist League in 1905. Haeckel was by then but a father figure for the League, as he was aged over seventy. The very diverse membership of the League reflects the breadth of Haeckel's influence, as it numbered distinguished naturalist authors like Wilhelm Boelsche (the author of the lyrical account of the evolution of love life in nature), eugenicists, feminists and socialists. Haeckel believed that observation of nature could provide evolutionary laws to solve ethical, social and ecological problems. He provided a framework for a popular anti-establishment ideology of biological reform. Public concern with the social question made popular biological tracts relevant to debates on social welfare reforms. The civic and individualist tenets of liberal economic theory, derided as vulgar *Manchestertum*, gave way to nationalist collectivism. A minority of Social Darwinists were critical of the extension of social welfare and of therapeutic medicine as preserving unfit generations. An influential group of eugenically-minded doctors urged a transition from individual patient-oriented medicine, to the doctor as a state official. Professional groups allied with the state were to superintend the health of the 'social organism'.

In its attack on revealed religion, monism sought to provide natural guidelines for biologically based social behaviour, psychology and art. Haeckel's popularity coincided with the fashion for the natural forms of the *art nouveau* and secessionist movements. Not only did Haeckel's drawings of marine organisms become a success in their own right, his organicist ideas influenced authors, artists and dancers.[103] The eurythmic dances of Isadora Duncan were inspired by Haeckel's theory of the recapitulation of animal movements.[104] Boelsche's lyrical account of the evolution of sexuality sought to liberate emotions from stifling bourgeois conventions and restore them to the instinctive realm of nature. Biology retained an emancipatory and liberating potential.

The monist movement suggests that Darwinists were subject to tensions between modernist demands for personal and social reform, and imperialism and racism. The toning down of the political radicalism of such as Vogt and Virchow meant that organicism was used to promote social reforms designed to consolidate national unity, and to create a more sympathetic mood to welfare issues. Political factions and interest groups attempted to float diverse forms of Social Darwinism as an objective basis for national unity and social progress. The mass sales of

---

[102] E. Haeckel, *Die Lebenswunder* (Stuttgart, 1904).

[103] E. Haeckel, *Kunstformen der Natur* (Leipzig, 1899–1904).

[104] I. Duncan, *Der Tanz der Zukunft* (Leipzig, 1903); Duncan, 'The Dance and Nature', (1905 essay), in *The Art of the Dance* (New York, 1928).

popularizations of biology testify to the popular interest in nature and in the demand for a naturalistic world view. Socialists such as Bebel and Kautsky drew on the positive certainties of Haeckel's biology, and biological popularizations were among the most popular reading matter among German workers during the 1880s.[105] Haeckel avoided pinning his evolutionary world view to a specific political party. He reacted strongly against bourgeois commercialism of the 'railway fever' and condemned socialist materialism.[106] He endeavoured to establish biology as a popular and participatory science, and as providing objective standards beyond the limitations of all parties whether liberal, socialist or conservative. Science was thus a surrogate for civic values and party political activism. His distinctive position is intelligible within the context of Wilhelmine intellectual imperialism; as critical of the repressive old regime, and yet concerned to develop revitalized forms of national power. Biology was used to offer a form of corporatist social thought that was nationalist but detached from either popular anti-semitism or Gobineau's aristocratic Aryanism. The theory of the social organism corresponded to the integrating needs of Wilhelmine imperialism. Biology was to take a leading role in social and psychological affairs. The expectation was that it would be emancipatory and objective, dissipating superstition and patriarchal prejudice.

Although Haeckel sought public support for monism, his views were hierarchical and authoritarian. But his aims and ideals were attractive to the Wilhelmine middle class, who were searching for a secure basis for their status and needed a *Weltanschauung* that could make sense of the rapid upheavals of industrialization.[107] Darwinism was looked to as an objective basis for nationalism and as an ideology of social integration. The centrality of biology in national political culture arose from the expectation that if one could understand the basic developmental laws for such primitive organisms as the *Gastraea* or the first germs of mental life in cell souls, then laws for higher and more complex mental and social organisms could be ascertained. Haeckel's monism resisted reduction to the categories of technological efficiency and mechanization, as monists envisaged a humane and civilized *Kulturstaat*. Haeckel's importance as a Darwinian demagogue lay in the shift away from party political activism to an organicist vision of a reformed society through applying biology in such areas as education and the anti-alcohol campaign. As the new breed of thrusting professionals in medicine, imbibed such biology, they also absorbed positivistic formulations of social concepts and a sense of mission to prescribe measures for the health of the social organism and of future generations. Scientific positivism replaced civic freedoms. Leading twentieth-century biologists, such as Richard Hertwig, Hans Spemann and Hans Nachtsheim, the Trotskyist biologist Julius Schaxel and sexual reformers

[105] A. Kelly, *The Descent of Darwin* (Chapel Hill, 1981), p. 130.
[106] Uschmann, *Ernst Haeckel*, pp. 157–8.
[107] H.-U. Wehler, 'Sozialdarwinismus im expandierenden Industriestaat', in I. Geiss and B.J. Wendt (eds.), *Deutschland in der Weltpolitik des 19. und 20. Jahrhunderts* (Düsseldorf, 1974), pp. 133–42.

such as Hirschfeld and Hodann were inspired by Haeckel's organicist Darwinism. Biological research on topics such as sex determination was regarded as crucial to a range of social issues as the removal of the penal codes against homosexuals, and disadvantaging women. Racial hygienists, such as Ploetz and the zoologist Plate were profoundly influenced by Haeckel's monist philosophy, from which they derived specific programmes for boosting the status of the nation's biological elite. That the rapid advances in biology and cellular pathology were triggered off by historical and political philosophies meant that the life sciences provided guiding social principles. It was left to a younger generation to take the initiative and apply the laws of biology to social and sexual problems.

SCIENTIZING RACE

Liberal anthropology

From the 1860s Darwinian anatomists and doctors took the lead in a public movement for anthropological studies. Liberal ideals of development and individualism were projected into studies of the diversity of physique, skull shape and cultural morphology of the inhabitants past and present of the lands that formed modern Germany. Ideas of fixed racial types and a vital essence or *völkisch* character were rejected by the first generation of Darwinian anthropologists. Aryan racial theories and colonial schemes were condemned by the liberal leaders of anthropology.

The politically radical scientists, Virchow and Vogt, were key figures in founding associations and organizing excavations and publications. Virchow dramatically showed the liberal hostility to aristocratic and chauvinistic theories of an ancient Germanic or Aryan race in 1872 at the Berlin Anthropological Society. He rebuffed the nationalist attack by the French anthropologist, Armand de Quatrefages, that German unification in 1870 was 'an anthropological error':

Ought we, as we construct our state, ask everyone what their ancestry and racial origins are? No, Herr de Quatrefages, we will not undertake such policies. Modern *Deutschland* is not the old *Germania*. It is fortunately no longer the Holy Roman Empire of the German nation, and that means France should not fear an intention to establish a universal state.[108]

De Quatrefages suggested that the 'Prussian race' was corrupted by dark Mongoloid Finnish and Slavonic elements, and differed from the 'true German race' in other regions; barbaric and deceitful Finno-Prussians had in 1871 bombarded Paris; the true Aryan aristocrats were the French and Southern Germans. This biological materialism contrasted to the emancipatory, organicist and liberal type of biology and politics that Virchow stood for. Virchow argued that it would be absurd if state formation depended on ethnological characteristics.

---

[108] R. Virchow, 'Ueber die Methode der wissenschaftlichen Anthropologie', *Zeitschrift für Ethnologie*, vol. 4 (1872), 300–20.

He divorced the state as a politically constructed entity from evolutionary biology, or the idealization of the glories of mediaeval German history.[109]

Virchow and his liberal associates carried out a survey of the diverse physical characteristics of the Finns and German-speaking peoples so as to refute de Quatrefages. The Freiburg anatomist and anthropologist, Alexander Ecker, gained the support of the state of Baden for a national anthropological survey. In 1871 Ecker suggested to Virchow that the planned survey on skull form should be extended to include such physical qualities as height and hair and eye colour in order to assess whether particular skull types were small or large in stature, and fair or dark in complexion.[110] These suggestions were taken up by Virchow in his directive to the survey commission. Although the Prussian War Ministry would not release material on the stature of military recruits, the state education administrations co-operated in every respect. Questionnaires were sent out to school teachers, and reports were received on fifteen million school children. The findings were intended to settle the issue of whether there had been intermingling of the Asiatic 'Aryans' with an aboriginal European population. The results of the surveys in Baden and Prussia were processed by the Prussian Statistical Office under the auspices of the medical officer, Albert Guttstadt. The results showed that there were many different physical types in Germany. Among the Jews, 11.17 per cent had blond hair and many were blue-eyed. Racial stereotypes did not correspond with national cultures. Given that the Reich established an impressive range of liberal rights, Germany seemed to be on the brink of an age of enlightened liberal freedoms and tolerance. Science was a guarantee of natural rights and justice.[111]

The biological unity of mankind

Darwinian biology set out to explain human origins and the causes of human variations, while accepting that there was a single human race derived from a common progenitor. Anthropology emerged in the context of radical challenges to aristocratic privilege. Biology scientized the meaning of race and transformed it from aristocratic and moralistic concepts 'of good breeding' and 'of pure blood' to the bourgeois science of anthropology. Nations and cultures were evaluated by anthropologists and medical experts according to biological concepts.[112] Anthropologists applied techniques of comparative anatomy and biology, and physiological measurement to the problems of human physique and culture. Individuality was removed from the moral sphere, and redefined in scientific terms with the individual subsumed in a 'race' (a category equivalent to a biological sub-species). During the 1780s the German anatomist, Johann Friedrich Blumenbach, had the

[109] Ackerknecht, *Virchow*, pp. 207–19.
[110] C. Andree, *Rudolf Virchow als Prähistoriker* (Cologne and Vienna, 1976), II, p. 77.
[111] L. Poliakov, *The Aryan Myth. A History of Racist and Nationalist Ideas in Europe* (London, 1974), pp. 262–8; Ackerknecht, *Virchow*, pp. 207–19.
[112] W. Conze, 'Rasse', in O. Brunner, W. Conze and R. Kosseleck (eds.), *Geschichtliche Grundbegriffe* (Stuttgart, 1984), V, pp. 135–78.

idea of measuring skull form. He instigated a tradition of anatomical studies of physical anthropology that gathered force during the following century. He used this to establish the existence of five main races: the Caucasian, Mongoloid, Ethiopian, American and Malayan, which he regarded as descended from a single human type. These races were not fixed and static, but fluid categories that could be altered by human behaviour. In 1845 the Swede, Anders Retzius, introduced a cephalic index for measuring skull shape as an indication of mental quality and racial origins. The technique was extended, especially in France to studies of brain anatomy, and of other physical characteristics such as hair or complexion. At the Anthropological Society of Paris there prevailed a view that cultural differences were physically and physiologically determined. The politically radical scientist, Paul Broca, made brain anatomy central to anthropology. The French anthropologists co-operated with Vogt, as they shared free-thinking, materialist and republican commitments, and some were doctrinaire positivists.[113] In 1861 there was a meeting of German anthropologists to establish a general method of craniometry.[114] This meeting was responsible for organizing anthropology as a national science. Those involved were all professors of medicine. Most anatomists and zoologists were keen physical anthropologists whose institutes had extensive collections of skulls and other human artefacts.[115] The close links between anatomy and anthropology suggest that questions of human origins lay behind many comparative anatomical and zoological investigations. As anatomy was fundamental in medical education, generations of medical students acquired a grounding in anthropology. Racial concepts became an integral part of medical thinking in connection with issues of physique and the immunity of populations to diseases.

Whereas biological anthropologists of the 1860s emphasized how mankind was a single species, ethnological studies of language and customs gave a sense of the great rift between 'primitive' cultures and European civilizations. Philologists unearthed an Indo-Germanic family of languages. The term 'Aryan', deriving from the Sanskrit word *arya*, meaning noble, was applied to all peoples speaking such languages.[116] The materialist anthropologists distanced themselves from philology and dilettante studies of cultures. Adolf Bastian, Virchow's longstanding second in command in the Berlin Society, saw thoughts as biological entities, developing in ways similar to cells. Studies of 'prehistory' focused on human palaeontology and formed a vital link between physical anthropology and the history of civilizations. All were part of the enterprise of the 'history of life',

[113] J. Harvey, 'Evolutionism Transformed: Positivists and Materialists in the *Société d'Anthropologie de Paris* from Second Empire to Third Republic', in D. Oldroyd and J. Langham (eds.), *The Wider Domain of Evolutionary Thought* (Dordrecht, 1983), pp. 289–310.
[114] J.W. Spengel, 'Zur Craniometrie', *Zeitschrift für Ethnologie*, vol. 9 (1877), 129; C. Blankaert, ' "Les Vicissitudes de l'Angle Facial" et les Débuts de la Craniométrie (1765–1875)', *Revue de Synthèse*, 4 series (1987), 417–53.
[115] A. v. Frantzius to R. Virchow, 28 April 1874, quoted in Andree, *Rudolf Virchow*, II, p. 181.
[116] Poliakov, *Aryan Myth*, pp. 255–61.

although there were conflicting interpretations of the interdependence of physical and mental characteristics.[117] Environmental conditions, ageing and diseases were seen in evolutionary terms. The grimey skin of industrial workers was the first stage of degeneration to animal life; the child's mind was equated to the primitive intellects; and 'natural' peoples were healthier.[118] Whereas philology was divisive, biology was a unifying force. Biological concepts of science were deployed to press for liberalizing and humanitarian measures.

Anthropology between the French Revolution and late-nineteenth-century imperialism was subject to political polarization over the issues of slavery and the decline of a natural aristocracy. In the first half of the century critics of slavery used race as a moral and physiological category for the humanitarian end of condemning slavery as violating the natural laws of human equality. Following Blumenbach many anatomists were convinced that there was a single human race. Differences were due to morals and education. Darwin shared this conviction, and it was widespread among liberal-minded Germans. Scientists imposed standard definitions by applying biology and medical science to anthropology.[119] Biological anthropology was dedicated to the liberal aim of proving the existence of a single human race, whereas cultural, linguistic and historical evidence was used by ethnologists to prove that ethnic differences were permanent. The French Restoration was a spur to the development of racial theories to support an insecure aristocracy. The idea of the mediaeval Frankish kings as heirs to Germanic racial virtues was mooted. Approaching the racial question through history rather than biology, Joseph Arthur de Gobineau, an Alsatian count and diplomat, attempted to synthesize such ideas. Gobineau's treatise on human inequalities, published between 1853 and 1855, established race as the driving force of history.[120] He argued against the liberal ideas of physical anthropologists in order to prove that there were several pure archetypal races. The 'Aryan race' was supreme and constituted an aristocratic caste. He attributed the achievements of the Chinese and Western civilizations to the Aryans. A precondition was 'purity of blood'. Degeneration was the result of intermarriage. Racial interbreeding was condemned as polluting the inner psychological essence rather than interpreted in biological terms. He argued that there was a hierarchy of languages corresponding to a hierarchy of races. The white race possessed superior beauty and intelligence and was threatened by the 'semitizing' of European civilization.[121]

Gobineau had virtually no impact on the bourgeois Paris anthropologists, who

---

[117] M. Hammond, 'Anthropology as a Weapon of Social Combat in the Late Nineteenth-century', *Journal of the History of the Behavioral Sciences*, vol. 16 (1980), 118–32.

[118] G. Weber, 'Science and Society in Nineteenth Century Anthropology', *History of Science*, vol. 12 (1974), 260–83.

[119] N. Stepan, *The Idea of Race in Science: Great Britain 1800–1960* (London, 1982).

[120] M.D. Biddiss, *Father of Racist Ideology. The Social and Political Thought of Count Gobineau* (London, 1970); E.J. Young, *Gobineau und der Rassismus. Eine Kritik der anthropologischen Geschichtstheorie* (Meisenheim, 1968).

[121] M.A. de Gobineau, *Essai sur l'inégalité des races humaines*, (Paris, 1853–55), I, pp. 176, 394, IV, p. 337.

preferred to use comparative anatomy to the vagaries of history.[122] Although Georges Vacher de Lapouge, an aristocratic lawyer and university librarian, reformulated Gobineau's theories in terms of biology, Lapouge was a marginal figure for the radical Parisians. German support for Gobineau was initially restricted to reactionary aesthetes.[123] Alexander von Humboldt was quick to condemn Gobineau for his arrogance and misunderstanding of German literature.[124] Gobineau was critical of Darwin and Haeckel as exponents of liberal biology. There was a conceptual, methodological, political and social chasm separating Gobineau from the Darwinian anthropologists. Bourgeois progress and .democracy were to Gobineau causes of degeneration. He was disinterested in skull measurements or in evolutionary biology. His aesthetic and psychological concept of fixed racial types was diametrically opposed to the Darwinian concept of continuous variation. From the outset Gobineau hoped to have an impact in Germany. He dedicated his treatise on racial inequality to George V of Hanover, as uniting the roots of the German and British races. The Aryan theory appealed to the cultural aesthetes of the Bayreuth circle during the 1880s. In 1882 Richard Wagner introduced Ludwig Schemann to Gobineau, and Schemann was to found a Gobineau Society. But there were few followers in Germany until the 1890s.[125] There was a religious rift between the anti-Catholic Haeckel and Gobineau's clerical sympathies that could only be bridged after Lagarde and Houston Stewart Chamberlain's ideas on Germanic Christianity gave a nationalist interpretation of Gobineau's caste theory. Leading academic anthropologists, such as Virchow in Berlin and Johannes Ranke in Munich, remained staunch critics of Aryan racial theories.

Anthropology as a popular movement

German anthropological science developed as an autonomous public forum, owing its growth to bourgeois initiative rather than to state patronage or to reactionary aristocrats. Interest arose in the origins and development of the German peoples and in the question of whether there was a distinct 'Germanic type'. Initially, archaeology was the dominant approach to these questions. The culture of the early Celtic, Slavonic and Teutonic settlements was debated with regards to modern German characteristics. The expectations of national unity were a major stimulus. In 1868 an Ethnographic Museum in Munich and an anthropological section in the Zoological Museum in Dresden were established. There followed the foundation of the German Society for Anthropology, Ethnology and Prehistory in September 1869.[126] This encouraged the founding of local societies such as those in

[122] J. Harvey, 'Races Specified. Evolution Transformed: the Social Context of Scientific Debates Originating in the Société d'Anthropologie de Paris', PhD thesis, Harvard University, 1983.

[123] G.L. Mosse, *Toward the Final Solution. A History of European Racism* (London, 1978), pp. 50–62.

[124] K.-R. Biermann, *Alexander von Humboldt* (Leipzig, 1980), pp. 104–5.

[125] Mosse, *German Ideology*, pp. 90–1.

[126] *Deutsche Gesellschaft für Anthropologie, Ethnologie und Urgeschichte.*

Freiburg, Göttingen, Munich, Würzburg and Vienna. The year of 1869 saw the foundation of the Leipzig Museum for Popular Culture[127] by a committee of professors, publishers and bankers, convened by the doctor Hermann Obst; the Berlin Anthropological Society[128] was launched in November 1869.[129] Liberals as well as radicals such as Vogt were prominent organizers of anthropology, and Schulze Delitzsch supported the Leipzig Museum.[130] Virchow took the lead among Berlin anthropologists, and presided over the meetings of the society for thirty years. Vogt organized the national society. Liberal enclaves such as the one in Baden produced vigorous public and state support for anthropology.[131] While university professors were dominant, other active members were doctors or businessmen, one notable example being Heinrich Schliemann, the excavator of Troy. Anthropological inquiries were sent to consulates and traders overseas. By the 1880s the Anthropological Society was one of the largest and most active scientific societies in Berlin. Membership peaked in the early 1890s with over 600 members; a decline set in due to the rise in subscriptions as a result of the cutting of state subsidies.

In contrast to Britain and France, German states were remarkably slow to institutionalize anthropology as a university discipline. From 1872, societies were offered state grants (for example, from the Prussian *Kultusministerium*), numerous state purchases were made on the advice of the Berlin Society, and the naval and railway administrations granted research facilities. Municipal support resulted in the establishing of the Märkisches Museum in Berlin.[132] In Berlin in August 1880, a national exhibition of German anthropology and archaeology was organized with the support of the conservative *Kultusminister*, Robert von Puttkamer. Its aim was to show the great regional differences and variations existing in Germany. Here was the chance to demonstrate unifying cultural characteristics of remote rural areas like the Oberlausitz in the East with its prehistoric tombs or the lake dwellings of the South. The Neanderthal skull and other prehistoric remains revealed that Germany was the cradle of modern mankind. Virchow, in keeping with his localistic liberalism, regarded the exhibition as an opportunity for expressing civic pride in the *Heimat*.[133] This paved the way for state subsidies, a charter and the opening of a *Museum für Völkerkunde* in Berlin in 1886. Bavaria established a museum for prehistory and anthropology in 1889. From the late 1880s there was a

[127] *Leipziger Museum für Volkskunde.*   [128] *Berliner Gesellschaft für Anthropologie.*

[129] T.K. Penniman, *A Hundred Years of Anthropology* (London, 1935), pp. 365–6.

[130] D. Drost, *Museum für Völkerkunde in Leipzig. Wegweiser durch Geschichte und Ausstellungen* (Leipzig, 1971).   [131] Ecker to Virchow, in Andree, *Rudolf Virchow*, II, pp. 74–7.

[132] C. Andree, 'Geschichte der Berliner Gesellschaft für Anthropologie, Ethnologie und Urgeschichte, 1869–1969', in *Hundert Jahre Berliner Gesellschaft für Anthropologie, Ethnologie und Urgeschichte, 1869–1969* (Berlin, 1969), pp. 23–7. C. Eser, 'Berlins Völkerkunde-Museum in der kolonialära', *Berlin in Geschichte und Gegenwart* (1986) 65–94.
(1881–91), Zedlitz-Trütchler (1891–92), Bosse (1892–99), Studt (1899–1907), Holle (1907–09), Trott zu Solz (1909–17), Schmidt-Ott (1917–18).

[133] R. Virchow, 'Die Ausstellung prähistorischer und anthropologischer Funde Deutschlands zu Berlin', *Verhandlungen der Berliner Anthropologischen Gesellschaft*, (1880), 260–88.

plan for a German National Anthropological Museum inspired by the Nordic Museum in Stockholm.[134] In 1889 a museum for German Folk Costume was financed by the banker, Alexander Meyer-Cohn and the businessman, Franz Görke. Meyer-Cohn underwrote a joint stock company to buy antiquities for the society. Even on the popular commercial level, displays such as the *Panoptikum* and the *Passage-Panoptikum* kept the society supplied with dwarfs and other human anomalies for examination. Anthropology relied more on public enthusiasm and commercial sponsorship than on state support. Plans for a national museum and for national surveys using medical facilities were to be taken up by eugenicists.

Despite vigorous commercial and public patronage, state-sponsored professionalization was a slow process. The first university chair of anthropology was established in Munich in 1879, and was occupied by a physician, Johannes Ranke, who had trained as a physiologist.[135] Berlin lagged behind: Felix von Luschan, who had also first qualified in medicine, was appointed as professor (*Extraordinarius*) in Berlin in 1900, and achieved a full chair (*Ordinarius*) in 1909. He supported the idea of 'applied ethnography'.[136] The attitude of the state authorities is revealing given that the professorship of anthropology was regarded as valuable for the solution of the problems of degeneration in cities.[137] Luschan's appointment marked a turning-point for anthropology; instead of a liberal cataloguing of human variation, it became a state-organized applied discipline. Luschan had extensive duties with the colonial administration and he became involved in the Racial Hygiene Society, although he enraged many eugenicists because of his philo-semitism.

Anthropology constituted a type of national cultural anatomy. University professors of anatomy offered courses in anthropology as a free-lance activity. The public was gripped by a fever of measuring, mapping and digging in the cause of science and national identity. Anthropology was a public and participatory field of study. Karl Hagenbeck, the circus entrepreneur, arranged for displays by ethnic groups such as Sinhalese, or the Bella Coolla and Sioux Indians. The public enjoyed the entertainments and the anthropologists had the opportunity to measure and photograph physique. The societies prided themselves on their ability to organize co-operative researches, and on the involvement of priests, teachers and doctors at meetings and as gatherers of material. By the 1880s, excavation of prehistoric sites was so popular that the state attempted to regulate activities by issuing permits. The public mind linked the unity of mankind and the animal world with the politics of national unification. The nation was the culmination of the evolution of life from simple to complex organisms, and anthropology offered insight into the formation of German culture and physical types.[138]

[134] R. Virchow, 'Festrede', *Verhandlungen der Berliner Anthropologischen Gesellschaft* (1894), 497–512.
[135] A. Geus, *Johannes Ranke (1836–1916). Physiologe, Anthropologe und Prähistoriker* (Marburg, 1987).
[136] S. Westphal-Hellbusch, 'Hundert Jahre Ethnologie in Berlin, unter besonderer Berücksichtigung ihrer Entwicklung an der Universität', in *Hundert Jahre Berliner Gesellschaft*, pp. 157–183.
[137] ZSTA M Rep 76 Va Sekt 2 Tit IV Nr 46 Bd 18.
[138] W. Waldeyer, 'Eröffnungsrede', *Correspondenzblatt der Deutschen Anthropologischen Gesellschaft*, vol. 34 (1903), 67–71.

Haeckel and Virchow typify the growing aspirations of biologists to dominate historical and social studies. Virchow accepted human history as an autonomous process. He regarded the main aim of anthropology as recording threatened human cultures. By way of contrast, Haeckel subordinated history to a cosmic law of cause and evolution that stretched from inorganic nature to human culture. He saw anthropology as a branch of zoology, and psychology was an off-shoot of physiology. To understand psychology, it was necessary to make comparisons with 'lower' forms of intellectual life: 'children, the mentally defective, the mentally ill, and lower human races – and their mental life must be compared with that of the highest animals'. He proclaimed a new science of 'comparative animal psychology'. This would explain the origins of all state and social formations: 'the differences between the highest and lowest humans were greater than those between the lowest humans and the highest animals.'[139] This contrasted to Darwin's view of the minimal intellectual differences between human races.

Virchow recognized the high cultural level of the early Slav settlers in areas such as his native Pomerania. With Robert Koch in 1875 he excavated a walled hill fort. Virchow visited the Caucasus in 1881 and 1894, and denied that it was the cradle of the white race. While not racist in the sense of emphasizing innate racial differences, Virchow's medical and biological approach led him to see races as pathological variations. Disease was part of the evolutionary process. The predominance of doctors in anthropology meant that anthropology reinforced medical theories accounting for differences in stature and in the incidence of disease. The committee of the Berlin Anthropological Society was appropriately dominated by medical professors such as Virchow and the anatomist Wilhelm Waldeyer.

A major preoccupation for anthropologists was atavism and pathology, and their relations to human variation. Like Darwin, Virchow rejected the notion of 'higher' and 'lower' races. None of the living races was lower than another.[140] Race was 'hereditary variation'. Virchow thought it unlikely that racial types were permanent. He condemned the view that pathological variations such as microcephaly were atavistic reversions.[141] While regarding certain races as 'pathological' variations from the parent type, the crucial distinction between peoples was cultural. Virchow distinguished between *Naturvölker* and *Kulturvölker*. Rather than the search for a single 'missing link' between ape and man as demanded by such Darwinians as Haeckel, it was necessary to scour the earth for human remains and cultural artefacts to show the immense potential for human variation. Anthropology amounted to a type of scientific liberalism.

Anthropology was a powerful weapon in the secularizing campaigns against clerical dominance. Darwinian studies in botany or zoology conveyed an implicit message about the natural origins of human culture. Roman Catholicism was the prime target of the emnity of German biologists. The Catholic church was accused

[139] E. Haeckel, *Prinzipien der Generellen Morphologie der Organismen* (1866, reprinted Berlin, 1906), pp. 418–21.   [140] Ackerknecht, *Virchow*, p. 203.

[141] F.B. Churchill, 'Rudolf Virchow and the Pathologist's Criteria for the Inheritance of Acquired Characteristics', *Journal of the History of Medicine*, vol. 31 (1976), 117–48.

of being an alien cultural force that undermined German unity and sapped national energies. Positive science was a secularizing weapon that would generate the spirit of unity and industry. There were strong anti-papal feelings among the more fervent nationalists. Anti-Catholicism and not anti-semitism was the major obsession of the first generation of German Darwinians. Scientific objectivity was a weapon against papal infallibility. The struggle against Roman Catholicism had many dimensions. It was claimed that papal doctrines of infallibility and absolute power violated national unity. Anti-Catholicism was also tied to anti-Polish sentiments, with concerns over the large Polish population in the East. Above all, Bismarck's resentment of the confessional Centre Party launched the *Kulturkampf*. *Kultusminister* Adalbert Falk established state schools free from clerical influence, and Jesuit institutions were dissolved in 1872.

Anti-Catholic prejudice can be seen in private letters of Darwinian biologists. They supported universities in predominantly Catholic and border areas such as Strasburg,[142] Bonn and Breslau[143] as bastions of German culture. They were scornful of popular religious ceremonies and festivals as 'primitive' and 'superstitious'. Haeckel was outspoken in *Anthropogenie* (1874), a book on human origins. He proclaimed embryology as the 'heavy gun' in the struggle of science and religion in cosmic terms: 'the trumpets of this gigantic struggle signal the dawn of a new day and the end of the long night of the middle ages'. Under the 'enlightened banner of science' there were the forces of 'tolerance and truth, culture and reason, development and progress'. These opposed the 'black flag of the Hierarchy', standing for 'subordination and lies, irrationality and vulgarity, superstition and backwardness'. Whole libraries stuffed full of 'clerical wisdom and anal philosophy'[144] would 'melt into nothing as soon as we illuminate this with the sun of embryology'.[145]

Haeckel's colourful phraseology reveals the significance of the energies of and commitment to evolutionary biology. He believed that human progress would arise from competitive selection in culture, economics and politics. This struggle would rid society of the burden of priests and despots. Selection was a guarantee of constant human progress. He did not envisage war as a positive selective process, and nor did he identify the category of race with that of the nation. From Blumenbach's five basic racial types, Haeckel developed a hierarchical scale of twelve human races. He divided these into thirty-six human races. He correlated physical characteristics with culture. The four lowest racial types were classed as 'woolly haired' (*Ulotriches*). Among the lowest of these were Australian aborigines and Hottentots. He considered that no woolly-haired race had ever been of historical significance. The different human species were grouped into four classes: the wild, the barbarians, the civilized, and the cultured. The leading nations of Europe had reached the rank of *mittlerer Kulturvölker*. The highest stage of culture was not yet attained: its characteristics would be state organization to provide

---

[142] Strasbourg.   [143] Wroclaw.   [144] *Afterphilosophie*.
[145] E. Haeckel, *Anthropogenie oder Entwicklungsgeschichte des Menschen* (Leipzig, 1874), pp. xi–xv.

economic support for education, arts and sciences. Armies, duelling and compulsory church attendance would disappear. Haeckel continued to regard German justice, administration and education as steeped in barbarism.[146] Haeckel's Social Darwinism did not seek to brutalize politics or to glorify imperialism in its militarist form. It expressed a type of cultural imperialism, in which Germany had a civilizing mission to the rest of mankind.[147]

Virchow continued to dominate academic societies for anthropology and prehistory. He insisted on autonomy between human culture and evolution, in contrast to Haeckel's monistic philosophy of man and nature. The anthropologists' opposition to colonial imperialism and anti-semitism demonstrates their liberal stance. They were concerned that anthropology should catalogue the immense variation among mankind. Indeed, they condemned colonization as threatening the survival of many cultures and as costly, risky and useless. Anthropologists argued that although Europeans might acclimatize to tropical climates, they could not survive over several generations. Moreover, they suggested that the more advanced the culture, the less resistance there was to infections.[148] That the relations with the German Colonial Society were frosty during the 1880s shows how liberal anthropology initially opposed colonialist ventures and the efforts to whip up public support for imperialism. A vociferous group of doctors overseas responded in 1886 to requests by the German Colonial Society for evidence on acclimatization. A transition in medical sympathies from liberalism to imperialism is shown in the fact that while in 1889 there were 144 doctors who were members of colonial societies, by 1893 this figure had climbed to 826.[149] The strong current of liberalism within the medical profession was subject to rising tensions between racially minded imperialists and social reformers.

The racializing of anti-semitism

The idea of a separate 'Jewish race' figured only sporadically in liberal German anthropology of the 1870s. Many anthropologists and ethnologists, who associated with Virchow, were Jews. Yet since the 1840s there was an undercurrent of anti-semitism in Germany that replaced religious discrimination with secular concept of the Jews as a separate race.[150] In 1881 Eugen Dühring drew the conclusion that the

[146] R. Winau, 'Ernst Haeckels Vorstellungen vom Werden menschlicher Rassen und Kulturen', *Medizinhistorisches Journal*, vol. 16 (1981), 270–9.

[147] P. von zur Mühlen, *Rassenideologien. Geschichte und Hintergründe* (Bonn, 1977), p. 81.

[148] Max Bartels, 'Culturelle und Rassenunterschiede in Bezug auf die Wundkrankheiten', *Zeitschrift für Ethnologie*, vol. 20 (1888), 169–83.

[149] S. Parlow, 'Über einige kolonialistische und annexionistische Aspekte bei deutschen Ärzten von 1884 bis zum Ende des 1. Weltkrieges', *Wissenschaftliche Zeitschrift der Universität Rostock, mathematisch-naturwissenschaftliche Reihe*, vol. 15 (1964), 537–49.

[150] L. Poliakov. *The History of Anti-Semitism* (Oxford, 1985); P. Massing, *Rehearsal for Destruction: A Study of Political Anti-Semitism in Imperial Germany* (New York, 1949); P.J. Pulzer, *The Rise of Political Anti-Semitism in Germany and Austria* (New York, 1964); R. Rürup, 'Emancipation and Crisis. The "Jewish Question" in Germany 1850–1890', *Leo Baeck Institute Yearbook*, vol. 20 (1975), 13–25.

key characteristic of Jewry was not religious but common descent.[151] The term 'anti-semitism' was invented by the Hamburg journalist, Wilhelm Marr, to convey the idea that Jews were a distinct semitic race. Baptism considerably eased the path for Jews wanting careers in academia or state service. Even the historian, Treitschke, one of the leading anti-Jewish campaigners in the 1880s conceded that once baptized, 'a Jew was no longer a Jew'. Anti-semitic groupings from the late 1870s tried to capture the ground of the left-liberals and socialists.[152] Anti-semites stigmatized Jews as part of an attack on secular culture and economic upheavals resulting from liberal capitalism.

In 1879 Adolf Stoecker, a court pastor reacting against popular irreligion and the urban squalor of Berlin, organized a Christian Social Party that was anti-liberal, anti-socialist and strongly anti-semitic. In 1880 Stoecker proclaimed a struggle of 'race against race'.[153] It marked the beginnings of organized political anti-semitism, but it was independent of Social Darwinism and other variants of organicist social theory. When there was a mass petition to the Prussian Assembly organized by Bernhard Förster against the Jews in 1880, Virchow protested that it confused religion and race. In 1881 Virchow and Stoecker were rival candidates for the Reichstag in the same constituency in Berlin. A number of Christian doctors resented the awarding of such posts as Poor Law doctors to Jews.[154] Berlin was the centre of an anti-semitic student movement during the 1880s.[155]

By 1890, Berlin's Jewish population has risen to 45,000 in a rapidly expanding population of 1.5 million. The trend was for Jews to move to the cities and in particular to Berlin so that by 1914 one quarter of Prussian Jews were concentrated in this metropolis. Stoecker was attempting to capitalize on growing antagonism to the success of Jews in all walks of life. Medicine was no exception. It was a popular field of study for Jewish students. While a career in one of the more prestigious branches of medicine such as surgery was difficult, the recently qualified generation of Jewish doctors often found a niche in the less attractive fringe specialisms of dermatology and venereology, or in the more arduous and less socially prestigious activity of Poor Law medicine. Certain Jewish practitioners combined practice in industrial suburbs with political radicalism. This is well shown by Zadek and Blaschko who, as medical students in the mid-1870s, made friends with leading socialists such as Eduard Bernstein. During the 1890s they agitated for a municipal health policy in Berlin. There were many Jewish pioneers of a radical social medicine.[156]

[151] Conze, 'Rasse', pp. 173–7.
[152] R.S. Levy, *The Downfall of the Anti-Semitic Political Parties in Imperial Germany* (New Haven and London, 1975), pp. 16, 265, 268.
[153] W. Kampmann, *Deutsche und Juden* (Frankfurt-on-Main, 1979), pp. 244, 247.
[154] W.F. Kümmel, 'Rudolf Virchow und der Antisemitismus', *Medizinhistorisches Journal*, vol. 3 (1968), 165–79.
[155] N. Kampe, 'Jews and Anti-semites at Universities in Imperial Germany (II). The Friedrich-Wilhelms-Universität of Berlin: a Case Study on the Students' "Jewish Question"', *Leo Baeck Institute Year Book*, vol. 32 (1987), 43–101.
[156] F. Tennstedt, 'Arbeiterbewegung und Familiengeschichte bei Eduard Bernstein und Ignaz Zadek', *IWK*, (1982), 451–81.

Stoecker made the most of the resentment against Jewish medical practitioners in his anti-semitic and anti-liberal campaign. Anti-semites delighted in using medical rhetoric to add force to their arguments. They declared that as long as there was no way of transfusing Aryan blood into the veins of Jews there would be a Jewish problem. During the second wave of anti-semitism in the early 1890s, Virchow used his position as Rector of the university of Berlin to denounce its inexplicable irrationality:

Our time, so sure of itself and of victory by reason of its scientific consciousness, is as apt as former ages to underestimate the strength of the mystic impulses with which the soul of the nation is infected by single adventurers. Even now it is standing baffled before the enigma of anti-Semitism, whose appearance in this time of the equality of right is inexplicable to everybody, yet which, in spite of its mysteriousness, or perhaps because of it, fascinates even our cultured youth. Up to the present moment the demand for a professorship of anti-Semitism has not made itself heard; but rumour has it that there are anti-Semitic professors.[157]

Virchow's condemnation indicates that at this time biological anthropology and anti-semitism were fundamentally opposed, just as liberal anthropology took a stand against colonial imperialism. It endorsed the authority of intellectual superiority, justifying the scientist as arbiter of social affairs. A liberal combination of scientific and patriotic interests inspired a widespread public enthusiasm for anthropology. Yet there were social forces that Virchow's individualistic liberalism could not comprehend. By the 1890s a generation armed with strong imperialist convictions was changing the complexion of anthropology, as most of the founders from the 1860s died. State support was withdrawn from anthropology by *Kultusminister* Gustav von Gossler. One aspect of the change was the emergence of a synthesis of racial anti-semitism, imperialism and science as a product of the sense of social crisis of the 1880s. The bourgeoisie attempted to adapt to industrial growth, urban expansion and to intense competition within the overcrowded professions for jobs and status. Biological social values were still distinct from Gobineau's Aryanism. As social convictions became more hereditarian and collectivist, anthropology was to be a major support for racial hygiene.

---

[157] R. Virchow, 'The Founding of the Berlin University and the Transition from the Philosophic to the Scientific Age', *Annual Report of the Board of Regents of the Smithsonian Institution to July 1894* (Washington, 1896), pp. 681–95.

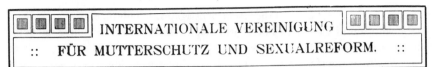

AUFRUF

AN MÄNNER UND FRAUEN ALLER KULTURLÄNDER.

Leben heißt Sichentwickeln. Aller Entwickelung Sinn und Ziel ist Vervollkommnung. Kraft der natürlichen Gesetze hat ein gewaltiger Aufstieg des organischen Lebens sich vollzogen und im „Menschen" seine höchste Staffel erreicht. Aber nicht seinen Abschluß! Auch der Mensch, unterworfen den Gesetzen der Entwickelung, ist der weiteren Vervollkommnung fähig. Seine Einsicht lehrt ihn, diese Gesetze zu ermitteln; Verstand und Wille fordern, sie nutzbar zu machen für seine eigene Entwickelung: in sozialem Zusammenwirken, zielbewußt, die organisch-geistige Vervollkommnung seiner Rasse zu erstreben und damit den festen Boden zu schaffen für eine höhere menschliche Kultur, für edlere und zugleich glücklichere Lebensverhältnisse.

Die erste Vorbedingung aber einer stetigen, aufwärts leitenden Entwickelung ist die Gesunderhaltung der Rasse. Ihr vornehmstes Mittel ist die in der Gattungsfortpflanzung sich vollziehende Auslese. Diese stark, gesund und rein zu erhalten, sie dem Ziele der Vervollkommnung anzupassen und so das Geschlechtsleben des Menschen zugleich dem Wohle der Lebenden und dem Aufstieg der Gattung dienstbar zu machen, ist die höchste Aufgabe der fortschreitenden Zivilisation.

Von dieser Warte betrachtet, zeigt gerade

das geschlechtliche Leben der Gegenwart

Erscheinungen, welche den Fortschritt nicht nur hemmen, sondern aufs schwerste gefährden; welche in schärfstem Widerspruche stehen nicht nur zu der glänzenden Außenseite unserer Kultur, sondern auch zu den durch die Wissenschaft vermittelten Einsichten in die Bedingungen unserer Entwickelung.

Wir sehen das heutige Geschlechtsleben in allen Gesellschaftskreisen beherrscht von der offenen und heimlichen Prostitution, der wahllosen geschlechtlichen Hingabe um materieller Vorteile willen. Wir sehen es durchseucht von Geschlechtskrankheiten, welche am Mark des Volkes zehren und in zahllosen Ehen die Erfüllung ihrer höchsten Zwecke im Dienste der Gattung vereiteln. Und während wir der Macht der Sexualität, die unser Blut durchflutet, mit heuchlerischer Verheimlichung begegnen, üben wir gegenüber ihren Schäden ein System der Vertuschung, das den besten Nährboden ihres Wachstums bildet.

Auf dem für die Geschlechtsauslese wichtigsten Gebiete der Eheschließung macht eine die Entwickelung schwer belastende Verquickung von „Geld" und „Liebe", eine verhängnisvolle Abhängigkeit der Gattenwahl vom wirtschaftlichen Interesse, auf Kosten der Gesundheit und Lebenstüchtigkeit der Nachkommenschaft, sich geltend. Die Ehe selbst, als wahrhafte,

---

2 'International Association for Protection of Mothers and Sexual Reform. Appeal to Men and Women of all Civilized Countries'. Among those supporting the Association were Helene Stöcker, Eduard Bernstein, Havelock Ellis, August Forel, Sigmund Freud, Rudolf Goldscheid, Ernst Haeckel, Carl Hauptmann, Magnus Hirschfeld, Käthe Kollwitz, Eduard Mach, Wilhelm Ostwald, Wilhelm Schallmayer, Bernhard Shaw, Frank Wedekind and H.G. Wells. The Association demanded a reform of marriage as a means of promoting self-fulfillment and of combatting venereal diseases and prostitution.

2

Between utopianism and racial hygiene

Depression and repression

Darwinism in the 1860s formed part of an enthusiastic outburst of faith in liberalism, economic progress and national culture. After national unification the effects of industrialization prompted a reversal of this liberal optimism as Darwinists pointed to the risks of degeneration resulting from industrial, urban and 'overly civilized' life. The sharp reversal of opinion occurred when confidence in social and economic progress was shaken during the economically depressed years between 1873 and 1879. Although rapid industrial growth resumed, there remained the sense that the basis of prosperity was fragile and had to be defended against the threat of socialism. By the 1880s a critical reaction to the physical and psychological degeneration arising from industrialization and rapid urbanization had begun to gather force. There were striking developments in the organization and ideology of socialism. In 1875 doctrinal and sectional differences among workers' associations were overcome, and the Social Democratic Party (SPD) was founded. Socialists rapidly gathered support in the cities and industrial areas, provoking the alarm of Bismarck. Using the pretext of an assassination attempt, Bismarck turned against socialists and liberal supporters of free speech. At the same time as economic expansion occurred the state imposed repressive policies with anti-socialist laws which lasted from October 1878 until October 1890. Not only did socialist groups survive, but discontented bourgeois intellectuals were sympathetic towards socialism in the repressive climate.

Symptomatic of the social dislocation were the high mortality and emigration rates during the 1880s. As faith wavered in economic progress as the means of social improvement, there was growing alienation from the artificiality and elitism of high culture.[1] Socio-economic upheavals and political repression generated a critical reaction which found expression in movements of international socialism,

---

[1] R. Harmann and J. Hermand, *Naturalismus* (Berlin, 1968).

imperialism, anti-semitism and *Lebensreform*. In an attempt to overcome the contradictory aims of these movements, elements from these were blended on a Darwinian basis by the group, who became the nucleus of the racial hygiene movement. Their concern over the survival of natural racial vigour was transmuted into a programme for a scientifically reformed lifestyle. How the German eugenics movement came to contain contradictory beliefs that resulted in internal tensions can be seen by tracing the sequence of responses of the eugenicists to the broader ideological currents.

There grew up a counter-philosophy of *Lebensreform* with agitation for a reformed lifestyle and for social organizations to guarantee natural values. Utopian ideals and natural laws of the right of every person to a healthy existence were guidelines for a return to natural purity. While critical of soul-destroying mechanistic science, an alternative type of science was cultivated. Its aim was to recover a holistic sense of nature that would regenerate the primitive racial vigour and sense of community that were threatened by industrialization. There arose a synthesis between *Lebensreform* and medical arguments for the eradication of racial poisons such as alcohol, meat and tobacco. The *Lebensreform* movement had offshoots in the vegetarian, clothing reform and anti-alcohol movements which demanded a transformation of lifestyle with rejection of unbridled consumerism and commercialism.[2]

The agitation for reformed lifestyle expressed the alienation of a younger generation, rebelling against the repressive moral conventions and lack of career prospects. Enthusiasm for the creative arts, and for philosophical speculations on the nature of life combined with plans for social reform. Modern industrial society was criticized for its physically and morally degenerative effects, for its destruction of human life and its soul-destroying mechanization of existence. Naturalist authors and artists portrayed the social reality of life in the new nation as that of corrupt decadence resulting from brash prosperity, or of degrading squalor of the burgeoning urban proletariat. Youthful dissidents formulated social plans to cure the degenerative effects of modern civilization. Moral and political remedies were not enough: it was necessary to purify the cultural and scientific structures that had been so debased by industrialization. Biology and health were central to the reformist strategy. There was revulsion from liberal economic progress and civic freedoms as having produced 'the social problem' to which liberal individualism offered no solutions. Convictions grew that industrial society required collective institutions for guaranteeing the physical basis of existence through adequate diet, housing and health care. Science and medicine supported demands for a society that would maintain individual fitness and health. More radical still was the belief that life could best be regenerated in a healthy and invigorating natural environment of overseas colonies.

Behind the enthusiasm for *Lebensreform* lay the complex social forces that were turning Germany from a predominately patriarchal and rural society into an

---

[2] W. Krabbe, *Gesellschaftsveränderung durch Lebensreform* (Göttingen, 1974).

industrial and world power. The political and cultural discontents of the late 1870s gave rise to a network of patriotic associations for disseminating German culture and solving social problems by establishing colonies. In 1878 Friedrich Fabri, an organizer of overseas missions, published a tract on the social benefits of colonies, and an Association for Commercial Geography and for German Interests Abroad was founded.[3] In 1882 the German Colonial Association was established,[4] and in 1884 Carl Peters founded a populist version of the colonial society, and urged East African colonization as a solution to poverty. In 1884–85 Bismarck conceded the establishment of colonies in West Africa and the Pacific. Instead of losing population as a result of emigration, colonies would strengthen the German nation throughout the world. Such societies supported a broadened view of the *Volk* as an ethnic unit defined by language and culture.[5] These organizations included academic enthusiasts such as tropical and ships' doctors, geographers and statisticians.[6] The Berlin statistician, Richard Boeckh, combined nationalist agitation with applying his expertise in statistical studies of the distribution of expatatriate German-speaking population groups, monitoring population movements, morbidity trends and mortality. The geographer, Friedrich Ratzel, welcomed this colonial policy as a means of renewing the National Liberal Party as well as the German nation.[7] He coined the term *Lebensraum* to express the concept of Germany as an organic and territorial unity.[8] Schools became a nationalist flash-point when in 1881 the General German Schools Association[9] was founded in order to strengthen German culture to counter ethnic minorities such as the Poles, and to reinforce German identity outside the Reich. Demands for colonies expressed the social insecurities of an economically hard-pressed middle class that also found outlets in the movements for *Lebensreform*, and anti-semitism. These various currents of disenchantment sought to dislodge the dominance of the aristocratic-Junker ruling elite, correct the narrowly economic individualism of liberalism, and enlarge the scope for nationally minded activities. This background of cultural crisis, colonialism, state interventionism and political repression was the starting-point for youthful protests.

The utopian circle

The concern to prevent racial degeneration inspired a group of adolescents to form a League to Reinvigorate the Race in 1879.[10] Their aim was to restore German

---

[3] *Zentralverein für Handelsgeographie und deutsche Interessen im Auslande.*
[4] *Deutscher Kolonial Verein.*
[5] R. Chickering, *We Men Who Feel Most German. A Cultural Study of the Pan-German League 1886–1914* (London, 1984), pp. 29–38.
[6] Parlow, 'Über einige kolonialistische und annexionistische Aspekte bei deutschen Ärzten', pp. 537–49.
[7] G. Buttmann, *Friedrich Ratzel, Leben und Werk eines deutschen Geographen 1844–1904* (Stuttgart, 1977), pp. 25–9, 81–93.
[8] R.E. Dickinson, *The German Lebensraum* (Harmondsworth, 1943).
[9] *Allgemeiner Deutscher Schulverein.* [10] *Bund zur Ertüchtigung der Rasse.*

peoples to the purity and vigour that they had possessed in their first millenium. They would unite all Germans in a world state. The leader of this schoolboy gang was Alfred Ploetz, and the *Bund* included Carl and Gerhart Hauptmann. They swore a midnight oath of blood brotherhood at an oak outside Breslau, their Silesian home town. They planned a utopian colony. Ploetz was to be President, Carl Hauptmann the Minister of Science, and Gerhart Hauptmann the Minister of Culture.[11] Ploetz was to take a central role in launching the German eugenics movement. He pursued his ideals with a remarkable organizing vigour and crusading fervour. He was an impetuous traveller, going wherever necessary for the pursuit of eugenic schemes. He tempered his Greater German sense of national identity that led to frequent visits to Switzerland and Austria with an internationalism that led him to seek his fortune in the United States and to benefit from German investments in Argentina. He had a wide-ranging intellect that related philosophy and social sciences to an obsession with heredity and race. He cultivated life-long friendships and recruited disciples to the ideals of the movement that he named 'racial hygiene'. He would sign effusive letters 'Dein alter Ploetzlich' ('your old Ploetzlich' – a pun on the word *ploetzlich* meaning sudden) and 'ein alter Kosmosbummler' (an old dreamer). Science was to weld socialism and nationalism into a coherent ideology of biological social reform, and be the weapon in the struggle to regenerate the race.[12]

While the youthful oath of blood brotherhood was an adolescent escapade, there lay behind it a fashionable enthusiasm for nature and a significant transition in German nationalism. Racial ardour was fuelled by a youthful fascination with Darwinism and the idealization of German national culture. Between 1870 and 1914 many adolescent renegades read Haeckel and revelled in the adventures of natural history collecting. Enthusiasm for natural history went with a fascination for 'primitive' racial prowess as in adventure stories glorifying German history. Favourite books were tales by the Breslau historian and writer, Felix Dahn, about Nordic warriors – the theatrical *Kampf um Rom* of 1867 and *Odins Trost* combining Germanic myths of a struggle of Teutons and Jews with ideas of harmony with nature and the universe.[13] This nationalist culture reflected the disappointed hopes of 'Gross-Deutsche' idealists hoping to incorporate Austria into Bismarck's Germany. National cultural regeneration and the stream of writings on the need to solve social problems by German colonies had common sources in the alienation from restrictive and repressive elite values.

Such programmes of racial imperialism appealed to the economic concerns and political ideals of the offspring of manufacturers and small businessmen. They

---

[11] Ploetz was later uncertain as to the year. See Gerhart Hauptmann papers, Ploetz to Hauptmann, 18 August 1935, 19 December 1935, 12 October 1936.

[12] For a biographical sketch see W. Doeleke, 'Alfred Ploetz (1860–1940). Sozialdarwinist und Gesellschaftsbiologe', med. Diss., University of Mainz, 1975.

[13] Carl Hauptmann papers, Ploetz to Carl Hauptmann, 6 October 1893. G.L. Mosse, 'The Image of the Jew in German Popular Culture: Felix Dahn and Gustav Freytag', *Leo Baeck Institute Yearbook*, vol. 2 (1957), 218–27.

Table 1. *The first generation of medically qualified racial/social hygienists*

	Date of birth	Father's occupation
Baur	14.iv.75	Apothecary
Blaschko	4.iii.58	Physician
Bluhm	9.i.62	Army Officer
Crzellitzer	5.iv.71	Manufacturer
A. Fischer	12.xii.73	Manufacturer
E. Fischer	5.vi.74	Commerce
Gottstein	2.xi.57	Commerce
Grotjahn	25.xi.69	Physician
Gruber	6.vii.53	Physician
Hirsch	3.i.77	Commerce
Hueppe	24.viii.52	Official
Kaup	11.i.70	Commerce
Krohne	29.v.68	Manufacturer
Lenz	9.iii.87	Landowner
Ploetz	22.vii.60	Manufacturer
Rüdin	19.iv.74	Commerce/teacher
Schallmayer	10.ii.57	Manufacturer
Weinberg	25.xii.,62	Commerce
Woltmann	18.ii.71	Carpenter

supported the medical education of their offspring who, once qualified, were discontented with the limited prospects of medical practice. Of the families of the racial hygienists, Ploetz's father had been manager of a soap factory, and the Hauptmanns were sons of an inn-keeper. The father of Ernst Rüdin was a teacher who became a buyer in the knitting industry. Several other eugenicists were also from the *Kaufmannstand*. Most of the others came from families in which the bourgeois tendency to limit fertility to two or three children was already evident (as in the case of Ploetz and Rüdin).[14]

There were a few exceptions to this type of background. Fritz Lenz came from a landowners' family, and Agnes Bluhm (one of the very few women involved) was the daughter of an officer employed in Turkey. But as table 1 indicates, commerce (to a greater extent) and the academically educated professions (to a lesser extent) supplied most of the founders of the eugenics movement.

There was a contradiction between personal dependence on the family as a sustaining economic unit, and unease with the family as degenerate and repressive. Eugenics was to be a means of resolving this tension between the personal and the ideal. On the death of his father, Ploetz's resolve to pursue plans for social reform hardened. The contrast between the occupation of Ploetz's father as a soap

---

[14] Eugenicists with several siblings were rare; Muckermann, born in 1877 and the son of a shoemaker, was one of twelve children, and Schallmayer was one of eleven.

manufacturer, and his sense of professional mission as a racial hygienist typifies the generation gap between commerce and professionalism on the basis of health.[15] These youthful dissidents were caught in a dilemma. On the one hand they believed commercial and industrial expansion to be poisoning the nation's cultural and social traditions. On the other they resented the narrowness of an academically educated society with its limited career prospects. Initially, they saw a solution to the contradiction between sustaining personal wealth and national cultural identity in the establishing of colonies for health rather than commercial profit. This utopian vision combined commercial entrepreneurship with cultural elitism, expressing the aspirations of university-educated young intellectuals. Such economically frustrated youth sought opportunities in emigration, or in the utilization of scientific ideals to open up spheres for the exercising of professional expertise.[16]

Lebensreform prompted the group of youthful renegades to assume defiant and distinctive clothing. The Ploetz circle dressed in the sanitary woollen reform clothing of the doctor and zoologist, Gustav Jaeger. This clothing expressed the 'Darwinian' conviction that as man was a mammal, he ought only to wear clothing made out of mammalian fibres. Such garments would give the body immunity from infection from newly discovered microscopic germs.[17] The clothing was meant to improve mental health, Jaeger being convinced that fear and nervousness were caused by the build-up of waste products in the body. Together with improved nutrition – particularly the consuming of less fatty foods – Jaeger's wool regime amounted to a form of lay self-help.[18] A general concern with health came before an interest in biology.

The adolescent malcontents of the Ploetz circle encountered rapid urban and industrial growth, and mass poverty, and were outraged at the police repression in Germany. Their home city of Breslau, and the university towns of Jena and Zürich were all in the grip of rapid industrial and population growth. During the 1870s Breslau was the third largest German city with a population of over 200,000; by 1900 the population had climbed to 500,000. The substantial Polish population and traditions of social protest predisposed the city to becoming the birthplace of racial hygiene. With the rise of the precision optical industries of Zeiss and of the Schott glass manufacturers during the 1870s and 80s, Jena grew from an isolated, rural university town to an industrial centre. The rapid expansion of higher education was a remarkable feature of German industrialization. At Breslau, Jena and more generally at the German universities, there was an unprecedented boom in student numbers during the 1880s. The universities, stigmatized as 'teaching factories',

---

[15] Carl Hauptmann papers, Ploetz to Carl Hauptmann 6 October 1893.
[16] Analysis of social composition and careers will be found on pp. 148–9 below.
[17] G. Jaeger, *Seuchenfestigkeit und Konstitutionskraft* (Leipzig, 1878); Jaeger, *Selections from Essays on Health-Culture and the Sanitary Woollen System* (London, 1884).
[18] E. Kaufmann, *Gustav Jaeger, 1832–1913. Arzt, Zoologe und Hygieniker* (Zürich, 1984), pp. 29–38.

rapidly ran into the problem of producing more graduates than could be readily absorbed in the professions.

Student radicals

Ploetz began to study economics at Breslau out of his sense of a mission to solve the nation's social problems. Many of those with whom Ploetz associated made successful careers in science-based professions such as engineering and medicine. But as students, Ploetz and his fraternity were outraged by prevailing social conditions. They studied socialist writings on population growth. Karl Kautsky's writings on population, in which the need for contraception was urged, led to an interest in Marx and scientific socialism. The mathematics student, Heinrich Lux, was impressed by Kautsky, and Simon turned to the biology of sexuality in nature as the topic for his doctorate.[19] Since the early 1880s Lux had been in contact with Breslau socialists. While Lux at first supported socialist agitation, he soon acquiesced in the others' view that a new society should be founded on the basis of scientific socialism in the free world. The group's priorities were utopian. On 1 November 1883 they established a society called *Pacific*. Ploetz and its secretary, the musician Karl Max Müller, registered this with the police in the belief that they would not contravene the Anti-Socialist Laws. The term, *Pacific*, betrayed the influence of Charles Fourier's socialist utopia of *Democracie Pacifique*. Enthusiasts included on the scientific side included the medical students, Julian Marcuse and Ferdinand Simon (the latter an advocate of temperance who in 1891 would marry the daughter of the German socialist August Bebel), Karl Steinmetz, an engineer who was to make a brilliant career with the American General Electric Company[20] and Wolfgang Heine, a member of national student organizations before becoming a leading socialist lawyer and later Prussian Minister of the Interior. The group established offshoots in Jena, Berlin and Zürich. In addition to the Hauptmanns, the circle embraced artists and authors such as Jan Kaspowicz (a Polish patriot and poet), Otto Pringsheim (the son of a Breslau banker) and the artist Hugo Schmidt.[21] In 1884 Käthe Kollwitz was entranced by the vitality of the artists in the group, whom she visited in Berlin.[22]

Radical politics was combined with admiration for science and literature. Indeed, it was hoped that art, science and social organization could all be given real power by establishing their basis in natural laws. At Breslau the Ploetz circle was impressed by the botanist, Ferdinand Cohn, who in 1876 was one of the first

---

[19] F. Simon, 'Die Sexualität und ihre Erscheinungsweisen in der Natur. Versuch einer kritischen Erklärung', Diss., University of Jena, 1883. H. Lux, *Die Prostitution* (Berlin, 1892).

[20] K. Kautsky Jnr., *August Bebels Briefwechsel mit Karl Kautsky* (Assen, 1971), pp. 281–3.

[21] *Die Geschichte der Breslauer Sozialdemokratie* (Breslau, 1925), pp. 207–212. My thanks to F. Tennstedt for this reference.

[22] K. Kollwitz, *Ich sah die Welt mit liebevollen Blicken* (Wiesbaden, nd), p. 270.

academics to recognize the brilliance of Koch's discoveries on bacteria as a cause of disease. Cohn, one of very few Jewish professors, combined positive support for experimental hygiene with anti-Catholicism, Darwinism and the evolutionary sociology of Schäffle and Spencer, providing a blend of ideas on the organism as a cell state that were to be later synthesized in Ploetz's racial hygiene.[23] The more the budding social reformers became immersed in their studies, the greater their urge became to apply science to the solution of social problems. Many of the *Jugendbund* proceeded to the University of Jena, where Carl Hauptmann matriculated in 1880.[24] Until 1884 they were in contact with Haeckel, and enthused over evolution as a basis for social reform. They formed the nucleus of a student scientific society in Jena. On behalf of the society of Darwinian enthusiasts, Wilhelm Breitenbach wrote an enthusiastic letter to Darwin, and Haeckel and Eduard Strasburger became honorary members.[25] The circle came to include Plate, a radical student of zoology, Johannes Walther, the geologist, and Carl Duisberg, the chemist. They benefited from contact with Richard Semon, a biologist who developed the 'mneme' theory of inherited memory and of culture as subject to Lamarckian laws of heredity. Initially they admired Haeckel's struggle to place German politics and culture on sound national lines. Science was to justify individualism and social progress. In 1883 Hauptmann completed a dissertation which used cell theory and Haeckel's biogenetic law as the basis for examining the origins of individualism and the process of reproduction.[26] Lux's dissertation of 1883 on sexuality in nature corresponded to the circle's broader interests in the biological basis of social processes. Evolutionary biology offered an alternative to Hegelian dialectics as a route to scientific socialism. The group became critical of Haeckel's descriptive morphology as too static. Hauptmann aimed at a unified theory of life and ethics based on physiological and psychological laws. Ploetz sought to implement a revolutionary ethics based on science.[27]

They maintained a strongly idealistic approach to Darwinism and social science. They cultivated the Platonist philosopher, Rudolf Eucken, who developed a philosophy of the totality of 'Life', and popularized idealism as an antidote to the technical and economic culture of the Reich. Inspired by Eucken's plans for the resurrection of the German tradition of idealist philosophers, the circle's reading encompassed the seventeenth-century pantheist Jacob Boehme, and explored the ideas on human perfectibility of utopian writers such as Plato, Thomas More,

[23] F. Cohn, 'Der Zellenstaat', *Deutsche Rundschau*, vol. 27 (1881), 62–80.
[24] C. Hauptmann papers, Ploetz to Carl Hauptmann, Breslau, 30 December 1881; C. Hauptmann, *Leben mit Freunden, Gesammelte Briefe* (Berlin, 1928), pp. 13–14, 24–6, 143, for letters to Haeckel.
[25] University of Cambridge Library, Darwin Letters Project, W. Breitenbach to Darwin, 10 February 1880, Darwin to Breitenbach, 13 February 1880. Breitenbach became a noted monist, publisher and a member of the *Fortschrittlichen Volkspartei*.
[26] C. Hauptmann, *Die Bedeutung der Keimblättertheorie für Individualitätslehre und den Generationswechsel* (Jena, 1883).
[27] A. Stroka, *Carl Hauptmann's Werdegang als Denker und Dichter*, (Wroclaw, 1965); W. Goldstein, *Carl Hauptmann, Eine Werkdeutung* (Breslau, 1931).

Tommaso Campanella and Robert Owen. The socialist Kautsky alerted Ploetz to the economic roots of the crisis in modern society, and the wave of naturalist writers and social critics deepened awareness of the commitments of how the creative artist could articulate the effects of industrial social conditions on the personality and on family life. Henrik Ibsen and Emile Zola set challenging standards in the literary portrayal of how social conditions resulted in degeneration of the family. The Ploetz circle discussed problems posed by Haeckel's monist philosophy, such as that of unifying the metaphysical with the physiological. They felt that they were looking for building materials for a regenerated social structure. Friedrich Nietzsche's *Also sprach Zarathustra*, recently published (1883–4), was considered. Although rejected by Ploetz as unsuitable, his first treatise on racial hygiene was to cite Nietzsche's aphorism on progress from the species to the super-species ('von der Art hinüber zur Ueber Art'), and on the risks of degeneration resulting from egoism. The group regarded biology as a means of social prophecy and regeneration.[28]

In order to create a model community the Pacific Society collected 3,100 marks with which it sent Ploetz to the United States to make arrangements for the colony. The others joked that in the meantime they expected to be banished to Siberia for their radicalism.[29] Ploetz visited Chicago in 1884 where he delved into the literature on utopias. He found the most suitable to be the Icarian colony in Iowa, where he then worked for several months. The colony had been founded by Etienne Cabet and was inspired by Fourier's utopian socialism and the principle of the right to work. Ploetz was dismayed to find the colony in dissolution. It convinced him that egalitarian idealism was not enough. He drew up a 'Constitution of the Freeland Society' which placed socialism on racial principles. For the German race to survive it was necessary to found elite colonies where racial purity could be maintained. Good health would be a condition of admission to such a colony.

Simon and Lux were furious when Ploetz returned. They felt that the rather academic conclusions that he had drawn about egalitarianism failed to solve the pressing need for a form of collective organization to counter the social misery of unbridled individualism. An indication of the political adventurousness of their thinking was the arrest of thirty-eight Icarians in Breslau in 1887. Lux, Marcuse and Kaspowicz were among those prosecuted, the others being workers. When Gerhart Hauptmann was sent a copy of Ploetz's utopian constitution, he burned it, fearing police arrest under the Anti-Socialist Laws. Later, in fact, he was interrogated by the police.[30] Lux became a socialist journalist and analysed virtues of utopianism in a tract on Icarian communism.[31] Such incidents convey the

---

[28] Doeleke, 'Ploetz', pp. 8–13.
[29] C. Hauptmann papers, C. Hauptmann to Ploetz, 6 January 1884.
[30] K. Jarausch, *Students, Society and Politics in Imperial Germany* (Princeton, 1982), pp. 340, 357; note that Lux is the 'Lutz' mentioned on p. 340.
[31] H. Lux, *Etienne Cabet und der Ikarische Kommunismus* (Stuttgart, 1896). A. Bebel, *Charles Fourier* (Leipzig, 1978).

genuine radicalism and confrontation with authority of this group of scientific reformers of society.

Medical regeneration

The *Jugendbund* embraced Jewish, socialist and Polish enthusiasts within the overall project of a racial utopia. The German universities with which the Ploetz circle were associated in the early 1880s, Breslau and Jena, were exceptional for their lack of student anti-semitism.[32] Ploetz prided himself on his cosmopolitanism. Their radicalism spurred migration to Zürich in 1885. This was a mecca for students and intellectuals alienated by the anti-socialist laws in Germany. Here was one of the very few universities to admit women, and to attract substantial numbers of Russian and American women medical students. A female element was added to the utopian group. Ploetz immersed himself in socialist circles, as he gathered ideas that he could use to construct his ideal society. Ploetz accompanied Simon on visits to Bebel at his holiday villa on Lake Zürich. Bebel had common interests in biology, in reform of the family and in utopian social visions: he planned a society reliant on solar energy and electricity, which would enable a shorter working day and more humane and hygienic working conditions. Ploetz continued to supply student colleagues, such as Lux and Marcuse in Breslau, with socialist literature; he sent Bebel's *Woman and Socialism*, and socialist and anarchist journals.[33]

Ploetz planned that his dream child – the Pacific colony – would have a socialist economy. Its aim was not to implement the Marxism of the SPD but to strengthen the race. Lux and Ploetz looked forward to armed struggle for a socialist republic. They absorbed a wide range of influences, and their socialism was combined with scientific planning and naturalistic sensibilities. The group retained a fascination for esoteric experiences, such as moonlight mountain walks and telepathy; but biology and medicine came to dominate their interests. Their mentor was the professor of psychiatry and expert on the social life of ants, August Forel. He instilled in the group the ideals of a world without alcohol and with equal sexual rights. Ploetz switched his course of studies from economics to medicine. This change was significant in showing that his reformist ideas were to be based not on economic reform but on biological engineering of the human constitution.

As an economics student Ploetz encountered a number of organicist social theorists. Influences on Ploetz included the economist Albert Schäffle, who between 1875 and 1878 published on the construction and nature of the social organism. Forel and Ploetz enthused over Schäffle's tract, *Quintessenz des Socialismus*.[34] This elaborated a Spencerian theory of the social organism emphasizing organic integration rather than struggle. It incorporated such

[32] Kampe, 'Jews and Anti-semites at Universities in Imperial Germany', pp. 38–46.
[33] K.R. Calkins, 'The Uses of Utopianism: The Millenarian Dream in Central European Social Democracy Before 1914', *Central European History*, vol. 15 (1982), 124–48; Carl Hauptmann papers, Ploetz to C. Hauptmann, 31 August 1897 on Simon and Bebel.
[34] Forel papers, Ploetz to Forel, 25 October 1887.

biological concepts as the 'cell state', and the integrative action of the nervous system which were taken as proving that collectivism was a natural form of social organization. Whereas Spencer placed his faith in the higher instinct of altruism, Germans looked to interventionist state agencies to engineer social reforms. The catalyst in Ploetz's change from political economy to biology was the anti-alcohol movement. Ploetz was impressed by the vigorous crusade against alcohol abuse. This movement was led by a group of reforming university professors. In 1885 the Baltic-German physiological chemist, Gustav von Bunge, denounced alcohol as a threat to health and heredity. He was a convinced vegetarian and anti-smoker, and must be regarded as taking the lead in injecting elements of *Lebensreform* into medical science.[35] Bunge had recently moved from Dorpat to Basel; he aroused the enthusiasm of Forel and of the physiologist Justus Gaule in Zürich, as well as impressing his students such as the youthful physiologist, Emil Abderhalden. Alcohol was perceived as a medical threat to heredity, and condemned as a cause of physical degeneration, moral depravity, crime, prostitution and a range of other pathological forms of behaviour. Drunkenness resulted in seduction, VD, unwanted pregnancies and criminal abortion. Eradication of alcoholism was regarded as the means of raising productivity, enhancing emotional stability and curing a broad range of social ills. The penchant of Swiss peasants for exceptionally strong spirits justified the conviction that alcohol was a major cause of human misery. Urban mortality statistics showed that the rising consumption of alcohol was a significant cause of death.[36] The causes of and cures for social deprivation were diagnosed in medical and biological terms.

The university professors led a crusade against alcoholism which was aimed not only against the debaucheries of student life, but also for reform of public morality. The anti-alcohol campaign inspired convivial forms of sociability such as orchestras, choirs and alcohol-free hotels and restaurants. The campaign was an evangelizing means of inculcating orderly behaviour in the masses. While the anti-alcohol movement of the 1880s also appealed to Christian moralists, the campaign led by the university professors was materialist and secular in outlook.[37] Forel admired the American abstinence league, the Knights Templars,[38] because of its secular tone. He became president of the Swiss section. Forel saw the campaign as a means of preventive medicine, given that alcoholism caused mental illness and led to casual sex when VD could be contracted. He also regarded it as a curable disease. He opened the first clinic for alcoholics in Zürich in 1888.

Ploetz was impressed by the experimental hygiene of Louis Pasteur and Robert Koch who argued for eradication of pathological germs, and by Forel's biological approach to mental illness. Forel's statistical studies of insanity carried out from 1881 indicated that four-fifths of cases of mental illness were due to heredity. This influenced the Zürich bacteriologist Edwin Klebs, who extended Forel's work to studies of the inheritance of abnormalities and diseases in families. The lectures on

---

[35] E. Graeter, *Gustav von Bunge. Naturforscher und Menschenfreund* (Basel, nd).
[36] See yearly volumes of *Statistisches Jahrbuch der Schweiz*.
[37] *100 Jahre Blaues Kreuz Basel 1882–1982* (Basle, 1982).   [38] *Guttempler Orden*.

pathology of Klebs included genealogical statistics of the inheritance of diseases in families.[39] Hidden biological forces held the key to unlocking the mysteries of personal and social life. Deeply committed to Forel's combination of Darwinism and psychiatry as a basis for socialism, Ploetz was converted to the abstinence movement. Now aware of the root of all human misery, he persuaded his fellow utopians – the Hauptmanns, Lux and Simon – to make vows of abstinence.[40] The next step was to organize a secular league against alcohol. Ploetz founded in 1890 an International Association to Combat Alcohol Consumption with the lawyer Otto Lang and the ophthalmologist Adolf Fick, who became its chairman. Members included Forel, the psychiatrist Bleuler, the physicians Simon and Rudolf Wlassek, and the medical student Max Bircher (who was to discover the nutritional value of muesli).[41] They sought to base the anti-alcohol crusade on science and medicine, replacing Christian and moral justifications. It was one of a number of international reforming associations to which Ploetz would devote his energies. The abstinence movement was given a racial motive by such Pan-Germanists as the ophthalmologist Fick, who saw abstinence as a means of recreating the vigour of the German race. The anti-alcohol movement thus combined biology and medicine with social reform and racial idealism, so providing a fertile basis for the growth of eugenics. That other leading social hygienists such as Alfred Grotjahn and psychiatrists such as Emil Kraepelin developed their views on the social role of medicine through the abstinence movement shows how it initiated a collectivist spirit in medicine with the doctor as hygienic Führer of the *Volk*.

The anti-alcohol campaign brought Ploetz into contact with Ernst Rüdin, a schoolboy from the Swiss town of St Gallen who was also inspired by Forel.[42] Ploetz convinced Rüdin that alcohol and tobacco were not only damaging to individual health but they also poisoned the fitness of future generations. Rüdin can be regarded as the co-founder of German eugenics. The group of budding eugenicists were bonded together by a shared enthusiasm for biology, which inspired a reformed lifestyle and its projection onto wider society. In 1890 Ploetz married Rüdin's sister, Pauline, who was studying medicine. Ernst Rüdin established an abstinence association, *Humanitas*, for Swiss grammar schools. Rüdin was imbued with reformist ideals similar to those of Ploetz and the Hauptmanns. Rüdin and his fellow schoolboys reinforced their abstinence by adventurously reading Bebel on women and socialism (the SPD's Party Congress was held in St Gallen in 1887), medical tracts by Forel and Bunge, and the utopian writings of Edward Bellamy.[43] There was a virtual epidemic of utopianism.

The linking of utopianism and *Lebensreform* was a stimulus to biological research. Also from the canton of St Gallen (from Toggenburg) came the budding physiologist Emil Abderhalden, who became concerned with improving the

[39] E. Klebs, *Die Allgemeine Pathologie* (Jena, 1887), pp. 42–53.
[40] Forel papers, Ploetz to Forel, 11 July 1889.
[41] *1. Jahresbericht des Vereins zur Bekämpfung des Alkoholgenusses in Zürich (1890–1891)* (Zürich, 1891).
[42] R. Meier, *August Forel* (Zürich, 1986).   [43] *Die Junge Schweiz*, vol. 16 (1941), 104–5.

conditions of the working class. While in his final year at school he wrote an essay on *La vie en l'an 2222*. He planned a utopian meritocracy. There should be social solidarity with the working class engendered by shared work and culture.[44] He was convinced of the medical and moral dangers of alcohol, and sought to replace alcoholic beverages with milk as the people's drink.[45] Abderhalden was to take a leading role in German population policy, in campaigns for sexual enlightenment and in research on the racial basis of heredity. Another youthful product of St Gallen was the geneticist, Carl Correns, who re-discovered the Mendelian laws. While a schoolboy (he gained his *Abitur* in 1885) he assembled an outstanding collection of mosses, and while convalescing from TB, he studied Darwinian authors.[46] That the generation born in the 1860s and 70s produced the future leaders of hereditary biology shows how intensely this generation perceived the tensions between nature and the corrupting effects of industrial society, and suggests that science was a means for resolving this conflict.

Ambitions and love

The utopian circle at Zürich embraced a broad range of unconventional young intellects who were grappling with the problems of social evolution and sexual instincts. The group was united by their hostility to repressive bourgeois morality. Literary self-expression was for some a solution to the dilemmas of achieving personal development in a repressive environment. Opposition to Ploetz's plans for racial regeneration was voiced by Frank Wedekind, an author concerned with expressing the elemental and natural force of youth. From 1886 until 1888 Wedekind was publicity chief of Julius Maggi, the manufacturer of ready-made soups from meat and vegetable extracts which were so tasteless that he concocted a recipe for fluid spice. Maggi hoped his soups would reduce infant mortality by improving protein deficiency and would save mothers' time and money. This was immortalized in an advertising jingle by Wedekind: 'Das wissen selbst die Kinderlein: Mit Würze wird die Suppe fein'.[47] Wedekind's friends included the authors Max Halbe and Karl Henckell, who in June 1887 founded a society called *Das junge Deutschland* to fight for truth and a free and modern morality. The Hauptmanns joined their discussions of literature, philosophy and politics. Simon and Ploetz supported the Hauptmanns' radical naturalism, whereas Wedekind was sceptical of their scientific presumptions. Wedekind was amused by Hauptmann's attempt to write an autobiographical novel containing schoolboy sexual experiences; that its hero was called Franz Loth suggests that it contained the germ of his first successful play. Wedekind himself was interested in sexual questions; he had visited the psychiatric clinic in Munich, and began to study works on the

---

[44] E. Abderhalden, 'Zum Abschied', *Ethik*, vol. 14 no. 6 (1938), 241–69.
[45] E. Shoen, 'Das Soziale Wirken Emil Abderhaldens', in *Emil Abderhalden* (Halle, 1952), pp. 36–8.
[46] M.S. Saha, 'Carl Correns', PhD dissertation, University of Michigan, 1984.
[47] 'Little children know that spice makes soup taste nice.'

psychology and physiology of the emotions by Jean Martin Charcot and Krafft-Ebing. In a dramatic fragment, *Elins Erweckung* of 1887, and in the drama *Frühlings Erwachen* (Spring Awakening) written between 1890 and 1891, he focused on the lack of sexual knowledge among school children. These works initiated a literary genre, the *Kindertragödie*, expressing hostility to the authority of adults over children. Children represented natural innocence and an elemental and uncorrupted vitality, which was opposed to the repressive influence of parents, teachers and pastors. Hauptmann had incorporated Wedekind's family situation into his 1890 drama, *Das Friedensfest*, much to Wedekind's annoyance. The group applied their remedies for human misery to their own situations. Standing at the threshold of a conventional career, marriage and family responsibilities, they sought escape into a naturalistic utopia and literary expressionism.[48]

What had been a *Männer-* or *Jünglingsbund* encountered the problem of the opposite sex. Zürich was the leading centre of women's medical studies. Ferdinand Simon took up the cause of female emancipation. Ibsen's *A Doll's House* that condemned marriage as repressing women had a deep impact when first staged in 1879. Emotional attachments posed problems for the cohesion of Ploetz's group since marriage seemed to be an act of disloyalty – especially when the proposed partner was judged to be of inadequate racial quality. The marriages of the Hauptmanns and of Ploetz all provoked stormy controversies.[49] Moreover, Carl Hauptmann, though now married, fell in love with a Polish student, Josepha Krzyzanowski, who diverted him from science to literature.

Ploetz's search for a suitable wife entailed not only an emotional choice, but adherence to his scientific ideals. His wife had to be a healthy, Germanic type who would provide him with children, and she would have to understand the importance of his scientific projects. Ideally, she should have the financial means to support him, so that he could pursue scientific research dedicated to the cause of human improvement. The choice was agonizingly difficult. In the summer semester of 1885 his emotions were first stirred by Pauline Rüdin in the lectures on organic chemistry. In the winter semester he fell in love with Agnes Bluhm during anatomical dissection. There followed a turbulent period of vacillation between Agnes ('Nestel') and Pauline. He was briefly engaged to Agnes in the spring of 1887, and dallied with an American medical student, Mary Sherwood, studying hypnotism with Forel. Carl Hauptmann persuaded Ploetz of the need to be happy in the present rather than only to calculate for the future plans for humanity. In the spring of 1888 Ploetz decided to sacrifice financial security and to marry Pauline.[50] They married in 1890 just before Pauline completed her doctorate on extra-uterine pregnancy.[51] Ploetz retained the life-long friendship of Agnes Bluhm, and she aligned herself with Ploetz's racial hygiene in feminist groupings. She was the third

---

[48] A. Kutscher, *Wedekind* (München, 1964), pp. 51–52; H. Wagener (ed.), *Frank Wedekind. Frühlings Erwachen* (Stuttgart, 1980).   [49] G. Hauptmann, *Abenteuer*, II, pp. 336, 349.
[50] Ploetz papers, autobiographical notes; Carl Hauptmann papers, Ploetz to Carl Hauptmann, Berne, 8 May 1888.
[51] P. Rüdin, *Beitrag zur Extrauteringravidität und deren Behandlung* (Zürich, 1890).

woman doctor in Berlin (the first six all studied at Zürich) and in the Racial Hygiene Society from 1906. Her own research concerned heredity and alcohol.[52]

Although Ploetz acquired Swiss nationality, his German nationalist convictions also intensified. In the physiological laboratory of Gaule, where he was completing his dissertation on heredity, worked the fellow abstinence-campaigner Fick, who was a hybrid between a democrat and a fervent Pan-German nationalist.[53] On qualification, Ploetz and his wife decided to emigrate with the aim of earning enough money to allow them to devote themselves to scientific research. He dreamt of combining farming with scientific research on animal breeding. The rapid increase in numbers of newly qualified young doctors meant that a university career was impractical. Fick persuaded them that they could earn well in South Africa where he had spent five years. Ploetz looked forward to being able to study bush men as among the lowest human races. However, the couple finally abandoned their African plans and decided on the United States, where they went in 1890 armed with introductions from Forel.[54] The Ploetzes emigrated just as Fick launched a publicity campaign in June 1890 denouncing the exchange of Zanzibar for Heligoland, with the backing of other German doctors resident in Zürich as the pathologist Otto Lubarsch. This culminated in the founding of the Pan-German League.[55] Ploetz encountered a strong current of nationalism although he chose not to become active in Pan-Germanist agitation.

In New York their first contact was the physician and philanthropist, Christian Herter, who was an admirer of Forel (and later a patron of Paul Ehrlich). He proved to be unresponsive to the Ploetzes' schemes, and they settled in Springfield, Massachusetts, where they opened a medical practice and bred chickens.[56] They later moved to Meriden, Connecticut. These years were a hard personal struggle to survive. Ploetz complained of the drunkenness and the prejudices of the population against a German doctor. For their part, doctors were seen as exploiters charging for excessive visits to patients since they could do virtually nothing against infections other than offer diagnosis. The couple were plagued by intense home-sickness, and a sense of intellectual isolation. They felt frustrated because they could not openly proclaim their hostility to Christianity and alcohol, and their sympathy for socialism.[57] They were becoming disillusioned with Forel's anti-alcohol crusade. Yet this was a fruitful period for Ploetz. He used his free time to write a book on the potential of 'our race' and on problems of social welfare.[58]

Ploetz hoped to convince émigré German socialists that there was a way to refute Darwinist criticisms of socialism. He was in touch with Jacques Loeb, a radically

[52] H. Rohner, *Die ersten 30 Jahre des medizinischen Frauenstudiums an der Universität Zürich* (Zürich, 1972). [53] 'Die Familie Fick', *ARGB*, vol. 14 (1922), 159–75.

[54] Carl Hauptmann papers, Ploetz to C. Hauptmann, 31 August 1897.

[55] O. Lubarsch, *Ein bewegtes Gelehrtenleben* (Berlin, 1931); Chickering, *Men*, p. 49.

[56] M.H. Frisch, *Town into City. Springfield Massachusetts and the Meaning of Community, 1840–1880* (Cambridge, Mass., 1972).

[57] Carl Hauptmann papers, Ploetz to Carl Hauptmann, Meriden, 19 January 1892.

[58] H.H. Walser (ed.), *August Forel – Briefe, Correspondance 1864 – 1927* (Berne, 1968), pp. 258, 281–2; Forel papers, 22 April 1891.

minded German biologist, who had emigrated because of opposition to social conditions. Ploetz had contacts with the Springfield Socialist Party, and with socialist journalists in New York. Through his Zürich comrade, the anarchist and Nietzschean John Henry Mackay, Ploetz struck up a friendship with a socialist carpenter, Adolph Gerecke, who wrote a treatise on the futility of moralism and was a contributor to German naturalist journals.[59] Ploetz was not an orthodox socialist. He stood for a non-Marxist critique of modern society. His aim was to reconcile socialism with Darwinism. Drawing on his dissertation research on variation in the frog, he emphasized that the recognition and cultivation of good variations was the only way forward for humanity. This could render the inhumane struggle for existence unnecessary. Control of reproductive variations seemed better than party politics and what Ploetz condemned as the recitation of empty slogans of Marx. Biological engineering was to substitute for changes in the political economy.

Ploetz continued to be an enthusiast for studies in physiology and hygiene. His medical treatment of children's diseases convinced him of the force of heredity, and he believed that he could predict a baby's sex and hereditary quality prior to birth. He considered that specialization as a paediatrician would enable him to combine medicine and biological research on heredity and variation.[60] He planned breeding experiments, and collected genealogies for the study of variation in families. By 1892 he had 325 genealogies of 2,430 persons out of a hoped for 5,000 genealogies. He hoped to use contacts with a German secret lodge in Connecticut to obtain the genealogies of its 20,000 members. Having formulated his programme for racial and social reform, his main objective was to conduct research into heredity and promote awareness of how sexual selection could be the basis of human improvement.[61] He was convinced that the main task of hygiene was to be the control of good and bad variations.[62] He wished to return to experimental animal-breeding when his work on human variation was finished. Ploetz hoped that, as with Koch, his scientific discoveries would cause a sensation and result in enough money to found a research institute.[63]

Sanitary utopias

Ploetz's choice of such an apparently unpromising place as Springfield might be explained by the presence of the utopian author, Edward Bellamy.[64] Bellamy edited a newspaper in Springfield and wrote the utopian novel, *Looking Backward 2000–1887*, which seized the imagination of a vast readership. It was published in 1888, translated into German in 1889, and was popular among socialists. Perfection

---

[59] Carl Hauptmann papers, Ploetz to Carl Hauptmann, 6 October 1893.
[60] Forel papers, Ploetz to Forel, 16 January 1892, 10 November 1892.
[61] Ploetz papers, letter to Carl Hauptmann, 5 September 1892.
[62] Gaule Papers, Ploetz to Gaule, 16 January 1892.
[63] Carl Hauptmann papers, Ploetz to C. Hauptmann, 14 January 1892, 26 August 1892.
[64] However, the archivist responsible for the Bellamy papers at Harvard informs me that there was no correspondence between Bellamy and Ploetz.

was the antithesis of urban Boston of 1887: there was to be a socialist society based on merit rather than wealth as the main spur to human endeavour. Bellamy condemned the chaos of liberal self-interest as resulting in 'a horde of barbarians with a thousand petty chiefs'. There should, instead, be established an orderly society 'as compared with that of a disciplined army under one general – such a fighting machine, for example, as the German army under von Moltke'. State socialism was placed on a medical and biological basis. The guide to Bellamy's revitalized Boston was a physician, Dr Leete. He compared the model society to 'one family'. Marriage was to be based on love and fitness, and the congenitally deficient would be banned from marriage. Bellamy admired Galton's 1873 work on 'stirpiculture' (a term pre-dating 'eugenics' first used by Galton in 1883).[65] The popularity of Bellamy's eugenic utopia coincided with Ploetz's formulation of a scientific method for its realization. Many German socialists responded enthusiastically to Bellamy's vision as offering the basis in evolutionary terms for a classless world community or *Volksgemeinschaft*.

Bellamy typified how political utopias were reformulated in biological terms. Social reformers were convinced that if science and medicine were judiciously applied, utopia was within mankind's grasp. Ploetz constructed a biological utopia from elements of state socialism, sanitary reform and Darwinism. Scientific positivism was to be linked with collectivist social philosophies. There was a division of opinion over the most effective type of utopian medicine. One line of thought argued for clearing away polluting filth with the assumption that an environment of clean air and pure water would guarantee health. This was expressed by the physician and sanitary reformer, Benjamin Ward Richardson, who in 1875 had outlined his vision of *Hygeia, a City of Health*. This was planned on sanitary principles with an emphasis on a clean environment as well as personal fitness. Ward's scientific approach to hygiene – which included housing and nutritional reform, bicycling and temperance – was an influential model. He proposed 'little colonies' to restore the tubercular to health by fresh air and exercise.[66] Health was a key element of such plans for colonies, land reform and the construction of totally planned urban communities. An economist, the Austro-Hungarian Theodor Hertzka, wrote on the laws of social evolution and on land reform in 1886. In 1890 he published a utopian novel, *Freiland*, which inspired efforts at its practical realization.[67] Hertzka combined Marxism and Darwinism, arguing that outworn social forms should be replaced in the struggle for survival. He planned a colony in Africa where doctors would be state officials, providing free medical treatment and sanatoria and where women's primary role would be to care for children, the sick and the aged.[68]

Ploetz's utopianism drew inspiration from bacteriology and hereditary biology

[65] S.E. Bowman *et al., Edward Bellamy Abroad* (New York, 1962), pp. 151–9; A.E. Morgan, *Edward Bellamy* (New York, 1944), p. 158.
[66] B. Ward Richardson, *Hygeia – A City of Health* (London, 1876).
[67] T. Hertzka, *Freiland: Ein soziales Zukunftsbild* (Leipzig, 1890).

as offering the means for control and eradication of polluting germs. The environmental and sanitary approach to health was seen as limited, with the growing realization that health and disease depended on control of hidden germs. At Zürich, Ploetz would have heard Klebs' advanced exposition of the bacteriological and hereditarian approach to hygiene. Utopians continued the endeavour of combining the movement for self-improvement in health with sport, diet and exercise. When the further step was taken of placing utopian sanitary reforms on a biological basis, the result was that instead of being wholly environmentalist, educational and egalitarian, the eugenic colonies were elitist and selective. The link between eugenics and utopianism can also be seen as an impulse for Galton who in 1910 outlined a utopia called Kantsaywhere where emphasis on hereditary biology was combined with a healthy lifestyle, energy and a courteous disposition. Such utopias endorsed ideas of the natural superiority of a biological elite of experts with outstanding mental and physical qualities.[69]

The biological and medical strands of utopianism were part of an increasingly popular counter-culture. In 1888 Wilhelm Boelsche and the socialist Bruno Wille established the influential naturalist group of authors and philosophers at Friedrichshagen near Berlin. They reacted against socialist egalitarianism as strongly as against the repressive ruling hierarchy. In 1893 Wille offered a Darwinian critique of the SPD Party programme, arguing for a *Sozialaristokratie* of creative intellectuals. Potent literary works by Ibsen and Nietzsche were used by Wille to promulgate theories of individual freedom and of superior personal qualities. This was the basis for an attack on the egalitarian socialism of Bebel. Ibsen's drama, *An Enemy of the People*, was taken as a manifesto for the superiority of the creative individual over the people who were like 'herd animals'. With the cult of the individual went faith in superior powers of the creative medical and scientific researcher. Ibsen's play was relevant in that its hero was a doctor who discovered how capitalism allowed society to be morally and biologically polluted.[70]

The outburst of utopian social protest took contradictory artistic, Germanic *völkisch*, or technocratic directions. Nature was a refuge for social radicals, who desired to intensify their experience of life. Carl Hauptmann withdrew to the rural isolation of Schreiberhau in Silesia. He tried to express how nature was a flowing unit, and he abandoned his mechanistic biological approach for a lyrical expressionism. He was a close friend of the Worpswede artists, whose community sought to develop an art true to nature in protest against the artificialities of bourgeois conventions. The diversity of utopian impulses can be seen in the growing interest in land reform with the founding of the *Bund deutscher Bodenreformer*, in promoting rural settlement to revitalize the nation and in the

---

[68] F.E. Manuel and F.P. Manuel, *Utopian Thought in the Western World* (Oxford, 1979), pp. 765–8; W.M. Johnston, *The Austrian Mind* (Berkeley, 1983), pp. 361–2.

[69] Compare P. Weingart, 'Eugenic Utopias – Blueprints for the Rationalization of Human Evolution', *Sociology of the Sciences*, (1984), 173–87.

[70] R.H. Thomas, *Nietzsche in German Politics and Society 1890–1918* (Manchester, 1986), pp. 9–15.

garden city and housing reform movements. Ploetz's efforts to promote the regeneration of humanity were paralleled in the 1880s by attempts to found Teutonic utopias abroad. Bernhard Förster (Nietzsche's brother-in-law, a leading anti-semite, and a disciple of Gobineau) emigrated because of hatred of the 'educated, liberal and humane values' that prevailed in Germany. With his wife, Elisabeth Förster-Nietzsche, he established a colony, *Nueva Germania*, in Paraguay in 1885 where the as yet unspoiled German peasants and artisans might find a refuge from corrupting tobacco, drink, meat, consumerism and science.[71] It was an experiment that ended in Förster's suicide when a scandal of financial corruption broke. Yet by the 1890s there was a change of mood. It was felt that Germany was not so much over-populated as under-populated, and that the positively healthy aspects of rural life should be preserved and emulated. Germany should be revitalized from within. The Land Owners' League, and liberal rural reformers such as Heinrich Sohnrey, campaigned for acceptance of the countryside as the natural source for revitalizing the *Volk*. In 1896 Franz Oppenheimer gave up his medical practice, convinced that agrarian settlement was the antidote to the physical degeneration resulting from urban squalor.[72]

The European communes sprouting up from the 1880s were based on ideas of positive health. Notable examples were the vegetarian colonies *Heimgarten*, founded in 1892, and *Eden*, in 1893, which survived by producing health foods and drinks. '*Eden* Reform-Butter' was a prototype of margarine. The physician, Raphael Friedeberg, underwent a metamorphosis from adviser to sickness insurance funds and SPD member in the 1890s to anarchism and *Lebensreform* in the 1900s. He replaced materialism by a creed of 'psychism', and conventional medical therapy by nature therapy. His settlement at *Monte Verità* near Ascona pioneered the first 'air huts' or *Lufthütten* for fresh air and nature therapy. The colony's vegetarianism and anarchism attracted such visitors as Bakunin, Kropotkin, Lenin, and Trotsky.[73] In Berlin in 1900 a sanatorium at Schlachtensee was used for a colony called the *Neue Gemeinschaft*. Here, intellectuals such as Martin Buber (the Jewish mystic), Gustav Landauer (the anarchist), Franz Oppenheimer (the doctor and social scientist) and Magnus Hirschfeld (the sexual reformer) discussed the ethics of Nietzsche and the anarchism of Max Stirner and Leo Tolstoy, the latter of whom had assumed the life style of a peasant as a gesture of asceticism. The Schlachtensee circle planned to reform sexual morality by improving the legal status of homosexuals and single mothers.[74] Oppenheimer drew up detailed plans for rural settlement programmes.[75] Reacting against capitalism and the repressive norms of Wilhelmine morality, they sought regeneration through a spirit of

---

[71] Levy, *Downfall of the Anti-semitic Political Parties*, pp. 29–30, 271–2.
[72] J. Reulecke, *Geschichte der Urbanisierung in Deutschland* (Frankfurt-on-Main, 1985), pp. 140–7.
[73] F. Tennstedt, 'Sozialismus, Lebensreform und Krankenkassenbewegung. Friedrich Landmann und Raphael Friedeberg als Ratgeber der Krankenkassen', *Soziale Sicherheit*, vol. 26 (1977), 210–14, 306–10, 332–6. U. Linse (ed.), *Zurück o Mensch zur Mutter Erde. Landkommunen in Deutschland 1890–1933* (Munich, 1983).   [74] C. Wolff, *Magnus Hirschfeld* (London, 1986), pp. 46–50.
[75] A. Löwe, 'In Memoriam Franz Oppenheimer', *Leo Baeck Institute Yearbook*, vol. 10 (1965), 137–48; also vol. 11 (1966), 336–7, on the influence of L. Gumplowicz.

harmony between humans and between the human race and nature. The programme of the German Garden Cities Society,[76] established in 1902, aimed to realize a natural lifestyle, removed from industrial pollution.[77] At the experimental settlement of Hellerau near Dresden, gardens and fresh air were supplemented by the eurythmic dancing of Isadora Duncan. The schemes were based on ideas of positive health as preventing disease and as part of physical, social and psychic development.[78] The nation was to be spiritually revived by naturally based social organizations.

An increasing number of utopian colonies involved eugenic and racial schemes. The spirit of utopias changed from optimistic idealism to the sense that their organization had to be in accordance with natural laws which were without pity for the weak and for individual preference. Although Ploetz and his comrades abandoned utopian idealism for scientific eugenics, they retained a commitment to radical social reform. They began with an idealistic and nationalist conviction of racial purity. Studies in biology, and medical training gave Ploetz and Rüdin a sense of professional identity and a conviction that the natural constituents of race could be moulded by environmental and human intervention. The result was a scientific and medical concept of race. Biological influence upon utopian convictions was widespread. Many eugenicists felt that utopia could not be achieved simply by harmonious co-operation, but required an adaptive and evolutionary process which might take many generations. Darwinian-inspired novels gave grim warnings of what the future might hold. Novels, dramas and philosophies publicized the reforming implications of medicine and biology. They prophesied degeneration if industrial and urban development continued to disregard the laws of heredity and health. They emphasized the physical and psychological limits to human perfectibility. The concern with alcohol as a 'racial poison' indicated the power of the biologistic diagnosis and prescriptive cures for social misery. During the 1890s the problem preoccupying Ploetz became not so much the establishment of an ideal settlement outside the mainstream of German society but the reformation of society itself.

THE PSYCHIATRY OF DEGENERATION

The transition in science and medicine from emancipatory liberalism to state-oriented expertise was most evident in psychiatry. Liberal psychiatrists advocated humane policies of no-restraint, cure and education, which were a force for reform during the 1850s and 60s. The adoption of the objective standards of the natural

---

[76] *Deutsche Gartenstadt-Gesellschaft.*
[77] U. Druvins, 'Alternative Projekte um 1900', in H. Gnüg (ed.), *Literarische Utopie-Entwürfe* (Frankfurt-on-Main, 1982), pp. 236–59.
[78] K. Bergmann, *Agrarromantik und Grossstadtfeindschaft* (Meisenheim, 1970); K. Hartmann, *Deutsche Gartenstadtbewegung: Kulturpolitik und Gesellschaftsreform* (Munich, 1976); I.B. Whyte, *Bruno Taut and the Architecture of Activism* (Cambridge, 1982).

sciences initially had a liberating effect as science was seen as a means of dispelling arbitrary ethical and political constraints. That the Prussian state devolved responsibility for the administration of asylums to the provinces during the 1860s arose from the conviction that the problem of humane and modern care could be solved through contact with the citizenry.[79] By the 1870s these humanitarian impulses gave way to a programme for the identification of the pathologically incurable and socially deviant. Liberal ideas of progress were replaced by the fear of degeneration.[80]

The optimism of enlightened rationalists that deviant individuals could be re-educated evaporated during the traumatic social changes of industrialization and urbanization of the 1870s. The idea of a social and individual pathology became conceptualized in terms of scientific anthropology and hereditarian psychiatry. This reflected the emergent professionalism of psychiatrists, as well as the growing bourgeois *Angst* of the criminal, diseased and riotous masses. The more the bourgeoisie gained authority and wealth, the more medical strategies to eradicate deviancy such as crime grew in appeal. A high proportion of psychiatrists were the sons of civil servants, and this added to a concern with social order among psychiatrists.[81] Positivistic explanations of deviancy were linked to scientific authoritarianism.

Initially, evolutionary biology pointed to the adverse social environment as a cause of both physical and psychic degeneration. Environmental factors ranging from climate and seasonality to individual age and morality were seen as causes of 'mental alienation'. Education, economic prosperity and liberal social reforms were thus cures for mental disease. But from the 1850s a shift of values from free will, moral responsibility and justice to the naturalist categories of biological evolution occurred: biological heredity rather than the social environment was seen as the cause of pathological behaviour. Psychiatrists argued that abnormality was to be explained in biological and positivist terms of an evolutionary throwback or reversion to a primitive state of savagery. Darwinism could be used to support theories of mental and physical degeneration.[82] Economic progress was seen as weakening the natural vigour of nations. Crime and mental disease furnished evidence of the depraving effects of industrial society. By the 1890s the liberal optimism of advocates of no-restraint and education had been transmuted to the interventionism of grandiose plans to monitor the hereditary health of families. At this time rejection of environmental explanations for degeneration occurred, resulting in a strictly hereditarian social pathology.

The shift to degenerationist psychiatry was first evident in France where republican and liberal psychiatrists were alienated by the Second Empire of Napoleon III. The state was hostile to their efforts, and asylums were overcrowded.

---

[79] D. Blasius, *Der verwaltete Wahnsinn* (Frankfurt-on-Main, 1980), pp. 38–45.
[80] K. Doerner, *Madmen and the Bourgeoisie* (Oxford, 1981), p. 270.
[81] Doerner, *Madmen*, p. 272.
[82] E. Chamberlin and S. Gilman (eds.), *Degeneration. The Dark Side of Progress* (New York, 1985).

Psychiatrists became pessimistic as to the capacities of cure, and they changed to custody and clinical observation. They sought a theory of morbid heredity in researches on pathological anomalies. The ideas of hereditary pathology were developed by the psychiatrist, Benoit-Augustin Morel. During the 1840s he advocated no-restraint treatment of the insane; but in the 1850s he began to correlate pathological lesions found in autopsies with nervous diseases. He attributed their development to a process of degeneracy. In 1857 he compiled an atlas demonstrating the prevalence of physical, moral and intellectual degeneracy.[83] Morel was one of a cluster of psychiatrists in the 1850s who combined environmental with hereditarian explanations for degeneration.[84] A range of diseases such as epilepsy, cretinism and hysteria, as well as deviant behaviour, were ascribed to the mysterious power of heredity. As a similar alienation of young psychiatrists occurred in Germany from the 1880s, degenerationist ideas became influential.

Among the first to make a link between organic disease and social deviancy was Cesare Lombroso, an Italian psychiatrist who gathered evidence on the evolution of criminality from animals to the habitual criminals and prostitutes of cities. He correlated mental and physical characteristics to prove that degenerates were evolutionary throwbacks. As poverty and harmful environmental conditions were major factors in causing degeneration, Lombroso supported social reforms. His positivistic views on criminal anthropology can be interpreted as part of the liberal movement for social order and progress, and by the 1890s Lombroso's scientific materialism led him to socialism.[85] His *L'uomo delinquato*, first published in 1876, achieved a wide readership in Germany, when his works were translated in the 1890s. Lombroso offered topics for empirical investigation by anthropologists and brain anatomists. German anatomists dissected the brains of murderers to see whether there was some pathological anomaly. A movement for criminal biology arose during the 1890s seeking to prevent crime by scientific rather than moral and educational means. Degenerationist ideas contributed to technocratic administration and research, and became part of a philosophy of revitalized conservatism. Lombroso's ideas reached the German public through the weekly journal, *Die Zukunft*. Its editor, Maximilian Harden, was a lapsed actor, a convert to Bismarckianism, and a relentless critic of Wilhelm II and the political policies of the 'new course'. His journal devoted a substantial amount of coverage (generally one article per issue) to considering the psychological and social implications of Darwinism, and of medical advances. Expositions of Lombrosian theories were in line with contributions by Arthur James Balfour, Büchner, Haeckel, Huxley, Tille

---

[83] B.A. Morel, *Traité des dégénérescences physiques, intellectuelles et morales de l'espèce humaine* (Paris, 1857).

[84] I. Dowbiggin, 'Degeneration and Hereditarianism in French Mental Medicine 1840–1890: Psychiatric Theory as Ideological Adaptation', in W. Bynum, M. Shepherd and R. Porter (eds.), *The Anatomy of Madness* (London, 1985), I, pp. 188–232.

[85] L. Bulferetti, *Cesare Lombroso* (Turin, 1975); D. Pick, 'The Faces of Anarchy: Lombroso and the Politics of Criminal Science in Unification Italy', *History Workshop Journal*, issue 21 (1986), 60–86.

and Wallace on Darwinism, by Emil Behring, Ferdinand Hueppe, Koch and Paul Ehrlich on infectious diseases, and by Albert Eulenburg, Albert Moll and Schweninger on psychiatry and medical affairs. The journal provided a forum for debating the natural basis of social progress, and pointed to how not only liberal parliamentarianism was a thing of the past, but also how the liberal science and medicine of Darwin and Virchow was being reappraised as part of a broader process of the restructuring of nationalist politics. The new organicism was subsumed in the integrationist social philosophies of Friedrich Naumann and Schäffle, and symbolically linked to the causes of Bismarck and the agrarian lobby through Harden's critique of the Kaiser's politics.[86] Harden's journal provided later medical commentators on Social Darwinism as Ploetz and Hertwig with a wide range of political and philosophical theories. Biology was part of the public discourse on social change. It gave not only a sanctimonious superiority to the compilers of lurid accounts of crimes, sexual perversions and corruption, but provided an authoritative basis for evaluating the ebb and flow of political and intellectual change.

The transition from liberal politics and psychiatry to hereditarianism was encapsulated by the work of the German psychiatrist, Wilhelm Griesinger. A gifted biologist and associate of Virchow, he took the ideas of 'medical reform' into the domain of psychiatry. Griesinger was one of the medical reformers campaigning for history and philosophy to be replaced by physics in the medical curriculum. The combination of natural science and liberalism served to advance a social programme for free treatment of the mentally ill poor in out-patient clinics, public asylums and colonies for the rehabilitation of the sick. At the same time the professional and intellectual status of psychiatry was to be raised to a branch of scientific medicine. Once irrationality was located in physiological processes, it could be treated. As pathological mental conditions like feeble-mindedness and idiocy were identified, the scope of psychiatry enlarged. Griesinger's liberal programme was the basis for a liberal professional dominance, comparable to that of the pathologist and sanitary reformer, Virchow. Psychiatrists still placed the health of the individual above the need to protect society from deviants. This position was later to be reversed as psychiatrists claimed to be guardians of the health of society and of future generations.[87] Griesinger discovered 'neuroses' which were prevalent among the bourgeoisie and particularly among young female governesses and teachers. Such stigmatizing of an emancipating group warned that hereditary predisposition to mental disease could undermine the self-

[86] W. Waldeyer, 'Das Gehirn des Mörders Bobbe', Correspondenzblatt der deutschen anthropologischen Gesellschaft, vol. 23 (1901), 140–1; B.U. Weller, Maximilian Harden und die 'Zukunft' (Bremen, 1970) and H.F. Young, Maximilian Harden. Censor Germaniae (The Hague, 1959) deal with the political rather than intellectual values of Harden; A. Eulenburg, 'Lombrosos Weib', Die Zukunft, vol. 5 (1893), 407–20; C. Lombroso, 'Der Antisemitismus und die Juden', Die Zukunft, vol. 6 (1894), 470–4; Lombroso, 'Die Theorie der Genialität', Die Zukunft, vol. 8 (1894), 551–7; P. Lombroso, 'Aus dem Leben meines Vaters', Die Zukunft, new series vol. 3 (1895), 333–7.
[87] Doerner, Madmen, pp. 269–88.

confident success of the bourgeoisie. In contrast to the eugenicists of the next century, he regarded beggars and vagabonds as mentally healthy. But he came to support the concept of an 'hereditary predisposition' in his *Mental Pathology and Therapeutics* of 1861.[88] The concept was still couched in terms of an individual predisposition that could be overcome by ceasing to suppress a neurosis. He extended this to sexuality, and dealt with the conflict between the ill-effects of sexual over-indulgence and repression.[89]

Richard von Krafft-Ebing, the Viennese psychiatrist, developed degenerationist theory into sexual pathology. He linked sexual 'perversions' with crime and nervous degeneration. His *Psychopathia Sexualis* of 1886 diagnosed modern civilization as the primary cause of the release of instinctual drives that led to such illnesses as alcoholism, epilepsy, venereal disease and sexual perversions. Carl Westphal in Berlin provided evidence for the physical degeneration of the nervous system. Degenerationist theories had a major impact on forensic psychiatry. What had once been judged in civil terms as a crime became explicable in scientific biology as a pathological variation from the normal. Psychiatry was placed on evolutionary foundations. There occurred a shift away from the individual's ethical outlook, to a correlation of mental with neurological and physiological symptoms. A further stage was to study patients' families with the idea that mental disturbance was inherited. The aim was a pathology of the family.

The medical approach to mental illness had institutional ramifications. While at Zürich, Griesinger urged the need for a new psychiatric hospital. Known as the Burghölzli, it was opened in 1870. Griesinger regarded such institutions as 'hospitals for brain diseases'. He combined this with a research programme for brain anatomy. His successors, Eduard Hitzig, Bernhard Gudden and Forel, were all brain anatomists, concerned with anatomical research. For Griesinger's generation, liberal medical science demanded modern hospitals that were to shed the images of prisons and workhouses. The professor was to conduct research but not to intervene in the life of the patient. At most there was to be active education for a free life. With Forel this was to change. He turned from anatomy to observation of patients. This resulted in a range of interventionist methods such as hypnosis (from 1886) and castration (during the 1890s), and the preventive anti-alcohol campaigns.[90] Forel was part of a movement that greatly extended the scope of medical science to hitherto moral spheres such as sexuality and crime. Ambitious programmes for building modern psychiatric hospitals, clinics and special schools meant the bed capacity of psychiatric hospitals trebled between 1870 and 1904 in Germany.[91] Once such a rapid expansion was under way, the costs of the hospitals began to be questioned. The scientific and medical empire-building of liberal medical reformers resulted in an extension of the power of bourgeois professionals.

---

[88] W. Griesinger, *Pathologie und Therapie der Psychiatrischen Krankheiten* (Stuttgart, 1861).
[89] Doerner, *Madmen*, pp. 284–5.
[90] *Zürcher Spitalgeschichte* (Zürich, 1951), II, pp. 377–419.   [91] Blasius, *Wahnsinn*, p. 69.

Eugenic psychiatry

Forel's change of heart occurred in the 1880s – just at the time that the Ploetz circle arrived on the scene. The psychiatric science of the 1880s was written in strictly clinical terms for doctors and lawyers. Yet it seized the imagination of a younger generation of medical students, including the early eugenic theorists Ploetz, Rüdin and Wilhelm Schallmayer. They became part of a movement of popularization of the biological scientific laws of health. They combined literary ambitions with a sense of mission as doctors to cure social ills and to impose healthy evolutionary laws for improving mankind. Psychiatric practice was crucial for a later generation of eugenicists. For example, the geneticist Erwin Baur had a brief period of experience as a psychiatrist, and the theoretician of social hygiene, Alfred Grotjahn, worked as clinical assistant in neurology during the 1890s. The Ploetz circle was influenced indirectly and Schallmayer directly by the psychiatrist, Bernhard von Gudden, whose change from non-restraint to custodial detention was to precipitate his death.

Gudden was an advocate of the liberal psychiatry of non-restraint and therapy. He had studied with Virchow, and shared his liberal convictions. While professor in Zürich from 1869 until 1872, Gudden had been a major influence on Forel. They shared progressive social views, and Forel followed Gudden to Munich and worked under him until 1879 when Forel was appointed professor in Zürich. Among Gudden's students was Schallmayer who assisted in the psychiatric clinic from 1883. While Schallmayer was writing his doctorate on the rejection of food by the mentally ill, Gudden mentioned to Forel in 1884 that he had proposed Schallmayer for an appointment as physician to Prince Otto von Wittelsbach, Ludwig II's brother. Gudden's opinion was decisive in the certification of Ludwig II as mentally deranged. It was a remarkable instance of the subordination of royalty to the norms dictated by bourgeois professionals. Gudden drowned in mysterious circumstances in 1886, along with his patient. Forel and Schallmayer were influenced by Gudden's therapeutic nihilism and his support for 'non-restraint' treatment of patients. Gudden's non-interventionism developed into the conviction that therapy only caused the weak to survive. He came to accept the force of heredity in mental illness as described by the French psychiatrists.[92] Clashes between political authority and professional powers were frequent as hereditarian psychiatry extended its domain.

Schallmayer looked to the positivist psychology of Théodule Ribot, an authority on the inheritance of diseases. Ribot argued for the hereditary transmission of diseases, crimes and passions. He admired English philosophy and drew on the evolutionary theories of Darwin, Spencer, and – significantly –

92 E. Kraepelin, *Lebenserinnerungen*, p. 14; Forel, *Briefe*, p. 176, letter of 13 August 1884; Schallmayer, *Die Nahrungsverweigerung und die übrigen Störungen der Nahrungsaufnahme bei Geisteskranken*, Med. diss, University of Munich, 1885.

Galton.[93] He was critical of Galton's statistical claims, but felt that Galton had established the inheritance of human psychology.[94] Ribot's work was one of the channels that communicated Galton's researches on heredity to the emergent German eugenics. Positivist psychology marked a transition from liberalism to professional elitism, once the medical profession claimed the power to decide who were the degenerates.

Schallmayer considered that the social implications of the use of hereditarian biology and medicine were collectivist solutions to social deviancy. His belief in doctors as medical officials, compulsory medical tribunals and health passports marked a positive attitude to the state that contrasted to the movements for deregulation of the mid nineteenth century. From about 1886 Schallmayer began work on a treatise on the problem of medicine and degeneration. He was inspired by Bellamy's utopian writings which depicted the doctor as the arbiter of social values. Schallmayer considered that the economic basis of medicine should be altered by appointing doctors as state officials. He proposed a system of health passports and of comprehensive registration of diseases. The experience of medical practice made him critical of the individualistic attitudes of doctors and psychiatrists. He condemned their concern for the welfare of individual patients, and their lack of regard for the social consequences of inherited psychiatric illnesses. He criticized Krafft-Ebing for recommending early marriage as a means of preventing mental disturbance. During the 1880s the psychiatrist, Kraepelin, accepted that patients with existing mental problems should be advised against marriage; but even where there was an hereditary predisposition to mental illness, marriage should not be advised against, as there was a statistical chance of only 30–40 per cent that illness would be inherited. Schallmayer regarded such 'humane' views as too soft. He was convinced that most mental illness was inherited, and that psychiatry was culpable in allowing the sick back into society where they might marry. He argued for laws to prevent the mentally ill from marrying and having children who would inevitably pose problems in the future. His view that 'the mad are a burden on the state' was to be a eugenic rallying cry in future years.[95]

The ideas of the Ploetz circle were evolving in directions similar to Schallmayer's. Forel demonstrated how the patients in the Burghölzli were ravaged by alcoholism and syphilis. He impressed on Ploetz the need to improve the reproductive quality of the human race. The scientific approach to social reform drove Forel to socialism and abstention from alcohol. He pioneered eugenic solutions to psychiatric problems by the mid-1880s, convinced that social misery and disease should be exterminated at their roots. During the 1890s Forel began to experiment with castrating patients as a means of controlling aggression. The aim

[93] T. Ribot, *Contemporary English Psychology* (London, 1873).

[94] T. Ribot, *Heredity: A Psychological Study of Its Phenomena, Laws, Causes and Consequences* (London, 1875), pp. 186–93.

[95] W. Schallmayer, *Über die drohende physische Entartung der Culturvölker* (Neuwied, 1895), pp. 13, 47–8, 103–4.

of biological control of deviant behaviour impressed Kraepelin, Ploetz and Rüdin, who studied how alcohol consumption led to vagrancy, crime, delirium tremens and epilepsy.[96] Hitzig and Kraepelin campaigned for the state to nationalize all psychiatric institutions in order to co-ordinate and rationalize costly measures against mental illness, with the result of a *Landtag* petition in 1896 for state control of psychiatric hospitals.[97] State mental hospitals and therapeutic experiments marked the transition from social radicalism to biologically based interventionism.[98]

Staging degeneration

The problem of degeneration reached the attention of a broader public through the works of naturalist authors. Ibsen's drama, *Ghosts*, created a storm of public controversy during 1882 with its dramatizing of the threat of congenital syphilis to the family. Zola's Rougon-Macquart cycle of novels (written between 1871 and 1893) depicted 'the natural and social history' of a family as it degenerated over generations. Such literary realism provoked a strong public reaction. Zola's novels demonstrated how alcoholism and mental disease led to crime, prostitution, cruelty and the political corruption of the Second Empire. Environmental degeneration influenced personal action, family circumstances and social customs. Zola borrowed from Haeckel's theories of recapitulation of lower evolutionary stages, from Lombroso's criminology, and from medical studies of the inheritance of disease. Such influences nurtured the naturalist movement in Germany. A spate of novels, pictures and plays depicted the brutalizing and depraving effects of current social conditions. Scenes of low life and violence abounded. Hermann Conradi's *Wenn die Isar rauscht* included a scene with a police doctor examining a prostitute. The concern was not so much with the moral or social stigma of poverty as with its depraving and pathological consequences in alcoholism, insanity and disease. The Haeckelian authors, Richard Voss and Wolfgang Kirchbach, wrote plays dealing with the ill-effects of degenerate parental behaviour. Wilhelm Boelsche published lyrical expositions of Haeckel's theories of the evolution of sexuality.[99] Naturalist periodicals such as *Die Gesellschaft* and *Die Freie Bühne* included articles on evolutionary biology and social reform. Biology was part of the public discourse on social reform. Despite the pessimistic conclusions drawn from evolution, there remained the hope that degeneration could be countered. Max Nordau, the expatriate Hungarian doctor and liberal who resided in Paris, contrasted the ill-effects of conventional religion, politics and economics with the

---

[96] E. Rüdin, *Über die klinischen Formen der Gefängnispsychosen* (Berlin, 1901).
[97] ZSTA M Rep 76 VIII B Nr 1849 Geisteskranke Verbrecher; E. Kraepelin, *Die psychiatrischen Aufgaben des Staates* (Jena, 1906).
[98] E. Kraepelin, *Lebenserinnerungen*, pp. 79–82; Forel papers, Rüdin to Forel, 11 December 1898.
[99] G. Schmidt, *Die literarische Rezeption des Darwinismus* (Berlin, 1974), pp. 132–8; R.J.V. Lenman, 'Censorship and Society in Munich, 1890–1914', DPhil dissertation, Oxford University, 1975, p. 56.

social freedom and solidarity that would result from the struggle for survival.[100] But he was disappointed in the naturalist authors whom he diagnosed as themselves degenerate. The works of Hauptmann and Zola were 'sewage exhalations' and 'filth'.[101]

Gerhart Hauptmann shows how the naturalist movement analysed the process of degeneration, in his own attitudes swaying between scientism and irrationalism, between self-restraint and passion. After his scientific enthusiasms in Jena, he had married in 1885 despite his friends' views that his bride was deficient in racial quality. In Berlin in the same year he wavered between the physiological positivism of Emil Du Bois-Reymond and the Christian nature mysticism of Boehme. He underwent a period of self-destructive alcoholic excess, which ended in the professor of clinical medicine and theorist of the organic personality, Friedrich Kraus, condemning his deviant *verfehlte Existenz*. He joined Ploetz in Zürich during the spring of 1888, and was converted by Forel's psychiatry, abstinence from alcohol and ventures in hypnosis. As a result of witnessing the miseries of mental illness at the Burghölzli asylum, Hauptmann abstained from alcohol. Johannes Guttzeit, an apostle of *Lebensreform* and vegetarianism, impressed Hauptmann with the power of the mystical and the irrational.[102]

Hauptmann channelled the conflict between scientism and mysticism, his emotions over his marital problems and his experiences with Ploetz into the 'social drama', *Vor Sonnenaufgang* (Before Dawn). This was first performed in Berlin by the naturalist 'Free Stage' company on 20 October 1889.[103] The play dealt with the conflict between personal emotions and the scientific laws of heredity. The central figure was a journalist, Alfred Loth, who was investigating living conditions of Silesian miners. Peasants who owned the land on which mines were sited had been corrupted by wealth, and were prey to alcoholism and a range of pathological traits. Loth fell in love with Helene, the daughter of a peasant drunkard. Loth was modelled on Ploetz, and Helene on Pauline Rüdin, Ploetz's first wife. The vivid scenes were rich in dialect, and the Silesian setting drew on Hauptmann's youthful knowledge of the region. As a student Loth had become convinced of the need to maintain the nation's racial purity. He vowed to abstain from alcohol, and to marry only into a healthy family. Loth had organized a colonization society of which a doctor and an engineer in the play had also been members. The society's aims were the 'propagation of a race sound in mind and body'. These features mirror the concerns of Ploetz and his circle of social reformers. *Vor Sonnenaufgang* focused on the pathological degeneration of Helene's family. The village doctor diagnosed her family as incurably degenerate: 'there is nothing but drunkenness, gluttony, inbreeding and, in consequence, degeneration along the whole line'. When the

---

[100] M. Nordau, *Die conventionellen Lügen der Kulturmenschheit* (Leipzig, 1883); Johnston, *Austrian Mind*, pp. 362–4.   [101] M. Nordau, *Degeneration* (London, 1895).
[102] G. Hauptmann, *Der Apostel, Bahnwärter Thiel* (Berlin, 1892).
[103] A. Lange, *Berlin zur Zeit Bebels und Bismarcks* (Berlin, 1972), pp. 705–9.

play was first performed the scenario of degeneration, with scenes of illicit sex, midwifery, jilting, hysteria and a final suicide, caused an uproar. In the tumult a pair of obstetric forceps was hurled onto the stage by the outraged journalist and physician, Isidor Kastan, as an act of protest. Nordau condemned the play as unconvincing as the daughter showed no signs of having inherited vice.[104]

Vor Sonnenaufgang can be regarded as the first major public statement in Germany on racial biology. It exposed the moral, emotional and social dilemmas arising from the use of the laws of heredity as a means of governing human behaviour. As a victim of degeneration, Helene is comparable with Osvald Alving in Ibsen's *Ghosts*, a victim of congenital syphilis. Although reformers could not endorse Loth's behaviour, he indicated the direction in which evolutionary science was pointing. Loth was criticized for not ascertaining whether Helene was really affected by an hereditary disease. Ploetz saw the play at the German theatre in New York, where he was touched by the love scene.[105] His verdict on Loth as a type of 'scientific Hamlet' was that his actions were 'ganz unsympathisch' (quite unsympathetic), although he acted according to the logic of a particular scientific point of view. Ploetz, whose own choice of spouse had involved years of vacillation, saw Loth as 'too free from inner conflicts' to be real.[106] Boelsche commented that Loth's conduct was cruel, selfish and scientifically mistaken in the refusal to take account of the higher instinct of altruism.[107]

The drama brought medical and sexual questions to the attention of the public. It indicated the human implications of a positivistic and biological approach to morality and social conditions. The naturalist movement pointed to deficiencies in the narrowness of conventional bourgeois morality, concerning marriage, property and the family. Naturalist literature aroused consciousness of how the miseries of industrial society could pollute marriage and the family, causing an inexorable process of degeneration. There were biological laws which dictated that human greed and indulgence would lead to unhappiness, sterility and death. Marriage and sexuality were key areas where either the paths of degeneration or of social progress could be chosen. The biological theorists and naturalist authors wished to break down prevailing taboos on the discussion of sexuality. It was hoped that by reconstituting codes of behaviour in accordance with the laws of human evolution humanity would be saved. Armed with science, racially 'superior' personalities pointed out the means of national salvation. Biology dictated a reform of social values before the dawning of a social era of sobriety and order.

[104] Nordau, *Degeneration*, pp. 523–5.
[105] Gaule papers, Ploetz to Gaule, 16 January 1892; Carl Hauptmann papers, Ploetz to C. Hauptmann, 14 January 1892.
[106] Ploetz papers, Ploetz to Carl Hauptmann, 26 August 1889; A. Ploetz, 'Trostworte an einen naturwissenschaftlichen Hamlet', *New Yorker Volkszeitung*, reprinted in *ARGB*, vol. 29 (1935), 88–9.   [107] W. Boelsche in *Die Gegenwart*, vol. 18 (1889) 234–6.

SEXUALITY AND SOCIALISM

Anxiety over chronic diseases and physical degeneration brought biological debates on heredity to the attention of the public at large. The utopians, socialists and *Lebensreformer* initially mounted their attack from outside established society, and accused capitalism and the Junker elite of causing deaths, disease and physical and moral degeneration. Some of these critics made common cause with medical reformers over the issues of health and welfare, and a small but vociferous group of socialist doctors emerged. Other more conservative biologists and doctors responded with scientifically-based solutions to national and racial ills. They pointed out the inadequacies of political and economic solutions to a range of social problems. Academic experts in biology and medicine claimed competence over psychological and social problems. The biological defence of the established social order appropriated ideas of a reformed lifestyle, and linked these to national survival.

The biological sciences achieved prestige with brilliant pioneering work in experimental cytology and embryology during the 1880s. At a time when academic radicalism was on the decline, biology disengaged itself from liberal politics, and became a source for drawing conclusions on society, psychology and disease. Heredity was revealed as a hidden factor shaping social life. Positive attributes such as commercial success and intelligence, or the social evils of crime and poverty, could all be ascribed to the predestinating force of heredity. Ideas of a natural aristocracy of outstanding physique and intellect were fused with the notion that inheritance was like acquired capital. As with land or money, physical qualities were passed on through the family. Biologists remarked that the term, 'inheritance' or *Erbmasse*, was the same as used in law for an inherited estate. Yet biologists were divided over the mechanisms of inheritance. The inheritance of acquired characters was at the centre of the controversy. The ensuing debate had overtones of being a secularized form of the theological controversy over free will and determinism as well as a political debate on individuality and the greater power of the organism. The salvation of the family, nation and human race was at stake. It was in this highly charged political and scientific atmosphere that new sciences of 'racial hygiene' and of 'sexual science' were formulated as intermediate positions between Marxism (with its economic critique of the bourgeois family) and aristocratic conservatism.

Microbiology revealed the hidden powers of heredity by demonstrating the effects of degenerative 'racial poisons' on the germplasm. Social misery was deemed to be the pathological product of alcohol on conception, of venereal diseases in causing sterility and congenital syphilis, and of female industrial labour resulting in the overstrain that brought on miscarriages, inability to breast feed and inherited malformations. Experimental embryology and studies of fertilization gave rise to a sense of being on the brink of discovering the cause of physical degeneration and a scientific means of excluding undesirable characters from society. By 1884 there was a consensus among biologists that the hereditary substance was located in the cell nucleus. The behaviour of chromosomes during fertilization and cell division was meticulously observed with the aid of improved microscopes and dyestuffs. The chromosomes were deemed to be the carriers of the hereditary properties. How hereditary germs determined sex, growth, and mental character were major concerns, and eugenicists suggested that such discoveries were imminent.

Control by hereditary powers in the nucleus excluded environmental effects on the protoplasm, which would be affected by such factors as nutrition and warmth. Such hereditary determinism reversed the liberal protoplasmic concept of the cell. This concept, introduced in the 1860s, had suggested that the protoplasm was the elemental vital substance, and that it was sensitive to the effects of the environment; as each protoplasmic cellular individual was like a citizen in the social organism, with continual processes of interaction between cells. However, the advocates of hereditarian explanations claimed that the totality of hereditary factors determined all factors in development, and that an immutable germplasm passed on by the chromosomes at each generation was the ultimate source of organic properties. The controversies over heredity and environment were regarded as of importance in settling what constituted differences between classes, nations and races. Questions of the rights of women could be solved by explaining the evolutionary basis of sexual differences, by determining the contribution of male and female to heredity, and by measuring how physiological and psychological capacities varied between the sexes. Biological observations were used to justify social roles. The fact that the sperm was observed to be active and mobile and that the egg appeared to be static in fertilization could be used to justify the view that the male ought to have an active social role, and the female a passively domestic one of child rearing. Biologists debated the reasons for the evolution of sex organs. Sexual division of labour seemed to represent a higher evolutionary stage, marked by greater differentiation between the physique, roles and character of the sexes. As these controversies raged during the 1880s and 90s, diverse scientific theories were promised to solve the social problems of industrial society.

The germs of heredity

Theories of heredity represented a shift from liberalism to authoritarian collectivism. During the 1860s Darwin had formulated a theory of inheritance in terms of particles, or 'pangenes'. These circulated freely throughout the body and then were concentrated in the reproductive organs. The pangenes could pass on characteristics acquired by an organism in its lifetime. It represented a liberal balance between inherited properties and individual exertions. This theory was refuted by Galton who was convinced that talent was inherited, and that improvements in the human race could be obtained by selective breeding.[108] In 1875 he criticized the inheritance of acquired characters. He suggested that a unit of heredity, the 'stirp' (from the Latin *stirpes* meaning a root), contained the sum total of the hereditary germs, and that these were concentrated in the ovum or sperm. He compared the stirp to a nation, and the germs which achieved development to its foremost men. It was an explicitly elitist theory. He darkly warned that diseases could arise from 'alien germs' just as there were aliens residing in any nation.[109] 'Stirpiculture' was used as an alternative term for eugenics. Galton's eugenics marked a turning point in the transition from liberal political economy to a biologically based authoritarian collectivism.

There was a similar rejection of acquired characters in Germany. In 1883 August Weismann, in an address to the University of Freiburg as pro-Rector, expressed doubts about the inheritance of individual exertions or environmental adaptation. Until this time Weismann shared opinions on society and Darwinism with his more radical colleague, Haeckel: both scientists were free-thinkers, anticlerical, and nationalistic, and they were ardent Darwinists even while accepting the inheritance of acquired characters. Like many biologists during the 1870s Weismann had joined in the search for the origins of reproductive cells: the recapitulation of the evolution of primitive 'Ureier' was a means of explaining sexual reproduction. But he was to reverse his views on evolution. He replaced the emphasis on the chain of continuity of individual sexual cells by claiming to have discovered the hidden substance of the hereditary material, which he called the 'germplasm'. It represented a transition from the individual cell to an immortal and immutable substance of which individuals were merely transitory carriers. It implied a shift from an individualistic theory of the cell as a creative person to a collectivist and authoritarian germplasm. Weisman argued that natural selection was all-sufficient to explain inheritance and evolution. In terms so similar to the stirp theory that Galton pointed out their common position, Weismann postulated an immutable reserve of hereditary material in the germplasm. This had 'conservative' characters which made it immune from environmental change. It was not non-use that caused degeneration of organs, but the cessation of selection. Natural selection held organisms at a peak when the full hereditary potential could be realized. If selection ceased to work then degeneration to rudimentary conditions would set in.[110] While the theory of the germplasm was accepted by socialists and conservatives alike, its inequalities posed problems for egalitarian socialists like Bebel. Its use by doctors for socialist ends – such as by advocates of social hygiene – had problematic authoritarian implications.

---

[108] R.S. Cowan, 'Nature and Nurture: the Interplay of Biology and Politics in the Thought of Francis Galton', *Studies in the History of Biology*, vol. 1 (1977), 133–208.

[109] F. Galton, 'A Theory of Heredity', *The Contemporary Review*, vol. 10 (1875), 80–95.

[110] F. Churchill, 'Weismann's Continuity of the Germ-Plasm in Historical Perspective', in K. Sander (ed.), 'August Weismann (1834–1914) und die theoretische Biologie des 19. Jahrhunderts', *Freiburger Universitätsblätter*, no. 87/88 (1985), 107–24.

Weismann's theory of an immutable germplasm challenged the evolutionary theories of Haeckel and Herbert Spencer, both of whom supported the inheritance of acquired characters. Denial of liberal ideas of self-exertion and individuality meant that during the early 1890s a debate flared up over heredity and adaptation in ant and bee societies. Spencer emphasized the role of nutrition in sex determination, an example being the differentiation of the queen bee from the drones. Other theorists suggested that light and temperature were factors in sexual dimorphism. Weismann argued that only natural selection could account for the development of sexuality and different social functions in state-forming insects. This view undermined democratic concepts of the insect-states of Büchner and Brehm, as well as Forel's socially oriented concepts which allowed for the learning capacities of insects.[111] Two biologists who were also National Liberals, Heinrich Ziegler and Hugo von Buttel-Reepen, employed Weismann's hereditary theories to provide an analysis of insect states in terms of inherited instincts. It typified the way the hereditarian biology of the 1890s was extrapolated into the realm of social theory; it amounted to a justification for a society dominated by an inherited elite with superior physical and mental qualities.

At the time of the Spencer-Weismann controversy, embryologists applied experimental techniques to explain inheritance and growth. Cells were destroyed with heated needles, and the effects of compression, mechanical shaking, and exposure to heat, light and chemicals were studied. During the 1880s the embryologist, Wilhelm Roux, proclaimed that his science of developmental mechanics was like placing a bomb in a factory: by destroying a part of the embryo, the role of each piece of machinery could be ascertained. Such mechanistic theories of development were opposed by Lamarckian theories of direct adaptation to the environment and of an inherent will-power in the organism. Other embryologists argued that injured embryos could regenerate damaged parts, due to formative powers in the whole embryo. Oscar Hertwig compared the multicellular organism to a cell state where each citizen had a social duty to respond to the needs of the organic whole. Natural selection violated such co-operative harmony. The testing of the effects of alcohol and other chemicals was an extension of this scientific work. Embryologists stressed that their researches were relevant to social questions such as inherited toxic poisoning by lead or the effect of drunkenness at conception and during pregnancy.[112] The new experimental biology paralleled the rising confidence in interventionist surgery and in such medical innovations as 'serum therapy'. A younger generation of doctors and biologists educated in the experimental biology during the 1880s and 90s set out to apply these biological laws and methods to re-shape the human constitution and society.

Two brilliant decades of research on heredity culminated in the re-discovery of the Mendelian laws of inheritance in 1900. The significance of the doubling of the

[111] D. Duncan, *The Life and Letters of Herbert Spencer* (London, 1911), p. 343.
[112] P.J. Weindling, *Darwinism and Social Darwinism in Imperial Germany* (Stuttgart, 1989), chapter 6.

chromosomal numbers as the egg and sperm fused at fertilization, and the subsequent reduction division of chromosomes was a major puzzle. The controversy over whether there was an equal contribution of male and female to heredity, raised the issue of whether there was equality between the sexes. It was debated whether double numbers of chromosomes meant that there was a hermaphroditic stage through which all higher organisms passed, before their sex was determined, and whether sex determination was the result of heredity or environment. Those scientists who believed that the chromosomes had a monopoly of hereditary substance argued that the cell nucleus had a controlling monopoly over the processes of growth and heredity. The idea of a dominant nucleus exercising control over cell protoplasm went with elitist social convictions.

Socialist Darwinism

The 1880s and 90s were dominated by debates on the extent that natural selection could be applied to nature and society. The scientific attacks on theories of environmental adaptation were accompanied by bitter refutations of socialism. Egalitarian principles of co-operation and integrated unity were pitted against theories of struggle for survival and dependent hierarchies. In 1883 Bebel published his *Die Frau und der Sozialismus*. By 1890 this popular anthropological tract for female emancipation had sold 15,000 copies in six editions. The lifting of the anti-socialist laws contributed to the popularity of Bebel's writings, and the 1890s saw growing support of women for the SPD.[113] When imprisoned during the early 1870s Bebel had read scientific works by Darwin, Haeckel, Büchner and Liebig, and he had remained interested in the anthropology and brain anatomy of French radicals such as Broca. Bebel's interest in Darwinism was symptomatic of a popular appetite for biological materialism which not only could explain the laws by which the body and mind operated but it was believed, could prophesy future social evolution. Bebel argued that as the struggle for survival intensified with industrialization, the position of women worsened. He considered the evolution of the family challenged partriarchal assumptions. Much physical and psychological ill-health was due to the repressive nature of bourgeois society. Venereal disease was a consequence of the repressive bourgeois family which reduced the woman either to being a reproductive machine (*Gebärapparat*) in the family or to prostitution outside it. It was necessary to evolve a socialist form of the family in which there could be free expression of the sexual instincts necessary for physical and mental health.[114] Bebel argued that Darwinism was essentially a democratic science, which proved the need for equal opportunities for men and women. The struggle for survival expressed itself in class struggle, and would result in more

[113] E. Bernstein, 'Vorwort', in A. Bebel, *Die Frau und der Sozialismus* (reprint of 1929 edition, Bonn-Bad Godesberg, 1977), pp. ix–xvi.

[114] Bebel, *Die Frau*, pp. 96, 124; A. Kelly, *The Descent of Darwin* (Chapel Hill, 1981), pp. 105, 125–39.

evolved political and social institutions. The laws of Darwinian evolution had to be publicized to promote a general awareness of their force in social life. Socialism was in harmony with the underlying natural mechanisms operating in animal societies, and was a higher stage in the evolutionary process.

Bebel's confidence in socialism as consistent with Darwinism was not shared by most biologists and doctors. Weismann's rigorous selectionism made Bebel's belief in adaptive evolutionary progress seem dated. Bebel used the opportunity of new editions of his best-seller for making revisions to take account of his biological critics. The eugenicists, Forel, Ploetz, Schallmayer and Woltmann, were concerned to reconcile the contradictions between socialism and Darwinism. Their solutions removed some of the harsher aspects of class struggle and of the struggle for survival. In the social sphere, national unity was substituted for class struggle, and the biological instincts of altruism and mutual aid were emphasized. Ploetz and Schallmayer were impressed by how organicist theories of the cell state legitimated a state with social insurance and welfare benefits. These socially concerned biological experts thus wished to take the Marxist sting of revolution and redistribution of wealth out of the body of socialist doctrine and at the same time overcome the contradictions of capitalist economic growth.

Schallmayer typified the attempt at formulating a collectivist social philosophy, and the expectation that medical science could solve social problems. Civil and economic categories were evaluated in biological terms. Human life was not to be considered in terms of productive capacity, but as biological capital. He suggested in 1891 that state socialism and social medicine could alter the meaning of marriage. The selection of partners ought not to be made by criteria of wealth but by intelligence and physique. Physical qualities were the inheritance of generations and ought not to be squandered. Therapy for the individual could do little to improve the conditions of the next generation, since environmentally induced variations could not be inherited. Weismann's criticisms of hereditary theories based on individual variations found its medical equivalent in the eugenic refutation of the value of therapy for the individual.[115]

Within the SPD there was a major debate on birth control, over-population and on the social implications of Darwinism. The reading of materialist biological works of Büchner, Haeckel and Vogt had long been popular among German workers. There was an element of truth to Virchow's accusation in 1877 that Haeckel's Darwinism nurtured socialism. Kautsky studied the evolutionary theories of Haeckel, and in 1882 approached Haeckel and the University of Jena in the hope of having his study of marriage and the family accepted as a doctoral dissertation. This was shortly before the advent of the Ploetz circle in Jena.[116] Kautsky's Malthusian tract on the effects of population increase impressed Ploetz

---

[115] Schallmayer, *Entartung*, pp. 23–8.
[116] G.P. Stenson, *Karl Kautsky 1854–1938* (Pittsburgh, 1978), p. 24. K. Kautsky, *Erinnerungen und Eröterungen* (The Hague, 1960), pp. 517–21.

and his utopian circle. Kautsky favoured family limitation to improve the economic and nutritional conditions of the working class.[117] He became interested in Schallmayer's proposals for the socialization of medical care. The SPD's Erfurt programme of 1891 demanded free medical care. Recognizing common ground between socialism and eugenics, he reviewed Schallmayer in the official party journal, *Die Neue Zeit*, in 1892.[118] His verdict was that the medical facilities that Schallmayer justified on the basis of Darwinian natural selection, should be provided on a socialist basis so as to aid the poorer classes.[119] The comment well shows how there were rival collectivist strategies for socializing medicine – one eugenic and the other Marxist. Schallmayer was opposed on evolutionary grounds to therapeutic improvements, whereas Kautsky demanded free and improved therapy.[120] He considered that just as industrialization necessitated the mass organization of technology in the factory, so modern therapy required large-scale organization in hospitals. Socialists were at that time locked in controversy with state authorities over questions of therapy and the administration of tuberculosis hospitals. The state and municipalities vied for control over the expanding medical institutions. It was an era when medical science buoyed up the expansion of welfare facilities and hospitals.

The Freiburg phalanx

The major opposition to socialist demands for increased welfare and to the socialist interpretations of Darwinism by Bebel and Kautsky came from a Baden group of academics centred at the University of Freiburg. Weismann's theory of the germplasm was fully articulated in a monograph of 1892. It offered a basis for examining the racial consequences of heredity. The group consisted of university professors: the zoologist Heinrich Ernst Ziegler, the gynaecologist Alfred Hegar, and the philosopher and anthropologist Ernst Grosse who held lectures on 'the developmental history of the family'. They shared a common interest in the evolution of social instincts. Students of biology and medicine imbibed the hereditarian theories of Weismann. The anthropologist, Eugen Fischer, met the botanist, Baur, at the university ski club. (Baur conducted systematic experiments to prove the suitability of skis in high alpine regions.) A protégé (and co-author of their famous text book on eugenics) was the medical student, Fritz Lenz. Two independent men of letters promulgated more extreme racial theories. One was the engineer, Otto Ammon, who lived in Karlsruhe in Baden but had substantial contact with Freiburg: on behalf of the *Karlsruher Altertumsverein* he conducted

[117] U. Linse, 'Arbeiterschaft und Geburtenkontrolle im Deutschen Kaiserreich von 1891 bis 1914', *Archiv für Sozialgeschichte*, vol. 12 (1972), 209.

[118] K. Kautsky, 'Medizinisches', *Die Neue Zeit*, vol. 10 part 1 (1891/2), 644–51.

[119] A. Labisch, 'Das Krankenhaus in der Gesundheitspolitik der deutschen Sozialdemokratie vor dem ersten Weltkrieg', *Medizinsoziologisches Jahrbuch*, vol. 1 (1981), 130.

[120] Kautsky, 'Medizinisches', p. 648.

anthropological surveys and wrote extensively on racial problems, introducing Galton's ideas into Germany. Ammon illustrates the transition from liberalism to racial anthropological thought. He bought the National Liberal *Konstanzer Zeitung* in 1869; by the 1890s he used his experience as a journalist to buy the *Badische Landeszeitung*, which he transformed from a liberal into an anti-semitic newspaper.[121] The other racial researcher was Ludwig Schemann, a Freiburg resident from 1898, who established a society to propagate the Aryan racial theories of Gobineau. Schemann was drawn to Freiburg by the university, and he enjoyed friendly relations with such as Grosse and Fischer.[122] Gobineau's theories of race were regarded as static and unscientific. But by the early twentieth century Ammon and Schemann were in broad sympathy with each other indicating how racial theories achieved respectability in anthropology by the twentieth century.

The Freiburg group fused French degenerationist theories, British Social Darwinism and distinctive German biological and social concerns. Weismann was especially keen to project his views on Darwinism to an English readership.[123] Benjamin Kidd visited Weismann in 1890 in order to prepare a major review of his theories.[124] In 1894 Kidd published a social theory derived from Weismann's principle that death was a mark of higher evolution, and only the lowest organisms were immortal. He used Weismann's principle of immutability of the germplasm to refute socialism. He argued that the more complex an organism, the shorter its life, but the greater its capacity to accumulate hereditary improvements. Progress depended on constant selection. Kidd's use of this theory to endorse social altruism was a concession to Spencerian views.[125] Weismann arranged for Kidd's work to be translated, for which he wrote a foreword pointing out that socialism contravened the law of natural selection.[126] He was especially interested in Kidd's extension of evolution to human society, commenting: 'I think that you are quite right in contributing to religion a great part of the developmental process of society. I do not doubt that the principles of Christianism had an enormous effect in this regard.'[127] Kidd suggested that religion could have a selective effect in improving the working class. Eugenics was to be a form of surrogate religion as a civilizing and disciplining creed.

Weismann's efforts to promote discussion of the social consequences of Darwinism were shown by his preface to the work of the physiologist, John Berry Haycraft, on *Darwinism and Race Progress*.[128] Haycraft elaborated extreme

---

121 B. Berblings-Ammon, *Das Lebensbild eines Rassenforschers* (Halle, nd); E. Fischer, 'Otto Ammon', *Der Erbarzt*, vol. 10 (1942), 267–72.
122 L. Schemann, *Lebensfahrten eines Deutschen* (Leipzig, 1925).
123 B. Kidd, 'Darwin's Successor at Home: Our Scientific Causerie', *Review of Reviews*, vol. 2 (1890), 647–50.
124 Weismann papers, Kopierbuch I, Bl. 739, 784, 803; D. Crook, *Benjamin Kidd* (Cambridge, 1984), p. 38.   125 G. Jones, *Social Darwinism in English Thought* (Brighton, 1980), pp. 84–5.
126 B. Kidd, *Soziale Evolution mit einem Vorwort von Professor Dr August Weismann* (Jena, 1895).
127 Weismann papers, Kopierbuch 2, Bl. 682; 3, Bl. 9–10.
128 J.B. Haycraft, *Natürliche Auslese und Rassenverbesserung* (Leipzig, 1895).

individualist views on the need to allow natural selection to work throughout society, and to dismantle all social welfare institutions. Weismann encountered degeneration in his personal life. When he discovered that his wife was a morphine addict, he separated from her (after attempts at a cure) in 1903. Weismann was severely handicapped by a chronic eye ailment which prevented him from working with a microscope. Comments in his work on the physical degeneration resulting from civilization – for example short-sightedness – had a personal poignancy. He pointed out that the sight of domesticated animals such as dogs was also deteriorating. The only social group immune from such deterioration in Germany were the peasantry. The first edition of Weismann's work on 'The Evolution Theory' of 1892 pointed out that many diseases might not be inherited, but be caused by infection carried by the sperm to the egg at fertilization. He considered that the transmission of syphilis from a mother to a developing child could be a model for how tuberculosis and even epilepsy were passed on at fertilization.[129] The combination of personal and social convictions meant that by the second edition of his lectures on heredity, Weismann readily incorporated the work of social anthropologists such as Ammon and Galton into his theory of heredity. He regarded civilized races as prone to degeneration: muscles, mammary glands and bone strength were all deteriorating among the higher classes. He regretted that the weak and degenerate were allowed to procreate. While Weismann was reticent about Mendelism, he aligned his biology with racial hygiene.[130] He concluded that continuous competition and selection were necessary to maintain physical and mental qualities.

The implications of socialism and Darwinism for the maintenance of the family were at the centre of the 1890s debate on social evolution. In 1891 Ammon published a Darwinian tract attacking socialism.[131] In 1892 Haeckel emphasized that socialism was opposed to the evolutionary view of a monistic unity of man and nature. In 1893 Ziegler savaged Bebel in a treatise on 'Science and Social Democracy'. Ziegler had studied in Freiburg and in Strasburg. He had been assistant to Oscar Schmidt who in 1878 criticized socialist uses of Darwinism. Ziegler became assistant to Weismann from 1887, when Weismann and others were undertaking fundamental research on the reduction division of chromosomes during fertilization. Ziegler was also interested in the biological bases of social psychology. In 1892, speaking to the Society of German Naturalists and Doctors, he extended Weismann's hereditary theory to explain instincts as inherited in the germplasm. He set out to classify inherited nervous reactions. In 1893 he addressed the Society of German Zoologists on the relations of biology to sociology. His aim was to correct the idealist utopian Darwinism of Bebel, and to pursue sociology as a

---

[129] E. Posner, 'August Weismann and the Genetics of Tuberculosis', *Tubercle*, vol. 48 (1967), 166–9.
[130] A. Weismann, *The Evolution Theory* (London, 1904), II, pp. 144–7; Weismann, *Vorträge über Deszendenztheorie*, (Jena, 1913), II, pp. 134–5.
[131] O. Ammon, *Der Darwinismus gegen die Socialdemokratie* (Hamburg, 1891).

type of comparative anatomical ethnology.[132] During the 1890s Ammon, Ziegler and Weismann used the *Naturwissenschaftlichen Verein Freiburg* as a base for disseminating anti-socialist human biology. For example, Ammon lectured on 2 June 1893 on class formation and race.[133] These hereditarian biologists were vehement popularizers and marked a decisive break with the liberal tradition of the Baden government.

Ziegler, a National Liberal, focused on Bebel's conviction that Darwinism proved the truth of social egalitarianism. Ziegler criticized male and female equality, and equal educational opportunity as idealist rationalism. Instead, he invoked Darwinian evolution to justify hereditary inequalities. The biological principle of division of labour was extrapolated to human society as composed of differentiated castes. He argued that evolutionary development and sexual differences were the result of a physiological division of labour. Hereditary inequalities arose from inherited reflexes, and underlay cultural diversity. Intellectual differences were inherited. The family was the natural elementary unit of social organization; the woman's role was to give birth to and care for children and the man's was to feed and protect the family.[134] Ziegler rejected the theory of the non-monogamous and matriarchal origins of the family of Morgan and Friedrich Engels, invoking reproductive physiology and observations on animal behaviour. He defended Malthusian theories of selection and struggle. The struggle for survival in war was to prevent social and moral degeneration. Yet within groups like families, tribes and peoples the struggle for survival did not operate, being replaced by social instincts of common interests. The authority of the state thus had biological roots. The state had evolved from more primitive social forms, the germs of which could be seen in animal life. Ziegler concluded that natural differences were immutable, and that the only means to improve humanity was through selection. In human societies selection was justified to eliminate criminals, mental illness and epilepsy.[135]

The Baden group pioneered a conservative type of Darwinian social anthropology. Ammon undertook extensive social surveys to investigate racial degeneration. His starting point was Galton's theory of the social distribution of hereditary quality as expressed in *Hereditary Genius* of 1869 and *Natural Inheritance* of 1889. Between 1887 and 1894 Ammon examined 27,719 military recruits with the aim of assessing the racial qualities of Baden's population. This survey had Virchow's investigation of the physique of school children as a model. Whereas Virchow's conclusions amounted to a refutation of Aryan racial theory, Ammon supported the idea of a German race that was threatened by degeneration. He was more

[132] H.E. Ziegler, 'Über die Beziehungen der Zoologie zur Sociologie', *Verhandlungen der Deutschen Zoologischen Gesellschaft*, vol. 3 (1893), 51–5.

[133] 'Die Bedeutung der Staendebildung für das Menschengeschlecht'.

[134] H.E. Ziegler, *Die Naturwissenschaft und die Socialdemokratische Theorie. Die Verhältnisse dargelegt auf Grund der Werke von Darwin und Bebel* (Stuttgart, 1893).

[135] Ziegler drew on R. Leuckart, *Ueber den Polymorphismus der Individuen oder die Erscheinungen der Arbeitstheilung in der Natur* (Corhessen, 1851).

cautious than the French ideologues of Aryan superiority such as Gobineau and Vacher de Lapouge. For example, he denied the existence of a pure Aryan racial type and divided the population into Germanic long heads and Asiatic round heads. While Lapouge's thesis of a 'de-nordification of France' was unpopular, his work on racial and social selection of 1888, *L'hérédité dans la science politique*, was well regarded by German conservatives including Ammon. Lapouge was a vehement scourge of Catholicism, democracy, Jews and negroes. He gave expression to the Aryan ideal through anthropological and biological statistics, drawing on the work of Galton. Consequently, he appealed to the medically minded German anthropologists in a way that Gobineau could not. Ammon and Lapouge became linked as pioneers of social anthropology.[136]

Ammon considered that the long heads predominated among officials and academics, and had a superior capacity for work and idealism. The round heads were calculating and complacent. Socialists and Catholics were round heads, whereas Bismarck and General von Moltke were long heads. The biologically lowest social group was the unemployed whose existence was being eliminated by the struggle for survival. He agreed with Schallmayer that therapeutic medicine benefited the individual rather than the race. Like Galton and Lapouge, he feared that the highest social group was producing the least children. The tone of Ammon's work was strongly anti-socialist and critical of Bebel. In 1891 he published a pamphlet specifically attacking socialism.[137] Ammon's racial anthropology drew the conclusion that there should be selective breeding of those with superior mental qualities.[138]

Anthropology had an impact not only on theories of reproduction but also on gynaecology. Hegar, professor of obstetrics at Freiburg since 1864, combined concern with inheritance and the family with innovative operative techniques made possible by antiseptic surgery. He was renowned for his diagnostic skills, his innovative use of metal dilators in uterine examination, and for 'Hegar's sign' in the uterus as an indicator of early pregnancy. His ideas and clinical practice show how medicine was affected by the hereditarian biology of Hegar's colleague Weismann. Hegar considered that not just an isolated diseased organ, but the whole organism and constitution of the patient had to be taken into account. He was concerned with the physical anthropology of the patient as well as with family background. Hegar's operative gynaecology was the counterpart of degenerationist psychiatry. Hegar, like the hereditarian psychiatrists, was vehemently opposed to alcohol and tobacco as 'racial poisons'.[139] Gynaecology was thus extended into the social and moral spheres.

Advances in antiseptic surgery meant that from the 1870s major gynaecological

[136] E. Seidler and G. Nagel, 'Georges Vacher de Lapouge (1854–1936) und der Sozialdarwinismus in Frankreich', in G. Mann (ed.), *Biologismus im 19 Jahrhundert* (Stuttgart, 1973), pp. 94–107.

[137] O. Ammon, *Der Darwinismus*.

[138] Ammon, *Der Darwinismus*, pp. 271, 280, 297; F. Tönnies, 'Ammons Gesellschaftstheorie', *Archiv für Sozialwissenschaft und Sozialpolitik*, vol. 19 (= n.s. 1) (1904), 88–111.

[139] A. Mayer, *Alfred Hegar und der Gestaltwandel der Gynäkologie seit Hegar* (Freiburg, 1961).

operations such as ovariotomies became possible. In 1872 Hegar carried out and publicized an operation for the removal of ovaries. (This was at the same time as an American surgeon Robert Battey performed the operation.)[140] They regarded ovariotomy as a cure for asthma and epilepsy and for various types of women's neuroses such as hysteria. This replaced the reflex theories of neurosis current in the early nineteenth century with a theory that neuroses were rooted in the degeneration of organs, especially the sexual organs. Thus an associationist and environmentalist theory was replaced by an organicist theory that could be developed in terms of an hereditarian predisposition.[141] Between 1885 and 1894, 139 operations for female 'castration' were carried out at Hegar's clinic.[142] Hegar insisted on caution in undertaking ovariotomies, in that when the reproductive organs were healthy the operation should not be carried out. He conceded that the operation had aroused a storm of criticism, owing to the lack of caution shown by others. But his approach represented a broadening of medical explanations of mental disorder. More than just 'brain disease', sexual neuroses and deviant behaviour such as morphine addiction could be explained and cured by attention to pathological signs throughout the body. During the 1890s Hegar's operation was recommended by psychiatrists like Westphal for cases of hysteria, even though there were no degenerative signs in the ovaries.[143] The ovariotomies of the 1890s had a counterpart in castration as a therapy for criminality. Such surgical interventionism was a preliminary for the eugenic programmes of the next decades.

Hegar joined the chorus of scientific refutations of Bebel. In 1894 he published an attack on Bebel which concentrated on the question of the sexual instincts. He condemned Bebel for undermining the woman's sense of duty to the family and society. A woman must not, as Bebel suggested, fulfil her personal sexual instincts, but subordinate these to the higher interests of society. Hegar's sense of moral indignation was vented when he spat in disgust at a performance of Ibsen's *Ghosts*. He advocated sterilization and castration as the best means of preventing inherited mental disease. He feared that the increase in the degenerate would result in a society in which the fit merely worked to provide for the degenerate. Symptoms of degeneration were two-child families and abortion. In 1894 he, like Ammon, advocated methodical selection and planned breeding to improve the race. His emphasis on the inherited constitution was the gynaecological counterpart of Weismann's germplasm theory.[144] The biologically based power of ancestral traditions was invading the territory of sexuality and reproduction.

[140] R. Battey, *Normal Ovariotomy* (Atlanta, 1873).
[141] A. Hegar, *Der Zusammenhang der Geschlechtskrankheiten mit nervösen Leiden und die Castration bei Neurosen* (Stuttgart, 1885).
[142] H. Liesau, 'Der Einfluss der Castration auf den weiblichen Organismus mit besonderer Berücksichtigung des sexuellen und psychischen Lebens', med. Diss., University of Freiburg, 1896.
[143] E. Shorter, 'Medizinische Theorien spezifisch weiblicher Nervenkrankheiten im Wandel', in A. Labisch and R. Spree (eds.), *Medizinische Deutungsmacht im sozialen Wandel* (Bonn, 1989), in press.
[144] A. Hegar, *Der Geschlechtstrieb. Eine social-medizinische Studie* (Stuttgart, 1894); A. Mayer, 'Die Bedeutung der Konstitution seit Alfred Hegar', in *Alfred Hegar zum Gedächtnis* (Freiburg, 1930), pp. 9–20.

The brave new science of *Sexualwissenschaft*

In reaction to the scientific onslaught on Bebel, there was a re-grouping of progressive doctors and biologists. They wished to salvage certain of Bebel's principles and bring these into line with Weismann's advances in biology and with the urgent need for public health reforms. Ploetz returned from the United States to find the biologists' attack on Bebel at its height. Ploetz's seminal treatise on racial hygiene of 1895 marked an attempt to reconcile the opposing camps. Ploetz went to Berlin because it was a centre for avant-garde thought on the social and psychological significance of medicine and biology. A group of Berlin doctors focused on social aspects of medicine such as venereology and the biological basis of sexuality. This group included Blaschko and Iwan Bloch, two venereologists, who sought more generally to improve the lot of mankind. Other physicians such as Albert Eulenburg, Grotjahn, Hirschfeld and Albert Moll considered the evolutionary and medical implications of sexuality. From 1893 Eulenburg campaigned against the theory of the deficient sexuality of woman. Hirschfeld agitated for a medical and biological understanding of homosexuality rather than the treatment of it as a crime. These doctors were impressed by such recent discoveries in biology as that sexual organs were not differentiated in the early stage of embryological development, and that there was a 'hermaphroditic' stage at conception. Such facts suggested a biological basis for variations in sexual behaviour in later life. These doctors laid the foundations of sexology or *Sexualwissenschaft*. They were active in public associations, as for the repeal of criminal statutes against homosexuality, and in popularizing scientifically based theories of sexuality. Sexual reformers developed a type of reforming and liberal eugenics; the link became explicit when in 1913 doctors founded the *Berliner Gesellschaft für Sexualwissenschaft und Eugenik*.

The sexual reformers had similar backgrounds to the racial hygienists in that as neurologists and venereologists they were on the margins of the medical profession. Sexual reform emerged during the 1890s, at the same time as racial hygiene, and figures such as Forel were part of both movements. There were additional features: many were Jewish (e.g. Blaschko, Bloch and Hirschfeld) and had migrated from eastern areas of Germany to Berlin; some (such as Blaschko and Hirschfeld after 1918) had socialist sympathies. As a medical student in Berlin from 1876 until 1881 Blaschko had combined studies in anatomy, physiology and hygiene with socio-political interests.[145] He typified the transition from an economic to a biological approach to social medicine. At first he was concerned with the way working conditions damaged health. Blaschko used his thriving insurance-based practice as a dermatologist in Berlin as the basis for extensive medical research. He endeavoured to apply and communicate the latest medical

---

[145] F. Tennstedt, 'Alfred Blaschko – das wissenschaftliche und sozialpolitische Wirken eines menschenfreundlichen Sozialhygienikers im Deutschen Reich', *Zeitschrift für Sozialreform*, vol. 25 (1979), 513–23, 600–14, 646–67.

science as a basis for preventive medicine and social hygiene. By 1914 he was a leading expert on legislative and educational prevention of VD. Pre-dating his public activity was his concern with inherited diseases. In 1890 Blaschko wrote to Weismann requesting guidance on the role of disease in evolution. Weismann replied that although he had occasionally considered the issue, he did not regard diseases as true acquired characteristics.[146] In 1894 Blaschko published an article reviewing Weismann's 1893 attack on Spencer. He was concerned over the persistence of mistaken Lamarckian theories of use and disuse in lay circles.[147] Blaschko sought to establish a progressive social philosophy on the basis of Weismann's reformulation of Darwinism.[148] The transition from an economic and environmentalist outlook to a biological and hereditarian analysis of the spread of diseases gave rise to eugenic theories, and allowed doctors to claim authority over social questions.

Blaschko developed a social biology on a non-racial basis. He reviewed Ammon's work on human selection for the socialist periodical, *Die Neue Zeit*. He disagreed with the use of Weismann's concept of 'panmixia'. This theory denoted the degeneration of an organ, character or instinct due to a cessation of natural selection. Blaschko accused Ammon of wrongly extrapolating Weismann's panmixia to sexual selection. To Ammon, interbreeding between different social classes and races represented a process of degeneration. Ammon had naively over-extended the concept to all human affairs, although he accepted that the higher classes had greater hereditary reserves of intelligence and other inherited qualities. Any attempt to breed an aristocratic elite of physically and mentally superior humans, like thoroughbred race horses, could not succeed. Aristocratic families became sterile after a few generations. Instead, Blaschko considered that industrial society's degenerative effects should be prevented. Factors such as poverty inhibiting the growth of children, causing mental illness, alcoholism and occupational diseases ought to be countered. It was an open question as to whether eugenicists such as Schallmayer were right in their assertions of the degenerative effects of hygiene and whether an irreversible degeneration had set in, or whether from the European proletariat a race could develop with superior mental and moral qualities.[149]

Similar to his colleague Blaschko, Iwan Bloch regarded Weismann's theory of the germplasm as providing a scientific basis for his studies of sexuality. He considered that Weismann had established the principle of the continuity of life, and the evolutionary necessity for sexual reproduction and individuality. Bloch's survey of the abundant varieties of sexual life began with an account of fertilization as the fusion of two cells. As with Haeckel and Boelsche, he saw this fusion as

---

[146] Weismann papers, Kopierbuch I, Bl. 765, 10 May 1890.
[147] Dr A. Bl. (= Blaschko), 'Bemerkungen zur Weismann'schen Theorie', *Die Neue Zeit*, vol. 13 (1894), 19–23.
[148] For Blaschko's copies of Weismann and Ammon, see the History Faculty Library, Oxford.
[149] A. Blaschko, 'Natürliche Auslese und Klassentheilung', *Die Neue Zeit*, vol. 13 (1894/5), 615–24.

representing an outburst of elemental emotional forces. He typified the shift towards a biological and medical account of sexuality, in contrast to Bebel's political and economic analysis. Bloch's biology was neither hereditarian nor racial in its ultimate aims. He criticized Krafft-Ebing's hereditary determinism, arguing that sexual perversions were acquired rather than inherited characteristics.[150] He was concerned with the hereditary consequences of diseases such as VD, but his aim was individual happiness in present and future generations. He extracted these elements from the accounts of racial hygiene by Hegar and Ploetz. He was only interested in that part of racial hygiene which was termed 'reproductive hygiene' and dealt with sexual selection, health and inheritance. While the economic aspects of marriage had been criticized as a cause of racial degeneration, Bloch did not wish to challenge marriage as an institution. His aims were natural love and healthy children. Degeneration followed when neither were achieved.[151]

The third sex

Magnus Hirschfeld was to take a lead in political agitation for repeal of criminal statutes against homosexuality. He too based his reforming strategies on biological premises. Like Blaschko, Hirschfeld came from a family of East Prussian Jewish physicians and liberals. When Virchow examined his doctorate in 1892, he recognized Hirschfeld as the son of a fellow liberal and sanitary reformer. Like Ploetz, Abderhalden, Rüdin and Grotjahn, he had as a schoolboy indulged in utopian speculations – in his case about a universal language. From 1895 he was involved in the utopian *Neue Gemeinschaft* for the cultivation of an alternative naturalistic lifestyle, and supported their plans for a garden suburb. He had contacts as a student with Bebel, was impressed by Ibsen's *Ghosts*, and was acquainted with Wedekind. He also gravitated from medicine to journalism and he visited America where he was impressed by nature therapy. He was active in the campaign against alcohol abuse which he saw as leading to mental disease and prostitution. Like Grotjahn, he was influenced by the liberal Berlin neurologist, Emanuel Mendel, and, like Grotjahn, he opened a medical practice in Berlin in 1896. He was innovative in establishing a fund (*Hausarztkasse*) for annual payments by families to practitioners. But he soon found his main vocation – the medical treatment and understanding of homosexuality.[152] Hirschfeld illustrates the transition from utopianism to social biology.

Hirschfeld regarded homosexuality as a 'natural sexual variation'. He attempted to reverse the psychiatrists' view that homosexuality was linked to sickness by reviving the 'third sex' theory of Karl Heinrich Ulrichs.[153] By 1897 he was

[150] I. Bloch, *Beiträge zur Archaeologie der Psychopathia Sexualis*, 2 vols. (Dresden, 1902–3).
[151] I. Bloch, *Das Sexualleben unserer Zeit* (Berlin, 1907), pp. 744–81.
[152] C. Wolff, *Magnus Hirschfeld* (London, 1986), pp. 21–51.
[153] H.C. Kennedy, 'The "Third Sex" Theory of Karl Heinrich Ulrichs', *Journal of Homosexuality*, vol. 6 (1981), 103–11.

promoting a 'Scientific and Humanitarian Committee' for repeal of the laws on homosexuality. On 1 December a petition was handed to the Reichstag. The tone was medical and liberal with a preamble mentioning the tolerant views of liberal doctors such as Virchow and Langenbeck on homosexuality in 1869.[154] Its leading signatories included Bebel and Kautsky, as well as such doctors as Krafft-Ebing, and young eugenicists such as Grotjahn and Paul Näcke.[155] There followed an even larger petition in 1898 with the names of leading authors such as Gerhart Hauptmann and Wedekind. At the same time Hirschfeld began to observe homosexual life. He was accompanied on expeditions to Berlin's underworld of bars and brothels by the Saxon psychiatrist and director of the Colditz mental hospital, Paul Näcke, who was to lead a campaign for the sterilization of criminals. From 1899 Hirschfeld edited a *Yearbook for Sexual Gradations*,[156] which applied anthropology and evolutionary biology to promote a medical understanding of sexual variants. Hirschfeld was also interested in 'female hermaphroditism and homosexuality' as aspects of the women's movement. In 1903 he sent questionnaires to students of the Technical University so as to establish the incidence of homosexuality, but was successfully prosecuted by right-wing students. In the following year a survey of 5,000 metal-workers met with a sympathetic response. He was deeply concerned about the suicide of F.A. Krupp in 1902, and suspected that the Kaiser's devotion to Krupp was a sign of the Kaiser's repressed homosexuality.[157] Other psychiatrists were less tolerant. Rüdin condemned homosexuality as leading to racial degeneration.[158] Over the next decade medical opinion became polarized between those arguing that homosexuals were normal and entitled to an equal share in public life, and those psychiatrists arguing that homosexuals were degenerates with such pathological characteristics as cheating and lying.[159]

The biology of sex

The hope of progress to a reformed and more noble sexuality was shared by Forel. The rapid population growth in Zürich had aroused his concern not only with alcoholism but also with the associated issues of prostitution and rising illegitimacy rates. In 1892 he founded a cantonal association to improve morality, and in the mid-1890s waged a campaign against brothels.[160] In 1898 he retired from his post as director of the cantonal psychiatric hospital, and began work on a popular treatise on 'the sexual question'. Avowedly a socialist, Forel sought to publicize the facts of sexuality, and to produce a medical substitute for Bebel's *Woman and Socialism*. Like Bloch, Forel wrote from the perspectives of evolutionary biology.

[154] J.D. Steakley, *The Homosexual Emancipation Movement in Germany* (New York, 1975).
[155] Wolff, *Hirschfeld*, pp. 445–9.   [156] *Jahrbuch für sexuelle Zwischenstufen.*
[157] Wolff, *Hirschfeld*, pp. 32–65.
[158] E. Rüdin, 'Zur Rolle der Homosexuellen im Lebensprozess der Rasse', *ARGB*, vol. 1 no. 1 (1904), 99–109.   [159] Wolff, *Hirschfeld*, pp 83–5.   [160] Meier, *Forel*, pp. 85–94.

Yet unlike Bloch, he sought to impose codes of behaviour based on a rigorously deterministic evolutionary biology. Forel also differed from those using Weismann as a basis for their social biology in that he relied on Semon's neo-Lamarckian theories of inherited memory. Ancestral energies could be combined with environmental stimuli that could be either positive or degenerative. Whereas Bloch, Hirschfeld and Moll had tolerant views on issues such as homosexuality and masturbation, for Forel these were part of a hereditary pathology of degeneration and waste. Forel hoped that the priorities of racial hygiene would replace political economy, just as ethics had been made redundant by science. It was senseless to punish criminals when their acts were determined by inherited pathological traits, and doctors ought not to censor patients for abnormal behaviour. Forel concurred with the view that human virtues and sound biological qualities could only be maintained by sexual selection.[161] Forel's widely distributed tract was symptomatic of how far liberal values of individual moral responsibility had been eroded.

The Bebel-Ziegler dispute had generated a wide range of intermediate positions. These were in many ways scientifically more sophisticated than what Bebel or even Ziegler could offer. Moreover, the younger generation of sexual reformers was well versed in social theory, and appreciated that there were a range of psychological and sexual problems that required more sensitive solutions than earlier commentators had suggested. The privacy of family life and sexual behaviour were being subjected to professional scrutiny by biologists and medical reformers.

REGENERATING THE RIGHT

Aristocratic renewal

While utopianism, *Lebensreform* and socialism represented challenges from outside the established social order, there were efforts to revitalize the ruling elite from within. Racial theories constituted a type of aristocratic *Lebensreform*. Cultural elitism, and hostility to liberalism, materialism and socialism, were spurs to developing ideas of a regenerated ruling elite. A few renegade academics such as Tille and Houston Stewart Chamberlain campaigned for a revived social aristocracy and national leadership. Chamberlain joined forces with the disciples of Gobineau, Nietzsche and the composer Wagner, and glorified the historical role and cultural traditions of the aristocracy. Associations for specifically 'German' types of culture were founded and were allied to the ultra-nationalist Pan-German League. Claiming to be the true custodians of German national culture, their racial nationalism appealed primarily to the *Bildungsbürgertum*. At the same time certain astute politicians, notably the Kaiser's close but manipulative friend, Philipp Eulenburg, seized on the ideas of Gobineau, Schemann and Chamberlain in seeking to reinforce the authority of the hereditary ruling elite. The Kaiser, the Junker-

---

[161] A. Forel, *Die sexuelle Frage* (Munich, 1905).

elite, heavy industry and the *Bildungsbürgertum* were to be dragooned into an alliance, with racial ideology as an intergrating force.

Despite their high-minded nationalist ideals, racial ideologists were pedantic, petty-minded and querulous, and were often isolated figures; they were neither scientists directing research institutes nor professional men. They turned their isolation into an advantage by claiming that their status as *Privatgelehrte* allowed them to stand above party politics and academic disciplines. There remained a considerable rift between the Aryan mythology of Gobineau and the biologistic hereditarianism of Weismann, Hegar and Ziegler. Among the first German enthusiasts for Gobineau's theories had been the Wagner circle in Bayreuth.[162] Gobineau first met Wagner in 1876 and became close friends with the composer. Gobineau admired Wagner's music as a testimony of Germany's racial genius. Wagner used Gobineau's theories of racial inequality to give a scientific gloss to his enthusiasm for a racial theory of culture. Wagnerism became synonymous with nationalist condemnation of liberalism and materialism. Until her death in 1930 Cosima Wagner endeavoured to fuse anti-semitism and ideas of Aryan superiority.[163] In 1894 Schemann established the Gobineau Society while at the Kaiser's favoured summer retreat at Wilhelmshöhe near Kassel. He dedicated his life to translating Gobineau and publicizing his gospel of racial inequality. The society's membership lists show that it aimed to racialize history and culture rather than biology and medicine. Of seventy-eight members and patrons in 1895 there were only two physicians (the Zürich psychiatrist Anton Delbrück, who worked with Forel, and Rudolf Götze from Leipzig). Indeed, Schemann had much sympathy for hydrotherapy.[164] Most members of the Gobineau Society were aristocrats, philologists or artists – the Bayreuth circle being the most distinguished grouping. Early members included Cosima Wagner, Chamberlain, and the widow of the Germanic theologian, Paul Lagarde. In the next year the Society was joined by French monarchists such as the author, Paul Bourget, and Edouard Schure, who in 1902 formed the militant *Action française*.[165]

During the 1890s, the political profile of the Gobineau Society was aristocratic and elitist. There was a link to the Kaiser's court through Philipp Graf zu Eulenburg-Hertefelde, who was an influential member of the Society's steering committee. Since the 1870s Eulenburg had been a devotee of Gobineau and Wagner, and was on intimate terms with both. After first meeting Gobineau in 1875, they were effusive correspondents.[166] Schemann republished Eulenburg's memoir of Gobineau.[167] From the early 1890s Eulenburg was a key figure in high

[162] W. Schüler, *Der Bayreuther Kreis von seiner Entstehung bis zum Ausgang der wilhelminischen Ära* (Münster, 1971), pp. 235–51.

[163] E. Newman, *The Life of Richard Wagner* (Cambridge, 1976), II, p. 654.

[164] Schemann, *Lebensfahrten*, pp. 238–40.

[165] *Gobineau-Vereinigung 1894–95. Verzeichnis der Mitglieder, Gönner und Förderer.*

[166] Philipp zu Eulenburg-Hertefelde, *Aus 50 Jahren* (Berlin, 1925), pp. 49, 59; J.C.G. Röhl, *Philipp Eulenburgs politische Korrespondenz* (Boppard, 1976), I, pp. 35–6, 111, 115.

[167] P. zu Eulenburg-Hertefelde, *Eine Erinnerung an Graf Arthur Gobineau*, (Stuttgart, 1906). Schemann papers, Eulenburg to Schemann November 1905.

political intrigues and in the appointment of ambassadors and chancellors. He tried to increase both the power of the Junker-conservative bloc and the personal authority of the Kaiser. Eulenburg was the go-between in bringing about the liaison between Gobineau's Aryanism and the imperial establishment, and it was said that the Kaiser slept with Gobineau's works at his bedside. While it is not possible to specify how Gobineau's Aryan mythologizing influenced the political premises of Eulenburg, the admiration of Gobineau can be seen as part of a belief in German cultural superiority. Since his youth Eulenburg was an enthusiast for Nordic mythology, spiritism and the arts. Aryanism was more of an elite aesthetic rather than a biological creed: its romanticized, Teutonic mythology contrasted to the social realism of naturalist authors and artists.

Eulenburg fell from grace in 1906 upon revelations of his homosexual relations with Count Kuno von Moltke, the *Stadtkommandant* of Berlin. The accusations by the journalist Maximilian Harden about the 'sick and degenerate' in the Imperial entourage were calculated to force Eulenburg to withdraw from politics.[168] The resulting court cases were regarded as symptomatic of the moral decay at the heart of Wilhelmine society.[169] Conservatives were outraged at Magnus Hirschfeld's evidence that homosexuality was inborn, and was neither a crime nor scandalous. Fears of moral degeneration, and the resolve to revive the ruling elite, meant that certain key administrators and politicians placed great value on the ideas of Gobineau as an inspiration for regeneration of the German aristocracy.[170]

Eulenburg's role in cementing the cohesion of an aristocratic and Aryan elite was also apparent in his close relations with Chamberlain. Eulenburg arranged a meeting between Chamberlain and the Kaiser in 1901. Chamberlain's scientific and historical convictions convinced the Kaiser that he should undertake a Germanic mission to revitalize the race. During two days' discussions about Aryan racism, Chamberlain suggested that racial regeneration was the Kaiser's special destiny. They agreed that ultramontanism, materialism and Jews were symptoms of decadence, and that a sense of Aryan racial mission would regenerate the nation. Chamberlain swayed the Kaiser towards faith in a racist Germanic Christianity.[171] Aryan racism boosted illiberal imperialism. Chamberlain was flattered by the Kaiser's interest in his ideas from 1899 when the bulky volumes of the *Foundations of the Nineteenth Century* were published. Chamberlain informed the Kaiser how academics were abandoning Virchowian liberalism in favour of a national, racial and hereditarian outlook.[172] A conflict resulted as to whether ideologies of racial

---

[168] Wolff, *Hirschfeld*, pp. 68–85.
[169] A. Hall, *Scandal and Social Democracy. The SPD Press and Wilhelmine Germany 1890–1914* (Cambridge, 1977).
[170] K.-D. Thomann, 'Auf dem Weg in den Faschismus. Medizin in Deutschland von der Jahrhundertwende bis 1933', in B. Bromberger, H. Mausbach and Thoman, *Medizin, Faschismus und Widerstand. Drei Beiträge* (Cologne, 1985), pp. 15–185.
[171] G.C. Field, *Evangelist of Race* (New York, 1981), pp. 248–61; I.V. Hull, *The Entourage of Kaiser Wilhelm II 1888–1918* (Cambridge, 1982), p. 74. Schemann papers, Eulenburg to Schemann 1901.
[172] H.S. Chamberlain, *Briefe* (Munich, 1928) II, p. 151.

purity, or medically and biologically based techniques of social reform should predominate. Eulenburg's strategy of racial elitism based on aesthetics and political manipulation was discredited after his fall from power. After 1900 there was a change from the aristocratic elitism of Eulenburg to more broadly based racial idealism. Links were established between the Gobineau Society and the Pan-German League and with anti-semitic propagandists such as Theodor Fritsch. By way of contrast, contacts between racial ideas and the positivist-minded academic establishment were strained. The Navy League, founded in 1898, had extensive support from Admiral Tirpitz and the government as well as a much larger public membership than the Pan-German League. In November 1899 professors took the lead in a Free Union for Naval Lectures. Professors of biology, such as Weismann, Ziegler and the Hertwig brothers, supported the Navy League, but were critics of *völkisch* racism.[173] The situation of racial enthusiasm but diversity created the opportunity for schemes to unify the racially minded nationalists. Chamberlain's popularity was a sign of a rising tide of anti-liberal sentiments among the *Bildungsbürgertum.*

Popularizing racial culture

Chamberlain concocted an influential fusion of biology, racism and German historical mythologizing. He had been interested in the movement of sap in plants, and between 1889 and 1890, he completed a botanical dissertation, which he submitted to the botanist Julius Wiesner in Vienna. Chamberlain believed that he had established the existence of a life force. He regarded this as placing him in the religious and prophetic tradition of German science with such forebears as Paracelsus and Johann Wolfgang von Goethe. He then abandoned hope of a scientific career and became a disciple of Wagnerism. That he dedicated the *Foundations of the Nineteenth Century* to Wiesner showed Chamberlain's scientific pretensions. Yet he wrote as an opponent of narrow academic specialization, arguing that rather than confining attention to microbiology or histology, a philosophical outlook was needed to understand the formative role of race in history.[174] As with Gobineau's racial use of philology, Chamberlain's work was essentially a compelling historical mythology. Chamberlain attacked Virchow's concept of racial equality, craniometry and physiological concepts of race as resulting in confusion over the idea of race and over whether there was actually an Aryan race. Chamberlain relied on his personal intuition as the basis for a 'self-evident' concept of Aryan and Jewish races.[175] Biological and scientific concepts of race were not in keeping with the philosophical and idealistic tradition of German *Wissenschaft* on which Chamberlain based his claims to a prophetic insight into

---

[173] W. Marienfeld, *Wissenschaft und Schlachtflottenbau in Deutschland 1897–1906* (Berlin, 1957), pp. 46–8, 110–15; Eley, *Re-Shaping*, p. 99.

[174] H.S. Chamberlain, *Die Grundlagen des Neunzehnten Jahrhunderts* (Munich, 1912), pp. x–xi.

[175] Chamberlain, *Grundlagen*, pp. 310–20; Chamberlain, *Arische Weltanschauung* (Berlin, 1905).

Germany's racial destiny. Chamberlain struck up friendships with some other biologists and philosophers who were also ardent Wagnerians. The circle of biological reactionaries included the environmental theorist, Jakob von Uexküll, the *Gestalt* philosopher, Christian von Ehrenfels, and the pioneer of hereditary hygiene, Ferdinand Hueppe.[176] It was significant that Ehrenfels, Hueppe and Uexküll had reputations as wild speculators who strayed from the paths of legitimate scientific theorizing, taking racial theory into the spheres of philosophy, biology and medicine. They attempted to formulate a nationalist type of science and medicine based on idealist philosophy. Chamberlain and Schemann, despite their scientific pretensions, did not count as reputable scientists. Eulenburg's spiritism meant that he was distrusted by the medical establishment, which was generally hostile to nature therapy. With the Kaiser prone to nervousness, his physician Rudolf von Leuthold feared that Eulenburg might introduce quack therapies.[177] The medical profession's hostility to spiritism went with scepticism of the wilder variants of Aryan ideology. The Wagner circle challenged the experimental basis of medicine by crusading against vivisection and vaccination.[178] Such traits illustrate how Aryan racism was in its origins distinct from academic biology and the liberal bourgeois values that supported it.[179]

During the 1890s biology and anthropology provided links between Aryan ideas and the Pan-Germanist movement of dissident radical bourgeois patriots. Ammon, the pioneer of social anthropology, took an intermediary position between the biological and ideological racists. He was on cordial terms with both Schemann and Weismann. The anti-liberal Darwinist polemics of Tille and of the Freiburg phalanx were taken up by nationalist pressure groups. Ammon, Schemann and Tille supported the Pan-German League, which they regarded as a vehicle for practical implementation of their racial theories. The League enthusiastically popularized nationalist versions of racial anthropology.[180] It sought to use the popularity of Chamberlain's and Gobineau's theories to revive its flagging fortunes when after 1902 there was official disapproval of the League.[181] From 1902 the Pan-German League joined the Gobineau League and took a lead in the dissemination of Aryan racial theories. By 1906 other ultra-nationalist organizations had joined: the *Deutschnationale Handlungsgehilfen-Verband*, and the *Deutsche Ostmarken-Verein*.[182] The Gobineau Society provided an ideological back-bone to the ultra-nationalist organizations, and they shared an interlocking membership and aims. Ammon and Wilser, the racial anthropologists, rallied to

---

[176] Field, *Evangelist*, pp. 94–105.
[177] Hull, *Entourage*, pp. 70–3, 112–13.
[178] I am grateful to Mark Almond for advice and material on the Wagner circle.
[179] Compare Chickering, *Men*, pp. 239–40 for a view of Chamberlain as advocate of a scientific theory of race and as central to the eugenics movement.
[180] Schemann papers, Ammon to Schemann, 27 November 1899.
[181] Chickering, *Men*, p. 212.
[182] *Gobineau–Vereinigung. Februar 1905 – Dezember 1906. Verzeichnis der Mitglieder, Gönner und Förderer.*

the crusade for racial purification. The linking of Aryan theories with the ultra-nationalist and anti-semitic right was achieved in the decade prior to 1914.[183] Although the Freiburg university academics and medical theorists of degeneration did not support these moves, the Pan-German League had a sizeable medical phalanx. Between 1894 and 1914, 8–10 per cent of all local Pan-German chairmen were doctors, and from 1906 to 1914, about 9 per cent of the membership consisted of medical men.[184]

Tille exemplifies an attempt to fuse Nietzscheanism, Darwinism and an individualistic conservatism. He left the strictly academic camp and became a general publicist; he favoured natural selection and opposed socialism and social welfare. While in an academic post teaching German philology at Queen Margaret College Glasgow, he wrote in 1890 his essay *Sonnenaufgang*. This was a reply to Hauptmann's drama, with Tille defending Loth's concern for future generations. He adopted Schallmayer's views on the degenerative effects of welfare and therapy in 1893.[185] Tille preached the necessity of a German morality based on a combination of Darwin, Haeckel and Nietzsche. An elite of the biologically fittest was needed to replace the degenerating aristocracy. In the following decade he elaborated his creed based on marriage restrictions and allowing free functioning of natural selection.[186] Tille was like Schallmayer, Ammon and Haycraft in welcoming high infant mortality as a means of racial improvement. He seized on the example of London's East End as a 'Nationalheilanstalt' or national curative institution. His was a type of free market Darwinism that ran counter to the welfare campaigns that gathered force from the 1890s. Yet, his sometime lover, Helene Stoecker, linked the combination of Nietzsche and Darwin to radical feminism and the demand to extend welfare to unmarried mothers. Nietzsche's ideas were venerated with a mystic awe, and were claimed as panaceas to social and psychological problems. As with the movements for *Lebensreform* and biological values, Nietzscheanism was politically ambivalent: it could inspire personal and sexual liberation, but also reinforce authoritarian and elitist social structures.[187] Tille's social elitism also established an institutional base. In 1900 Tille was forced to leave Glasgow as a result of anti-German feeling in the Boer War and he became friends with the industrialist Carl Friedrich Freiherr von Stumm Halberg. As a result Tille joined the *Deutsche Reichspartei* and took up contacts with leading industrialists.[188] Tille's Aryan enthusiasms and antagonism to social welfare kept him aloof from eugenic organizations after 1900. He was elected to the committee of the Pan-German League in 1900, and worked for a number of industrialist organizations such as the *Zentralverband deutscher Industrieller* until 1903, and then

---

[183] Chickering, pp. 237–45.
[184] S. Parlow, 'Über einige kolonialistische und annexionistische Aspekte bei deutschen Ärzten', pp. 537–49.   [185] A. Tille, *Volksdienst – Von einem Sozialaristokraten* (Berlin and Leipzig, 1893).
[186] W. Schungel, *Alexander Tille. Leben und Ideen eines Sozialdarwinisten* (Husum, 1980).
[187] R.H. Thomas, *Nietzsche in German Politics and Society 1890–1918* (Manchester, 1986).
[188] A. Tille, *Aus Englands Flegeljahren* (Dresden and Leipzig, 1901).

for the Saarbrücken Chamber of Commerce and for the south-west group of the Association of German Iron and Steel Manufacturers. He opposed the social welfare measures of the *Kathedersozialisten* such as Lujo Brentano, and criticized the burden of social insurance on the fit. Tille argued against hereditary wealth and power as degenerative and favoured an elite government based on achievement. At the same time he argued for the superiority of the Aryan race. Tille's attempt to fuse Darwinism, national culture and the conservative manufacturing interests was paralleled by other attempts to float a science-based nationalism. Darwinism reversed its social function from being liberal and reformist to assisting the popularization of broad-based conservative nationalism.

The Krupp Prize

The twentieth century opened with a venture in placing politics on scientific foundations. On 1 January 1900 a competition was announced for an essay on the application of the laws of evolution to society. The aim of the competition was to use science to secure a theoretical basis for the unifying of 'progressive' social forces. The prize was announced at a time when there were plans for a broad coalition of the right against socialism. From 1897 such leading national figures as the Prussian Finance Minister Johannes von Miquel and Admiral Alfred von Tirpitz attempted to develop twin policies of internal social cohesion and imperialist *Weltpolitik*. Nationalist pressure groups such as the Navy League encouraged university academics to vent their opinions on social issues. The prize represented an attempt by a coalition of Bebel's critics to broaden the debate on social evolution. They attempted to re-cast biology so as to provide a nationalist basis for collectivist politics. Scientifically and historically proven laws of social evolution were to rally agrarian, industrial and middle-class interests of property and culture in a call for a united and strong nation. In 1900, the Chancellor Chlodwig Hohenlohe-Schillingsfürst expressed the hope that biology could provide guidance in the management of national affairs. Having once believed in progress he confessed:

I must now admit that this belief has been somewhat shaken in recent years. The struggle for existence imposed upon us by nature has of recent times assumed a character and a direction which reminds us of its conduct in the animal world, and gives us grounds to fear that progress may be retrogressive.

He wished that heroes of the intellectual battlefield could provide a bastion against material interests. Yet the ranks of biologists were less solid than the Chancellor might have hoped.[189]

The zoologist, Ziegler, who was one of Bebel's major scientific critics, conceived the plan to unite diverse factions of biologists. In 1895 he hoped that the

---

[189] C. Hohenlohe-Schillingsfürst, 'Speech to the Prussian Academy of Science', in F. Curtius (ed.), *Memoirs of Prince Chlodwig of Hohenlohe Schillingsfuerst* (London, 1906), II, p. 478.

Society of German Naturalists and Doctors could provide a platform for a novel type of scientific and medical sociology. That Ziegler and Hueppe began to take prominent roles in this public forum for science indicated a shift away from liberal reformism. Ziegler wrote to Ploetz of his hope that social biology could be used to secure legislation to solve the problems of alcoholism and of the rising numbers of hereditary degenerates by controls on reproduction.[190] He recognized that powerful political and industrial support was needed for such a programme. He attempted to win the support of business interests. He overcame the animosity between Haeckel and Weismann, when Haeckel supported his candidacy for a professorship of phylogeny in Jena in 1898. The chair was endowed by the Swiss businessman, Paul von Ritter, who obliged the incumbent to give public lectures. Ziegler welcomed the opportunity to take his campaign for national biological values on to the public stage. He lectured on the social life of animals. His research was on the socially relevant issue of the effect of alcohol on marine organisms.[191] Haeckel and Ziegler opposed both the Catholic Centre Party and socialism as posing a threat to science and the social order. Haeckel's public agitation for monist philosophy with its strongly anti-Catholic overtones reinforced the attempt to check Catholic intervention in biology. Protestant agitation to materialist Darwinism culminated in the *Kepler Bund* which was established to resist monism; the Jesuit biologist Erich Wasmann opposed the evolutionary views of Haeckel and Ziegler's Darwinian studies on instinct. Ziegler was anxious to counter the ultramontane accusation that science furthered socialist materialism. He condemned the socialism of Marx and Bebel as being as dogmatic as ultramontanism. He was also hostile to revisionist socialism, and to the welfare-oriented *Kathedersozialisten*, accusing the latter of aiding socialism. Instead, Ziegler favoured a more industrially geared social theory and system of welfare.[192]

Ziegler felt that his nationalist social biology required support which would be powerful enough to combat Catholicism and socialism. He negotiated with a Belgian industrialist, Albert Samson, for an institute for psychological and ethical studies, which he hoped to attract to Jena. This plan had backing from Forel, the anatomist and anthropologist Waldeyer, the physiologist Hermann Munk, and the psychiatrist Paul Flechsig.[193] Massive resources for popularization of Darwinism for political ends were provided by the industrialist, Friedrich Alfred Krupp. As his father, Krupp was an enthusiastic advocate of workers' welfare schemes, and continued to extend the by now legendary model housing colonies for Krupp workers. The housing colonies went with a range of welfare provisions that catered for all events in the family from birth to death. Instead of communal institutions, workers were given a new degree of domestic privacy with the introduction of the

---

[190] Ploetz papers, Ziegler to Ploetz, 1 July 1895.
[191] Haeckel-Haus, Jena, Letters of Ziegler to Haeckel, 22 September, 5 October, 10 October, 3 December 1898.   [192] Haeckel-Haus, Ziegler to Haeckel, 6 February 1895.
[193] Haeckel-Haus, Ziegler to Haeckel, 30 August 1900.

Wohnküche.[194] Frau Krupp engineered the extension of medical care for workers. Welfare measures were a means of securing a stable and loyal workforce. During the 1890s Krupp came to appreciate how his love of science could solve the nation's problems. As a youth in the 1870s, Krupp had been a passionate botanist, but his iron-willed father forbade this pursuit as effeminate. Krupp's wife drew his attention to Haeckel's *Natural History of Creation*, an early work of Darwinist popularization, in which the idea of competition as necessary for social improvement was clearly articulated. Krupp then read Haeckel's later writings, and admired *The Riddles of the Universe* on its appearance in 1899.[195] These visions of co-operative and hierarchical evolution provided the scientific counterpart to industrial welfare schemes. It is in the context of the search for an antidote to socialism that Darwinism promised to be an efficacious remedy.

Krupp was the most influential businessman in the Kaiser's entourage. Although his friendship with the Kaiser was based on patriotism and profits from armaments, they shared interests in German culture and technical progress. The link between Krupp and Haeckel was forged by Ziegler in association with Eberhard Fraas, a palaeontologist from Stuttgart. Fraas became curator of Krupp's mineral collection. From 1898 until 1902 he gave lessons in the natural sciences to Krupp and to his personal assistant, Justizrat Korn. Evolutionary biology thus entered into Krupp's broader social calculations. Fraas encouraged Krupp to undertake research in deep-sea marine zoology. Convalescing from asthma and high blood pressure, Krupp lavishly equipped two yachts for research. From his villa in Capri, he sought from May 1898 to establish good relations with the Naples Zoological Station of Anton Dohrn. The immunologist, Emil Behring, who also settled on Capri, encouraged Dohrn to assist Krupp's research on plankton. Dohrn remained a liberal Darwinist and personally preferred more politically liberal industrialists such as Abbe of the Zeiss works at Jena, or Werner and Carl von Siemens. At this time innovative concepts of partnership between industry and science were proposed. In 1898 Krupp established a chemical and physical institute for experimental research. By 1902 this had developed a prototype of a submarine. In 1899 an association to publicize science to the Krupp workers was established. Krupp was an enthusiast for large-scale biological research institutes. He offered Dohrn 100,000 marks for rebuilding the Zoological Station as well as the facilities of his yacht, the Puritan.[196] Krupp also donated money for a freshwater biological institute at Plon, where he enjoyed admiring the aesthetic forms of freshwater plankton.[197] He identified numerous species of fish, marine worms, plankton and

---

[194] E. Führ and D. Stemmrich, '*Nach gethaner Arbeit verbleibt im Kreise der Eurigen.*' *Bürgerliche Wohnrezepte für Arbeiter zur individuellen und sozialen Formierung im 19. Jahrhundert* (Wuppertal, 1985), pp. 131–49.

[195] E. Haeckel, *Natürliche Schöpfungsgeschichte* (Berlin, 1868); Haeckel, *Die Welträthsel* (Bonn, 1899).

[196] T. Heuss, *Anton Dohrn* (Stuttgart and Tübingen, 1948), pp. 341–2; G. Wendel, *Die Kaiser-Wilhelm-Gesellschaft 1911–1914* (Berlin, 1975), p. 47.

[197] Otto Zacharias, 'Zur Würdigung der Verdienste Friedrich A. Krupp's um die zoologische Wissenschaft', *Anatomischer Anzeiger*, vol. 26 (1902), 113.

crustaceans.[198] A monument to Krupp's enthusiasm for marine biology was a hefty zoological dictionary; it was originally compiled as a reference manual for Krupp by Fraas and Ziegler, and then became a standard reference work.[199]

From 1887 Krupp became active in politics and an enthusiast for an expanded navy. He was involved in moves for founding a national party from 1892, and opposed the Centre Party. In nationalist associations such as the Navy League he met academics like the historian (and Pan-Germanist supporter) Dietrich Schäfer. Krupp earnestly wished to show that his interests in promoting military and naval expansion were more than just for his firm's profits from armaments manufacture. He wished to make his mark in biological research and popularization, believing that patronage of science with its objective and universal values was a means of demonstrating disinterested motives.[200] Krupp's patronage of academic marine biology and Darwinism contrasted to the Pan-Germanists' taste for *völkisch* racial theories.[201]

In 1897 negotiations began for a substantial prize on social applications of evolutionary theory. Fraas acted as intermediary for Krupp and Haeckel from 16 December 1897.[202] Ziegler's move to Jena cemented the bonds between Haeckel and Krupp. On 30 July 1899, Fraas wrote to Krupp that he had suggested a meeting about the competition.[203] Krupp invited Ziegler and Fraas to visit him to finalize the competition details on 20 August 1899 – and to view his workers' housing estates and other social institutions. On arrival they were faced by an extensive memorandum drafted by Krupp. This was the genesis of the prize manifesto.[204] Krupp stressed the themes of heredity and adaptation. He emphasized a people's inheritance in the form of institutions and laws, and the need for gradual evolutionary change. He relied on the combined effects of heredity and adaptation without drawing attention to scientific doubts about direct adaptation. His draft was therefore more Lamarckian and historicist than the published version. It argued explicitly against the unnaturalness of sudden change as opposed to 'healthy progress'. Competitors were asked to deal with topics close to Krupp's heart: the threat of socialist revolution, and the stagnation of conservatism and ultramontanism. This early draft amounted to a political manifesto by Krupp in the hope of producing a formula for revitalizing conservatism. It contrasted with the published manifesto which had been re-worked by Ziegler, Fraas and two of Krupp's managers. Ziegler and Haeckel had previously discussed how to keep science separate from history. To muddle them up would open the door to unscientific

---

[198] W. Manchester, *The Arms of Krupp 1587–1968* (London, 1969), p. 263.

[199] H.E. Ziegler and E. Bresslau, *Zoologisches Wörterbuch* (Jena, 1912).

[200] G. Eley, *Reshaping*, pp. 49, 144.

[201] This point draws on Chickering's distinction between the social recruitment and strategies of the Navy and Pan-German Leagues. Chickering, *Men*, pp. 14–15, 198.

[202] Haeckel-Haus, Best A Abt 1 Nr 1354/1.

[203] Historisches Archiv Friedrich Krupp, Essen, F.A.H. III C 62 S. 12.

[204] G. Heberer (ed.), *J. Walther, Im Banne Ernst Haeckels. Jena um die Jahrhundertwende* (Göttingen, 1953), p. 93; H.E. Ziegler, *Der Begriff des Instinktes einst und jetzt* (Jena, 1920), pp. 196–7.

racial theories of history. Ziegler submitted a draft emphasizing the natural sciences, but his approach was rejected. Yet Fraas and Ziegler at least managed to secure a separation of 'natural inheritance' from the 'inheritance of tradition'.[205]

The published announcement offered 30,000 marks for a scientific answer to the problem: 'What can we learn from the principles of evolution for the development and laws of states?' Competitors were asked to keep in mind the role of hereditary instincts, whether relating to the individual, family or society. The inequality of natural predisposition was highlighted. It was suggested that a people's constitution could be changed either by natural selection or by direct inheritance of acquired characters. Adaptation and tradition were stressed as factors in social evolution. Civilization was seen as causing a series of changes in social and political life. Institutions had to correspond to the 'flesh and blood' of people's traditions in order to retain their value. The first section of each entry was to be scientific, and the second section historical. Current political tendencies in Germany were to be considered in a concluding section. Competitors were asked to combine a scientific analysis with a generally accessible style – in the popular tradition of German science.[206]

To the public, the prize seemed to originate from Haeckel rather than Krupp, whose role as instigator was posthumously revealed. It was therefore called the 'Jena Prize Competition'. Ziegler felt that Haeckel should not publicize the prize only in his name. It was issued in the name of 'The Prize Commission', consisting of Haeckel, the Halle economist Johannes Conrad, and Fraas. Krupp determined the composition of the organizing panel. Fraas was selected, so that he could inform Krupp about the progress of events; Conrad was chosen in October 1899 as a respected economist who could judge the historical and socio-political aspects of the prize.[207] The manuscripts were to be sent to Haeckel, and the panel of judges was to consist of Schäfer, Conrad and Ziegler. The closing date was 1 December 1902. The competition was advertised in historical, social science and zoological journals.[208] On 4 December 1901 Haeckel wrote, much to Krupp's delight, that he had already responded to 300 inquiries about the prize on politics and evolution.[209] Haeckel visited Krupp from 4 to 8 August 1902. By this time Krupp was embroiled in a moral scandal that culminated in his death on 22 November 1902.[210]

There were sixty entries. Forty-four came from Germany, eight from Austria, four from Switzerland, two from Russia and two from the United States. Already published works, such as an entry submitted by Ammon, were disqualified. The first prize of 10,000 marks was awarded to Schallmayer on 7 March 1903. There

---

[205] Historisches Archiv Friedrich Krupp, W.A. IX d 244, Niederschrift von F.A. Krupp.
[206] Historisches Archiv Friedrich Krupp, W.A. IX d 244, Veröffentlichung der Preisaufgabe.
[207] Haeckel-Haus, Ziegler to Haeckel, 5 September 1899; Best A Abt 1 Nr 621/ 1–7, Haeckel to Conrad.
[208] *Schmollers Jahrbuch*, vol. 24 (1900), 826. It was also to appear in: *Zoologischer Anzeiger, Historische Zeitschrift*; and in Conrad's *Zeitschift für Sozialwissenschaft*.
[209] Historisches Archiv Friedrich Krupp, F.A.H. III D 159 S. 2–3.
[210] Haeckel-Haus, Ziegler to Haeckel, 5 August 1902.

were three second prizes, with 18,000 marks divided between the social scientists Arthur Ruppin, a leading Zionist,[211] Heinrich Matzat, and Albert Koch-Hesse, who was a statistician and evolutionary sociologist.[212] Further prizes were awarded to Ludwig Woltmann, a lawyer Hermann Friedmann, Curt Michaelis a writer educated in oriental philology and psychology,[213] and the Zürich philosopher Abroteles Eleutheropoulos.[214] Some small consolation prizes were awarded: one thousand marks went to the sociologist Ferdinand Tönnies, and to F. Lüthenau, a lawyer.[215] Six more unsuccessful entrants can be identified. These were Heinz Potthoff, who was elected to the Reichstag in 1903 to represent the *Fortschrittliche Volkspartei*; Erich Schalk, an American industrialist;[216] Walther Haecker, employed at a teacher's seminary;[217] a physician from Breslau, Alfred Methner;[218] the lawyer and conservative Aryan ideologue, Ludwig Kuhlenbeck; and Hermann Rehm, a professor of law from Strasbourg.[219] These entrants represented a broad ideological spectrum ranging from Ruppin's Zionism to Kuhlenbeck's Aryan racism, and politically the candidates ranged from socialism to conservatism.

The award sparked off heated controversy. Different interests involved in the prize sought to use the entries to endorse varieties of social biology. Ziegler supervised publication of nine entries in a series *Natur und Staat*, appearing between 1903 and 1907 and provided a concluding volume on heredity in biology and sociology.[220] Ziegler's introduction analyzed the entries. Most approved of a moderate state socialism. There should be an extension of social insurance, and welfare benefits as well as of state custodial institutions for criminals and the mentally subnormal.[221] A third of the entries favoured far-reaching state socialism, but only one had any Marxist sympathies. The entries showed that natural selection and social welfare measures were not inevitably opposed. Schallmayer's winning monograph blended Weismann's selectionist biology with the demand for state intervention. Ziegler criticized Schallmayer's 'socialist tendencies'; but as Schallmayer was a socialist only in that he considered that biology dictated collectivist forms of social organization, his entry was indeed in the spirit of the prize.[222] The

---

[211] A Beir, 'Arthur Ruppin: the Man and his Work', *Leo Baeck Institute. Year Book*, vol. 17 (1972), 117–42.

[212] A. Ruppin, *Darwinismus und Sozialwissenschaft* (Jena, 1903); H. Matzat, *Philosophie der Anpassung* (Jena, 1903); A. Hesse, *Natur und Gesellschaft* (Jena, 1904).

[213] C. Michaelis, *Prinzipien der natürlichen und sozialen Entwicklungsgeschichte des Menschen* (Jena, 1905).

[214] A. Eleutheropoulos, *Soziologie* (Jena, 1904).

[215] F. Lüthenau, *Darwin und der Staat. (Preisgekrönt in Jena, Krupp'sche Stiftung)* (Leipzig, 1905).

[216] E. Schalk, *Der Wettkampf der Völker mit besonderer Bezugnahme auf Deutschland und die Vereinigten Staaten von Nordamerika* (Jena, 1905).

[217] W. Haecker, *Die ererbten Anlagen und die Bemessung ihres Wertes für das politische Leben* (Jena, 1907).

[218] A. Methner, *Organismen und Staaten* (Jena, 1906).

[219] Seventeen entrants can therefore be identified.

[220] Based on Ziegler, *Die Vererbungslehre in der Biologie* (Jena, 1905).

[221] H.E. Ziegler, 'Einleitung zu dem Sammelwerke *Natur und Staat*', in *Natur und Staat: Beiträge zur naturwissenschaftlichen Gesellschaftslehre*, vol. 1 (1903), p. 14.

[222] H.E. Ziegler, in *Deutsche Literaturzeitung* (19 March 1904), 686.

prize at this stage seemed to fulfill Krupp's dream of fusing conservatism with nationalist-oriented social reformism.

Schallmayer was critical of party politics as partial and divisive, and hoped that generative ethics could provide the basis for national consensus.[223] He emphasized that he had obtained an assurance from Haeckel that the quality of scientific opinions rather than political allegiancies was to be the criterion for the judges. Schallmayer did not write in Krupp's historicist vein; nor did he subscribe to Haeckel's Lamarckism. Instead he used Weismann's theories to formulate a code of 'generative ethics'. Hereditary biology was to supply the basis for social reform. It was the state's responsibility to provide the conditions of existence for the population. This would result in a powerful state, capable of competing in the international struggle for survival. He favoured measures to prevent the 'unfit' from reproducing. The degenerate included the insane, the feeble-minded, the alcoholic, those infected by TB and VD, and criminals. Ultimately, fitness and degeneracy were to be determined by hereditary science, but in the meantime biological value would depend on the social contribution being made. He concluded his work with a section on public health and social hygiene.[224] His ideas found some favour with social hygienists and with socialists who were concerned with the degenerative effects of poverty and who considered a modified form of *Sozialeugenik* to be necessary.[225]

The prize did not serve to unite evolutionary biology, social science and nationalist politics, as Krupp had hoped. Krupp fell a victim first to blackmail threats and then to a public scandal over his homosexuality. Italian and then German newspapers charged him with homosexual and paedophile relations while staying on Capri. In October 1902 Frau Krupp received anonymous letters about her husband's homosexuality. She asked the Kaiser for advice. He apparently suggested that Krupp be declared insane. Instead, Admiral Hollman (a close friend and until 1897 Secretary at the Navy Office) intervened on Krupp's behalf by casting doubt on Frau Krupp's mental health. Krupp reacted by attempting to have his shocked wife certified as insane by the psychiatrists Forel, Otto Binswanger, Oscar Vogt and Fritz Pahl. Frau Krupp was incarcerated at Binswanger's asylum in Jena. The furore ended when Krupp died in November 1902.[226] Although the doctors pronounced that this was due to a stroke, suicide was suspected. Krupp's identity as the benefactor of the 'Jena Prize' was not known. His involvement with the prize was revealed only during the bitter quarrels that later erupted.

Disgruntled Aryans

The award to Schallmayer aroused most dissension among the ultra-nationalist right. Racial anthropologists were indignant that the winner opposed Aryan racial

[223] S.F. Weiss, 'Race Hygiene and the Rational Management of National Efficiency: Wilhelm Schallmayer and the Origins of German Eugenics 1890–1920', PhD dissertation, Johns Hopkins University, 1983, pp. 166–7.   [224] Weiss, 'Race Hygiene', pp. 170–6.
[225] O. Olberg, 'Rassenhygiene und Sozialismus', *Die neue Zeit*, new series vol. 25 no. 1 (1907), 882–7.
[226] Hull, *Entourage*, pp. 170–1.

theory. They supported the complaints of the winner of the fourth prize, Ludwig Woltmann.[227] He refused a prize, regarding fourth place as an insult, and demanded the return of his manuscript for publication. Woltmann had studied medicine and philosophy, obtaining doctorates in philosophy and medicine from Freiburg in 1896. This was at a time when the Bebel–Ziegler dispute was at its height. In July 1898 he specialized as an ophthalmologist in Barmen. He then taught hygiene and biology at a teacher training college, until he established a journal for political anthropology in 1902. He attempted to reconcile evolutionary theory with socialism. His activism in the SPD between 1892 and 1898 contrasted with the detached positions of Grotjahn, Ploetz and Schallmayer. Grotjahn, who in the 1890s moved only on the intellectual fringes of the SPD, described Woltmann as his 'most intimate opponent' (*intimsten Gegner*).[228] Woltmann, Grotjahn, Franz Oppenheimer and Koch-Hesse (the winner of the second prize) had attended social science seminars in Berlin during 1893–94.[229] Woltmann allied himself to the revisionist evolutionary gradualism of Eduard Bernstein and the patriotism of Joseph Bloch, the editor of the unorthodox periodical *Sozialistische Monatshefte*. This grouping was renowned for its imperialism and interest in such renegade philosophers as Nietzsche. Racial theories were an appropriate legitimation of imperialism.[230] Domestic politics was prone to a racial interpretation, once social problems of chronic diseases and the declining birth rate were highlighted.

Woltmann dramatically illustrates the trend away from political economy by his attempt to reconcile Marxism with Aryan racism and Darwinism. His metamorphosis from a Kantian and party political activist to Aryan racist was rapid. He was one of the first medical practitioners to espouse Gobineau's ideals. His entry for the Jena Prize, entitled *Politische Anthropologie*, developed theories of racial struggle as benefiting workers in nations as racially unified and cohesive organisms. He argued for Germanic racial purity. Race was the fundamental unit of human biology, which determined the rise and fall of cultures. There was a complex interaction of heredity, environment, climate, national history and economics. He hoped that there could be an inductive science for study of racial biology. He concluded that most European geniuses, even those in France and Italy, derived from the Nordic race.

On refusing the prize of 2,000 marks the manuscript was returned by Haeckel with a note stating that Ziegler and himself had requested a first or second prize for Woltmann, but that it had been blocked by the historian Schäfer on the grounds of factual error. As a result of receiving the returned copy, Woltmann wrote a letter of protest. He was outraged by Schäfer's marginal annotations that Woltmann was 'completely ignorant'. In July 1903 he confided in Haeckel that the winners of the

---

[227] W. Hammer, 'Leben und Werk des Arztes und Sozialanthropologen Ludwig Woltmann', med. Diss. 1979.   [228] *Politisch-Anthropologische Revue* (1907), p. 74.

[229] D. Gasman, *The Scientific Origins of National Socialism: Social Darwinism in Ernst Haeckel and the Monist League* (New York, 1971), p. 148; G. Lichtheim, *Marxism* (London, 1964), pp. 192–4.

[230] R. Fletcher, *Revisionism and Empire. Socialist Imperialism in Germany 1897–1914* (London, 1984), pp. 111–12, 133, 164.

second prize (the social scientists) were 'scientifically deficient'. He accused the economist Conrad of favouritism in the awards to his ex-students Koch-Hesse and Ruppin. Conrad prosecuted Woltmann for libel for which he was fined 300 marks.[231] Woltmann tried to persuade Haeckel to intervene on his behalf by publishing the judges' opinions.[232] Haeckel for his part supported Woltmann's criticisms of Schäfer, whom he regarded as backsliding from evolutionary anthropology.[233]

The racial anthropologists rallied to Woltmann's cause. Ammon, the pioneer of racial surveys, was impressed by Woltmann's heroic refusal of a prize.[234] The Gobineau disciples, Vacher de Lapouge, Schemann and Ludwig Wilser, supported Woltmann's complaint that the winner had not faced up to questions of racial anthropology. Schallmayer roundly criticized Gobineau's Aryan racism as unscientific. A protracted controversy occurred between Schallmayer and Schemann over the validity of the concept of race.[235] It expressed the clash between Schallmayer's eugenics, as a technocratic approach to social problems, and the Aryan racial ideology. Ammon confided to Schemann that Schallmayer's admiration for the Chinese really got on his nerves, and that his work was devoid of any sense of a hereditary racial psyche.[236] In the second edition of *Vererbung und Auslese* of 1910, Schallmayer attacked the followers of Gobineau for their naive Nordic racism.[237] Woltmann's and the other racist entries by Kuhlenbeck and Lüthenau were published independently. Woltmann's journal, the *Politisch-Anthropologische Revue*, provided a forum for the racial anthropologists. He enlisted their support for critical reviews of Ziegler's edition of the prize entries. The prize thus divided Aryan racism from those with hygienic and biological priorities.

Failure and fragmentation

Ploetz profited by his lack of public involvement in the prize. All sides courted him as an impartial observer. Woltmann confided in Ploetz in March 1903 that Haeckel and Ziegler regarded his entry as deserving the first prize, but that Schäfer's historical pedantry had triumphed. Woltmann considered that Schallmayer's work was devoid of anthropology or history, and that scientifically it was unoriginal.[238] By July 1904 the controversies were so bitter and extensive, that the identity of Krupp had become known to Ploetz and Woltmann. The more Woltmann cultivated Haeckel, the more Schallmayer attempted to distance

---

[231] Haeckel-Haus, Woltmann to Haeckel, 15 and 22 July 1903, 20 January 1905.
[232] Haeckel-Haus, Woltmann to Haeckel, 30 April 1904.
[233] L. Woltmann, 'Nachschrift zu Lapouges Kritik des Jenenser Preisausschreibens', *Politisch-Anthropologische Revue*, vol. 3 (1904/5), 313–14.
[234] *Politisch-Anthropologische Revue* (1907), p. 34.
[235] Schemann papers, Schallmayer to Schemann, 21 April, 27 August 1912.
[236] Schemann papers, Ammon to Schemann, 7 May 1912.   [237] Weiss, 'Race Hygiene', p. 197.
[238] Ploetz papers, Woltmann to Ploetz, 20 March 1903, December 1903.

himself from Haeckel's biology and social thought. He emphasized the importance of the anonymity of the donor. Ploetz, however, recommended to Haeckel a public announcement as to Krupp's identity.[239] By 1904 Schallmayer was under such fire from the racial anthropologists Wilser, Ammon, Lapouge, Woltmann and Hueppe, that he turned to the social hygienist Grotjahn for support as having favourably reviewed Schallmayer's entry. Schallmayer testified to Grotjahn that although he was not an orthodox SPD supporter, he was a socialist and a democrat. He opposed egalitarianism and the belief that economic improvements could benefit the race without eugenic control of fertility, and he regarded socialism as providing the best circumstances for implementing hereditary hygiene.[240]

Publication of the entries from 1904 provoked further controversy. Journals for the social sciences carried extensive reviews, evaluating the social relevance of biology. The establishment-oriented *Preussische Jahrbücher* criticized the publications as an 'Haeckelian series', and as lacking in understanding of history.[241] A Nietzschean breeding of a race of supermen through state regulation of reproduction belonged to the category of scientific superstition of such as the positivist historian, Karl Lamprecht and Chamberlain. This accusation added to the confusion as the Aryan racists were in fact critical of Schallmayer's reproductive hygiene. Despite Schallmayer's opposition to Aryan racism, his work did not find favour among social scientists. The most substantial critique was contributed by Tönnies, in the social science journal, *Schmollers Jahrbuch* in lengthy reviews of what could now be termed the '"Krupp" Prize'. Tönnies had a longstanding interest in evolutionary theory, and had himself submitted an entry which received a commendation and 1,000 marks. In the 1880s he had drawn on the works of Haeckel, Carl Naegeli, George Romanes, Spencer and Schäffle, in his analysis of the categories of race, *Volk*, community and society. The resulting treatise, *Gemeinschaft und Gesellschaft*, was published in 1887. Since then he had become critical of Ammon's social anthropology, and of the Nietzsche cult. He maintained links to developments in evolutionary social thought, for example, from 1892 through his student Grotjahn.

Tönnies censured Schallmayer's demands for compulsory controls on marriage. He compared Schallmayer unfavourably with Galton's voluntaryism.[242] Yet he doubted Galton's views on the inheritance of mental qualities. He condemned both Schallmayer and Galton as utopian, and criticised the use of analogies between biological and social organisms.[243] Biologically, there was a weakness in that all

[239] Haeckel-Haus, Ploetz to Haeckel, 17 July 1904.
[240] Grotjahn papers, Schallmayer to Grotjahn, 10 November 1904, 4 November 1918.
[241] E. Daniels, review of *Vererbung und Auslese, Preussische Jahrbücher*, vol. 116 (1904), 342–7.
[242] A. Tönnies, 'Zur naturwissenschaftlichen Gesellschaftslehre', *Schmollers Jahrbuch*, vol. 29 (1905), 27–101, 1,283–321; vol. 30 (1906), 121–46; Tönnies, 'Zur naturwissenschaftlichen Gesellschafts-lehre. Eine Replik', *Schmollers Jahrbuch*, vol. 33 (1907) 487–552; W. Schallmayer, 'Selektive Gesichtspunkte zur generativen und kulturellen Völkerentwicklung', *Schmollers Jahrbuch*, vol. 30 (1906), 421–69.
[243] A. Tönnies, 'Eugenik', *Schmollers Jahrbuch*, vol. 29 (1905), 1089–106.

entries seemed to support Weismann, whose theories Tönnies regarded as unproven. Socially, he regarded the biologists as offering a crudely unhistorical reductionism. Tönnies' comments were further supported by French sociological criticisms of Social Darwinism. He concluded by denouncing the bankruptcy of 'biological politics' on the one hand, and of Conrad's economic superficialities on the other.[244] At least Woltmann's racial anthropology showed greater originality. Ziegler was furious with Tönnies' even-handed condemnations.[245] The psychologist Alfred Vierkandt joined Tönnies' defence of the social sciences against social biology. His review of Schallmayer was called, 'An Invasion of the Humanities by the Natural Sciences?'. He considered that Schallmayer's faith in Weismann was an unreliable basis for the reconstruction of society. Vierkandt defended psychology and sociology against what he regarded as crude biological reductionism.[246]

The attempt to organize patronage of a major collection of Social Darwinist works by heavy industry exposed disunity among the Social Darwinists and social scientists. The assumption of a close correspondence between the views of Krupp, Haeckel and Schallmayer cannot be supported by the organizing of the prize, or by later responses. Schallmayer was always at pains to deny any links between his views and the sponsors of the prize. Although the prize was initially called the 'Jena Prize', Haeckel's direct participation was limited. He neither drafted the prize manifesto, and nor did he influence the judges. Although Krupp provided the original draft of the manifesto, this was less biological than Haeckel or Ziegler would have liked, and so was modified. Yet the panel of judges had a bias towards social science and history, as Conrad and Schäfer could out-vote the biologist Ziegler. Because Ziegler's biology was primarily based on Weismann, there was no support for racial anthropology of the type so often assumed to have been furthered by the Krupp Prize. Ziegler emerges as a major figure in the instigation, organization, and subsequent publication of the results. Although both Ziegler and Schallmayer preferred Weismann's determinism to Haeckel's adaptive Lamarckism, Schallmayer was opposed to Ziegler's rabid anti-socialism. The prize did not unify disparate Social Darwinists, but provoked and publicized dissension among the various groupings of social evolutionists. It left Ziegler, Schallmayer and Woltmann rather isolated figures, and the social anthropologists did not actively support Ploetz's campaign to establish racial hygiene as a science.

The prize marked a turning point in the development of eugenics. Hitherto, all advocates of eugenics had written as individuals without an institutional basis. After the prize a number of formalized groups were to emerge. The prize had been part of an attempt to secure a biological ideology for Krupp's strategy of *Sammlungspolitik*. Expectations of this ideology took two directions. One was

[244] Tönnies, 'Zur naturwissenschaftlichen Gesellschaftslehre', p. 551.
[245] Tönnies papers, Ziegler to Tönnies, 10 February 1905; Woltmann to Tönnies, 27 June 1905.
[246] A. Vierkandt, 'Ein Einbruch der Naturwissenschaften in die Geisteswissenschaften', *Zeitschrift für philosophische Kritik*, vol. 127 (1906), 168–77; Vierkandt, review of *Vererbung und Auslese*, *Archiv für die gesamte Psychologie*, vol. 7 (1906), 183–5.

science-based, with Schallmayer's programme for a 'national biology'. The other went towards glorification of the Aryan race. Just as the mobilization of public support for the Navy League exposed differences between elite groups in the government and popular nationalist expectations, so the Krupp Prize exposed similar divergences between the elite of university academics and Aryan propagandists. Although it had failed to establish any consensus over the biological basis of social evolution, it provoked some theorists such as Ploetz to attempt to direct and organize public opinion in the direction of a distinctive synthesis of 'racial hygiene'.

Racial hygiene

During the 1890s Ploetz took a middle course between socialism and the ultra-nationalist ideologues. He hoped to demonstrate how biological theories of selection could provide a basis for reconciling socialism and Darwinism. He maintained contacts with Bebel as well as with racial anthropologists. The concept of 'racial hygiene' provided a means of overcoming the differences between the political left and right. While the science of racial hygiene was conceived as a politically neutralizing force, it expanded the social role of a scientifically expert elite. Political conflicts were to be defused by science.[247]

In 1895 Ploetz published his monograph on racial hygiene, establishing his credentials as founder of an academic discipline and a method of social reform. The book opened with an aphorism of Nietzsche: 'the way forward led from being a species to a super species, but egoism was degenerate'. This must have struck Ploetz as expressing the problem of how to ensure evolutionary progress without relying on unbridled individualism. He attacked individualistic 'Manchester liberalism'. Capitalism produced diseases and social misery on a scale so large that this cancelled out the benefits of any selective value that the mortality of the economically vulnerable might have had. Poverty caused such high mortality that it prevented the race from being replenished.[248] Ploetz was impressed with how Alfred Russel Wallace had posed the problem of reconciling social welfare with Darwinism in 1890. Theories of the inheritance of acquired characters meant that education, hygiene and social improvement had been regarded as beneficial. But the refutation of Lamarckism by Galton and Weismann meant that faith in economic and social progress as a means of assisting human evolution was no longer tenable. Ploetz added that Schallmayer had established the degenerative effects of therapeutic medicine.[249]

---

[247] A. Ploetz, 'Rassentüchtigkeit und Socialismus', *Neue Deutsche Rundschau. Freie Bühne*, vol. 5 no. 10 (October, 1894), 989–97.

[248] A. Ploetz, *Die Tüchtigkeit unsrer Rasse und der Schutz der Schwachen. Ein Versuch über Rassenhygiene und ihr Verhältnis zu den humanen Idealen, besonders zum Socialismus* (Berlin, 1895), pp. 151, 168, 188.

[249] A.R. Wallace, 'Menschheitsfortschritt', *Hardens Zukunft*, vol. 8 no. 48 (1894), 145–58; Ploetz, *Tüchtigkeit unsrer Rasse*, p. 3. Ploetz papers, Wallace to Ploetz 10 June 1895.

Ploetz abandoned socialism and land reform as utopian. He criticized Marx and Bebel for regarding natural resources as so great as to be able to support any level of human population. The social liberalism of land reformers like Hertzka was mistaken in their allocation of land to individuals on a non-selective basis.[250] Galton's solution of state controls on marriage was too elitist and presupposed a competitive society. It would benefit only the most gifted but not raise the level of average ability.[251] Ploetz praised Wallace as 'the first true socialist on a Darwinian basis'. Wallace recommended women's freedom of choice in marriage, giving women the power of sexual selection. To the idealistic Wallace, it was inconceivable that the lazy, the selfish, the sick and the feeble-minded would ever be chosen to procreate. The survival of the fittest meant the elimination of the unfit. Humanitarianism towards the weak and the sick was a barrier to racial improvement. A future society would best combat the selfish, common and cruel by allowing the feelings of women to determine the choice of their partners.[252] Ploetz had reservations over Wallace's plan for sexual selection. He feared counter-selective dangers; as less educated and refined women, for example, might choose inadequate husbands. But Wallace was right that it was necessary somehow to combine humane ideals with Darwinism.

Ploetz's strategy of selective breeding was based on his medical and scientific qualifications. His technocratic solution to social ills avoided the conflicts and omissions of political economy by developing the science of racial hygiene. Although he claimed that this would promote the welfare of the human race, he limited his humanitarianism by identifying the interests of the human race with that of the Western Aryan race. This was the *Culturrasse par excellence*. He invoked the analogy of the cell state in order to suggest that national and racial organisms depended on the health of individual cellular components. It was necessary to understand the laws of variation and to apply these to improving the quality of offspring. The more one could prevent the reproduction of poor variants, the less the exterminating process of the struggle for survival would be necessary. Bebel had also looked for an acceptable socialist equivalent to natural selection. As a means of artificial selection, he hoped that education could produce equivalent effects to selective breeding.[253] The gynaecologist, Hegar, had appreciated that a strong race would be produced by education and change of the external environment, so affecting the variations in the next generation. Selective breeding was a common interest of both the left and right.

Ploetz suggested that every improvement in hygiene, therapy and welfare had to be compensated for by improving the quality of the racially fittest groups. It was necessary to obtain the equivalent improvements which would have resulted from selective processes under natural conditions. A promised second volume on the 'hygiene of reproduction' was to show how variation could be favourably

---

[250] Ploetz, *Tüchtigkeit unsrer Rasse*, pp. 201–2.   [251] Ploetz, *Tüchtigkeit unsrer Rasse*, pp. 210, 215.
[252] A.R. Wallace, 'Menschliche Auslese', *Hardens Zukunft*, vol. 8 no. 93 (7 July 1894), 10–24.
[253] Bebel, *Die Frau* (1892), p. 199. Ploetz papers, Bebel to Ploetz 11 December 1895.

manipulated. Reproductive hygiene was the science of how to influence the selection of reproductive cells. Ploetz's solution was to transfer the processes of selection and survival of the fittest from the level of whole organisms to that of the reproductive cells.[254] Given the proliferation of welfare institutions, Ploetz argued that reproductive hygiene was urgently needed to counteract the non-selective effects of welfare. He expected that the next few years would see further steps towards socialism and the welfare state. Whether the advance of welfare was in a democratic, state or Christian socialist manner was immaterial. Its development was accompanied by a Malthusian tendency to limit family size which proved a threat to the survival of the race. Although Ploetz argued for scientific solutions to social problems, his beliefs remained utopian in that the scientific basis for an effective reproductive technology did not actually exist. But he expected an imminent breakthrough in establishing the science of reproductive hygiene. Its achievement was inevitable as it did not differ from the reliable methods of scientific observation and experiment. He concluded his work – begun with a challenging Nietzschean declaration – with Haeckel's slogan of 'fearless advance' in science as the means of realizing social progress.[255]

THE NEW SCIENCE

The transformation of racial hygiene from an anti-establishment ideology to an organized science and public association involved a number of crucial steps. Racial hygiene had to be popularised and converts won in the right social circles. It had to have all the hallmarks of a genuine science: a special vocabulary, a journal, an association, congresses and lectures, and the support of leading academics. The ultimate aims were technical – creating a national institute for monitoring the health of the population and analyzing genealogies – as well as ideological – infusing racial consciousness in those families deemed to be of high racial quality. The movement combined characteristics of a national association, a scientific society and a professional pressure group. As racial hygiene assumed the character of a professional middle class ideology of social improvement, it came to be affected by structural changes in the medical profession at the turn of the century. The public debate on social conditions and imperialism left its mark on the embryonic science. The Racial Hygiene Society was not open to all and sundry, but exclusively for those assessed as possessing high mental and physical qualities.

   Much of the energy and inspiration behind the growth of the racial hygiene movement was supplied by Ploetz. He steered a course between Aryan enthusiasts and socialist Darwinists, established the major scientific journal in the field, and organized a racial hygiene society. Yet although he had a clear idea of these aims in the early 1890s, their realization confronted him with many obstacles and difficult choices in his personal life. He agonized over whether he could best advance racial

254 Ploetz, *Tüchtigkeit unsrer Rasse*, pp. 229–31.   255 Ploetz, *Tüchtigkeit unsrer Rasse*, pp. 237–9.

hygiene as a journalist, university academic or medical practitioner. Ploetz's return to Berlin on 18 May 1895 was followed by an unsettled decade. He was frustrated with conventional medicine and yearned for a broader field of activity.

Economic problems confronted any doctor opening a practice in a metropolis where there was already a high percentage of doctors per head of population; there were complaints that medicine was becoming 'overfull' as a profession. Ploetz joined the ranks of recently qualified doctors who were disenchanted with contemporary medicine; they hoped to solve their problems by professional imperialism – by colonizing social spheres related to health and reproduction in the name of 'social pathology'. Struggling young doctors who took an interest in various forms of eugenics during the 1890s included Blaschko, Bluhm, Adolf Gottstein, Grotjahn, Hirschfeld, Max Marcuse and Franz Oppenheimer, all in Berlin, and Franz Müller-Lyer, Rüdin, Schallmayer, Wilhelm Weinberg, Wilser and Woltmann in other parts of Germany. They sought to apply medical approaches to solve social ills. For example, in 1896 Grotjahn opened a practice in Berlin, and attempted to make ends meet while undertaking studies of the degenerative effects of alcoholism and occupational diseases. In the first two years of practice, venereal disease accounted for the largest number of patients. Experience of urban health confirmed theories of degeneration.[256] Grotjahn was exposed to formative influences similar to those which acted on Ploetz. Grotjahn was inspired by the naturalist writings of Zola and Hauptmann, and by Hertzka's *Freiland* scheme for an African colony.[257] Oppenheimer left medicine and worked as a journalist for *Welt am Montag*, the same weekly that Ploetz had helped to found, while establishing his reputation as an expert on land reform. Bluhm was among the first women practitioners in Berlin, and survived by working for the sickness insurances. Weinberg also had a large panel practice in Stuttgart. Other Berlin physicians like Bloch and Moll established themselves as writers on moral and sexual questions. The pattern was repeated elsewhere in Germany: Wilser abandoned medicine in 1897 to settle as a social anthropologist in Heidelberg, Schallmayer gave up his medical practice in 1897, and Woltmann in 1900.

Ploetz was frustrated by his experience of medical practice as it left unsatisfied his scientific ambitions and hampered his schemes for social reform. Gerhart Hauptmann arranged for Ploetz's treatise on racial hygiene to be published early in 1895 by S. Fischer, a leader in the publication of naturalist authors and periodicals. Ploetz wrote to Forel that Berlin seemed to offer the best prospects for himself and for his wife who was herself established in medical practice.[258] Although Ploetz did not abandon his interest in heredity, between December 1895 and April 1897 he worked as political editor for the *Welt am Montag*, 'an independent magazine for

---

[256] P.J. Weindling, 'Medical Practice in Imperial Berlin', *Bulletin of the History of Medicine*, vol. 61 (1987), 397–410.

[257] D.S. Nadav, *Julius Moses und die Politik der Sozialhygiene in Deutschland* (Gerlingen, 1985), p. 63; D. Tutzke, *Alfred Grotjahn* (Leipzig, 1979).

[258] Forel, *Briefe*, p. 305, Ploetz to Forel, 28 June 1895; Forel papers, Ploetz to Forel, 15 July 1895.

politics and literature'.[259] Ploetz did not take to pure journalism, and was disturbed that the two other editors were Jews. He resigned and began to search for other sources of support for himself and for his scientific research. As the financial settlement with the newspaper guaranteed two years' income, he resumed study of human heredity, and set out to finish one hundred genealogies in a Rhine village.[260] The second, more scientific volume of his treatise on racial hygiene hung over Ploetz as needing completion. He planned that the second volume would contain a comprehensive analysis of scientific data on human variation and the individual's role in racial hygiene, and that a third volume would cover public and social aspects. Then he decided that what was needed was an altogether new book which would deal with the physiology, pathology and hygiene of race. These plans were always hampered by the incompleteness of the scientific data.[261] Ploetz became caught in the 'technological fix' that the only solution to the partial scientific data was yet more research.

The period was personally unsettling for Ploetz, and ended in separation from his wife Paula in September 1898. He wished to have children, and accused Paula of deliberately avoiding pregnancy.[262] By April 1898 he was friends with Anastasius Nordenholz (or 'Stasius'), a social scientist, and he married his sister, Anita. That she was the daughter of a wealthy Bremen merchant, meant that Ploetz could look forward to a substantial inheritance. On 18 March 1900 Ploetz proudly announced the birth of his first of three children, Ulrich, so-called in honour of the chivalrous Reformation poet, Ulrich von Hutten. There was something of the religious reformer and intellectual crusader in Ploetz.

Ploetz was determined to gain scientific credentials and to establish racial hygiene as a legitimate branch of medical science. He approached Albert Neisser, the Breslau dermatologist who at the time was under attack for human experiments, with regard to qualifying in dermatology.[263] Ploetz's aim was to return to his home city of Breslau in order to conduct a series of animal experiments so as to provide the scientific basis for racial hygiene, and to attain the right to practise medicine in Germany. Neisser was surprised that Ploetz, whom he considered to be the creator of a new branch of scientific research with immense relevance to social problems, should consider being his assistant. He advised that in time Ploetz would attain a justly deserved recognition, and that he should not be diverted from his course. After visiting Neisser on 9 January 1900, Neisser recommended that Ploetz write to Siegfried Czapski (a relative of Neisser and a friend of Abbe, the physicist directing Zeiss optical manufacturers in Jena) to intercede with the scientific publisher Gustav Fischer in Jena, for the publication of his second volume. Ploetz requested a loan from Fischer of between 15,000 and

---

[259] Felix Holländer was the literary editor, and Ruhemann, the publisher. The publisher was later to change to Martin Langen.   [260] G. Hauptmann papers, Ploetz to G. Hauptmann, 2 April 1897.
[261] Ploetz papers, 'Einleitung' II Bd R.H.   [262] Ploetz papers, diary 31 January 1908.
[263] Gerhart Hauptmann papers, Ploetz to G. Hauptmann, 1 November 1900, 16 March 1901, 11 May 1901.

20,000 marks, so that he could continue his researches on the causes of degeneration and of variation. By this time he had compiled 11,000 genealogical tables.

Ploetz was tempted during March 1901 by a Red Sea expedition with the zoologist Plate (a favourite of Neisser); Ploetz wished to accompany the expedition as an anthropologist. He unsuccessfully approached the Berlin anatomist Waldeyer with the project of researching on the relation between the brain and the shape of the head. He obtained a generous loan from Neisser, so tiding him over for the next three years. In return Neisser asked Ploetz to persuade Gerhart Hauptmann to sit for a portrait by Fritz Erler; he wished to hang this by the portrait of Richard Strauss so that he should possess pictures of the greatest artistic geniuses of the age. For (as Ploetz wrote to Hauptmann), Neisser was not an average Jewish professor but a man of the highest culture.[264] At the end of this period set aside for finishing his book, Ploetz decided that he would publish a monthly journal of research and publicity concerning racial hygiene.[265]

Ploetz maintained contact with literary circles containing figures such as the Hauptmanns and Boelsche, the naturalist, poet and popularizer of Darwinism. They discussed plans for journals where biology and literature could be combined, as well as technical problems in zoology. Boelsche required scientific guidance for his monumental work-in-progress *Love Life in Nature*.[266] The zoologist Plate (a supporter of the liberal *freisinnige Volkspartei*, a fervent nationalist and anti-semite) formed part of the group. On 11 May 1901 Ploetz agreed with Gustav Fischer that there should be a monthly journal for racial hygiene. However, Ploetz was to be disappointed in Fischer, whom he condemned as 'worse than a Jew'.[267] The plan for a journal re-surfaced on 5 December 1902 when Ploetz was with Stasius. They began to seek sources of support, both financial and academic.

Family finances were crucial to the success of the venture. As Ploetz had the support of his brother-in-law, Stasius, he could sink some of the Nordenholz's wealth into the scheme. They each contributed 12,500 marks to the *Archiv-Gesellschaft*. The zoologist Plate became engaged in April 1902 to Hedwig von Zylinski, the daughter of a Prussian general, so that Plate could also contribute financially to the journal. Ploetz scouted around for additional capital. Haeckel recommended Friedmann, a lawyer who had won one of the smaller 'Krupp' prizes, as someone who could finance the journal.[268] On 19 October 1903 Ploetz could announce to Haeckel that the *Archiv* was founded as a campaigning force on the side of Darwinism and the modern *Weltanschauung*.[269] Prospective contributors were approached. Forel was offered 160 marks *pro Bogen*. On 26 January 1904 the first issue appeared.[270]

---

[264] Ploetz papers, Neisser to Ploetz, 24 November 1900 (two letters), Ploetz to Czapski, 12 December 1900, Czapski to Ploetz, 3 January 1901; Ploetz to Waldeyer, 9 February 1901; Ploetz diary, 9 January 1900.   [265] G. Hauptmann papers, Ploetz to G. Hauptmann, 11 May 1901.
[266] Ploetz papers, Boelsche to Ploetz, 15 November 1900, 2 May 1902.
[267] Ploetz papers, Rüdin to Ploetz, 11 February 1908.
[268] Haeckel-Haus, Ploetz to Haeckel; Ploetz papers, Haeckel to Ploetz, 30 April 1903.
[269] Haeckel-Haus, Ploetz to Haeckel.   [270] Ploetz papers, diary 'per sheet'.

In 1904 the journal underwent further changes. In mid-January 1904, Friedmann withdrew. Ploetz was uneasy with the discovery that Friedmann was Jewish. Rüdin appealed to Forel for an additional editor. He should be young, progressive and have plenty of money. The anthropologist, Richard Thurnwald, was enlisted in December 1904.[271] Rüdin was paid 200 marks to do editorial work and to contribute, a position he held until 22 June 1911 when Ploetz took sole control of the journal.[272] By April 1905 the journal's future seemed assured, as publication was taken over by the scientifically reputable Teubner Verlag of Leipzig. This coincided with the founding of the Racial Hygiene Society in Berlin. The *Archiv* became the organ of the Society. A recurrent risk in Ploetz's strategy, that the *Archiv* should be scientific in orientation, was that a popular journal would be established by rival racist ideologues. Ploetz managed to prevent the first attempt when Ulrich Patz (a pharmaceutical manufacturer) and Rüdin proposed a popular journal in 1907.[273]

Defining racial hygiene

An important function of the *Archiv* was to demarcate the territory of racial hygiene. This involved reaching a suitable readership, but also excluding rival projects. Ploetz was in competition with Woltmann who in 1903 had established a monthly journal, *Politisch-Anthropologische Revue*. Woltmann's aim was to unite political economy, anthropology, physiology and hygiene, to make these sciences intelligible for the public, to examine human history from the perspectives of natural history and to establish biological and anthropological principles for application to social questions. Woltmann failed to recruit his friend Eduard Bernstein as a contributor. The contributors to the first volume included Ludwig Gumplowicz the sociologist, Hegar the gynaecologist, Robert Kuczinsky the demographer, Friedrich Naumann the Christian social politician, Schallmayer and Wilser, the doctor and racial anthropologist. The second volume included contributions from the vitalist philosopher Hans Driesch, Forel, Gustav Fritsch the anatomist and anthropologist, Haeckel, Willy Hellpach the psychologist, Koch-Hesse, Lanz-Liebenfels the Austrian racial propagandist, Lombroso, Rüdin, and Wiedersheim, the anatomist. Woltmann's strategy was to unite left and right on the basis of racial anthropology, and with a legacy of influential political contacts, he achieved a prestigious list of contributers. By the end of the first year the journal claimed to have 2,000 subscribers.[274]

Ploetz held himself aloof, despite being pressed by Woltmann for contributions. He pursued a different strategy to Woltmann's all-inclusive approach. Rüdin

[271] Ploetz papers, diary 1905.   [272] Ploetz papers, diary.
[273] Ploetz papers, diary 4 August 1907.
[274] L. Woltmann and H.K.E. Buhmann, 'Naturwissenschaft und Politik. Zur Einführung', *Politisch-Anthropologische Revue*, vol. 1 (1902), 1–2; W. Hammer, 'Leben und Werk des Arztes und Sozialanthropologen Ludwig Woltmann', med. Diss, University of Mainz, 1979 pp. 26–29.

criticized Woltmann for an overly personal tone.[275] Ploetz encouraged contributions from biologists and social scientists, but his *Archiv* attacked prophets of Aryan racism. He solicited Schallmayer's support on 1 December 1905 as an ally against the *völkisch* racists. Ploetz stated that despite their disagreements the *Archiv* was broadly based. For Schallmayer had criticized the racial anthropologists Lapouge, Wilser, and Woltmann. Woltmann's *Revue* survived Woltmann's death in 1907, and although it continued until 1922, it lost its prestigious contributors and was a refuge of Aryan utopians. By way of contrast, the *Archiv* attracted articles based on hereditary biology and the medical sciences.

The scientificity of Ploetz's approach can be seen in the *Archiv's* dedication to Haeckel and Weismann on their seventieth birthdays. While scientists might differ in their theories of heredity, the *Archiv* intended to promote diverse views of Darwinism and Lamarckism. Contributors to the first volume included many distinguished biologists and doctors: Abderhalden writing on parthenogenesis, Correns, the geneticist, Julius Grober, professor of clinical medicine at Jena, writing on hereditary diseases, Valentin Haecker, the zoologist, Ferdinand Hueppe on infectious diseases and TB, Friedrich Ratzel, the Leipzig geographer and ideologist of *Lebensraum*, contributing on the Indo-Germanic race, and Paul Uhlenhuth, professor of hygiene at Strasburg, on human and ape blood. Ploetz cultivated potential contributors. For example he wrote to the leading British Darwinist and biometrician, Karl Pearson, who submitted a paper on heredity in 1906.[276]

Ploetz used the *Archiv* as a platform for his programme of racial hygiene as a means of reform. In a foreword, dated January 1904, he declared his aim to be the welfare of the family and the *Volk*, and suggested that their salvation could be attained through science. Such a science should combine logic, experiment, and racial and social categories. Racial biology was to describe the inner and external conditions of racial development, and should establish the optimal conditions for the maintenance and improvement of the race. It should draw on history, social and economic science, law, philosophy and psychology.[277]

He considered how the category of race should be related to society and the state. Societies could form within a race or be multi-racial. Societies competed in a struggle for survival, and within a society different elements competed. Organisms should be understood in the light of social laws, but he rejected organicist analogies and any simplistic transfer of biology to society. These comments suggest that the concept of a civic society was weak, and that Ploetz preferred to apply racial biology directly to human problems. From these empirically cautious beginnings, Ploetz went on to develop his view of racial biology. He declared his aim to be the monistic unity of the physical and the psychic. Race and life were synonymous.

[275] Ploetz papers, Rüdin to Ploetz, 12 August 1905.
[276] Ploetz papers, Ploetz to Pearson, 21 July 1904 and Pearson to Ploetz, 6 August 1904, 9 March 1906.
[277] A. Ploetz, 'Die Begriffe Rasse und Gesellschaft und die davon abgeleiteten Disciplinen', *ARGB*, vol. 1 (1904), 3.

Biologically, race gave immunity against bacteria. Yet at the highest metaphysical level race found expression in ethics and poetry. Racial hygiene was preventive therapy against alien bacteria and against cultural phenomena like the declining birth rate. Racial hygiene was to protect and improve the quality of future generations. In order to counteract the lack of natural selection in modern societies, social hygienic measures were to be substituted for natural, evolutionary processes. Life had evolved from a primal struggle of cells against bacteria, to cell states resisting racial poisons. He invoked the theory of the cell state in terms of Haeckel and Schäffle. Ploetz was thus working very much in the mould of Haeckel's Darwinism with additions from the hereditarian critique of bacteriology.[278]

The reaction against the liberal medicine of Virchow and Pettenkofer was expressed by an attack on individualism. Ploetz dealt with the distinctions between 'individual hygiene', 'social hygiene' and 'racial hygiene'. He saw a fundamental conflict between individual hygiene as opposed to racial or social hygiene. For individual hygiene conflicted with the racial priorities of the elimination of undesirable characteristics. Racial and social hygiene thus had to counter the harmful effects of individualism. Racial hygiene could function by both private or public methods. There could be voluntary abstinence from sexual reproduction, or state-enforced marriage laws. Above all, it was necessary to locate and eliminate dangerous hereditary cell substances. Yet the most altruistic and humane method was to control reproduction. Ploetz concluded that if no more weaklings were bred, then they need not be exterminated.[279]

Monism

The monist movement bridged the gap between the founding of a journal to advance racial hygiene as an academic discipline and the founding of a society to advance racial hygiene as a means for reforming lifestyle. The success of racial hygiene drew on monist and Darwinian strains in philosophy, anthropology and social thought. The popularity of Darwinism meant that art, politics and social thought all bore some form of Darwinian imprint. The climate of biologically inspired thought meant that the relations between academic science and biologistic beliefs were fraught with tensions. The free thought and monist movements of the early twentieth century claimed the authority of Darwinism as authentic proof of their validity. Yet these cultural forms differed greatly in the depth of awareness of biological theories of heredity. Advances in biology meant that evolutionary theory was rapidly changing. Although Haeckel continued to publicize evolutionary theories, these were scientifically dated, and could earn the scorn of dilettantism from the scientific community. While racial hygiene drew on the popularity of Haeckel's monism, it sought a more advanced scientific basis than Haeckel's dated theories of phylogenetic recapitulation.[280]

---

[278] Ploetz, 'Begriffe', pp. 2–20.   [279] Ploetz, 'Begriffe', pp. 23, 26.
[280] Compare D. Gasman, *The Scientific Origins of National Socialism* (London and New York, 1971).

Not only had Ploetz learned much of his biology from Haeckel, he continued to cultivate support from Haeckel for his journal and society. He noted with pride that Haeckel had complimented him on the *Archiv für Rassen- und Gesellschaftsbiologie*. Ploetz was a frequent visitor to Jena, and he made sure that he attended when Haeckel spoke in Berlin.[281] Ploetz also maintained contacts with Haeckel's disciples such as Heinrich Schmidt and Boelsche.[282] The foundation of Ploetz's journal coincided with the institutionalizing of Haeckel's campaign for naturalist ethics in the Monist League. It arose from a suggestion made by Haeckel in Rome in September 1904, and was formally established in 1906. Monism contrasted to the professional elitism of racial hygiene in its broader basis of public support. By 1912 the League numbered approximately 7,000 members in forty-three groups. Lectures and meetings were universal in scope, spanning the origins of the universe to pacifism. Biology and eugenics were merely a fragment of a greater whole. The Monist League took a part in the dissemination of biological values, and in campaigning for such eugenic and medical demands as non-sectarian hospitals, sex education and voluntary euthanasia, but it cannot be regarded as a specifically eugenic organization.[283] Its public role was to disseminate a scientific approach to ethics and politics.[284] Haeckel recruited Forel and in 1911 the Nobel Prize-winning chemist Wilhelm Ostwald as leaders of the League.[285] Whereas Haeckel's popularizations resonated with pantheistic rhetoric, Forel and Ostwald wished to pursue a more scientific and materialistic direction. There emerged an open split between what Ostwald referred to as 'monism' and 'Haeckelism'.[286] Forel criticized Haeckel as full of mysticism, secret allusions and metaphysical 'Klimbim'. Forel's programme of moral reform based on positive science was allied to socialist materialism.[287]

Although Ploetz attempted to use monism as a basis of support for racial hygiene, there were forces in monism opposed to racial concepts. Ploetz maintained links with Haeckel. In 1902 he reverently measured Haeckel's head. He took Haeckel's advice in the founding of the *Archiv*, and linked his concept of race to monism.[288] He joined the League on 14 February 1906.[289] Anxious to secure the blessing of Haeckel, the Monist League was joined by such biological reformers as Goldscheid, Müller-Lyer, Plate, Ploetz, Schallmayer and Ziegler. The League published a eugenic pamphlet by Schallmayer but Ploetz remained a marginal figure. The split between Haeckel and Forel had repercussions in that Forel became suspicious of Ploetz's racial hygiene as embodying an alien metaphysical strain in

---

[281] Ploetz papers, diary, 14 and 15 February 1905.
[282] Ploetz papers, diary, 19 April 1905.
[283] W. Mattern, 'Gründung und erste Entwicklung des Deutschen Monistenbundes, 1906–1918', med. Diss., FU Berlin 1983.   [284] Luebbe, *Politische Philosophie*, pp. 168–70.
[285] Forel, *Briefe*, p. 375, Haeckel to Forel, 17 November 1904.
[286] Forel, *Briefe*, p. 420, Ostwald to Forel, 18 November 1911.
[287] Forel, *Briefe*, pp. 414–6, Forel to Unna, 9 November 1911.
[288] Ploetz, 'Begriffe', *ARGB*, vol. 1 (1904), p. 3.
[289] Ploetz papers, Ploetz to Haeckel, 14 October 1903, 14 February 1906.

the concept of race. Forel would have been an important convert for Ploetz given his work, *The Sexual Question*, published in 1905. His aim was to communicate 'the facts' of reproductive biology to the public, and to encourage self-conscious attitudes to child rearing. He compaigned against the parasitic burden of the degenerate and the chronically and mentally ill on the fit and industrious. While refusing to accept moral stigmas such as 'illegitimacy' or sexual inequalities (provided women recognize their natural function of child bearing), he wished for ethics and social hygiene to be equivalent.[290] Ploetz in vain attempted to convince Forel of the validity of the racial concept.[291] Forel distanced himself from Ploetz, and never joined the Racial Hygiene Society. On 3 November 1908, he spoke on racial degeneration and improvement in Berlin. This was the preliminary for the founding of an International Order for Ethics and Culture with Forel, Grotjahn and Semon among the members.[292] Forel came to the conclusion that he preferred 'the social' to 'the racial', and he criticized the tendency to refer to societies as organisms.[293] Forel was a eugenicist insofar as he believed in the improvement of the human race but he was not concerned with racial differences among humans. He accepted the vice-presidency of the International Scientific Congress on Eugenics in London in 1912. The divergence between Ploetz and Forel was to be echoed by crucial divisions among German eugenicists in the 1920s. By that time, Forel was a convert to the supra-confessional world religion of the Baha'i faith.[294]

Anthropology

'Racial hygiene' represented an attempt to ally hygiene with anthropology. Ploetz was active in anthropological circles in Berlin, particularly at the University and at the Berlin Anthropological Society. Under the influence of imperialism, anthropology had been transformed to include the physique and culture of overseas races with an eye to their suitability as colonial subjects, the evaluation of the Germans regarding their capability of settlement abroad, and assessment of whether the transition of Germany from a predominately rural into an urban and industrial nation could have ill-effects on the physical and mental constitution of the people. Darwinian evolutionary concepts pervaded both physical and cultural anthropology. German anthropology had been slower to develop as a university discipline than in Britain or France. Althoff came to appreciate that anthropology would be of value in assessing the changes in social conditions, and supported the campaign for university chairs. From 1898 the Strasburg anatomist and anthropologist, Gustav Schwalbe, campaigned that there be a national network of

---

290 A. Forel, *Sexual Ethics* (London, 1909).
291 Ploetz papers, Ploetz to Forel, 12 April 1905 and 12 December 1905.
292 Ploetz papers, diary, 3 and 8 November 1908.
293 Forel, *Briefe*, pp. 423–6, Forel to Roesler, 30 April 1912.
294 J.P. Vader, 'August Forel Defends the Persecuted Persian Baha' in 1925–27', *Gesnerus*, vol. 41 (1984), 53–60.

anthropologischer Stationen based in clinics and anatomy institutes. These would collate data on living populations as part of a national survey. This scheme represented a crucial transition from Virchow's collection of data on physique to a more biological approach.[295] It was a crucial period for institutional expansion and scientific methods. In Imperial Germany the dominant method was that of physical measurement, especially of head shape. Physical anthropology predominated, and here anatomists controlled the field. There was an innovative biological approach to anthropology with the application of the Mendelian laws of inheritance to explain human variation. This kindled interest in eugenicists' theories of human heredity. Eugenicists such as Ploetz were well versed in the skills of craniometry.

Among the anthropological institutions providing manpower for racial hygiene were the Museum für Völkerkunde where Thurnwald was employed from 1901, and the Berlin Anthropological Society. Ploetz joined the Berlin Anthropological Society on 21 February 1903.[296] Rüdin joined in 1905. With its high proportion of medical men as members, the Society was a favourable recruiting ground. In 1905 the chairman of the Society, Abraham Lissauer, was a physician, and 184 out of 507 individual members were medical men. Those anthropologists who were attracted by Ploetz's racial hygiene appreciated the socio-political dimensions of their subject.[297] Ploetz shared with Thurnwald the political conviction that there should be a German-dominated Central Europe, free from Roman Catholicism and the Habsburgs.[298] Important converts to racial hygiene were the ethnologists Paul Traeger and Luschan. Luschan was departmental director of the Museum für Völkerkunde in Berlin, and was the first professor of anthropology at the University of Berlin. He was concerned with the problems of degeneration and industrialization. He compared the effects of domestication on animals to the condition of the *Kulturrassen* or civilized races. Like Ploetz he believed that the higher priorities of national duty and the race were in conflict with individualism and sentimentality. He regarded the weak as parasitic on the strong, the pure and the healthy.[299] He consequently represented a type of anthropology more oriented to social issues than to ideas of Aryan racial ideology.

Ploetz spoke on 'Race and Society' at Luschan's colloquium on 18 February 1904. He continued to participate in lively colloquia debates on subjects such as the anarchist Kropotkin's symbiotic theory of mutual aid in nature, and on anthropological techniques.[300] Other anthropologists who joined the Racial Hygiene Society were Max Kiessling, a geographer; and Wilhelm Filchner, an

---

[295] E. Fischer, 'Gustav Schwalbe', *Zeitschrift für Morphologie und Anthropologie*, vol. 20 (1917), i–viii.
[296] *Verhandlungen der Berliner Gesellschaft für Anthropologie*, vol. 35 (1903), 337.
[297] Ploetz papers, diary, 18 January 1905; 'Berliner Gesellschaft für Anthropologie, Ethnologie und Urgeschichte. 1905', *Zeitschrift für Ethnologie*, (1905), 1–18.
[298] Ploetz papers, diary, 29 January 1905.
[299] Luschan papers, MS 'Die gegenwärtigen Aufgaben der Anthropologie', p. 205.
[300] Ploetz papers, diary, 16 April 1904 meeting with Martin, 7 July 1904, 19 January and 23 February 1905, 10 January 1907, 25 January 1908.

explorer. That Hans Virchow, the anatomist and son of Rudolf Virchow, joined indicated how even the Virchow family succumbed to the shift to racial biology. A number of doctors in the tropics also joined, including Philaletes Kuhn and Ernst Rodenwaldt. By 1910 there were differences between Luschan and Thurnwald within the Racial Hygiene Society.[301] While medicine itself was becoming racialized, there was no consensus over the classification and exact meaning of race.

The founding of the Racial Hygiene Society drew on contacts with anthropologists, biologists and physicians. Ploetz claimed that it occupied the middle ground between socialism and social hygiene on the one side, and Aryan ideologies on the other. Intellectually the aim was a synthesis of anthropology and medicine. Yet the society was more than an intellectual association. It carried the conversion experience of abstinence beyond the avoidance of such racial poisons as alcohol and tobacco to a total reform of lifestyle and sexuality. By this combination of science and a personal sense of responsibility to future generations of the race, an elite with supreme physical and scientific qualities would arise. Their ideas were to permeate medicine and welfare measures.

Aryan purity

The organizing of racial hygiene as an academic discipline and as a public movement coincided with Chamberlain's success in popularizing Aryan racial theories. Distinctions between positive science and racial ideology were difficult to maintain, as many anthropologists were becoming sympathetic to racial imperialism. Racial hygiene offered a convenient middle ground by insisting on rigorous academic criteria, while emphasizing the importance of racial factors in a wide range of medical and social areas. Racial hygiene offered anthropology the chance to modernize scientific approaches by utilizing the latest biological theories of heredity, rather than human measurements. Racial hygienists were faced with the problem that by absorbing racial enthusiasts and advocating Aryan superiority and such wilder schemes as polygamy for the breeding elite they would earn the enmity of influential scientists. Ploetz and Schallmayer felt this acutely, as they attempted to gain acceptance from academic social scientists and biologists. Preserving academic standards remained important to eugenicists as they embarked on attempts to convert other academic and professional groups to their theories, and to establish their own society. Racial ideologists and eugenic groups competed to bring academic and public groups round to their point of view. Thus eugenics or social or racial hygiene was always far greater than the sum total of members in any eugenics society. There were factions among eugenicists within eugenics organizations and in competition for the attention of other public pressure groups like the Monist League and women's organizations. The setting up of the *Archiv für Rassen- und Gesellschaftsbiologie* and the opinions expressed in its pages

---

[301] Ploetz papers, diary, 22 January 1910, 4 November 1911.

show Ploetz had to negotiate a series of compromises with competing groups of Aryan enthusiasts, monists, anthropologists, biologists, public health experts, social scientists and feminists.

Although racial hygiene was an offshoot from racist nationalism, eugenics was distinct from the ideology of an Aryan master race. While Ploetz was personally anti-semitic and sympathized with Pan-Germanist schemes for extending the borders of Germany, he suppressed his personal racial convictions as unsuitable for launching an influential social movement. His racial hygiene journal and society grew out of contacts with biologists and public health experts. Indeed, he can be seen as spearheading an attack on Aryan racial ideology on behalf of a group of professional experts. In the aftermath of the Krupp prize, the Aryan and social anthropologist camp supporting Woltmann generated propaganda against a narrowly scientific approach to eugenics. That Schallmayer was seriously wounded by the Aryan attacks was convenient for Ploetz in mounting a campaign for his own type of scientific racial hygiene.

Ploetz cultivated Aryan ideologists in private but criticized them in public. In 1904 Ploetz was in contact with a number of racial propagandists like Willibald Hentschel, Schemann and Woltmann. The balance between racist ideology and technocratic eugenics was precarious. In 1905 there appeared the critique of 'Modern Theories of Race' by the Austrian economist Friedrich Hertz. This was targeted primarily at Chamberlain and Aryan idologues.[302] The *Archiv* observed that Hertz criticized the Aryan evangelists for their lack of understanding of geographical milieu, social science and history, but that Hertz's understanding of biological heredity was deficient. This scientistic position was used by Ploetz to criticize both social scientists and Aryan ideologists.[303]

The case of Hentschel illustrates the ambivalence of racial hygiene. After studying with Haeckel at Jena and assisting the chemists Ostwald and Johannes Wislicenus (a founder of the Pan-German League), Hentschel published plans for an Aryan racial utopia named *Mittgart* in 1904.[304] The publisher was the Hammer Verlag of the anti-semitic propagandist and Gobineau enthusiast Theodor Fritsch, whom Ploetz also contacted.[305] Hentschel suggested a 'means of practical renewal of the German race', which was under threat from urbanization and social democracy. It was necessary to raise the rural birth rate. The solution was breeding colonies with one thousand women per hundred men, selected for the very best physiques. He attacked doctors as 'microbe hunters' who served only to keep more of the syphilitic and tubercular alive.[306] While sympathizing with Hentschel's aim

---

[302] F. Hertz, 'Moderne Rassentheorien', *Sozialistische Monatshefte*, vol. 6 (1902), 876–83; Hertz, 'Die Rassentheorie des H. St. Chamberlain', *Sozialistische Monatshefte*, vol. 8 (1904), 310–15.

[303] *ARGB*, vol. 2 (1905), 860–1.

[304] W. Hentschel, *Varuna: eine Welt- und Geschichtsbetrachtung vom Standpunkt des Ariers* (Leipzig, 1901); W. Hentschel, *Mittgart, ein Weg zur Erneuerung der germanischen Rasse* (Leipzig, 1904).

[305] Ploetz papers, diary, 14 February 1908. Fritsch was a member of the Gobineau Society.

[306] D. Löwenberg, 'Willibald Hentschel, seine Pläne zur Menschenzüchtung, sein Biologismus und Antisemitismus', med. Diss., University of Mainz, 1978; STA Dresden Ministerium für Volksbildung Nr 15385.

of reviving the primal force of the race, Ploetz regarded Hentschel as dangerous because of his advocacy of polygamy. On the one hand he allied with Hentschel against the eccentricities of the feminist, Ruth Bré, the founder of the *Bund für Mutterschutz*. Ploetz wrote to Hentschel that without his warning he would have become more involved with Bré.[307] On the other hand, Ploetz feared that Hentschel would also be a liability. The *Archiv* carried a series of articles condemning Hentschel for his lack of scientific understanding and for transferring the practices of his cow-shed to human reproduction and rearing.[308] The disapproval of Hentschel was confirmed, as when Lenz, Fischer and others from the Freiburg group of the Racial Hygiene Society debated Hentschel's Mittgart manifesto.[309]

Ploetz rallied to the defence of the German family when confronted by the breeding plans of Christian Freiherr von Ehrenfels, a professor of philosophy in Prague. In the 1890s Ehrenfels had laid the foundations for Gestalt psychology.[310] Between 1902 and 1915 he published a series of works on sexual morality, spurred on by the calamity of a declining Central European birth rate. He supported an aristocratic type of racial elitism. There was to be selection based on psychic qualities in order to produce men who disdained all economic and moral conventions in the struggle for a reformed social order. He accepted individual and sexual hygiene so long as they did not interfere with 'vital selection', on which the future progress of humanity depended.[311] He was critical of Ploetz's acceptance of monogamy, and shrewdly regarded Ploetz's hope of chromosomal engineering as utopian.[312] Ploetz sought to remain on good terms with Ehrenfels but he wished to disassociate racial hygiene as a science from Ehrenfels' idiosyncratic morality.[313]

Relations with Schemann, the apostle of Gobineau and founder of the Gobineau Society posed further problems. Whereas Schemann emphasized aesthetic and moral priorities in racial regeneration, Ploetz wished to see a biologically and medically based racial hygiene movement. At Freiburg, the anthropologist Fischer combined pioneering research in human genetics with a degree of sympathy for Schemann. For example, he wrote in 1910 that he found Schemann's work valuable, and that he hoped the 'idea of race' would triumph, even though it would

---

[307] Ploetz papers, Ploetz to Hentschel, 15 June 1905.
[308] A. Ploetz, 'Willibald Hentschels Vorschlag zur Hebung unserer Rasse', *ARGB*, vol. 1 (1904), 885–95; W. Hentschel, 'Zuschrift betreffend den Artikel von A. Ploetz "Willibald Hentschels Vorschlag zur Hebung unserer Rasse"', *ARGB*, vol. 2 (1905), 269–72; Ploetz, 'Entgegnung auf W. Hentschels Zuschrift', *ARGB*, vol. 2 (1905), 272–3.
[309] Lenz papers, Freiburg Racial Hygiene Society MSS, 19 June 1911, pp. 8–9.
[310] F. Weinhandl (ed.), *Gestalthaftes Sehen* (Darmstadt, 1974).
[311] C.v. Ehrenfels, 'Die konstitutive Verderblichkeit der Monogamie und die Unentbehrlichkeit einer Sexualreform', *ARGB*, vol. 4 (1907), 814.
[312] Ploetz papers, diary, 20 October 1911; R. Oppitz, 'Freiherr von Ehrenfels und die Entwicklung des "neuen Menschen" zu Beginn des 20. Jahrhunderts', med. Diss., University of Mainz, 1980.
[313] A. Ploetz, 'Bemerkungen zur Abhandlung Prof. v. Ehrenfels über die konstitutive Verderblichkeit der Monogamie', *ARGB*, vol. 4 (1907) 859–61; C. v. Ehrenfels, 'Erwiderung auf Dr A. Ploetz' Bemerkungen zu meiner Abhandlung über die konstitutive Verderblichkeit der Monogamie', *ARGB*, vol. 5 (1908), 97–112.

have to be in 'a greater form' (i.e. scientifically updated) than that envisaged by Gobineau.[314] The *Alldeutsche Blätter* contained a broad range of racial theories: the editor, Paul Samassa, admired Gobineau, and there were contributions by Hentschel, and Adolf Lanz von Liebenfels. Schemann maintained contact with a wide variety of writers on eugenics and in other academic disciplines, as well as with many nationalists. The Landowners' League also echoed the Social Darwinist convictions of Aryan racial superiority.[315] Ploetz disliked Walter Claassen, a statistician and from 1907 an official of the Landowners' League.[316] Moreover, the publicizing of theories of ethnic struggle against Jews and Slavs embarrassed Schallmayer and Ploetz – at least in public. In a protracted correspondence with Schemann, Schallmayer argued against the scientific validity of Aryan racial theories.[317] Privately, Ploetz elicited from Schallmayer that he was an anti-semite.[318] Ploetz enjoyed cordial but distant relations with Schemann, and did not join the Gobineau League. On 20 September 1910 Ploetz visited Schemann who hoped that the Racial Hygiene Society would be a corporate member of the Gobineau League; Ploetz put him off with empty promises.[319] The Freiburg group of the Racial Hygiene Society kept Schemann at a distance, and Ploetz rejected corporate membership of the Gobineau Society as a matter of policy, because he wished to avoid having Fritsch, Hentschel and Schemann as members of the Racial Hygiene Society.[320] It was a delicate balance to maintain the separation of racial hygiene from Aryan racism.

Social biology and sociology

As a combination of social science and hereditary biology, racial hygiene sought to influence the content and scope of the social sciences. The Krupp prize of 1900 showed the interest among social scientists in biology and hygiene. There was a reaction among social scientists against the liberal concept of social progress, as they sought an objective basis to give their studies status as an autonomous science and to provide a means of conceptualizing social cohesion while avoiding socialist materialism. To some social scientists, biology offered such a basis as it replaced hypothetical moral and legal categories with positive evolutionary certainties. Demography, studies of class differentials in fertility and disease, and health as a crucial feature of urban social problems were areas of common interest to social scientists and medical experts. Darwinism provided channels of communication

---

[314] M.D. Biddiss, *Father of Racist Ideology. The Social and Political Thought of Count Gobineau* (London, 1970); E.J. Young, *Gobineau und der Rassismus* (Meisenheim, 1968).

[315] Chickering, *Men*, pp. 238–42; H.-J. Puhle, *Agrarische Interessenpolitik und preussischer Konservatismus im Wilhelminischen Reich (1893–1914)* (Hanover, 1967).

[316] Ploetz papers, diary, 18 January 1905.   [317] Schemann papers, Schallmayer to Gobineau.

[318] Ploetz papers, diary, 14 January 1912.

[319] Schemann papers, Ploetz to Schemann, 19 September and 3 October 1910; Ploetz papers, diary, 20 September 1910 Ploetz used the expression 'Habe ihn vertröstet'.

[320] Ploetz papers, Ploetz to Gruber, 19 November 1911.

between medicine and social science, and organicist sociology continued to be innovative. This was demonstrated in France by René Worms' choice of Spencer and then Schäffle to preside over the International Institute of Sociology, established in 1893.[321] The concept of struggle was replaced by co-operation, which was given a biological formulation. In Worms' case, social organicism corresponded to the needs of republican solidarism. French intellectuals were gripped by a movement of solidarity, which used science to provide an organicist theory of social unity based on positive obligations. German organicist social theorising merits comparison with the French doctrines of solidarism and the 'new liberalism' in Britain, which between 1890 and 1910 shaped the provision of social services and welfare policies.[322] In Germany, although some of the most brilliant social scientists such as Ernst Simmel and Max Weber sought to establish social science in terms of autonomous criteria, collectivist concepts of a co-operative social organism continued to be a force in the development of sociology and applied social studies. This went with an interest in social planning by an expert elite. Statistics and human biology were regarded as important auxiliary techniques in the new enterprise of sociology, and eugenicists supported the development of a sociology which had biology at its core.

The links between eugenics and social science were controversial at a time when societies for sociology were being established. Advocates of social hygiene and demographic studies oriented to the European problem of a declining birth rate conflicted with those concerned primarily to establish sociology as an academic discipline. At the Sociological Society, founded in London during 1903, marriage, parenthood and demographic statistics were frequent topics of discussion.[323] The founding of the Eugenics Society in 1907 was partly the result of the failure of eugenicists to maintain their influence over sociology. In Germany, eugenics and other variants of social biology were of interest to critics of the economic and historical methods of the *Kathedersozialisten*. The Society for Racial Hygiene was a reaction against a social science orientation in public health such as that developed by Grotjahn. It was in areas of applied social science, such as state planning and the socio-economic implications of fertility, that eugenics influenced German social science. Grotjahn, Hans Kurella (the neurologist and criminal anthropologist), Ploetz and Schallmayer maintained cordial relations with such social scientists as Tönnies, Sombart and Rudolf Goldscheid. Eugenicists were contributors to the innovative *Zeitschrift für Sozialwissenschaft*, and journals such as the prestigious *Schmollers Jahrbuch* carried review articles on eugenics.[324] Ploetz never gave up

[321] L.L. Clark, *Social Darwinism in France* (Alabama, 1984), pp. 118–36.
[322] F.W. Coker, *Organismic Theories of the State* (New York, 1910); T. Zeldin, *France 1848–1945. Ambition, Love and Politics* (Oxford, 1973), pp. 656–60. For Britain, see M. Freeden, *The New Liberalism. An Ideology of Social Reform* (Oxford, 1978); G. Searle, *The Quest for National Efficiency* (Oxford, 1971).
[323] P. Abrams, *The Origins of British Sociology 1834–1914* (Chicago 1968); C. Klingemann (ed.), *Rassenmythos und Sozialwissenschaften in Deutschland* (Opladen, 1987).
[324] F. Tönnies, 'Eugenik', *Schmollers Jahrbuch*, vol. 29 (1905), 1089–106.

hope that he could win acceptance for racial hygiene among social scientists by presenting social biology as an area of common interest. Thurnwald and Vierkandt supported Ploetz's *Archiv*. For many years Ploetz maintained contacts with Werner Sombart in Berlin and with the Austrian sociologist, Goldscheid, who was also a member of the Monist League.[325] Sombart's classic study of Jews in economic life (published in 1911) analyzed the social relations of capitalism in biological and racial terms. Sombart considered that biological qualities of the blood might explain racial character.[326] Goldscheid developed the influential theory of the 'human economy', which he published in 1911. Goldscheid had protracted discussions with Ploetz on the topics of race and society, and they considered establishing a sociological society in Munich.[327] When Goldscheid established such a society in Vienna, it included a section for 'social biology and eugenics'. This was headed by the anatomist, Julius Tandler, and the secretary was Paul Kammerer, the zoologist.[328]

While remaining in a biologistic and monist framework, Goldscheid had a capacity for innovative theoretical analysis. He dedicated his study to the monist chemist, Ostwald. Eugenics fitted in with the prevalent distaste for Manchesterism and a market economy. Goldscheid suggested that social organization was to benefit the population rather than to produce profit. His aims were a healthy and productive population. He considered that a reinforcement of moral commitment to the social organism was necessary. He developed the Spencerian concept of social integration into a demand for a scientifically based socialism. Relating poverty to overpopulation, he believed that social problems could be solved by attention to the biological basis of society. He favoured *Mutterschutz* and welfare benefits for 'child rich' families, along with many other standard aims of social hygiene. The modern state was an *Ueberorganismus* (super-organism) that had to extend its responsibilities in response to social evolution. His exclamation of *Mehr Seele!*[329] contrasted to those seeking a value-free social science.[330]

Goldscheid's demand for the 'human economy' exerted an immense appeal on economists and state officials concerned with taxation. Yet there were alternative directions emerging. The demand for a value-free social science was attractive to those academics wishing to express detachment from imperialist society. But such *Wertfreiheit* (value neutrality) was *Wertblindheit* (value blindness) to Goldscheid. A climax came with the first congress of the German Society for Sociology[331] in October 1910. Tönnies placed the issue of 'the concepts of race and society' on the agenda, with Ploetz as speaker. It was one of only seven lectures. Ploetz considered

---

[325] Ploetz papers, diary, 5 November 1908, 12 February 1909.
[326] W. Sombart, *Die Juden and das Wirtschaftsleben* (Berlin, 1911); J. Herf, *Reactionary Modernism, Technology, Culture and Politics in Weimar and the Third Reich* (Cambridge, 1986), pp. 130–43.
[327] Ploetz papers, Goldscheid to Ploetz, 31 May 1910.
[328] Max Hirsch papers, Goldscheid correspondence, *Soziologische Gesellschaft in Wien, Sektion für Sozialbiologie und Eugenik*.   [329] More spirituality.
[330] R. Goldscheid, *Höherentwicklung und Menschenökonomie – Grundlegung der Sozialbiologie* (Leipzig, 1911).   [331] *Deutsche Gesellschaft für Soziologie*.

the relationship between sociology and racial biology. He presented an account of society in evolutionary terms, using the theories of Darwin, Galton and Haeckel to express ideas about the evolution of social instinct, altruism and the sense of social solidarity. Society was defined in biological terms as the category that maintains life. He outlined degenerative social influences such as alcohol and birth control, and proposed remedies concerning sexual selection or the control of degenerative reproductive cells.[332]

This type of social pathology provoked a clash between those interested in social biology, such as Goldscheid, Oppenheimer and Ploetz, and those concerned to establish sociology as an autonomous academic discipline. Weber rejected the validity of comparisons of biological organizations with social organizations on the grounds that they combined a number of precise concepts into a single vague one. In working on an industrial psychology project between 1909 and 1911 Weber had come to dislike hereditarian analyses of workers' psychology. Weber considered that 'with race theories you can prove or disprove anything you want'; the theory of 'inherited disposition' could not be evaluated scientifically.[333] Yet here Weber seems to have been criticizing academic imprecision and not the concept of race itself.

The majority of sociologists agreed with Sombart's defence of his friend Ploetz, that 'the strong opposition expressed against Dr Ploetz did not mean that the Society did not have an interest in biology. We *are* interested.'[334] Although few social scientists went to the extremes of racial hygiene or Ammon's racist social anthropology, social biology continued to be a major force in German social science. It offered a means of integrating demography, medicine and evolutionary biology in a flexible framework, and accorded with interest in 'the human economy'. The family, as the locus of conflict between rational social values and higher demands by the state and race, became the subject of moral propaganda and scientific study.

INSTITUTING THE RACIAL HYGIENE SOCIETY

The Racial Hygiene Society, founded in Berlin in 1905, was the first of the eugenics societies to be established. It represented an attempt by Ploetz to lay claim to the middle ground between the Pan-German Aryan ideologues on the one side, and the social hygienists and socialist doctors on the other.[335] The recruitment of the professionally qualified as members meant that the social elite of intellectuals and scientists was to be transformed into a racial elite. An exemplary healthy personal

---

[332] A. Ploetz, 'Die Begriffe Rasse und Gesellschaft und einige damit zusammenhängende Probleme', in *Verhandlungen des Ersten Deutschen Soziologentages* (Tübingen, 1912), pp. 111–36.

[333] Max Weber, *Economy and Society*, ed. G. Roth and C. Wittich, (Berkeley, Los Angeles, London, 1978), p. 398.   [334] Weber, *Economy and Society*, p. 398.

[335] Ploetz papers, Ploetz to Gruber, 19 November 1911, concerning Gruber's criticisms of an overly liberal membership policy.

lifestyle and commitment to having a large family went with attempts to solve social problems. The society was primarily the brain child of Ploetz, and until 1914 he was the major force in shaping its growth. Ploetz's activities show him cultivating anthropologists, physicians and social scientists in order to win support for the *Archiv* and the Racial Hygiene Society. He resisted all attempts to persuade him to relinquish either the Society or *Archiv* into the hands of others.[336]

The Racial Hygiene Society was an offshoot from the *Archiv*. Ploetz had suggested founding a society to Rüdin on 18 February 1905. He then discussed matters with Haeckel and Ziegler in Jena, and with the professor of internal medicine, Friedrich Martius, who was concerned with alcohol and racial degeneration.[337] After further conferring with Thurnwald and Rüdin on 23 April and 19 May, the first meeting of the society was held in Berlin on 22 June 1905. Ploetz, Rüdin, Thurnwald and Nordenholz were the founder members. The biologist, Ludwig Plate, was the fifth to join on 17 July. They were all involved with the *Archiv*. Ploetz's diary, and the membership lists and memoranda which he issued permit reconstruction of his evangelizing activities and of the social composition of the Society. The next to join were Ploetz's literary friends: Carl and Gerhart Hauptmann, Boelsche, and the landscape artist Erich Kubierschky along with their families. In October 1905 a group of scientifically distinguished honorary members were added: Bunge, Hegar and Haeckel. The biologists Konrad Guenther and Ziegler were also recruited. By December 1905 there were twenty-eight members, in 1906 a further twelve members, and in 1907 forty-four more members joined. Eighteen of the forty members in the society by December 1906 had a background in biology, these being nine doctors, six zoologists, and three anthropologists.[338]

Local groups

The growth of the Racial Hygiene Society was determined by Ploetz's extensive travelling and cultivating of individuals and organizations. The meetings of the society alternated between scientific discussions and either social evenings or such group outings as walking and cycling tours. In 1907 Ploetz moved to Munich where his mother-in-law lived. This provided the opportunity for the society's expansion. What had hitherto been just the *Gesellschaft für Rassenhygiene* was on 9 April 1907 formally constituted as the *Berliner Ortsgruppe* of the society. On 31 May 1907 Ploetz persuaded the professor of hygiene, Gruber, to be chairman of a Munich Society for Racial Hygiene, which was formally founded on 24 September.[339] The Munich society prospered. The Munich Anthropological

---

[336] Ploetz papers, Plate to Ploetz, 3 April 1910, Thurnwald to Ploetz, 27 May 1911.
[337] Ploetz papers, diary, 10 and 13 April 1905.
[338] Ploetz papers, MS 1907 membership list; E. Fischer, 'Aus der Geschichte der deutschen Gesellschaft für Rassenhygiene', *ARGB*, vol. 24 (1930), 1–5.
[339] Ploetz papers, diary, 31 May 1907.

Society urged amalgamation with the Racial Hygiene Society, and eventually they agreed to hold joint meetings.[340]

Until 1908 Ploetz could list in his diary every member who attended, each meeting attracting between three and twelve members. In 1909 numbers rapidly increased. Ploetz noted that forty attended a meeting in Munich held in July when Georg Sittmann spoke on 'Rasse und Volk'. When the biologist Franz Doflein spoke on heredity on 8 November 1909 there were over sixty members present; fifty to fifty-five attended the monist Johannes Unold's talk on 'Racial Hygienic Ethics' on 10 December 1909, and when Gruber spoke on over-eating on 16 January 1910 there were over one hundred members in the audience.

From the outset the society was intended to be a racial elite. On 11 January 1907 the anthropologist Luschan undertook to conserve the skulls and brains of members. In 1908 Ploetz began to use the category of 'founder member', *Gründer*, to denote those members who submitted to an anthropological examination. The results were sent to the society's central office. There was a second category of auxiliary members, *Förderer*, for those who merely wished to attend lectures. Physical examinations necessitated a special medical committee. The society encouraged members to subscribe to eugenic codes. Spouses and children were urged to join. Unmarried members were advised to undertake only to marry after the society had approved of a prospective partner. The society characterized itself as a breeding elite and as a biological order of chivalry. It was interested more in improving the quality of this elite, than in mobilizing a broad-based public enthusiasm for eugenics.

Freiburg's pedigree of having nurtured racially aware biologists made it an appropriate centre for a local group. Ploetz cultivated the anatomist and anthropologist, Eugen Fischer, who organized a local committee for anthropological investigations and set about establishing a local group spurred on by a visit from Ploetz in July 1908.[341] Fischer proudly wrote of how he included the society's ideal of qualitative improvement of the race in his lectures to medical students. The medical student Fritz Lenz was influenced by a combination of hereditary biology and the neo-Kantian philosophy of Alois Riehl and Heinrich Rickert. By 1907 he was convinced of the necessity of racial hygiene.[342] He fused Mendelism with *völkisch* idealism. Ploetz met Lenz first in 1909, secured for him the status as a founder member of the Freiburg society, and invited him to join the editorial board of the *Archiv* in 1913.[343] A local society was provisionally established in Freiburg on 24 June 1908 by Fischer, Doflein, Hegar and Konrad Guenther, a nationalist-minded ecologist. Fischer was about to leave for his important expedition to study inter-breeding among whites and natives in South-West Africa, an expedition

---

[340] Ploetz papers, Ranke to Ploetz, 29 November 1909; diary, 17–21 May 1909.
[341] Ploetz papers, Fischer to Ploetz, 21 May and 26 June 1908; 7 February 1909.
[342] F. Lenz, *Die Rasse als Wertprinzip, Zur Erneuerung der Ethik* (Munich, nd), p. 6.
[343] Ploetz papers, Lenz to Ploetz, 14 January 1910; Ploetz to Lenz, 23 April 1913; diary, 24 October 1911.

which resulted in his claim to have proved Mendelian inheritance in humans. Activities resumed in 1909 when Fischer had returned. In 1909 he was prevented from lecturing on 'racial hygiene' on the grounds that it interfered with the territory of the hygienists, and, taking his cue from Ammon, he lectured instead on 'social anthropology'. On 23 May 1909 Ploetz recorded how he joined an outing of the society with Ludwig Aschoff, Fischer, Lenz and Wiedersheim. The group was formally constituted on 21 July 1910.[344]

Although small – in 1910 it had only twenty-three members – the Freiburg group was of outstanding importance.The innovations in evolutionary biology and in medicine in Freiburg continued. As the group had an exclusively academic membership, it took a major role in establishing eugenics and anthropology on the basis of Mendelism. Other innovative scientists at Freiburg included the pathologist Aschoff and the psychiatrists Robert Gaupp and Oswald Bumke. From November 1910 the group arranged frequent meetings on such burning issues as inability to breast feed, mental degeneration, inherited diseases, social anthropology, and research into family life. There were close links with the local Society for Natural Sciences, and agitation for state resources for racial hygiene.[345] The text book of human heredity and eugenics by Baur (who had studied at Freiburg), Fischer and Lenz was a product of Freiburg eugenics, and was planned by 1914.

Expansion in Dresden came after it was agreed with Gruber and Rüdin on 4 May 1910 that the Racial Hygiene Society should participate in the International Hygiene Exhibition. Rüdin directed the preparation of a racial hygienic display. Ploetz characteristically dashed off to Dresden where he constituted a local group under the auspices of the psychiatrist, Paul Nitsche. Gruber and Rüdin produced a catalogue outlining major issues in reproductive biology, demography and racial hygiene. As the International Exhibition was visited by 5.5 million visitors, the society's display was of major importance. The catalogue was published by Julius Lehmann, who was to become the major publisher of eugenic literature.[346] The exhibition provided the opportunity for staging a general meeting of the society as an international eugenic congress. Nitsche guarded against infiltration by radical sexual reformers. Conflict erupted between family-oriented racial hygienists such as Gruber, and the radical sexual reformers (who like Stöcker and Adele Schreiber advocated contraception). Racial hygienists were outraged that feminists addressed the conference.[347]

A further local group was established in Stuttgart in 1910 by the doctor and medical statistician, Wilhelm Weinberg. There was consternation because Weinberg was a baptised Jew.[348] Local organizations necessitated a national

---

[344] Lenz papers, Freiburg MSS; Ploetz papers, Fischer to Ploetz, 10 March 1909.
[345] E. Fischer, *Sozialanthropologie und ihre Bedeutung für den Staat* (Freiburg, 1910).
[346] M. v. Gruber and E. Rüdin (eds.), *Fortpflanzung, Vererbung, Rassenhygiene. Katalog der Gruppe Rassenhygiene der Internationalen Hygiene-Ausstellung 1911 in Dresden* (Munich, 1911).
[347] Ploetz papers, Ploetz to Gruber, 19 November 1911.
[348] Ploetz papers, diary, 29 September 1904.

Deutsche Gesellschaft für Rassenhygiene. This was constituted on 12 March 1910.[349] Gruber was chairman from 1910 until 1922, and Ploetz was secretary until 1914 when he became vice-chairman. That Lehmann was the secretary, Lenz the vice-secretary, and Spatz the treasurer confirmed the dominance of the Munich group over the national society.

Social Composition

As can be seen from table 2 below, the Society initially expanded only slowly. The most rapid phase of growth was between January 1910 and March 1911 when the membership rose from 175 to 411. There was a surge in attendance at meetings during 1912. The psychiatrist Alois Alzheimer (famous for his observations on senility), lectured on the brain to an audience of 300 on 9 January 1912 for the Munich Racial Hygiene Society. Between 500 and 600 members and visitors attended a eugenics lecture by Fischer in Freiburg on 1 February 1912. By 1913,

Table 2. *The growth of the International Society for Racial Hygiene, 1905–1913*

	German members	non-German members	Total members
1905 December	18	2	20
1906 December	33	4	37
1907 December	75	10	85
1908 March	82	14	96
1908 December	134	16	150
1909 March	126	19	145
1909 December	175	57	232
1910 February/March	211	75[a]	286
1910 December	291	89[b]	380
1911 March	N/A	N/A	411
1913 December	425[c]	N/A	N/A

Notes:
N/A signifies not available.
[a] Includes 46 Swedes.
[b] Includes 58 Swedes.
[c] The membership list of December 1913 covers only the German Racial Hygiene Society. It included a small number (9) of Austro-Hungarian, Swiss or Romanian nationals, or Germans overseas in the colonies.
Sources: for 1905 and 1906: Ploetz papers – manuscript lists; for 1907–1910, and 1913, printed membership lists in Ploetz papers, G. Hauptmann papers, or lists of Eugen Fischer in Lenz papers; for 1911, letters of Ploetz to G. Hauptmann on 21 March 1911, G. Hauptmann papers.

[349] Ploetz papers, diary.

there were 425 members in Germany from the one national and four local groups, as well as from a Swedish group. These numbers were exceeded by the Eugenics Education Society in London, which in 1914 had 1,047 members and associate members. Germany was only able to match this figure in 1931 when there were 1,085 members, although by then the Eugenics Society membership was on the decline.[350]

The Racial Hygiene Society was initially an extension of Ploetz's social circle. Physicians and university teachers predominated, and there were a few writers and artists. This is reflected in the organization of recruitment drives for young members, especially students. Agnes Bluhm in 1909 was of the opinion that the women members of the society were too middle-aged; in order to have maximum effect members should be as young as possible.[351] In 1913 the social composition of the constituent groups of the society showed a dominance of the medically qualified.

Ploetz attempted to recruit among kindred groups of middle-class professionals. He attended a genealogical course offered by the psychiatrist Robert Sommer in Giessen and used this as an opportunity to publicize the Racial Hygiene Society among genealogists and those interested in criminal biology.[352] Racial hygiene was to defend the bourgeois social order and the family, and on this platform the Society hoped to recruit a great many women as members. The idea was that the society should form an elite breeding group, and that while receiving professional education, women should be made aware of their 'higher' duty to the race. Most women members did not have an occupation listed as they were wives or daughters. In 1913 there were seven women physicians: Bluhm, Selma Friedrich and Pauline Ploetz in Berlin, Maria von Eggelkraut and Mally Kachel in Munich, Jula Dittmar from Erlangen and Elisabeth Winterhalter from the Taunus. There was also a dental surgeon, Elisabeth Schenck-Böhmer, who came from Dessau. Ploetz opposed the admission of supporters of 'modern sexual ethics'.[353] The women members were expected to combat the ideas of radical sexual reformers such as Stöcker. For the constituent groups, the numbers of men and women were:

	Berlin	Munich	Freiburg	Stuttgart	Other	Total
men	103	68	39	10	94	314
women	45	25	8	2	31	111
total	148	93	47	12	125	425

Students and the youth movement of the *Freischar* and *Wandervogel* were other prime targets for recruitment. Ploetz frequently lectured to student societies such as the *Verein Deutscher Studenten* where he spoke on liberalism and race, and to the *Freie Studentenschaft* and *Freiland* societies.[354] He hoped that if the *Freischar* could be

---

[350] L.A. Farrell, *The Origins and Growth of the English Eugenics Movement 1865–1925* (New York, 1985), p. 210; G.R. Searle, *Eugenics in Britain, 1900–1914* (Leyden, 1976), p. 160.
[351] Ploetz papers, Bluhm to Ploetz, 2 April 1909.   [352] Ploetz papers, diary, 4–6 August 1908.
[353] Ploetz papers, Ploetz to Gruber, 19 November 1911, concerning rejection of Frau Musil-Hess.
[354] Ploetz papers, diary, 6 May 1909, 1 and 14 December 1911.

weaned away from pacifist ideals of international co-operation, they might form a chapter of the society.[355] As a medical student Lenz attempted to recruit among the Free Youth Movement (Freideutsche Jugend). The Racial Hygiene Society's message of fitness and duty to the race coincided with a rising tide of youth patriotism, and articles on racial hygiene frequently appeared in the student fraternity magazines.[356]

Officially the society had no political ties. Ploetz described himself as 'without party' in 1913. Ploetz refused to accept any social democrats or feminist sexual reformers as members, and informed Gruber that he had to deflect an application from Kautsky. However, the socialist sympathizers Blaschko and Grotjahn were accepted as members.[357] The society's members included many academics and professionals who had liberal or National Liberal sympathies, but were increasingly nationalistic. Examples of National Liberals were Aschoff, Otto Lubarsch, Weinberg and Richard Hertwig. The psychiatrist Ribbert referred to himself as 'liberal', the biologists Doflein and Plate were abandoning Virchowian liberalism, and Konrad Guenther was 'national' in outlook.[358]

The social composition of the society shows that racial hygiene appealed primarily to professional sectors of the *Bildungsbürgertum*. There was a distinctive blend of technocratic concepts of hygiene with the idea of Germanic chivalry. It showed how modern ideas were combined with the glorification of the medieval Germanic past. However much the society kept aloof from Pan-German ultra-nationalist leagues and from conservative politics, the lines of division were to be increasingly blurred.

International organization

In November 1908 the International Order for Ethics and Culture was founded by a free-thinking group in Berlin, which included Forel and Ploetz. Although Ploetz promptly resigned – judging the group as too materialistic – the establishment of an international association remained a priority for him. The project for an international society was implicit in the universality of the early 'Gesellschaft für Rassenhygiene', as shortly before its foundation Ploetz had agreed with Thurnwald that Europe needed a higher form of state organization with a federation of Germany, Austria, Switzerland, Scandinavia and Belgium.[359] The internationalism of the society became explicit only in 1907. Although Ploetz believed in a hierarchy of races, with the Australian aborigine as the lowest and the white Germanic or Nordic European as the highest, he recognized that degenerate elements were present in all races. He considered that as races were not limited to

[355] Ploetz papers, Ploetz to Gruber, 24 November 1911.
[356] L. Hoeflmayr, 'Rassenhygiene in Theorie und Praxis', *Burschenschaftsblätter*, vol. 26 (1912), 186–8.
[357] Ploetz papers, Ploetz to Gruber, 19 November 1911.
[358] For political affiliations, see H.A.L. Degener, *Wer Ist's* (Leipzig, 1912).
[359] Ploetz papers, diary, 29 February 1905.

Table 3. *The membership of the German Racial Hygiene Society in 1913, according to occupation*

Occupation	Berlin	Munich	Freiburg	Stuttgart	Other	Total	Per cent
Medically related occupations							
Physician	25	22	17	6	40	110	25.9
Medical student	10	11	13		2	36	8.5
Dental surgeon					1	1	0.2
Apothecary					2	2	0.5
Botanist/zoologist	2	3	3	1	3	12	2.8*
Anthropologist	4	1			2	7	1.6*
Non-medical academics							
Student (non-medical)	9	10	2		4	25	5.9
Geologist/mineralogist		1			1	2	0.5
Philologist	1					1	0.2
Philosopher					1	1	0.2
Geographer					1	1	0.2
Archaeologist					1	1	0.2
Economist/statistician	3				3	6	1.4
Teacher	7	3		1	2	13	3.1
Pastor					1	1	0.2
Lawyer	5	1			4	10	2.4
Architect	2	3			3	8	1.9
Engineer	3	2			3	8	1.9
Chemist		1	1		2	4	0.9
Librarian		1	1			2	0.5
Prof (unspecified)	1				3	4	0.9
Dr (unspecified)	4	1	3		3	11	2.6
Writers and artists							
Author/artist/composer	13	5			5	23	5.4

Miscellaneous							
Journalist	1	1			1	3	0.7
Bank employee	1					1	0.2
Landowner	2	2			3	7	1.6
Army officer	5					5	1.2
Official/privy counsellor/diplomat	5			1	3	9	2.1
Riding master	1					1	0.2
Politician			1			1	0.2
Municipal officer					1	1	0.2
Publisher		1		1	4	6	1.4
Commerce	7	3				10	2.4
Occupations unspecified							
Men	2				1	3	0.7
Women	21	35	6	2	25	89	21.0
Total (all categories)	148	93	47	12	125	425	100.0

Notes:

Note that the percentages have been adjusted to the first decimal point.

*A substantial proportion of these had medical degrees.

Source: Deutsche Gesellschaft für Rassen-Hygiene. Mitgliederliste vom 31. Dezember 1913, copy annotated by Eugen Fischer in Lenz papers. This statistical analysis should be compared to my analysis of the Racial Hygiene Society in 1910, published in *Zeitschrift für Sozialreform*, vol. 30 (1984) 675–87, and to the analysis of the Societies in 1907 and 1913 by Sheila Weiss, 'The Race Hygiene Movement in Germany', *Osiris*, 2nd series vol. 3 (1987), 209. Weiss gives a total membership of 407 for the Society in 1913.

national boundaries an international society was necessary.[360] Much planning went into the expansion of the society. On 8 April 1908 the committee composed of Ploetz, Gruber, Nordenholz and Rüdin discussed policy for non-German lands. There were three main areas of recruitment. Ploetz took charge of relations with Austria–Hungary and Britain, and Rüdin evangelized in Scandinavia and France.

Ploetz was *Grossdeutsch* in his ideals that unification of the German people was more important than the limited state established in 1870. For a time he took Swiss nationality, and resumed German nationality again only in 1913. Other leading eugenicists, although active in Germany, were Swiss like Rüdin, or Austrian like Gruber, Kaup, Luschan and Thurnwald. What had become the 'Deutsche Gesellschaft für Rassenhygiene' was defined as embracing those 'with German as their mother tongue'. From the outset there were two Swiss resident members, the doctor Beckmann and the physiologist Bunge (in origins a Baltic German) in Basel, but numbers grew to only four by 1910. Ploetz and Gruber set much value on contacts with Austria. Ploetz was recommended by Luschan to visit Graf Wilczek, who agreed to found an Austrian group.[361] Ploetz hoped that Austria would separate from Hungary and join a Greater Germany. He kept in with progressive thinkers like the sociologist Goldscheid. In February 1909 Ploetz recruited the agrarian economist Michael Hainisch and the professor of pathology, Anton Weichselbaum.[362] Other avant-garde Austrians regarded as prospective recruits were experts in social hygiene such as Julius Tandler. But such social hygienists did not join, and there were only five members in Austria in December 1913. A few Hungarians became enthusiasts for racial hygiene. The Hungarian consul in Berlin, Géza von Hoffmann, was a noted commentator on German and American eugenics. Ploetz made friends with Graf Paul Teleki, a geographer (and the future authoritarian political leader). Thus although Austrian and Hungarian eugenicists were few, they were to take leading political positions after 1918 when, for example, Hainisch became president of Austria from 1920 until 1929.

Ploetz venerated Scandinavia as the motherland of the *Germanen*. That Scandinavians responded to racial hygiene with the greatest enthusiasm reinforced the ideal of Nordic racial purity. But it was initially scientists and liberal progressivists who joined the society. Rüdin visited Norway and Sweden in March 1907, when he recruited seven members, and again on 7 May 1909 when twenty-six new members were acquired. The Norwegian chemist, Alfred Mjöen, underwent a transition from liberal and anti-alcohol campaigner to staunch enthusiast for Nordic ideals.[363] Swedes became keen eugenicists. In part this was because of concern over psychiatric disease among peasant populations. Pioneering use was made of genealogical records by the psychiatrist, Hermann Lundborg.[364]

[360] Ploetz papers, *Denkschrift über die Gründung der Internationalen Gesellschaft für Rassen-Hygiene*.

[361] Luschan papers, Ploetz to Luschan, 28 November 1908.

[362] Ploetz papers, diary, 12 and 15 February 1909.

[363] N. Roll-Hansen, 'Eugenics before World War II. The Case of Norway', *History and Philosophy of the Life Sciences*, vol. 2 (1981), 269–98.

[364] H. Lundborg, *Medizinisch-biologische Familienforschungen innerhalb eines 2232 köpfigen Bauernge-schlechtes in Schweden (Provinz Blekinge). Mit einer Vorrede von Max von Gruber* (Jena, 1913).

Ploetz, Gruber and Rüdin were impressed by his method of family research.[365] There were also controversies over national identity and ethnic composition, especially over the place to be accorded to Lapps and gypsies. Swedish academics tended to follow German scientific initiatives, and remained within the German cultural sphere. A *Svenskt Sällskap för Rashygien* was constituted on 27 January 1910 by Wilhelm Hultkranz, professor of anatomy in Uppsala. On 31 January 1910 its numbers had risen to fifty-eight; thirty-one of these were physicians or medical students.

Whereas countries with traditionally strong cultural ties to Germany were responsive to racial hygiene, attempts to forge links with Germany's major rivals, France and Great Britain, could not take the strain of the deteriorating international situation. On his way to Algiers in 1909 (where he was to study paralysis), Rüdin recruited in France. The distinguished statistician, Jacques Bertillon, joined the Racial Hygiene Society, as did the paediatrician Eugène Apert, the anthropologist L. Manouvrier and three residents in Algeria. When a *société eugénique* was founded in 1912, Apert was the first secretary.[366] But the French were more concerned with positive health and pro-natalism than the Germans.

Ploetz expended much energy in securing recognition in England. He sought Galton's support as honorary member of the International Society. He translated an essay by Galton for the *Archiv*. He wrote to Galton on 17 August 1905: 'We take the highest interest in your eminent and important Eugenics', and solicited his 'cool judgement' of his 1895 book on racial hygiene.[367] Although the Eugenics Education Society (EES) was founded in 1907, contacts were slow to develop. The EES was impressed by the sexual reform writings by Forel and Bloch. In 1909 there was only one German member of the EES, and Ploetz's International Society had only one member in England (Galton) and one in Scotland (John Henry Koeppern who had joined in Freiburg). Concerned that Pearson was not a member of the EES, he wrote on 21 May 1909 for advice and informed him of the International Society, which he claimed had been in existence for four years. He foresaw two potential difficulties. He reassured him that the location of the society would be transferred to Holland or Switzerland. With regard to the name 'Rassen-Hygiene', he explained that this was more immediately intelligible to the common man than the foreign term, 'eugenics', but of course there was considerable overlap.

In July 1909, Ploetz offered Galton the presidency of the International Society which Galton (recently knighted) accepted.[368] Galton was well aware that he was backing a practical movement, when he wrote: 'I shall await with much interest the publication of the details showing *how* the more suitable 1/4th of the population are to be appraised. Of course there will be less *practical* difficulties in doing so, than in framing exact scales. More especially, it will be difficult to ensure uniformity in the action of the different examiners. Still I see no insuperable obstacle to a fairly good

[365] Lundborg papers, Ploetz to Lundborg, 14 September 1911. My thanks to Gunnar Broberg for copies of letters from Ploetz to Lundborg.
[366] Luschan papers, Ploetz to Luschan, 7 May 1909.   [367] Galton papers, III B 545–6.303/4.
[368] Ploetz papers, Ploetz to Galton, 18 July 1909, Galton to Ploetz, 22 July.

and very useful selection being made.' Pearson had greater doubts and warned Galton: 'I think Ploetz is a sound man, and keen on eugenics. I should not, however, allow his "International" Society to absorb yours as a branch, which he may suggest'.[369] British eugenicists remained suspicious of German cultural imperialism. German eugenicists like Kaup maintained that their society had a greater interest in medical and biological research and thus offered the prospect of effective medical legislation for eugenic ends.[370]

In June and July 1910 Ploetz visited England where he spent much time with Galton, Pearson and members of the EES like Montague Crackanthorpe and the Secretary, Mrs Gotto. Although the EES held a reception in honour of Ploetz on 27 June 1910, it responded cautiously to Ploetz's overtures. At the Dresden Hygiene Exhibition of 1911, Ploetz negotiated with Mrs Gotto and H. Barnes as EES representatives when the International Society for Racial Hygiene met on 5–7 August.[371] Swedes and Germans far outnumbered the EES delegation. In October 1911 the Council of the EES accepted that there should be some form of co-operation with the International Society, pending election of an International Eugenic Council at the International Congress on Race planned for 1912.[372] There was much distrust of Ploetz's International Society, both on a personal and nationalistic level. Ploetz objected to an International Committee, as it threatened to rival his International Society for Racial Hygiene. Leonard Darwin wrote as President of the First International Eugenics Congress that the work of eugenics societies had to be primarily national, and that the EES could be affiliated with (but not be a subordinate to) the Racial Hygiene Society. It was suggested that the Racial Hygiene Society might meet concurrently with the congress.[373]

Ploetz attended the International Congress on race in London during August 1912. He spoke on 'The Bearing of Neo-Malthusianism on Race Hygiene', Bluhm on 'Racial Hygiene and Gynaecology'. The thirty vice-presidents of the Congress included Forel, Gruber, Ploetz and Weismann. Honorary members included Schemann and the geologist General von Bardeleben. (That Winston Churchill was also a vice-president was to be a source of mirth to Nazi eugenicists). Gruber and Ploetz planned tactics to secure German scientific leadership of the eugenics movement. Gruber recommended that Ploetz first obtain Charles B. Davenport and the Americans as allies, and then with Swedish backing try to gain the confidence of the EES. It would be necessary to agree to changes in the statutes to accommodate the EES.[374] The background of international diplomatic tensions meant that relations between the British and Germans remained cool. In a gloomy letter to the *Berliner Tageblatt* Ploetz explained that the results of the congress were

[369] Galton papers, IIIA, pp. 388–9.
[370] I. Kaup, 'Ueber die eugenische Bewegung in England', *Concordia*, vol. 18 (1911), 359–65.
[371] Ploetz papers, Mrs Gotto to Ploetz, 16 June 1911.
[372] Ploetz papers, Gotto to Ploetz, 5 October 1911.
[373] Ploetz papers, Leonard Darwin to Ploetz, 23 November 1911.
[374] Ploetz papers, Gruber to Ploetz, nd.

that: (1) it refused to recognise the Dresden meeting of 1911 as the first international eugenics congress; (2) there was a public rift between Pearson and the EES; (3) Berlin was rejected as the next meeting place in three years' time, in favour of Paris and then San Francisco. Ploetz criticized the London congress as too dominated by women which meant that the discussions were too lay and general.[375]

The International Society for Racial Hygiene had to be content with being a constituent member of the International Eugenic Committee. Only the Swedes continued to accept German leadership. The French founded a national society in 1912 after the London Congress and thereafter adhered more to Anglo-American models. Unlike either the English or German societies, it was primarily a scientific forum.[376] On 3 August 1913 Ploetz met George Darwin and Mjöen in Paris for a sitting of the International Eugenic Committee. Ploetz again was defeated when he suggested a congress in Germany and the founding of an International Association for Racial Hygiene. He consoled himself by drinking brotherhood with Mjöen, who was an ardent Nordicist.[377]

Despite the growth in the Racial Hygiene Society's size, Ploetz attempted to preserve the intimacy of the early meetings. Walks and cycle tours were a regular feature of the first years of the society, because physical fitness was fundamental to the eugenic creed. In February 1912 the utopian Freiland group in Munich agreed to amalgamate with the Racial Hygiene Society. The Nordic racists Riemscheider, Schmilinsky and Wollny urged this. Following an archery session on 23 April, it was agreed on 4 May to establish a secret Nordic cabal in the society to be called *Der Bogen* (The Bow). It was convened by Sittmann, Wollny, Schmilinsky, Ploetz and his wife.[378] By 1913 there were about fifteen members, including Lenz and Lehmann, and a club house with a library and reading room.[379] In a letter to Gerhart Hauptmann, Ploetz explained that the bow symbolized Nordic vitality. It was necessary to recover the primitive vigour of the early Indo-Germanic race in order to strengthen the *Volk*. The club was an opportunity to put racial hygiene into practice.[380]

Racial hygiene was intended to be a personal creed of faith in the Nordic race and its physical and moral ideals, as well as a scientific movement. Ploetz divided his time between Nordic rites and science. It meant maintaining a scientific front with the result that Ploetz cultivated academics and physicians. Yet bubbling beneath the surface was a fiery Nordic idealism. Ploetz's diary was punctuated by references to personal declarations of anti-semitism by acquaintances, notes on who was Jewish or half-Jewish, and exploits demonstrating physical prowess. There were

---

[375] Eugenics Society Papers, CMAC Wellcome Institute Eug/A.83.

[376] W. Schneider, 'Toward the Improvement of the Human Race: The History of Eugenics in France', *Journal of Modern History*, vol. 54 (1982), 268–91.

[377] Ploetz papers, diary, 3 August 1913; *6th Annual Report of the Eugenics Education Society*.

[378] Ploetz papers, diary, 9, 16 October and 16 November 1912.

[379] Ploetz papers, diary, 23 January 1913.

[380] Gerhart Hauptmann papers, Ploetz to G. Hauptmann, 24 December 1913. My thanks to Wilfrid Ploetz for showing me the bows.

discussions of the 'Jewish problem' with Schmilinsky on 9 February 1907, and with Schallmayer and Sombart on 2 June 1913. Ploetz published notes in the *Archiv* on Jewish emigration from Galicia.[381] He acknowledged that anti-semitic organizations had aims consistent with racial hygiene. He cited as examples the *Deutschbund* (founded in 1894 for the 'purity of Aryan, Germanic blood'), and the *Deutsche Erneuerungsgemeinde* of the anti-semitic propagandist, Theodor Fritsch.[382] Yet Ploetz held racial hygiene, as an organized scientific society, aloof from the Gobineau Society of Schemann and from extreme racial ideologues. The balance between scientific technocracy and racial ideology was precarious in Ploetz's case. It worked as long as the Racial Hygiene Society was a growing organization and relevant to debates on health, the family and the birth rate. But the upheavals of the First World War resulted in conflicts among the eugenicists as tensions mounted between welfare-oriented social biology and Aryan racist nationalism.

[381] A. Ploetz, 'Die Ausbreitung der Polen nach Osten', *ARGB*, vol. 1 (1904), 476; and Ploetz papers, diary, 16 February 1905, 14 February 1908 (visit to G. Fritsch), 14 January 1912; Gerhart Hauptmann papers, Ploetz to Hauptmann, 11 May 1901. *ARGB*, vol. 1 (1904), 476.

[382] A. Ploetz, 'Gesellschaften mit Rassenhygienischen Zwecken', *ARGB*, vol. 6 (1909), 277–80, 577–8; vol. 10 (1913), 403–7.

3

From hygiene to family welfare

Hygiene and professional authority

Fresh air, pure water, clean streets, food free of impurities and personal cleanliness were hailed by German liberals as the basis of civilized society. It was debated whether these hygienic principles were best maintained by sanitary authorities, or by personal prosperity and education. There were divergent strategies of public health administration. Imperial Germany inherited both a well-developed system of medical police, and a liberalizing movement for medical reform. The medical police system was a relic of the 'enlightened absolutism' of the eighteenth century when a growing population was considered to be a means of strengthening state power. The state was to prolong life by control of infectious and epidemic diseases, to promote cleanliness and assume the role of guardian of public morality.[1] Alternative liberal strategies valued health as the product of economic and educational improvement.[2] During the mid nineteenth century, state intervention was resented. Measures such as quarantine and police inspection interfered with free trade and violated property rights. Fierce rivalry persisted between the movements for state medicine and the liberal medical reform movement.[3] Reformers saw improvements in medicine as a means of benefiting individual welfare. Positive health could be enhanced by physical exertion. Gymnastics and sport were favoured by the liberal nationalists. Exercise gave physical expression to liberal ideas of individual self-exertion. Health was a genre of personal moral reform. With roots in the bourgeois culture of the pre-1848 period, nature therapies gained immense popularity. Examples were the hydrotherapy of Vincenz Priessnitz and the macrobiotic therapies of the physician Christoph Wilhelm

---

[1] H. Eulenberg, *Das Medicinalwesen in Preussen* (Berlin, 1874).
[2] U. Frevert, *Krankheit als politisches Problem 1770–1880* (Göttingen, 1984).
[3] G. Rosen, *From Medical Police to Social Medicine* (New York, 1974); P.J. Weindling, 'Was Social Medicine Revolutionary? Virchow on Famine and Typhus in 1848', *Bulletin of the Society for the Social History of Medicine*, no. 34 (1984), 13–18.

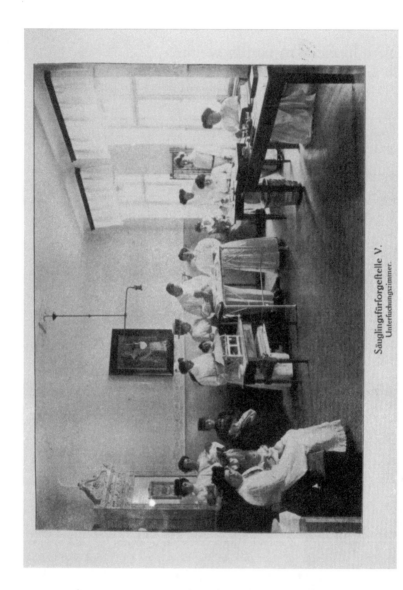

Säuglingsfürforgestelle V.
Unterfuchungszimmer.

3 'Infant Welfare Clinic 5'. Reproduced from *Die gesundheitliche Einrichtungen der königlichen Residenzstadt Charlottenburg. Festschrift gewidmet dem 3. internationalen Kongress für Säuglingsschutz im September 1911* (Berlin, 1911). The municipality of Charlottenburg pioneered model facilities for infant and child welfare. Adolf Gottstein took a leading role as the medical officer in organizing child health care measures. In 1919 Gottstein became Prussian Ministerial Director of the Department of Health.

Hufeland. Health care was provided for the poor in the form of policlinics and dispensaries.[4]

The 1848 Revolution unleashed a movement of medical reform which challenged state control and demanded that a doctor direct a national ministry of health. Rudolf Virchow campaigned for an autonomous medical profession, and for the removal of state controls on medicine. In public health he emphasized the need for municipal improvements in sewerage and drainage. Liberal values were combined with chemistry, physiology and technology in a new science of hygiene. The *Handbook of Hygiene* of Friedrich Oesterlen developed a utilitarian analysis of environmental causes of disease.[5] When in 1855 Max Pettenkofer, a Munich chemist, replaced lectures on 'medical police' by lectures on 'hygiene', this showed how science would replace the policing element with public health. This marked a transfer of authority from the state to the professional academic sphere. Pettenkofer was appointed to the first university chair of hygiene in 1865 and established the first hygiene institute in 1879. He justified scientific hygiene in economic terms (calculating costs of loss of work days) and referred to hygiene as 'the economy of health' (*Gesundwirtschaftslehre*). He assumed that economic progress would improve health. He investigated clothing, housing, heating and diet.[6] Following Liebig's demonstration of the high nutritional value of meat extract, he joined Liebig in a partnership and established a factory at Fray-Bentos in Argentina during 1865. His liberalism encouraged features such as municipal improvements, civic welfare associations ('a city must consider itself a family'), and education for the purpose of improving health.[7] Decentralization and individualization were the slogans of the 1850s and 60s.

It was in such a liberal spirit that in 1873 a National Society for Public Health was established as an offshoot of the German Association of Scientists and Doctors. Local public health societies were founded in industrializing regions such as the Ruhr. The liberal faith in economic improvement was reflected in the strong representation by engineers, builders and experts on water supply and sewers. Technology and health care were seen as closely allied. An introduction to the society's journal by Carl Reclam, a liberal-minded Leipzig police doctor, depicted the role of public health as raising the productive capacity or *Leistungsfähigkeit* of the individual and of the state. Reclam's emphasis was on self-government and the development of local authorities of which he regarded those in England as the most advanced. Professionalism was to be combined with reformist ideas by extending public health services.[8] To uphold public morals, Reclam favoured extension of

[4] A. Labisch, ' "Hygiene ist Moral – Moral ist Hygiene" – Soziale Disziplinierung durch Ärzte und Medizin', in C. Sachsse and F. Tennstedt (eds.), *Soziale Sicherheit und soziale Disziplinierung* (Frankfurt-on-Main, 1986), pp. 265–85.

[5] F. Oesterlen, *Handbuch der Hygieine der privaten und öffentlichen* (Tübingen, 1851).

[6] H. Breyer, *Max von Pettenkofer* (Leipzig, 1980).

[7] Max von Pettenkofer, *The Value of Health to a City. Two Lectures Delivered in 1873* (Baltimore, 1941).

[8] C. Reclam, 'Die heutige Gesundheitspflege und ihre Aufgaben', *Deutsche Vierteljahrsschrift für öffentliche Gesundheitspflege*, vol. 1 (1869), 1–5. The journal was published by the GDNA.

medical and policing powers by such means as supervising prostitutes and enforcing compulsory membership of a sickness fund.[9] Liberalism retained authoritarian elements. The next eighty years would see a shift of emphasis in medicine away from the individual to such collectivities as society and the race.

The liberal vision of hygiene was challenged in the 1880s. Instead of health being assessed in individualist economic terms as a worker's most valuable personal capital, the idea of a healthy society was postulated as a means of social integration. The liberal belief in the individual's responsibility for personal health became reformulated in collectivist terms of the health of the family and of future generations. Bismarck's sickness insurance system, inaugurated in 1883, was developed from the principle that economic gain was a way of securing resources in the event of future misfortune. Medical care was provided for the insured individual worker (but not for family dependents). Workers became a clientele for the expanding medical profession. While state legislation designated those categories of workers who were to be insured, the sickness insurance funds were to remain autonomous bodies. Workers and employers were represented on insurance funds, and there was an external state supervisory authority. Sickness insurance was organized on corporate principles: the medical profession was to be represented by a professional body, the *Ärztekammer*, and insurance funds became powerful vested interests in their own right. Once the SPD was restored to legality in 1891, socialists gained a sphere of influence as health administrators for sickness insurances. They arranged for additional benefits to be paid to workers and their families, and supported the development of social hygiene and preventive medicine. The medical profession mobilized against schemes for the socialization of health services, and the fear arose that the chronically sick represented a costly burden to the fit and healthy.

Bacteriology and the state

A challenge was posed to liberal values by the science of bacteriology as the means of overcoming the social miseries of industrial and urban society. There was official support and public enthusiasm for the promotion of scientific therapies and preventive medicine. These offered attractive alternatives to the political complexities of social reform. This technocratic strategy of medical science as a solution to social problems was grounded on the hope of rapid scientific advance in bacteriology during the 1880s. These hopes were not unrealistic. Robert Koch's 'germ theory' of disease postulated that each disease had a specific cause in a pathogenic micro-organism. His techniques for growing organisms in pure cultures meant that pathogenic organisms could be isolated, and that experimental proof could be supplied for their causal effects when the organisms were injected into healthy animals. Methods of microscopic observation developed by

---

[9] C. Reclam, 'Die Ueberwachung der Prostitution', *Deutsche Vierteljahrsschrift für öffentliche Gesundheitspflege*, vol. 1 (1869), 379–95.

Darwinian biologists for the observation of the simplest of organisms, *Protozoa* as the 'germs of life', were also helpful in the study of bacteria. Between 1873 and 1900 the causal organisms of a great number of the bacterial diseases were isolated. Koch's discoveries of the anthrax bacillus in 1876 and of the tuberculosis bacillus in 1882 initiated a wave of discoveries using his method of cultivating pure bacterial strains. Koch's assistants, Friedrich Loeffler and Georg Gaffky, proved how diphtheria and typhoid were caused by pathogenic bacilli in 1884. The typhoid bacillus was discovered by Carl Eberth in 1880 before being cultured by Gaffky, and the diphtheria bacillus was first observed by another researcher, Klebs, in 1883 before being cultured by Koch's assistant Loeffler. These illustrate how the discoveries of the 'Koch school' were the result of applying standard methods of cultivation and replication in order to supply experimental 'proof'. Occasionally the expectation of a discovery led to mistaken conclusions, as when Koch's assistant, Richard Pfeiffer, claimed to have discovered a bacterial cause for influenza in 1892. However, most of the discoveries of pathogenic bacteria occurred in Germany, or were by German trained researchers (see table 4).[10]

Despite the priority claims of Louis Pasteur, many successful Pasteurians such as Emile Roux and Alexandre Yersin deployed methods derived from bacteriology in Germany. Koch proved the supremacy of his biological understanding of bacteria when he discovered the 'comma bacillus' as the 'cause' of cholera in Egypt in 1884, in competition with a French team of researchers.[11] Many foreigners worked in Koch's Institute, such as the Japanese researcher Shibasaburo Kitasato who discovered the tetanus and plague bacilli. German methods of research on pure cultures were supreme in this period.[12]

Underlying advances in microbiology was the development of the precision optical industry, capable of mass-producing good quality but inexpensive microscopes. These became generally available to students and individual practitioners, and large numbers were supplied to the new public health laboratories. English microscopes were produced by craft methods with lenses ground by hand, and so were only affordable by the well-to-do amateur. Prussia invested in glass production of Schott at Jena, developing mass-produced glass of high quality without such optical distortions as the chromatic aberration.[13] Technical problems were overcome by the entry of scientists such as the Jena professor of physics, Ernst Abbe, into industry. By the 1890s, the Germans had developed microscopes with apochromatic and oil immersion lenses of outstanding optical qualities. The precision optics industry was sustained by the medical and natural sciences, and increasingly by military demands.[14] The artificial dye-stuffs industry provided stains which were used as colouring agents to identify bacteria

[10] Table 4 compiled from W. Bulloch, *The History of Bacteriology* (London, 1938), pp. 236–8.
[11] W. Coleman, 'Koch's Comma Bacillus: The First Year', *Bulletin of the History of Medicine*, vol. 61 (1987), 315–42.   [12] B. Möllers, *Robert Koch* (Hanover, 1950).
[13] S. Bradbury, *The Evolution of the Microscope* (Oxford, 1967), pp. 204–56.
[14] F. Auerbach, *Ernst Abbe* (Leipzig, 1922).

Table 4. *Discoveries in bacteriology*

Year	Discovery	Medical Researcher	Town/City	Nationality
1873	relapsing fever	Obermeier	Berlin	German
1876	anthrax	Koch	Wollstein	German
1879	gonococcus	Neisser	Breslau	German
1880	lepra	Hansen	Bergen	Norwegian
1882	tuberculosis	Koch	Berlin	German
	glanders	Loeffler/Schütz	Berlin	German
1884	cholera	Koch	Calcutta	German
	diphtheria	Loeffler	Berlin	German
	(diphtheria bacillus observed 1883)	(Klebs)	(Zürich)	(German)
	(typhoid bacillus observed)	(Eberth)	(Halle)	(German)
	staphylococcus and streptococcus isolated	Rosenbach	Göttingen	German
1885	proof that Neisser's gonococcus caused gonorrhoea	Bumm	Würzburg	German
	bacterium coli commune	Escherich	Munich	German
1886	pneumonia	A. Fränkel	Berlin	German
1887	malta fever	Bruce	Malta	British
	meningococcus	Weichselbaum	Vienna	Austrian
1889	tetanus isolated	Kitasato	Berlin	Japanese
	(tetanus bacillus observed by Nicolaier, 1884)			
1891	actinomycosis	Wolff/Israel	Berlin	German
1894	plague	Kitasato and Yersin	Canton Hong Kong	Japanese Swiss
1896	micrococcus catarrhalis	R. Pfeiffer	Berlin	German
1897	botulism	van Ermengem	Ghent	Belgian
1898	dysentry	Shiga (assistant to Kitasato)		Japanese
1900	paratyphoid	Schottmüller	Hamburg	German

and cellular constituents. Most of the aniline colouring agents were introduced by Paul Ehrlich for observation of tissues and minute organisms. His experimenting with stains led him to appreciate the therapeutic potential of dye-stuffs in their action on cellular constituents for promoting mechanisms of immunity. It paved the way to pharmaceutical research and production. Bacteriological techniques were a spin-off from industrialization.

When the Imperial Health Office[15] was founded in 1876, Pettenkofer was offered the post of director, the office being a supervisory and statistical agency designed to monitor rather than intervene in public health. This liberal policy changed with the rise of bacteriology. In 1879 laboratories for chemistry and hygiene were established, to which Koch was appointed in 1880. Military intervention accompanied the scientization of hygiene. The Prussian War Ministry paid for Koch to act as a veterinary inspector and ordered military medical officers to act as Koch's assistants. This ensured that as bacteriology invaded public health those in the forefront of research and administration had strong military ties. Military doctors taught courses in bacteriology for medical officers, and the Prussian medical department came to have a number of ex-military medical officers in leading positions, as when Martin Kirchner was appointed *Ministerialdirektor*.[16] The education official Friedrich Althoff and the Prussian Minister of Culture, Gustav von Gossler, were staunch supporters of the new experimental medicine. In the 1880s and 90s they defended animal experiments on behalf of German physiologists in the Reichstag. They cultivated good relations with Koch, Behring and Ehrlich, and established scientific chairs and research institutes. They hoped that hygiene would win German science and medicine international acclaim, and solve problems of public health. They overcame Virchow's resistance to chairs of hygiene when Virchow, a conservative in professional matters, joined forces with the conservative parties in 1884 and 1889 to oppose their foundation.[17] The authorities envisaged a Germany covered by a network of university and state hygiene institutes responsible for monitoring the natural and urban environment and for providing early warning of epidemics.

Bacteriologists allied with state and military authorities to challenge both Pettenkofer's liberal programme of hygiene and Virchow's cellular pathology. Many pathologists deserted the cellular study of organs and disease forms, and were among the first to lecture on bacteriology during the 1880s. From this time hygiene can be seen as divided between the physiological, chemical and sanitary approaches of Pettenkofer and the bacteriological methods of Koch. The divide between the municipally oriented Pettenkofer school and the state technocrats of the Koch school reflected the earlier divisions between liberal medical reform and state-oriented medical police. The rift was most pronounced in Prussia; other states balanced the two approaches. Most Prussian bacteriologists appointed to university

---

[15] *Reichsgesundheitsamt.*   [16] Möllers, *Koch*, pp. 130–3.
[17] N. Andernach, *Der Einfluss der Parteien auf das Hochschulwesen in Preussen* (Göttingen, 1972), pp. 147–9.

chairs between 1887 and 1900 had a military or naval background: von Esmarch's father was a military doctor, related to the Kaiser; Loeffler had military training and his father was a leading army doctor; Behring was seconded by the army to Koch's laboratory. While Koch and Fraenkel had non-military backgrounds, there were many points of contact with military authorities as a result of Koch's early researches on wound infections in 1878. The pattern of military education was repeated throughout Germany. For example, August Gärtner, the professor of hygiene at Jena, had military and naval experience before he was seconded to work with Koch. In addition to the universal experience of military service, many doctors and medical officers retained a rank as reserve officers. This meant that medical science and public health services could be moblized for military purposes. Ten professorial appointments were made between 1887 and 1900 in Germany of hygienists who had been trained either at Pettenkofer's institute or by the Munich physiologist Carl Voit.[18] While continuing to work on housing, ventilation and nutrition, some such as Hans Buchner and Flügge became adepts at bacteriology.[19] The intensity of the rift between the bacteriological and sanitary approaches can be illustrated by Koch's unpopularity while professor of hygiene at Berlin; when he resigned to take up an appointment at the Institute for Infectious Diseases in 1891, there was a switch to the Pettenkofer-Voit school with the appointment of Rubner, whose studies of the human metabolism introduced the concept of calories. The balance was restored when the bacteriologist Buchner succeeded Pettenkofer in Munich in 1894. Although Saxon public health institutions in Dresden and Leipzig were directed by Pettenkofer's pupils, Georg Friedrich Renk and Franz Hofmann, bacteriological laboratories were established in the early 1890s.[20] Certain bacteriologists became medical officers, one example being August Pfeiffer, a pupil of Koch and Flügge in Wiesbaden. The next generation of professors endeavoured to develop a science of hygiene as a biologically based synthesis of the physiological and bacteriological approaches. As a result there were competing strategies of social and racial hygiene, with social hygiene drawing on the environmentalist approach of Pettenkofer, and racial hygiene substituting hereditary biology for bacteriology.

Darwinian concerns with micro-organisms led to simultaneous advances in cell biology and bacteriology that were to lay the foundations for understanding of the immune defence systems of the body cells. When fertilization as fusion of cell nuclei and chromosomes was first observed by zoologists during 1875–6, Koch was conducting his observations on anthrax bacilli. First to appreciate Koch's work was a group of biologists and medical researchers in Breslau which included Cohn,

---

[18] Buchner, Flügge, Rubner, Ludwig Pfeiffer, Wilhelm Prausnitz, Dittmar Finkler, Gustav Wolffhügel, Karl B. Lehmann (brother of J.F. Lehmann), Renk and Joseph Forster.

[19] H.-H. Eulner, 'Hygiene als akademisches Fach', W. Artelt, *et al.* (eds.), *Städte, Wohnungs- und Kleidungshygiene des 19. Jahrhunderts in Deutschland* (Stuttgart, 1968), pp. 17–33.

[20] D. Tutzke, 'Das Sächsische Medizinalwesen um die Wende vom 19. zum 20. Jahrhundert', *Zeitschrift für die gesamte Hygiene*, vol. 29 (1983), 556–9.

Weigert and the young Ehrlich. Taxonomic classification of micro-organisms was an essential prerequisite for bacteriology, and Koch continued to work with the histological and microscopical methods of botanists and zoologists. Added to this was an experimental flair, necessary to prove that a particular species of micro-organism was indeed the causal agent of a disease. When during the 1880s an experimental approach became prevalent in the German life sciences, such as in embryology and neuro-physiology, medical scientists, and especially bacteriologists, became imbued with a conviction of their right to undertake animal and human experiments.

Technocratic medicine

The bacteriologists' scientistic perception of disease was accompanied by authoritarian political overtones. Virchow's influential classification of diseases was localist, and based on symptoms in the affected part of the body. Koch classified according to the causal agent. Before Koch's inauguration of germ theory, diseases were classified according to the locality in the body where they occurred. This corresponded to the localism of political liberalism. Different forms of tuberculosis were diagnosed as lupus of the skin, meningitis or hydrocephalus of the brain, scrofula of the glands, special diseases of the bones and joints, and phthisis or consumption of the lungs. Koch's discovery of the TB bacillus unified all these different forms as 'tuberculosis'. In 1890 he was pressurized by von Gossler, the Prussian *Kultusminister*, to make the sensational claim that he had developed a cure for TB, the injection of a glycerin extract which he called 'tuberculin'. Although then a therapeutic disappointment, it was recognized during the early twentieth century as a successful diagnostic test.[21] When it was revealed that 95 per cent of the population had traces of TB, the need for medical surveillance was established. Not only was TB a recently unified disease entity, it was virtually universally present. As comprehensive programmes of welfare and preventive medicine were necessary, bacteriology greatly enhanced the scope of state and professional responsibilities.

The germ theory opened the way to technocratic strategies for the control and cure of diseases. In 1890 there were plans to manufacture tuberculin as a state monopoly. In January 1891 it was suggested that Koch should vest the remedy *in der Hand des Königs*, and receive an annuity in return. (Such a royal monopoly would have resurrected the medieval tradition of the royal touch for scrofula.) Instead, Koch preferred to work directly with the aniline dye manufacturers, Hoechst, and arranged for special treatment centres. He obtained 150 beds at the Berlin municipal hospital of Moabit in 1890. A special hospital for tuberculin therapy was proposed by the Berlin *Magistrat* at Malchow. When the *Institut*

---

[21] The diagnostic use of tuberculin as a sub-cutaneous reaction was established by Clemens von Pirquet in 1907.

Pasteur was founded in 1888 as an institute purely for medical research, Prussia emulated this by establishing the Institute for Infectious Diseases for Koch.[22] Not only was an isolation barracks for tubercular patients included but the state co-operated with the Berlin city council for provision of joint facilities for clinical research at the planned fourth municipal hospital. This strategy of co-ordinating scientific, state and municipal facilities was to prove controversial.

Behring's discovery of a blood serum therapy for diphtheria in 1891 provided additional justification for expanding facilities for scientific therapies. The medical technology of serum and other injected therapies replaced the necessity for sanitary and welfare improvements. Behring's serum therapy confirmed that bacteriologists were at the forefront of developing laboratory-based therapies. In 1893 Behring launched a powerful attack on Virchow's view of social medicine and on his political liberalism. He argued that his view of contagious or 'catching' diseases spreading like a forest fire was in keeping with folk beliefs. By contrast, Virchow's environmentalist view was an artificial result of excessive rationalism. Whereas Virchow's recipe for preventive medicine was democracy and economic improvement, Behring argued that all that was needed was control of the infective organism. There was, however, a tension in the laboratory therapies between Behring's populist appeal, and a de-politicized view of public health that would result in a racial ideology attached to purity of blood, and a technical laboratory-based strategy of serum therapies and immunization.[23] In 1893, publicity campaigns instigated by newspaper publishers such as Mosse rallied the public into making donations for the treatment of poor children with a curative serum. For anti-TB measures, the state intervened in a strategy that linked public concern with well-publicized medical discoveries. Radicals feared that plans for a municipal health office would be jeopardized by Koch's Institute for Infectious Diseases.[24] The technocratic strategy for control of disease was an attractive option to military and state authorities.

TB and municipal resistance

While the localist and topographical approaches to epidemics were under attack from the bacteriologists, concern over tuberculosis provided an incentive for the development of municipal welfare institutions and for municipal planning regulations. Air, light and space became the priorities of architects, municipal officials and public health experts. This led to an intensification of the movement for environmental reform, to planning controls on housing densities, and, finally to intervention in the home and family life. It was best seen in the garden city

---

[22] *Institut für Infektionskrankheiten.*
[23] E. Behring, *Gesammelte Abhandlungen zur ätiologischen Therapie von ansteckenden Krankheiten* (Leipzig, 1893), pp. xix–xx.
[24] M. Stürzbecher, 'Rudolf Virchow: Über bakteriologische Untersuchungsinstitute (1896)', *Bundesgesundheitsblatt*, (1973), 306–9.

movement from the 1880s. Only few plans for garden cities or suburbs came to fruition; but there was awareness of the need for public amenities and planning regulations to control housing densities. Civic improvements were reinforced by a medical rationale. Parks were the 'lungs of the city'. Sports grounds, holiday colonies, swimming pools and public baths were provided by municipalities, philanthropists and philanthropic associations.[25] Housing surveys, *Wohnungs-Enquête*, linked TB to poor ventilation, damp and over-crowding, and emphasized the immorality and bad health associated with the renting out of beds on a shift basis. Under the rubric of *Wohnungshygiene* the concerns of public health experts and other reformers with aesthetic and socio-political motives were again amalgamated.[26]

Municipal amenities were intended to inculcate civic and national pride as well as to promote health. But their introduction was controversial. The case of Berlin illustrates tensions between the state policing authorities of the *Magistrat*, and the civic representatives. These tensions were evident in the controversy over tuberculin therapy. During the 1880s there had been pressure on municipal hospitals and welfare institutions. In 1888 the municipal health committee[27] discussed the establishment of a special 400-bed hospital[28] for pulmonary diseases. There was division of opinion between those public health officials who regarded the hospital as an urgent necessity, and others who maintained that cross-infection would result in excessive deaths. Demands for 'special hospitals' for pulmonary diseases became widespread. These were modelled on a scheme by Peter Dettweiler (a pupil of the politically radical Hermann Brehmer, the initiator of fresh air and nutritional treatment for TB), who opened a *Curanstalt* at Falkenstein in 1876, and the first public sanatorium or *Volksheilstätte* nearby in 1892. Hydrotherapy, nutritional and fresh air treatments were used, and the sanatorium was supported by an association for convalescents[29] and the municipality of Frankfurt-on-Main.[30] He popularized the idea of free public hospitals.[31] Ernst Leyden, professor of internal medicine in Berlin, gave prestigious support for sanatoria in 1889. Leyden's proposal resulted in a committee of Berlin doctors for establishing sanatoria, and his lecture at the International Medical Congress held that year proclaimed TB as curable with fresh air, good nutrition and moderate exercise. Berlin saw competing strategies of cure and prevention backed by the Reich, Prussia, and the municipality with its own internal divisions.

---

[25] 'James Simon, Industrialist, Art Collector and Philanthropist', *Leo Baeck Institute Yearbook*, vol. 10 (1965), 3–28.
[26] G. Asmus (ed.), *Hinterhof, Keller, und Mansarde. Einblicke in Berliner Wohnungselend 1901–1920* (Reinbek bei Hamburg, 1982).   [27] *städtische Deputation für Gesundheitspflege in Berlin.*
[28] *Heil- und Pflegeanstalt.*   [29] *Verein für Reconvalescentenanstalten.*
[30] H. Wasserfuhr, 'Aerztliche Gesichtspunkte bei Errichtung von Heilstätten für unbemittelte Brustkranke', *DMW*, (1892), 952–3; P. Dettweiler, 'Mitteilungen über die erste deutsche Volksheilstätte für unbemittelte Lungenkranke in Falkenstein i. T.', *DMW*, (1892) 1098–9.
[31] P. Dettweiler, 'Die Therapie der Phthise', *Kongress für innere Medizin* (Wiesbaden, 1887), VI, pp. 13–43.

The sharp antithesis between Koch's tuberculin therapy and advocates of a modified form of nature therapy in 1890 polarized opinions on municipal initiatives. The Malchow scheme for a tuberculin hospital provoked opposition from noted liberals such as Virchow and socialist advocates like Zadek of a public sanatorium. A *Volksheilstätte* in 1891 at Blankenfelde for *brustkranke Frauen* was due to the initiative of the trade union sponsored *Gewerks-Kranken-Verein*. When on 10 February 1891 Malchow was suggested by the *Magistrat* as a centre for tuberculin therapy, the proposal was resisted. The municipality wished to remain master of its house.[32] Instead, the demand arose that the institution be used as a general convalescent home for 'incurable' tuberculous patients from municipal hospitals, and not just for tuberculin therapy. The liberal position of the surgeon, Ernst von Bergmann, and of Virchow was that grouping the tubercular together would increase the risk of infection, and that a monopoly of Koch's tuberculin therapy was objectionable. The proposal outraged the *Gewerks-Kranken-Verein*, which refused to refer patients. The socialist doctor Zadek demanded a public sanatorium with natural methods of treatment on Dettweiler's model. Virchow was as critical of the socialist nature therapy as of Koch's 'injection-therapy'. Between 1891 and 1897 the Berlin municipal committee for tuberculosis continued to be a battleground between Virchow, Zadek and the Koch school.[33]

There was a growing lobby within the SPD advocating hospital expansion and free hospital care. Popular perceptions were that hospitals were disliked as workhouses, or, as with the boycott of the Charité state hospital during 1893, for their military discipline. But party policy was falling into the hands of technocratic experts, who placed faith in medical science. Bebel had welcomed the establishment of a state agency that could monitor deteriorating health conditions, although he hoped that it would have stronger powers in formulating legislation.[34] There was a small but influential lobby of socialist doctors, who reinforced a faith in scientific socialism with positive medical science. The Workers' Health Commission (*Arbeitersanitätskommission*), instigated by Zadek, was an autonomous socialist medical organization.[35] Its strategy of self-help gave way to collective organization directed by professionals. Hospital care was gaining in favour among leading socialists. Althoff regarded socialist pressure for modernization of hospitals as a convenient lever for raising money from official sources for state hospital expansion.[36] The sanatoria offered an ideal type of sanitized environment, where diet and other amenities were adequate. The surveys of housing and working

---

[32] 'Herr im eigenen Hause'.

[33] Stadtarchiv Berlin Rep 00/967 Verwaltungsbericht des Magistrats zu Berlin Nr xvii, Verwaltungsbericht über die Städtischen Heimstätten für Genesende 1887–1914; Rep 00/1969 Die Heimstätten für Genesende 1887–1900.

[34] A.B. (= August Bebel), 'Das Reichs-Gesundheitsamt und sein Programm vom sozialistischen Standpunkt beleuchtet', *Die Zukunft*, vol. 1 (1878), 369–83.

[35] A. Labisch, 'Selbsthilfe zwischen Auflehnung und Anpassung: Arbeitersanitätskommission und Arbeiter-Samariterbund', *Argument-Sonderband*, vol. 77 (1983), 11–26.

[36] Tennstedt, 'Alfred Blaschko', p. 604.

conditions can be seen as extending the interventionist collectivism of medical reformers into the domestic environment. The socialist administrator of the *Berliner Ortskrankenkasse*, Albert Kohn, sponsored surveys of housing and domestic living conditions, and made pioneering use of photography to show the lack of bedding, overcrowding, damp and lack of ventilation. All these factors were regarded as part of the aetiology of TB.[37] Ironically, the more socialists used urban disease as an indictment of social conditions, the more dependent they became on scientific and professionalized medicine.

War on germs

The alignment of bacteriologists with a militaristic state was reflected in the use of military analogies in observations on bacteria. In order to boost the public and professional image of bacteriology, Koch described how hordes of alien parasites invaded the body;[38] organisms were referred to as 'cell states', and as having defence mechanisms of 'antibodies'; with chemotherapy came the popular metaphor of drugs as 'magic bullets'. Bacteriology was glamorized with the comparison of laboratory researchers to soldiers in a battle against disease. Experimental methods were hazardous, and there were casualties among researchers. It was argued that medical research should be placed above the ethical codes of civil life. The image which bacteriologists cultivated was that of a 'warrior against disease'. The racial anthropologist, Ammon, glorified the doctor as a Germanic warrior. He classified the Aryan longhead as prepared to risk death and to work for a poor financial reward in order to attain a higher ideal. The scientificity of bacteriology boosted the social prestige of medical research. Medicine was to be based on scientific bacteriology and serum therapy. The German doctor was portrayed as slaying the alien beast of quackery, ignorance and evil. The spectacular advances in bacteriology during the 1880s and 90s greatly enhanced the public prestige of laboratory science. There was widespread adulation of Koch: thousands of handkerchiefs on which his face was embroidered were sold.

Bacteriology impressed Ploetz and his circle. Koch had early links to Cohn at the University of Breslau. Ploetz hero-worshipped this founding father of bacteriology and he hoped that his own discoveries on human heredity would make a sensational impact. As a student, Ploetz excitedly observed the recently discovered TB and cholera bacilli.[39] The Zürich circle included the bacteriologists Elias Tomarkin and Simon (the latter of whom was to die from septicaemia contracted while researching on a serum therapy for scarlet fever). When Koch's tuberculin became available, Ploetz wanted to obtain the 'Berlin lymph' for use in his recently opened Springfield practice.[40] Bacteriology and experimental biology inspired the

[37] Asmus, *Hinterhof*, pp. 45–222.   [38] *Scharen.*
[39] Gerhart Hauptmann papers, Ploetz to Hauptmann, 13 July 1885.
[40] Forel papers, Ploetz to Forel, 20 December 1890.

hope that degenerate germplasms could be located and prevented from reproducing. Just as pathogenic bacteria could be isolated, so it was hoped that the germs of psychopathic mental illness, criminality and feeble-mindedness could also be isolated.

While eugenicists admired bacteriology, they were divided over the benefits of therapy. Schallmayer criticized progress in individual therapy as enabling the degenerate to survive. Eugenicists regarded the TB bacillus as 'the friend of the race' in that it eliminated the unfit.[41] Yet others were concerned to maintain a humane balance between individual welfare, and racial priorities. They foresaw a eugenic role for such welfare institutions as the sanatoria that proliferated in Germany after 1890. Such institutions were a means of 'humane' custodial detention of the sick, so isolating the degenerate from the fit, and preventing reproduction. Racial hygiene first gained public acceptance in welfare organizations for the prevention of chronic diseases and the high rates of infant mortality.

Human experiments

Advances in bacteriology and serum therapy encountered serious opposition from among the medical profession and also from the public who were disappointed that the miracle cures promised by bacteriologists in the early 1890s had not materialized. Medical opinion objected to the over-simplification of the causes and course of diseases. Virchow criticized Koch's bacteriology as not being able to explain why a single bacteria could produce so many different forms of a disease. Virchow's localist pathology corresponded to his support for local initiatives in public health. He was convinced that diseases were spread by poor industrial and urban living conditions, whereas bacteriologists emphasized infection and contagion. Virchow condemned bacteriologists in the Prussian Assembly as 'poisoners and murderers' for their excessive use of animal experiments.

Powerful attacks were mounted on the ethics of experimental medicine. The anti-vivisectionist campaign was extended from opposition to the mass slaughter of animals in laboratories to opposition to human experiments. The first successes of the anti-vivisectionists during the 1870s had been based on an appeal to a morally superior elite. The agitation of Ernst von Weber against 'the torture chambers of science' impressed Wagner's Bayreuth circle.[42] That Weber was also an advocate of colonialism suggests that the crisis during the 1870s, which saw the emergence of demands for colonies, produced conflicting attitudes to science. Whereas Weber initially relied on support from notables (including Bismarck's wife) for an international movement, by the 1890s the anti-vivisectionists broadened their social basis of support. Campaigners like Paul Förster (the brother of Bernhard Förster, and also an anti-semitic leader) sought to mobilize popular support for

---

[41] The phrase comes from the physiologist John Berry Haycraft.
[42] E. v. Weber, *Die Folterkammern der Wissenschaft* (Berlin and Leipzig, 1879).

agitation against animal experiments. He successfully allied anti-vivisection with other campaigns such as those for nature therapy, vegetarianism and anti-vaccination and anti-semitism. Doctors were criticized for treating the poor in hospitals as no better than laboratory guinea pigs. Other vulnerable groups were children and the mentally ill. Doctors in the colonies became notorious for experimenting on native peoples, especially in the concentration camps where sufferers from sleeping sickness epidemics were herded. Scientific medicine became stigmatized as inhumane.[43] The attack on medical science was spearheaded during the 1890s by socialist newspapers, anti-vivisectionists and nature therapists, many of whom combed the medical press for evidence of scientific atrocities. Besides bacteriology, experiments in other surgical and physiological areas were condemned.[44] Examples were the transplantation of cancerous tissue, the deliberate implanting of worms in children, and the injecting of gonococci for the study of the resulting inflammation. The state was criticized for lack of controls on experiments and for the failure to invoke legislation against assault resulting from medical malpractice.[45]

A classic example of protests against human experiments was the row over the research by the dermatologist Neisser who in 1879 had identified the gonococcus as the cause of gonorrhoea. In 1895, inspired by Behring's successes with anti-diphtheria sera, he injected young prostitutes (the youngest aged ten) with a cell-free syphilis serum in the hope that this would provide immunity. Instead, the effect was to infect some with syphilis. In 1898 a scandal erupted over these experiments.[46] Medical colleagues such as the dermatologist Blaschko and the medical historian Julius Pagel rallied to Neisser's aid, as did state officials such as Althoff to whom Neisser owed his appointment.[47] As had been the case with animal experiments, professors were confident that the state would approve of their work. Althoff and his medical advisers were a significant lobby in support of the extension of clinical research. In the event, Neisser received only a formal censure from the state. Henceforth, he used Java apes for experiments on a state-funded expedition. In 1905 he was one of the first to observe the syphilis spirochete, and with August von Wassermann he developed a diagnostic test for syphilis based on analysis of blood serum. Neisser's prestigious supporters in the medical profession and public health administration argued that a certain amount of sacrifice was justified to maintain the forward march of science.[48]

43 H. Bretschneider, *Der Streit um die Vivisektion im 19. Jahrhundert* (Stuttgart, 1962); U. Tröhler and A.-H. Maehle, 'Anti-vivisection in Nineteenth-century Germany and Switzerland: Motives and Methods', in N. Rupke (ed.), *Vivisection in Historical Perspective* (London, 1987), pp. 149–87.
44 'Arme Leute in Krankenhäusern', *Münchner Freie Presse* (1 October 1898); *Haus der Abgeordneten* (11 March 1899).
45 ZSTA M Rep 76 Va Sekt 1 Tit X Bd 1 ärztliche Versuche an Menschen 1898–1900.
46 'Arme Leute in Krankenhäusern', *Vorwärts* (3 February 1899).
47 Althoff, in *Haus der Abgeordneten* (6 March 1900).
48 ZSTA M Rep 76 Va Sekt 1 Tit X Bd 1; B. Elkeles, 'Medizinische Menschenversuche gegen Ende des 19. Jahrhunderts und der Fall Neisser', *Medizinhistorisches Journal*, vol. 20 (1985), 135–48.

Darwinism and bacteriology transferred problems of health from the geographical and social environment to the microscopic levels of germs. The achievements of bacteriology impressed the public, which rapidly contracted 'bacteria phobia', and generally enhanced the authority of scientific medicine. There was a borrowing of medical imagery by anti-semitic extremists. This was evident in phrases such as 'the Jewish bacillus' which became a stock-in-trade slogan of anti-semites. Serum therapy raised the issue of purity of blood which could also be popularized by ideologists of racial purity. Attacks were made on the 'judaification of medicine'. The mentality of science was depicted as a calculating and materialist product of 'Jewish science'.[49] That Neisser was Jewish meant that veteran anti-semites such as Paul Förster were venomous in their denunciations of medical research. Förster's attempt to gain popular support against the cruelties of Jewish experimental medicine, which he attacked as the product of 'Jewish rationalism', shows how medical nationalists wished to appropriate the popular concern with health for anti-semitic campaigns. Anti-semites were divided in their reactions to bacteriology with Ammon typifying adulation of German science, and Förster abominating science as bourgeois and liberal. While the racial mythologizing of bacteriology was a concern only of fringe groups, scientists gave serious thought to problems of the inheritance of defence systems of immunity, and to relations between the inherited germplasm and diseases. Efforts began to be made to fuse the science of hygiene with hereditarian biology.

RACIAL POISONS

The disputes over the efficacy of tuberculosis and serum therapies shook confidence in the adequacy of bacteriology as a means of solving the problems of the nation's health. Even though infectious diseases such as cholera, typhus and typhoid were on the decline, there was alarm at widespread sickness and deteriorating physique in society. This pessimism led to speculations on the possibility of fusing hereditary biology with public health. Eugenicists recognized that chronic diseases were a greater threat to the nation's health than epidemic infectious disease. Alcoholism, tuberculosis and venereal disease were dubbed 'racial poisons', which it was feared were damaging the nation's hereditary stock. Hereditarian medicine was accompanied by political demands for 'state socialism'. This fused the traditions of medical reform and medical police. A public movement to combat what was referred to as the 'people's diseases' (*Volkskrankheiten*) was generated. State officials and doctors took a leading role in public health campaigns.

Constitutional hygiene

The germ theory of infectious disease was criticized as simplistic. Two lapsed bacteriologists, Adolf Gottstein and Ferdinand Hueppe, explained how disposition

---

[49] Tröhler and Maehle, 'Anti-vivisection', p. 177.

and inherited constitution made people susceptible to infections. They rejected the bacteriologists' assumption of the constant virulence of a specific causal organism. They accused the state of arbitrarily selecting certain organisms as causing specific types of diseases and maintained that the organisms and the diseases were subject to immense variation. They condemned bacteriology as relying only on animal experiments, in which artificial 'injected diseases' and not 'natural diseases' were studied. Critics argued that epidemics could be understood only by mass observation of human populations. Doctors turned to demography and social science to develop statistical epidemiology. These controversies were followed with interest by clinicians, who came to accept constitutional factors as a standard part of medicine. Gottstein, Hueppe and the clinician, Friedrich Martius, became renowned for the principle that resistance to infection was inversely proportional to the strength of a constitution. The importance of hereditary biology was greatly enhanced for clinicians. Medicine became susceptible to development in the direction of social and racial hygiene.

How eugenics became a central concern of liberal reformers can be seen in the case of Gottstein. He was an assistant doctor in Breslau at the time of Koch's discovery of the TB bacillus in 1882. He became expert in clinical bacteriology, but interrupted his scientific career when he married in 1883. He moved to Berlin where he opened a general practice, but continued to undertake laboratory research and to participate in liberal gatherings of social scientists. He was impressed by Hans Buchner's studies of the bactericidal powers of the blood, showing the importance of natural immunity to infections. This provided a biological rationale for the extension of welfare services. In 1893 Gottstein criticized Behring's views on diphtheria therapy, and turned from laboratory research to epidemiology. He became interested in acquired immunity as a racial characteristic, and took a lead in developing municipal welfare services in Berlin. In 1919 he became Prussian *Ministerialdirektor* of the Department of Health in the Ministry of Welfare, replacing the bacteriologist Kirchner. This appointment marked a reversal of official policy, as biological, social and epidemiological criticisms of bacteriology were accepted.[50]

Hueppe illustrates a conservative and nationalistic strain in hereditarian medicine. His career was initially that of an orthodox bacteriologist. He studied at the Academy for Military Medicine in Berlin, and in 1879 was seconded to the Imperial Health Office where he worked with Koch until 1884. In 1892 he used the opportunity of the devastating cholera epidemic in Hamburg to claim that he had invented a specific remedy for the disease. His treatment, based on internal disinfection, provoked a scandal because of the above-average fatalities that resulted.[51] In 1893 he caused a sensation at the Society of German Naturalists and

[50] 'Adolf Gottstein', in L.R. Grote (ed.), *Die Medizin der Gegenwart in Selbstdarstellungen*, (Leipzig, 1925), IV, pp. 53–91.
[51] R.J. Evans, *Death in Hamburg* (Oxford, 1987), pp. 334–6.

Doctors by criticizing the inadequacies of bacteriology.[52] He developed a theory of *Konstitutionshygiene*, which made hereditary biology central to hygiene.[53]

Hueppe's decisive break with liberal concepts of hygiene was accompanied by admiration for state socialism. He believed that the state ought to promote the health of future generations. Concern for the 'future generations' was to become a rallying cry of those supporting social welfare measures and of the eugenicists. This call was taken up by Buchner in Munich. That Buchner was Pettenkofer's successor, and a bacteriologist, underlined the break that occurred with sanitary liberalism during the 1890s. From 1896 until his death in 1902, Buchner supported measures to promote the natural resistance to infection and the vigour of the population. His belief that medical science could engender social unity culminated in a national movement for 'positive hygiene' (*Volkshygiene*). That his successor was the eugenicist Gruber shows how Munich encapsulates the transition from Pettenkofer's liberalism to the radical nationalism of racial hygiene.[54]

Hueppe went further than hygienic collectivism in that he fused hygiene with Aryan racism. When Ploetz published on racial hygiene in 1895, Hueppe responded positively with favourable reviews.[55] His academic publications bore the influence of the racial anthropologists, Ammon and Wilser. In 1897 he published a monograph on the racial hygiene of the Greeks as an Aryan race.[56] His 1899 textbook of hygiene introduced the discipline as enhancing the vigour of the race. He warned of the dangers of racial interbreeding. He attributed the lower fertility of the German Jews to their hybrid racial origins from semitic and hamitic roots, mixed with a small dose of Aryanism. He characterized the Jews as a degenerate race; by contrast, the Aryans were a rural *Naturvolk*.[57] Throughout his life Hueppe was a sports and gymnastics fanatic. When von Gossler, the Minister of Education, introduced gymnastics in schools in 1882, he turned to Hueppe for advice. But after Gossler lost his post, Hueppe was without official supporters. Hueppe initiated a *völkisch* strain in hygiene. He hailed hygiene as a means of Nordic and Germanic rebirth. He became unacceptable to the Prussian state and Althoff did not recall him from the Charles University in Prague where he was professor. Houston Stewart Chamberlain complained to the Kaiser that Hueppe, as Germany's most brilliant and patriotic epidemiologist, was unable to obtain a chair in a German university.[58] But Hueppe remained influential among the medical profession. The Society of German Doctors and Scientists established a TB

---

[52] F. Hueppe, 'Die Ursachen der Gärungen und Infektionskrankheiten und deren Beziehungen zum Kausalproblem und zur Energetik', *Verhandlungen der Gesellschaft Deutscher Naturforscher und Aerzte* (1893), vol. 1, pp. 134–58.

[53] 'Ferdinand Hueppe', in L.R. Grote (ed.), *Die Medizin der Gegenwart in Selbstdarstellungen* (Leipzig, 1923), II, pp. 77–138.

[54] H. Buchner and M. v. Gruber (ed.), *Acht Vorträge aus der Gesundheitslehre* (Leipzig, 1909).

[55] F. Hueppe, 'Soziale Hygiene', *Die Zukunft*, vol. 3 no. 50 (1895), 507–11. Hueppe, 'Ueber Sozial- und Rassenhygiene', *Die Zeit*, vol. 5 (1895), 63.

[56] F. Hueppe, *Zur Rassen- und Sozialhygiene der Griechen im Altertum und in der Gegenwart* (Wiesbaden, 1897).   [57] F. Hueppe (ed.), *Handbuch der Hygiene* (Berlin, 1899).

[58] H.S. Chamberlain, *Briefe 1882–1924 und Briefwechsel mit Kaiser Wilhelm II* (Munich, 1928), I, pp. 78–80, II, 195–6. Field, *Evangelist*, p. 214.

committee over which Hueppe presided. He believed that doctors should take the lead in abstinence from alcohol, and in nature therapy, gymnastics and nudism.[59] The common denominators in Hueppe's and Gottstein's views were state socialism and heredity.

Family diseases

During the early 1890s there was renewed criticism of the theory of contagion. In 1891 Ottomar Rosenbach, a relentless critic of medical science and specialization, published on the aims and limitations of therapy.[60] He pioneered preventive medicine for heart disease based on reduction of nervous stress. The shift from concern with contagion to an hereditarian approach meant that the screening of whole populations for hereditary defects was deemed necessary. This can be seen in the case of TB. With a massive proportion of the population believed to be infected, certain scientists went so far as to suggest that all humans were tubercular, but only some became ill. The idea of a hereditary disposition to TB in certain families was examined in terms of hereditary biology and genealogy. Air, sunlight and wholesome food were valued as effective in aiding recovery, and the loss of a healthy natural environment was blamed as bringing on TB. Deprivation from nature was added to the economic privations suffered by the proletariat. Official circles recognized that the problem of degenerative diseases needed radical solutions. They began to accept the theory that diseases were racial poisons, and to adapt elements of the *Lebensreformers'* and socialists' strategies of environmental improvement. Such hereditarian ideas coincided with popular criticisms of industrial society. During the 1890s, despite Koch's proof that TB was contagious the theory of a hereditary tuberculous disposition persisted. Hospitals continued to classify certain types of TB as hereditary. The assumption that the disease was inherited, prompted debate as to whether some human stocks were more prone to TB than others? If so, TB constituted a means of natural selection that could modify the inherited constitution of a race. Certain scientists, such as Louis Landouzy in France and Karl Pearson in Britain, maintained that TB was not hereditary but that the disposition to infection was. Children were born *bacillisés*. By contrast, the zoologist Weismann denied the inheritance of TB as an 'acquired character'. Instead he agreed with the suggestion that sperm might transmit tuberculosis. Yet autopsies of foetuses and infants under eight weeks failed to reveal signs of TB. Baumgarten carried out animal experiments such as the injection of TB bacilli into the testes of guinea pigs and rabbits. Although the offspring were not tubercular, their reproductive capacity seemed to have declined.[61] The point was made that

---

[59] 'Ferdinand Hueppe', Grote, *Die Medizin der Gegenwart*, pp. 77–138.
[60] O. Rosenbach, *Grundlagen, Aufgaben und Grenzen der Therapie* (Berlin, 1891); Rosenbach, *Ansteckungsfurcht und die Bakteriologische Schule* (Stuttgart, 1892).
[61] A. Reibmayr, *Die Ehe Tuberculöser und ihre Folgen* (Vienna, 1894); M. Heinemann, 'Ueber die bacïläre Heredität der Tuberkulose', Diss. Würzburg 1900; F. Lämmerhirt, 'Erblichkeit und familiärer Faktor bei den tuberkulösen Entwicklungen', *Politisch-Anthropologische Revue*, vol. 1 (1902/3), 789–98.

there was a difference between inherited diseases and congenital infections such as syphilis which were acquired in the womb or at birth.

The Prussian medical official, Martin Kirchner, expressed concern over TB in marriage. He accepted that TB could be inherited, but the problem was that it often lay latent until the later years of life – that is, until after marriage. Moreover, marriage intensified the 'consuming fire' of the disease. He cited the genealogical research of the Baden doctor, Alexander Riffel, on TB in 716 families: 25 per cent had a single tubercular parent, 15 per cent had both parents with TB, and 10 per cent had tubercular children.[62] His military experience demonstrated that TB of the urinary tract was rare and he concluded that infection was primarily through sputum rather than sperm. Kirchner recommended that the German home must become a castle and a bastion against infection.[63] These views were supported by the medical statistician Weinberg, who used local family registers in a study of TB in Stuttgart from 1873. He concluded that tuberculous adults were liable to infect children, and that once infected, TB was likely to recur later on in life. His findings were supported by the racial hygienist Gruber, although it was pointed out that the fertility of the tubercular was below average.[64]

There were renewed demands for marriage restrictions for those suffering from TB, VD and hereditary mental disease. During the 1890s there was concern over the effects of VD on population growth. Statistical studies of marriages revealed a high incidence of VD. The French study by Alfred Fournier of a single medical practice showed that 50 per cent of marriages were infected. Half the pregnancies from such marriages resulted in miscarriages, still-births, or in babies suffering from congenital syphilis, blindness, lameness, epilepsy and idiocy. One quarter of all cases of blindness were diagnosed as having been caused by VD. Fournier's immensely influential study provided detailed guidance on the circumstances under which doctors could permit those who had once contracted syphilis to marry.[65] These points were brought to the attention of the public in 1902 by the drama, *Les Avariées*, *(Damaged Goods)* about VD in the family. Eugène Brieux, its author, publicized the medical demand for a certificate of freedom from syphilis prior to marriage. The Berlin gynaecologist, Ernst Bumm, considered that 20–30 per cent of sterile marriages were due to gonorrhoeal infections. Berlin doctors encountered high rates of VD in the practices. Blaschko estimated in 1892 that 10 per cent of the population of Berlin was syphilitic. This was a low estimate; the eugenicist Lenz later pronounced that 40 per cent of Berlin's population was syphilitic. Blaschko calculated that 20 million marks per annum could be saved by

[62] A. Riffel, *Die Erblichkeit der Schwindsucht und tuberkulöse Prozesse* (Karlsruhe, 1893); P. Riffel, 'Alexander Riffel und seine Bedeutung für die Konstitutionsforschung bei Lungenschwindsucht und Krebs', *ARGB*, vol. 14 (1922), 425–9.

[63] M. Kirchner, 'Die Gefahren der Eheschliessung von Tuberkulösen und deren Verhütung und Bekämpfung', in Kirchner, *Hygiene und Seuchenbekämpfung. Gesammelte Abhandlungen* (Berlin, 1904), pp. 312–327. Paper given in May 1899.

[64] W. Weinberg, *Die Kinder der Tuberkulösen, mit einem Begleitwort von Obermedizinalrat Professor Max von Gruber* (Leipzig, 1913).   [65] A. Fournier, *Syphilis et Marriage* (Paris, 1890).

preventing VD. That students were the social group with the highest incidence of VD was a cause of especial concern to the middle-class reformers as students were meant to be the *Kulturträger* for future generations. Economic and social motives spurred on the campaigners against VD.

Distress as to the moral, social and racial consequences of alcoholism, VD and TB prompted the establishment of mass hygiene organizations to combat these diseases. Welfare organizations marked a step towards the realization of a welfare state, although they were not state bodies. Althoff, who had done so much to further the development of bacteriology and experimental biology in the universities, turned his attention to the social problems of diseases in the mid-1890s. The Prussian Finance Ministry insisted that family welfare was a matter for private philanthropy and beyond the responsibility of the state. This demarcation derived from the liberal constitutional principles that shaped the administration during the 1870s. Opposition to state interventionism was to be steadily eroded. When Wilhelm II became Kaiser, expectations of a 'new course' of social reform were initiated in the wake of the dismissal of Bismarck. In 1890 the Kaiser addressed the schools conference on the need to pay attention to the physical welfare of the coming generation. Certain influential state officials, aristocrats, and medical scientists believed that reforms were vital to combat the twin evils of poverty and socialism. Although the Kaiser's energy as a social reformer was short-lived, subterranean reformist impulses continued in official circles. The *Verein für Sozialreform*, supported by the reformist Hans Hermann von Berlepsch, who was Minister of Trade until 1896, took an interest in industrial working conditions.[66] Yet factory inspection and economic measures were costly, cumbersome and controversial. Expansion of medical and welfare services offered an area of activity which could be a focus for philanthropic and economic reformers. Welfare measures provided opportunities for state dignitaries, the medical profession and other concerned social groups to co-ordinate reforming efforts.

Welfare organization: from liberalism to corporatism

From the 1880s there was a rapid growth of welfare organizations to combat chronic diseases and to defend infant health. These mobilized the public, welfare experts and state officials in causes which had wide appeal and far-reaching implications as they attacked the problem of degenerating family health and welfare. Welfare organizations cemented the cohesion of the social groups organizing welfare. They represented intermediary stages in the shift from doctrines of liberal self-help in the 1880s to state intervention by the First World War. In many ways the anti-alcohol movement was a classic expression of self-help, combining moralistic with medical concerns. Doctors supported the

---

[66] U. Ratz, *Sozialreform und Arbeiterschaft. Die "Gesellschaft für soziale Reform" und die sozialdemokratische Arbeiterbewegung* (Berlin, 1980).

campaign against alcoholism as a way of extending professional power into moral and social spheres. Welfare organizations enhanced the importance of the doctor as an arbitrator of social issues and created opportunities for medical practice and direction of social affairs. Initially, this professionalism could be reconciled with an ideology of self-help; doctors had themselves campaigned for the de-regulation of medicine from the restrictions of state control.[67] Around the turn of the century campaigns such as those against tuberculosis and for infant welfare fused with currents of social imperialism, as doctors and eugenicists joined forces with national and local dignitaries in welfare work.

During the 1880s temperance reformers opposed legislative intervention by the state. The National Liberal, August Lammers, gathered together doctors, businessmen and the evangelical philanthropists of the *Innere Mission* to found the German Association Against the Abuse of Alcoholic Drinks in 1883. Lammers' strategy was to present it as a voluntary movement under royal patronage.[68] The growth of the anti-alcohol movement coincided with the 'new course' of social reformism in the 1890s, and involved leading political exponents of *Sammlungspolitik*, such as the Prussian Finance Minister, Johannes von Miquel. By 1914 there were 41,000 members in 240 local abstinence or temperance groups. Members included von Miquel, General von Moltke, the Darwinist Haeckel, the statistician Viktor Böhmert, social scientists such as Gustav Schmoller and leading psychiatrists and eugenicists. The famous joined as individuals to set a personal example and to give the temperance campaign respectability. It was patriotically hoped to reform moral standards of key social groups such as students and soldiers, and to break the connection between drink and poverty. Anti-alcohol reformers used their moral and scientific authority to alleviate a disease associated with industrialization.[69]

Alcoholism was a divisive issue for political parties and the state because of the entrenched interests opposing legislative remedies. Many landowners and commercial interests were dependent on revenues from brewing, and socialists did not wish to alienate party members or publicans who allowed meetings on their premises. The abstinence and temperance movements lacked co-ordination: radical abstainers from all alcohol clashed with moderate temperance reformers, and the religiously inspired were opposed by the secularist and medically motivated. Many different types of organizations were founded, such as the Knights Templars (*Guttempler-Orden*) introduced in the 1880s and the German Workers' Abstinence League in 1903.[70] Initially, medical officers regarded alcohol abuse as best left to voluntary initiatives. But at the turn of the century attitudes began to change and there was a substantial lobby among public health experts and

[67] P.J. Weindling, 'Hygienepolitik als sozialintegrative Strategie im späten Deutschen Kaiserreich', in A. Labisch and R. Spree (eds.), *Medizinische Deutungsmacht im sozialen Wandel* (Bonn, 1989), in press.

[68] *Deutscher Verein gegen den Missbrauch geistiger Getraenke.* J.S. Roberts, *Drink, Temperance and the Working Class in Nineteenth-Century Germany* (Boston, 1984), p. 53.

[69] Roberts, *Drink*, p. 64.   [70] *Deutscher Arbeiter Abstinenten Bund.*

psychologists opposed to alcoholism. In part this was due to medical reformers who correlated alcoholism with higher rates of TB and VD. The consumption of good quality milk rather than alcohol was urged as a means of reducing the incidence of TB.[71] There was increasing official support for anti-alcohol campaigns and welfare measures. Graf Hugo Sholto Douglas, a conservative *Landtag* representative and philanthropist, urged co-ordinated state action against alcohol abuse. In 1904 the Chancellor, Posadowsky-Wehner, opened an anti-alcohol exhibition in Charlottenburg. In 1906 a clinic for alcoholics was established in the Psychiatric Clinic of the *Charité* state hospital in Berlin. In 1909 a conference for the establishment of alcoholics' clinics was organized. By 1912 there were 48 asylums, and 158 outpatient clinics, or *Trinkerfürsorgestellen*. In 1908 the Prussian Medical Department began to distribute temperance propaganda. When in 1910 the Kaiser publicly condemned alcohol abuse, 85,000 copies of the speech were distributed to schools, and to the army and navy. By 1914, it was officially accepted that alcohol impaired the military and reproductive power of the *Volk*.

Measures against alcoholism conform to the transition in liberal welfare from individual philanthropy to the demand for state-supported medical controls. Pressure from the medical profession was crucial in changing official attitudes. Distinguished medical scientists and psychiatrists were active in the anti-alcohol movement. Gruber, the professor of hygiene, had been a *Temperenzler* since his days on the fringes of Viennese socialism. The Munich psychiatrist, Kraepelin, was a leading advocate of abstinence. Budding eugenicists like Grotjahn, Ploetz and Rüdin first became aware of the need for preventive measures against chronic diseases as youthful participants in the anti-alcohol movement. They made contact with senior medical figures through their concern with alcoholism. The organizations against alcoholism were the breeding ground for later, more comprehensive and centralized strategies of public health based on social and 'racial' hygiene. Despite the difficulties of enacting legislation, state medical authorities gave their support. The anti-alcohol movement then followed the institutional models which had been established for TB during the 1890s.

Sanatoria, clinics and social integration

The rise of socialist agitation on health was a spur to the state to co-ordinate a comprehensive welfare programme. National organizations under the patronage of royalty and establishment figures were ways of preventing socialist initiatives in welfare. TB was an issue which could be used to integrate and direct reforming efforts. The public sanatoria[72] provided fresh air and dietary therapies as natural cures for TB. By 1910 Germany had more public sanatoria than any other country, a result of insurance offices being prepared to fund buildings and TB treatment.

---

[71] ZSTA M Rep 76 VIII B Nr 1944 and 1945 Die Bekämpfung der Truncksucht.
[72] *Volksheilstätten*.

The main initiative came from welfare associations which were founded to support sanatoria, and in 1895 these were co-ordinated on a 'national' basis. The Prussian official, Althoff began to intervene in public health. He directed the efforts of reforming doctors such as Dettweiler and the Left Liberal Theodor Sommerfeld, insurance fund administrators and leading politicians.[73] The German Central Committee for the Erecting of Sanatoria[74] was founded on 21 November 1895. Althoff persuaded Chancellor Hohenlohe Schillingsfürst to become its president. The vice-president was initially Heinrich von Boetticher until he lost his position as Prussian Minister; he was succeeded by Posadowsky-Wehner, who remained in office until 1907. The society mirrored national politics as the presidency was taken over by Chancellor Bernhard von Bülow in 1900, until in turn he was succeeded by Theobald von Bethmann Hollweg.[75] Leading politicians, generals, bankers, industrialists and doctors – and especially their wives – joined forces in the organization of the anti–TB movement. Empress Auguste-Viktoria as patron confirmed that TB was a national priority. Associations were founded in each constituent state. The crusade against TB exemplifies a state-initiated organization to inculcate national values of health and fitness. It was the domestic counterpart to the Navy League as a means of mobilizing public support to strengthen the nation by promoting fit military recruits and industrial workers.

The *Heilstätte* movement appropriated radical initiatives and ideas, and directed them to nationalist ends. The emphasis on dietetic measures and hydrotherapy represented a broadening of scientific medicine. Nature therapy was popular among workers, as shown by the wide diffusion of the manuals of Bilz and Platen during the 1890s, as well as among dissident bourgeois *Lebensreformer*. It represented a critique of the values of the industrializing nation. Parallel to the officially sponsored sanatoria movement was the growing popularity of *Naturheilanstalten*. Kneipp's success began in the mid-1880s, and he developed a therapeutic village, Bad Wörishofen, from 1891; in 1887, the physician Theodor Lahmann founded the *Weisser Hirsch* sanatorium for 'scientific' nature therapy near Dresden. When the Berlin professor, von Leyden, came out in support of hydro- and nutritional therapy at this time, he was responding to a widespread popular movement. Elements of nature therapy were adopted by the ruling elite in the immensely prestigious national organization to combat TB. The anti-TB movement represented a concession to the critique of the narrowness of the 'nightwatchman state' as its liberal premises disclaimed responsibilities for alleviating social ills. While it was not possible to give state authorities powers to intrude into the realm of domestic hygiene – indeed, this would have aroused

---

[73] ZSTA Merseburg Rep 92 Althoff AI Nr 227 Central Comite der Errichtung von Heilanstalten für Lungenkranke 1895–1906. For reports on French dispensaries see ZSTA M Rep 92 Althoff AI Nr 227 Bl 53, and in 1903, Rep 92 Althoff AI Nr 225 Bl 1–27.

[74] *Deutsches Central-Komite zur Errichtung von Heilstätten für Lungenkranke.*

[75] E. Pütter, 'Wie ich dazu kam, vor 25 Jahren die erste Lungenfürsorgestelle in Halle a.S. zu begründen, und wie ich sie einrichtete', in K.H. Blümel (ed.), *Handbuch der Tuberkulose-Fürsorge* (Munich, 1926), pp. 1–4.

popular resentment – the anti-TB organization successfully extended the scope of welfare. However 'voluntary' it was, it was given much official support by state and municipal authorities. The Prussian Finance Ministry was outraged that state medical authorities encouraged municipal sanatoria instead of relying on the Poor Law.[76]

Socialists were integrated into the official welfare strategies. A novel feature was co-operation with the representatives and resources of sickness and invalidity insurance funds. In 1892 Gebhardt, the director of the *Hanseatische Anstalt für Invaliditäts- und Altersversicherung*, argued that therapy for the tubercular would save the costs of pensions. The Reich Insurance Office accepted this reasoning, and by 1897 the first insurance-financed sanatorium at Andreasberg in the Harz was opened. In 1896 the doctor and socialist, Friedeberg, organized a central commission of Berlin sickness insurances, and a national German committee for sickness insurances. In 1897 the *Invaliditäts-Versicherungsanstalt* combined with the Red Cross to open a sanatorium at Grabowsee for Berlin. TB measures thus extended the role of insurances as well as increasing their collective solidarity.[77] The combination of sickness insurance funds and a well-disposed ruling elite resulted in the rapid growth of public sanatoria:

year	numbers of public sanatoria	beds
1900	26	
1905	72	6,000
1911	97	11,000

As a German invention, these *Volksheilstätten* became the object of national pride. They provided the centrepoint of discussions at the first International Tuberculosis Conference held in Berlin in 1899. When French doctors criticized the efficacy of public sanatoria, German doctors took this as a slur on the nation.[78]

Yet the costs of TB sanatoria were high. The design of buildings had to be modified so that a barrack-like structure could allow maximum fresh air at a minimum cost. The other method was to establish welfare clinics to take the campaign for prevention into the homes of the sick. Sommerfeld, a liberal investigator of working conditions, submitted to Althoff plans for a system of clinic-based domiciliary care in 1898. In Halle the Poor Law medical official, Ernst Pütter, established a welfare clinic for the tubercular in 1899.[79] Pütter was supported by a welfare movement instigated by Boetticher, who had advocated the reforming 'new course' when Minister of the Interior. This ended in his dismissal and relegation to the ranks of provincial officials. Boetticher's support

---

[76] ZSTA M Rep 76 VIII B Nr 4155, Auskunfts- und Fürsorgestellen 1904–1907.
[77] F. Tennstedt, 'Socialismus, Lebensreform und Krankenkassenbewegung', *Soziale Sicherheit*, vol. 26 (1977), 210–14, 306–10, 331–6.
[78] G. Pannwitz, *Bericht über den Kongress zur Bekämpfung der Tuberkulose als Volkskrankheit, Berlin 24 bis 27 Mai 1899* (Berlin, 1899).
[79] K. Strubel, W. Tetzner and W. Piechocki, *Zur Geschichte der Gründung des Zweigvereins zur Bekämpfung der Schwindsucht in der Stadt Halle am 15. Juni 1899* (Halle, 1974).

indicates that the dispensary movement represented a surrogate for national legislation for welfare measures. Althoff sent delegates to inspect the French dispensary at Lille in 1901, and the Prussian *Kultusministerium* carefully drew up plans for organizing a modified form of TB welfare clinic.[80] The national importance of the TB clinic was underlined when in 1904 Althoff transferred Pütter to Berlin as director of the *Charité*.

Althoff quickly organized clinics for the metropolis. The Berlin committee included the expert on urban poverty, Emil Münsterberg, and the radical physician Rabnow. The secretary was Kayserling who established a TB museum in Charlottenburg. Berlin was divided into districts, each superintended by a clinic. Medical staff diagnosed and referred patients, but so as not to offend the medical profession, the clinics did not provide therapy. The dispensaries did supply milk stamps and dietary supplements, as well as crockery, bedding and spittoons. They co-operated with other welfare organizations on matters such as for soup kitchens[81] and with the German Society for *Volkshygiene*.[82] In the first eighteen months, 50,000 marks were raised. 8,200 homes were visited representing 15,661 patients; 1,000 children were sent to holiday health colonies and woodland convalescent settlements;[83] 465 beds were delivered; 3,923 marks were paid as rent supplements, and a further 11,805 marks for other welfare purposes. Pütter proudly concluded that the campaign enabled many families to move into healthy housing.[84]

The network of clinics rapidly spread. In 1904 there were 26 clinics. This number had risen to 321 by 1910 and by 1914 the number was 1,145. Clinics selected the sick for appropriate treatment, and distributed welfare supplements, toothbrushes and tooth powder, paper handkerchiefs and bedding. Althoff emphasized the educational role of the clinics or *Auskunfts- und Fürsorgestellen* as he called them, thus making it clear that their role was to provide information and welfare. Families were instructed in domestic hygiene. Taboos were imposed on coughing, spitting and kissing. The anti-TB campaign was an opportunity generally to raise standards of domestic and personal hygiene and to inculcate nationalist sentiments. As most TB victims were cared for at home, there was much attention to relations within the family: propaganda warned that a parental kiss could be fatal. Beds were a focus of attention. There was to be no sharing or renting out of beds to lodgers during the day, and bed linen had to be regularly changed. The hygienization of private life represented a solution to the worsening urban overcrowding and squalor. The TB 'Information and Welfare Clinic' was a model of organization adopted by the anti-alcohol, infant care, cancer and anti-VD

---

[80] For French developments see P. Guillaume, *Du désespoir au salut: les tuberculeux aux 19e et 20e siècles* (Paris, 1986), pp. 187–215; D. Dessertine and O. Faure, *Combattre la Tuberculose* (Lyon, 1988).
[81] *Volks-Küchen Verein.*
[82] ZSTA Merseburg Rep 92 Althoff AI Nr 225 Bl 1–298; Althoff B Nr 147 Bd 2 Bl 95–102; Althoff AI Nr 230 Auskunftsstellen. Poliklinik für Lungenkranke Berlin; Rep 76 VIII B Nr 4155; Auskunfts- und Fürsorgestellen für Lungenkranke, 1904–1907.   [83] *Kinderheil- und Walderholungsstätten.*
[84] 'Viele Familien haben durch unsere Hilfe gesunde Wohnungen beziehen können'.

campaigns. Clinics were a means of not only intervening in the domestic habits of the poor, but also of cementing cohesion among diverse social sectors of the wealthy. Philanthropy was a mechanism by which the newer commercial and professional groups could acquire status. Local officials were expected to direct 'voluntarily' the organization of the clinics. As a commentator observed: 'the nurses conduct home visiting, the doctors diagnose and the provincial official administers with the help of the mayor'.[85]

The Empress took a leading role in the Patriotic Women's League, the *Vaterländische Frauenvereine*. The League was affiliated to the Red Cross, and its purpose was to train women for military nursing. During the 1890s its responsibilities were extended to include welfare work. Voluntary women workers staffed many of the clinics in the infant welfare and TB organizations. Although socialist welfare organizations such as the Workers' Samaritan League offered a radical alternative, the Patriotic League was the largest women's organization in Imperial Germany with half a million members by 1910. Domestic welfare work such as nursing in children's and convalescent homes became an important sphere of voluntary – but officially directed – activity. Women were regarded as having a special national responsibility to set higher standards in domestic hygiene.[86] Local officials were expected to organize doctors and voluntary women helpers, and to co-ordinate their work with municipal welfare schemes. The crusade against TB and infant mortality made health a nationalist rallying cry. It meant that national values became fused with hygiene and that there were trained auxiliary forces to do nursing work in the event of war. Women's organizations became active on health issues.[87]

Venereal diseases and preventive medicine

The Society to Combat Venereal Diseases launched a public campaign to secure a reformed life style. The society was founded in 1902 after three years of careful planning by dermatologists whose preventive strategy required a broad base of public and official support. The society was a means for raising the status of dermatology as a medical specialism, as it highlighted VD prevention as a major national and international issue. Following international conferences, the *Société française de prophylaxie sanitaire et morale* was established in 1901 by French doctors who had close links with German colleagues. Neisser was the president of the German society, and Blaschko was secretary. Neisser was a National Liberal, and had the support of ministerial and police officials. Blaschko had good contacts with

---

[85] 'Die Schwestern besuchen, die Ärzte untersuchen, und der Landrat verwaltet mit Hilfe des Bürgermeisters'. W. zur Nieden-Rohwinkel, 'Die Tuberkulosefürsorge in den Landkreisen der Rheinprovinz', *Schmollers Jahrbuch*, vol. 37 (1913), 103–18.

[86] U. Frevert, 'The Civilizing Tendency of Hygiene. Working Class Women under Medical Control in Imperial Germany', in J.C. Fout (ed.), *German Women in the Nineteenth Century* (New York and London, 1984), pp. 320–44.

[87] ZSTA M Rep 76 VIII B Nr 1698 Die Vereine von Rotem Kreuz (vaterländische Frauenvereine).

socialist doctors and with sickness insurance officials. The steering committee had the support of feminist advocates of the abolition of police controls on prostitution.[88] In the first year the society acquired nearly 1,000 members, formed local groups and began its work of distributing millions of pamphlets. It campaigned for sex education in schools and for recognition of VD treatment for medical insurance purposes.[89] The society was welcomed by Chancellor Bülow, and received regular grants from Prussia and the Reich. Apart from filling an important social need, the society represented a useful pressure group against the Centre Party and ultra-conservatives.[90] These mounted a moral purity campaign from 1898 to regulate prostitution and control decadent art and literature. The aim of the anti-VD society was the reform of sexual morality. The hypocrisy of bourgeois morality was criticized as hypocritical; it was pointed out that taboos on sexuality resulted in men resorting to prostitutes. Earlier marriage was suggested as the best preventive remedy. There was much discussion of contraceptives as prophylactics against VD, health examinations prior to marriage and other methods to improve the health of families. Gruber, the Munich professor of hygiene, attacked the society's prescription of condoms as immoral.[91]

Innovative socialist administrators on sickness insurance funds such as Kohn extended their responsibilities into the realm of preventive medicine. This represented a more fully social approach to the problem of disease, compared with the calculations of individual contributions and risk factors on which the insurance funds had been established. As a political weapon the slogan of *Proletarierkrankheiten* had strong emotive appeal, and could be objectively supported by statistics on social differentials which correlated diseases with low income, overcrowding and dusty occupations. It could justify demands for higher income and shorter working hours. Friedeberg's emphasis on family welfare[92] went with a plan for the centralization of sickness insurance funds and the extension of socialized medicine. More than this, he wished to use sickness insurance funds and trade unions to arouse socialist consciousness. Yet while academic studies such as that by Sommerfeld correlated TB with occupational hazards, there was little done by the authorities in the way of interfering with the processes of industrial production. Compensation

---

[88] For example, Marie Stritt, Anna Pappritz and Wally Zepler.

[89] ZSTA M Rep 77 Tit 662 Nr 44 Beiakten 4 betr. die Deutsche Gesellschaft zur Bekämpfung der Geschlechtskrankheiten; Tennstedt, 'Alfred Blaschko'; 'Ein Brief des Herrn Reichskanzlers', *Mitteilungen der Deutschen Gesellschaft zur Bekämpfung der Geschlechtskrankheiten*, vol. 1 (1902/3), 45; U. Linse, 'Über den Prozess der Syphilisation – Körper und Sexualität um 1900 aus ärztlicher Sicht', in A. Schiller and N. Heim (eds.), *Vermessene Sexualität* (Berlin, Heidelberg, 1987), pp. 163–85.

[90] ZSTA M Rep 76 VIII A Nr 4151, Alfred Blaschko; *Zeitschrift für Bekämpfung der Geschlechtskrankheiten*, vol. 16 (1915/6), 333.

[91] 'Eingabe der Deutschen Gesellschaft zur Bekämpfung der Geschlechtskrankheiten an den Bundesrat und Reichstag, betreffend Abänderung des Krankenversicherungsgesetzes', *Mitteilungen der Deutschen Gesellschaft zur Bekämpfung der Geschlechtskrankheiten*, vol. 1 (1902/3), 81–92. *Mitteilungen der deutschen Gesellschaft zur Bekämpfung der Geschlechtskrankheiten*, vol. 1 (1902/3), 45, 82–9; ZSTA M Rep 76 VIII B Nr 2017.   [92] *Familienfürsorge*.

legislation for TB as an occupational disease was not introduced. Given that the disease was so widespread, it was medically debatable whether the disease was contracted at work. The recognition and extension of compensation for other fibroses of the lungs was painfully slow: specific occupations required specific diseases, as the recognition of silicosis as a distinctive (and thus compensatable) type of lung fibrosis was to show. Intervention in the home was preferable to intervention in the workplace. Socialist agitation against the chronic diseases of poverty and industrial work was deflected into the realm of a normative and positivistic social medicine. It was ironic that the funds gathered from labour by the sickness and invalidity insurances should have been diverted away from the workplace into measures to sanitise the domestic environment of housing and family life. Here medical intervention was far less controversial than it would have been in industry. Socialists moderated their views regarding the socialization of the medical profession, and were prepared to work with the ruling establishment and within the limitations of professionalized medicine. Zadek remained within the professional medical paradigm. His workers' health library pamphlet on TB accepted ideas of a tubercular physique and the inheritance of the disease, as well as the statistic that 90 per cent of the workforce were tubercular.[93] He recommended personal hygiene as self-help and a hygienization of relations within the family. He insisted that the sick belonged neither in the workshop nor at home but in special sanatoria.[94]

The rift between popular perceptions of sickness and the medical establishment continued because sickness and invalidity benefits were generally so inadequate as to deter workers from registering as sick. It was in a worker's interest to feign health. Suspicion of sanatoria persisted. There was awareness of the discrepancy of conditions between the dirt, damp and poor diet at home and in the sanatoria as an ideal hygienic environment; when back at work, medical advice on discharge to undertake 'light work' was futile. The sanatorium was to function as an educational institution by inculcating orderly and hygienic habits into patients. In 1902 Kayserling attempted to organize discharged patients from the Heilanstalt Belzig into a society of health educators who would spread the laws of hygiene among the people.[95] There was evidence that patients could build up collective resistance to medical science and perpetuate their own beliefs about disease and health. Patients' solidarity extended into the realms of politics. At the Heilanstalt Beelitz, there were lively socialist reading and discussion groups.[96] Clinics could also have their functions appropriated by radicals; the feminist doctor Adams–Lehmann, for example, used a clinic of the *vaterländische Frauenvereine* in Munich for carrying out abortions. Clinics became central to socialist welfare schemes.

The preventive strategies were based on a broadened and socialized concept of health care. This reconciled the divergent interests of the profession, the state, social

---

[93] *Arbeitergesundheitsbibliothek.*   [94] Tennstedt, *Vom Proleten*, pp. 481–4.
[95] 'Pioniere der Gesundheitspflege im Deutschen Volke'.   [96] Tennstedt, *Vom Proleten*, p. 462.

critics and patients. The campaigns provided opportunities for practitioners to seek new outlets for their skills. All interested parties used health as a means for reconciling conflicting interests and for adapting welfare to the needs of mass urban society. Groups deprived of the vote by a discriminatory political system, such as women and youths, could be mobilized in national and socially useful causes. Domestic welfare organizations were a highly innovative means of social imperialism. They had a broader basis of popular support than renegade patriotic groups such as the Pan-German or Navy Leagues and yet had the imperial, administrative and professional elite to provide guidance. Such welfare organizations could establish durable institutional structures with the patriotic aim of ensuring fit and healthy military recruits and of providing solutions to the social ills of industrial society. Association with leading dignitaries yielded honours and influence for a wide range of social groups, as well as creating a cohesive social structure.[97]

The anti-TB campaign offered the ruling elite a means of reaching parts of society where the state could not reach. The tentacles of welfare systems reached into the home and inculcated hygienic habits which could be equated with 'orderliness'. Disease prevention and control were outlets for the rising tide of nationalism and civic pride. The campaigns encouraged bourgeois and popular participation so ensuring homogeneity of a national life style. TB prevention was a model for a successful health strategy that united conflicting social interests on the basis of a broad social concept of health, including housing, nutrition and education. From the anti-TB campaign arose a network of institutions and a theory of social hygiene which could be applied to all aspects of disease and society. Clinics and preventive medicine were to justify the medical profession's acquisition of new powers and growing interventionism.

Heredity and hygiene

The move towards welfare organizations opened the door to eugenics and to concern with heredity as a factor in infectious and chronic disease. Emphasis on heredity stigmatized the inadequacy of 'individual' hygiene, and stressed the need for preventive measures and the gathering of data on social conditions and family ancestry. Racial and hereditarian ideas could readily be injected into the nationalist ideology of welfare organizations. Of the eugenicists, Bluhm, Grotjahn, Ploetz and his wife Paula, and Schallmayer were active in the anti-alcohol and anti-VD movements, although only Grotjahn took a part in anti-TB measures. Schallmayer was critical of anti-TB measures, seeing them as a means of keeping the unfit alive.[98] The eugenicists made influential contacts with leading medical experts in

---

[97] Compare G. Eley, 'Social Imperialism in Germany', in Eley, *From Unification to Nazism* (London, 1986), pp. 154–67.

[98] W. Schallmayer, 'Infektion als Morgengabe', *Zeitschrift für die Bekämpfung der Geschlechtskrankheiten*, vol. 2 (1904), 389–419.

welfare organizations. They cultivated university professors such as the psychiatrist Kraepelin, the bacteriologist Gruber, and the clinician Martius. Massive public membership provided a vast audience for hereditarian theories. In 1914 the national anti-alcohol league had 30,000 members.[99]

The organizations against alcoholism were the breeding ground for later, more comprehensive programmes of 'racial' and 'social' hygiene. The problem of alcoholism and degeneration was the focus for Grotjahn's first attempt to apply social science to medicine in 1898. He correlated alcoholism with a range of degenerative conditions such as obesity and heart disease, as well as prostitution and criminality. He constructed a hereditary pathology showing how social deprivation activated any pathological predispositions.[100] Ploetz found that the campaign against alcoholism was an effective channel for popularizing racial hygiene and winning over medical experts to the cause. The international congress against alcoholism which he helped to organize at Bremen in 1903 provided valuable contacts and a platform for racial hygiene.[101] He contacted the biologist, Weismann, for information on the hereditary mechanisms resulting in the degenerative effects of alcoholism.[102] Despite a personal dislike of the physiologist Abderhalden, who was a prominent member of the anti-alcohol movement, Ploetz was impressed with how he bred rats in order to test experimentally for the effects of alcohol.[103] Ploetz became a life-long enthusiast for breeding animals for the purpose of discovering the effects of alcohol over several generations, and Abderhalden became a convert to racial hygiene. Ploetz warned that alcoholism resulted in decreased fertility, weakened progeny and high rates of infant mortality. Ploetz continued to be active in the medical campaign against alcoholism, which he associated with a hereditary disposition to TB, nervous diseases, obesity, and degeneration of the heart, liver and kidneys. Ploetz recommended restrictions on marriage and the institutionalization of criminals and psychopaths.[104] At the Congress for Internal Medicine in 1905, Ploetz supported Martius' demand for state registry offices to identify alcoholics and all others suffering from hereditary defects.[105]

Rüdin shocked the Bremen congress of April 1903 with a radical analysis of the problem of alcoholism. He considered alcoholism as an exterminating factor in the process of racial evolution. Unfortunately it took many generations for a line of alcoholics to die out. He therefore recommended institutionalizing chronic alcoholics in order to prevent them from having children, and declared that eugenic abortion and marriage laws were necessary. If alcoholics wished to marry

---

[99] *Allgemeiner Deutscher Zentralverband zur Bekämpfung des Alkoholismus.*
[100] A. Grotjahn, *Der Alkoholismus nach Wesen, Wirkung und Verbreitung* (Leipzig, 1898).
[101] Ploetz papers, Ploetz to A. Delbrück, 13 January 1905.
[102] Ploetz papers, Weismann to Ploetz, 12 March 1903.
[103] Ploetz papers, Ploetz to Rüdin, 12 August 1904; Abderhalden to Ploetz, 13 January 1905.
[104] A. Ploetz, 'Der Alkohol im Lebensprozess der Rasse', *Bericht über den 9. internationalen Kongress gegen den Alkoholismus* (1904), 70–95; Ploetz papers, diary, 7–9 April 1904.
[105] Ploetz papers, diary, 12–13 April 1905.

they could consent to 'a little operation' of sterilization. This marked the beginning of a life-long crusade for sterilization of the degenerate.[106] Demands for networks of clinics and eugenic schemes for segregation and sterilization of degenerates were to remain linked.

The impact of the hereditarian analysis was substantial. Influential political support was given by Graf Douglas, who spoke on *erbliche Belastung* (hereditary burdens) and alcoholism in the Reichstag. The Association against the Abuse of Alcoholic Beverages[107] argued in 1905 that as alcohol-induced hereditary degeneracy resulted in economic losses and burdens on the Poor Law, the state ought to intervene. Since the state was responsible for the care of minors, the mentally subnormal, the deaf, the dumb and the blind, it ought to tackle these problems at root by controlling alcoholism.[108] State support for welfare clinics meant that a network was established to locate and select the diseased for institutionalization and treatment. Such clinics could be turned to eugenic ends.

Heredity was a major concern of the Society for the Prevention of VD. Leading figures such as Blaschko and Neisser were well versed in the hereditarian theories. Ploetz and Schallmayer warned that therapy might allow weaker, less valuable racial elements to procreate, whereas preventive measures would ensure a healthy racial stock in the future. The science of hygiene was itself changing in response to the challenge of youthful advocates of racial, social and cultural factors in hygiene. Leading researchers in hygiene were deeply impressed by criticisms that their work might lead to a weakening of racial fitness. Carl Flügge dealt with the Spencerian assertion that hygiene resulted in the multiplication of an enfeebled generation. He argued in his textbook of hygiene that 'weakness' in the hygienic sense related only to specific diseases. It did not represent a general enfeeblement of the population. He suggested that only the fitter families would take hygienic precautions and adopt hygienic remedies for infections.[109] Other researchers considered that susceptibility to infection was itself an indicator of a biologically degenerate constitution. There was a pronounced swing among certain bacteriologists towards racial hygiene by the turn of the century. Gruber represented a classic example of the transition, leaving bacteriology to become one of the leading advocates of racial hygiene in Munich. In 1896 he developed a diagnostic technique called agglutination using the clumping properties of bacteria in blood serum. He lost interest in a laboratory-based solution to prevention of disease, and turned to moral and educational measures to promote immunity. Other experts in hygiene followed the lead of Gottstein, Gruber and Hueppe away from bacteriology to an emphasis on the inherited constitution. Die-hard opponents of bacteriology, such as the pathologist David von Hansemann, emphasized the inherited physical constitution as the main factor for explaining differential responses to infective

[106] E. Rüdin, 'Der Alkohol im Lebensprozess der Rasse', *Politisch-Anthropologische Revue*, vol. 2 (1903–4), 553–66.   [107] *Verein gegen den Missbrauch geistiger Getraenke.*

[108] ZSTA Merseburg Rep 76 VIII B Nr 1944 and 1945 Die Bekämpfung der Trunksucht.

[109] C. Flügge, *Grundriss der Hygiene* (Leipzig, 1902), pp. 17–19.

organisms. The divide between bacteriologists and the sanitarian/physiological approaches to hygiene was unified by hereditarian biology.

In 1903 Gruber addressed the German Society for Public Health (*Deutsche Gesellschaft für Volkshygiene*) on whether hygiene caused racial degeneration. He considered the evidence of a decline in mortality and of infectious diseases. While improved health was mainly a result of improved living conditions, he recognized that medical advances had had an impact in certain fields, such as in the decline of smallpox. He considered the accusation that improved welfare meant a decline in the fitness of the race. It had been suggested that high mortality meant that efficient selection was occurring. Lower infant mortality rates would allow weaker offspring to procreate so sapping the hereditary vitality of the race. If hygiene really caused degeneration, then the feebler individuals must be sacrificed. For the individual was worthless when set against the welfare of a race. Gruber reassuringly argued that races suffering high infant mortality rates, such as the Eskimo, also had a high adult mortality. The ultra-Darwinian argument that high infant mortality was necessary to sustain a fit adult population (as was argued in relation to the peasantry) was untenable. However hardy a constitution, certain infections were inevitably fatal. As holiday colonies proved, the effects of an inherited weak constitution could be offset by improved food and environmental conditions. It was unscientific to separate the degenerate *Minderwertigen* from the fit *Vollwertigen* as such indicators of degeneration as sickness were ever present. Natural selection could not improve the race. Only a 'rational selection' at marriage combined with social improvements could be effective. He concluded that hygiene helped both the individual and the race.[110]

Gruber's speech was recognized at the time as a landmark. It showed how far racial categories had intruded into hygiene. His typified the effort being made to combine bacteriology, welfare measures and arguments for racial improvements. He was one of the first to use (even though critically) the concept *minderwertig* (literally, of lesser value) that became a major feature of the eugenic argument against the social and economic costs of degeneracy. The categories of 'less value', 'full value' and 'hereditary burdens' as applied to human life indicated how public health was developing into a scientistic surrogate for political economy. The speech had its critics among the defenders of therapeutic medicine, who considered that degeneration could be staved off.[111] But the repercussions for social policy of medical advance and natural selection could no longer be ignored, as demands arose that the state restrain the weak from reproducing in order to maintain the race.[112] That the racial hygiene movement made many converts from hygiene and

---

[110] M.v. Gruber, 'Führt die Hygiene zur Entartung der Rasse?', *MMW*, vol. 50 (1903), 1713–18, 1781–5.

[111] J. Orth, *Aufgaben, Zweck und Ziele der Gesundheitspflege* (Stuttgart, 1904); W. Kruse, 'Entartung', *Zeitschrift für Sozialwissenschaft*, vol. 6 (1903), 359–76, 411–34.

[112] E. Bleuler, 'Führen die Fortschritte der Medizin zur Entartung der Rasse?', *MMW*, vol. 51 (1903), 312–13; A. Gottstein, 'Entartung', *Nation*, (14 November 1903).

bacteriology, indicated how a shift was occurring in medicine which sought a scientific basis in a blend of evolutionary theory with bacteriology, and an institutional basis in state socialism.

FROM CRADLE TO BARRACKS

Saving infant lives

The increasing public concern with child health illustrates the transition in medicine from liberal political economy to biologically based social hygiene. Underlying the rise of paediatrics as a medical specialism from the 1870s was a combination of political economy, scientific expertise and liberal humanitarianism. The statistician Ernst Engel calculated the economic value of each life. This influenced the doctor Philipp Biedert to approach the question of whether infant mortality was a drain on the national economy. The infant health movement was a means of saving the nation's resources and strengthening its vitality.[113] The rising prosperity of the middle classes meant that specialist practitioners could make a living from treating children's diseases. Children's hospitals were supported by middle-class philanthropists; the introduction of asepsis meant that such hospitals were no longer 'gateways to death'. The strength of liberal sentiments reinforced the state's denial of responsibility for the family: it was felt that child care was a private sphere or at most a field for philanthropic endeavour. In 1868 a petition for university teaching in paediatrics was presented to the Prussian state but rejected. But by the early twentieth century, state medical officials took the lead in infant and child health. In 1869 a section for child health was established at the Society of German Scientists and Doctors. This became a fully-fledged professional association in 1883. Membership climbed from 98 in 1883 to 295 in 1910.[114] The child health movement conformed to the pattern of a liberal middle-class movement caught up in the wave of social imperialism and professionalization at the turn of the century.

Advances in serum therapy during the 1890s initiated a concerted effort by the state, philanthropists and medical researchers in the combatting of infectious diseases: the anti-diphtheria campaign established a model for a co-ordinated attack on a major health hazard. But infant welfare (as opposed to child welfare) became a major object of medical, public and state concern only in the early twentieth century. In the context of social imperialism, the saving of infant lives became a national issue, as well as a separate sphere for the exercising of medical expertise. The indifference to high rates of infant mortality gave way to an emotive and nationalistic campaign to promote infant health. The reversal of values was strikingly shown in the case of the babies of unmarried mothers. During the

---

[113] G. Lilienthal, 'Paediatrics and Nationalism in Imperial Germany', *Bulletin of the Society for the Social History of Medicine*, no. 39 (1986), 64–70.
[114] A. Windorfer and R. Schlenk, *Die Deutsche Gesellschaft für Kinderheilkunde* (Berlin, 1978).

nineteenth century the 'illegitimate' were the objects of neglect, moral censure and legal discrimination. By 1910 this hostility evaporated in the heat of enthusiastic campaigns for medical and welfare measures. Demands arose that the state should take over responsibility for improving the legal and economic status of the 'illegitimate'. Not only were there innovative concepts of guardianship on a commercial and professional basis, but one eugenicist, Max Hirsch, referred to the illegitimate as *Staatskinder* (state children) and urged central state supervision. Eugenicists remained divided over whether the 'illegitimate' represented a valuable national resource, or whether they were hereditarily inferior.[115]

The abundance of human resources in the mid nineteenth century accounts for the neglect of infant health. High rates of infant mortality were tolerated as a harsh fact of existence, just as high emigration rates were accepted as inevitable. The concern with infant and child health was related to the birth rate and the labour market: the higher the birth rate, the less worry there was about the persistently high rates of infant mortality. From 1870 rising life expectancy and high fertility resulted in rapid population growth. Between 1871 and 1910 the German population grew from 41 million to 65 million. By 1900, the demand for labour as a consequence of the growth of the economy meant that the view that the nation was overpopulated gave way to the fear that it was underpopulated. Although the population continued to rise, the birth rate fell by 70% between 1871 and the 1930s. There followed an emotive campaign to raise the birth rate with idealization of motherhood, of large families as 'child rich', and of nationalist appeals that Germany was a 'nation without youth'. Concern with infant health rose as the birth rate fell.

Population growth and the fall in the birth rate were primarily features of urban life. Whereas in 1870 a quarter of the population lived in cities, this proportion increased to one half by 1910. By 1907, 30% of the nation were industrial workers. But it was in the cities that the fall in the birth rate was most marked. Between 1880 and 1900 there was a 2% gain in fertility in rural areas of Prussia, but a 13% decline in towns. That Berlin was a pace-setter in the decline prompted especial concern. There was a 32% decrease of births in Berlin and a 42% decrease in neighbouring Charlottenburg. There were more first-born children, but 20% fewer second-born, 45% fewer third-born and 60% fewer fourth-born in Berlin during this time.[116] *Angst* arose that cities could not sustain their populations and were simply consuming healthy rural stock. It was only in 1901 that the decline in fertility began to slow down the nation's population growth. This prompted agitation against the 'two child system', and the selfish materialism of small families. Doctors were prominent in the debate on the birth rate. They felt that contraception and abortion were issues over which the doctor should have authority. There should also be

[115] G. Lilienthal, 'Max Taube, Ein Wegbereiter moderner Säuglings- und Jugendfürsorge', *Sozialpädiatrie in Praxis und Klinik*, vol. 8 (1986), 476–80.
[116] P. Marschalck, *Bevölkerungsgeschichte Deutschlands im 19. und 20. Jahrhundert* (Frankfurt-on-Main, 1983), p. 44.

medical intervention at childbirth and in the care of infants in the hope that this could reduce the high rates of infant and maternal mortality. The chronic diseases of urban life such as TB, VD and alcoholism were denounced as causes of sterility and weak or disabled offspring. The urban environment was condemned as posing serious threats to the health of families, and to the nation's population resources.

The causes of infant deaths

Despite the general decrease in mortality rates from the 1880s, infant mortality continued to show pronounced regional variations. A general downward trend for infant death rates began only between 1903 and 1906. Great power rivalry and the need to replenish the industrial labour force intensified medical and philanthropic concern with infant health in Germany. The infant mortality rate was higher in Germany than in the rival great powers of Britain and France; although Russian and Eastern European rates of infant mortality were far greater there was alarm at the rapid population growth of Slav populations.[117] Deaths showed marked class and regional variations. These were due to different local customs of infant care and feeding as well as to varying cultural attitudes and conditions of land tenure. It was hoped that saving infant lives would compensate for the fall in the birth rate. Medical experts encouraged the emergence of standard practices of child care and hygienic habits throughout Germany.[118] The reduction in regional differences in mortality rates was a sign of the emergence of a uniform national lifestyle and set of values.

High rates of infant deaths were linked with the numerous births that weakened maternal health, and were a counterpart to the high rates of abortion. That many unmarried mothers found their offspring an unwelcome burden is suggested by death rates of around 60 per cent for the 'illegitimate'. Those who genuinely cared for their babies encountered a society which was morally and economically hostile to single-parent families, even though in isolated rural localities such as in parts of Bavaria illegitimacy was accepted as normal because of the conditions of land inheritance and the need for extra helping hands.[119] Although infants were vulnerable in an age before hygienic precepts created a sanitized environment to shield the infant from infections, medical measures had only a limited effect. Smallpox vaccination was widespread by the 1840s as it was believed to be effective in curbing a major killer. The Prussian authorities hesitated in making vaccination compulsory for they were reluctant to usurp parental responsibility for children's

[117] The infant mortality rate per 1000 live births in 1905 in England and Wales was 128, in France 135, in Russia 272, and in Germany 205. Source: B.R. Mitchell, *European Historical Statistics 1750–1975* (London, 1981), pp. 140–1.
[118] R. Spree, 'Sozialisationsnormen in ärztlichen Ratgebern zur Säuglings- und Kleinkinderpflege. Von der Aufklärungs- zur naturwissenschaftlichen Pädiatrie', in J. Martin and A. Nitschke (eds.), *Zur Sozialgeschichte der Kindheit* (Freiburg and Munich, 1986), pp. 609–59.
[119] W.R. Lee, 'Germany', in Lee (ed.), *European Demography and Economic Growth* (London, 1979), pp. 144–95.

health. Vaccination encountered popular resistance as an unwarranted intrusion into the personal sphere of the body. Despite vaccination, infant deaths continued to rise, reaching a high point in the 1880s. Thereafter, improved vaccination procedures not only resulted in declining mortality from small pox, but offered the chance for doctors to advise mothers to breastfeed.[120]

Most infant deaths were due to mysterious convulsions or 'cramps'. A study in Berlin in 1910 suggested that three-quarters of all convulsions were caused by diarrhoeal diseases.[121] The main causes of death were digestive diseases, followed by infectious and respiratory diseases and congenital defects. A difficulty in determining the causes of infant mortality lay in knowing whether the convulsions were caused by airborne infections causing respiratory diseases, tuberculosis and whooping cough, or by water-borne infections resulting in typhoid, diarrhoea and the mysterious 'cholera infantum'. The reduction of mortality until 1933 was held to be due to the decline of diarrhoeal diseases to 10 per cent of deaths.[122] It was ideologically convenient to emphasize nutrition as the major cause of infant deaths. Poor diet and dirty homes could be blamed on maternal incompetence in household budgeting, cleaning and cooking, and negligent care of babies. The remedies were courses in mothercraft and the promotion of breast feeding; advice was reinforced by patriotic pro-natalism and condemnation of women going out to work.

Geographical and environmental factors predominated in studies of mortality until the 1890s. Demographers puzzled over the extent to which social factors such as religion and the economic status of parent, or factors like marital fertility related more to airborne or water-borne diseases. For example, it was suggested that Catholics were prone to airborne diseases because of overcrowding resulting from larger families.[123] It was observed that in cities with good water supply and sewerage before 1900, infant mortality remained high. The trend towards smaller families with the firstborn at a younger age of the mother was frowned on by contemporaries and yet would have contributed to a decline in infant mortality. Seasonal variations were also controversial. It was often said that there was a summer peak due to enteric diseases, and a rather lower winter peak due to respiratory diseases. There was much concern with the planning of cities and the flow of air. Arthur Schlossmann in Düsseldorf argued that the lack of ventilation was an essential factor in the summer peak. The Rhine in the old town centre ventilated the city ensuring cooler nights, whereas in the newer suburbs temperatures remained high. The reasons why infant mortality began to fall were complex and indeterminate. It was difficult to isolate a single causal factor. Analysis of rural and urban differences was inconclusive. It was clear that there were some

[120] C. Huerkamp, 'A History of Smallpox Vaccination in Germany: A First Step in the Medicalization of the General Public', *Journal of Contemporary History*, vol. 20 (1985), 617–35.
[121] H.J. Kintner, 'The Determinants of Infant Mortality in Germany from 1871 to 1933', PhD dissertation, University of Michigan, 1982, p. 142.
[122] Kintner, 'Determinants', pp. 157, 276. [123] Kintner, 'Determinants', p. 186.

cities with far higher infant mortality rates than others. Similarly, the high mortality among the peasant population of East Prussia contrasted with the low mortality in the West as in rural Westphalia. The large Westphalian peasant families with their low mortality were proclaimed as a national model.[124] The variations and uncertainties of infant mortality suggest that the infant welfare campaign was motivated more by imperialist ideologies than by objective evaluation of demographic data.

Public responses to infant deaths

There was a shift from a geographical and environmental approach to infant health to an emphasis on bacteriology and serum therapy during the 1890s. This marked the transformation of child health from a philanthropic and autonomous movement to medical measures overseen by state officials and dignitaries. State support for paediatrics in Prussia did not materialize until the advent of bacteriology. Paediatrics developed during the 1890s to supplement the bacteriologists' serum therapies. In 1894 Otto Heubner was appointed the first full professor of child health in Berlin after work with Behring on diphtheria serum. As in the case of hygiene, the university objected to the appointment of a professor of paediatrics. It argued that paediatrics was not a viable science in its own right.[125] But as with hygiene, societies and journals were established, giving the specialism academic credentials, while protesting against the restrictive conservatism of medical faculties and finance ministries. Althoff took a major initiative in the development of paediatrics during the 1890s, expecting that Behring's anti-diphtheria serum would revolutionize child health. But a separate discipline of infant health did not develop. Althoff had to resort to a special non-university institution for infant health (the Kaiserin Auguste Viktoria Haus), which the paediatricians resented as an 'infant palace'. Child health was still a weakling among the medical specialisms. In 1910 only twelve out of twenty universities possessed a children's clinic. Before 1914 university chairs in child health were established only at Berlin in 1894, Leipzig in 1896, Breslau in 1906, Strasburg in 1910 and Munich in 1912. But between 1919 and 1921 fourteen universities instigated chairs in the changed social climate of the Weimar republic.[126]

Bacteriology came under fire from Social Darwinists who argued that high mortality was a sign of effective natural selection. Better quality military recruits and less TB were expected. The eugenicist, Tille, depicted the high mortality of London's East End, as the nation's 'curative institution'. Karl Pearson correlated low infant mortality with a long parental life expectancy. Ploetz analysed the data

---

[124] W. Salomon, 'Säuglingskrankheiten', in A. Grotjahn (ed.), *Soziale Pathologie* (Berlin, 1923), pp. 211–35.
[125] ZSTA M Rep 76 Va Sekt 1 Tit X Nr 10, Lehrstühle für Kinderkrankheiten.
[126] H.-H. Eulner, *Die Entwicklung der medizinischen Spezialfächer an den Universitäten des deutschen Sprachgebietes* (Stuttgart, 1970).

from royal families, and concluded that infant and early paternal deaths could be correlated. Longevity was thus a hereditary quality.[127] A debate arose over whether societies with high infant mortality had a lower child and adult mortality. Among the degenerative factors was the inability to breast feed caused by inherited incapacity or alcoholism.[128] Syphilis, contracted at birth, was a major concern, as parental syphilis was considered to cause most of the cases of blindness and a substantial number of the mentally ill. These were suppositions about which there were no statistics but widespread conjecture.[129] As with other branches of medicine, a tendency to hereditarian thinking in paediatrics became evident. Convulsions were attributed to congenital weakness and inherited diseases, and were diagnosed as due to a hereditarily disturbed nervous condition. If babies suffering convulsions survived, it was held that they would grow into nervous and unstable children, and then into neurotic adults. Infant convulsions were seen as a major cause of idiocy, and of arrested moral development. Convulsions were a sign that pathological behaviour such as stealing and lying was to develop.[130] As paediatrics came to concentrate on an infant's nerves and digestion, the infant became seen in primarily biological terms.[131] As biology became less environmental and more hereditarian, child health became dominated by ideas of hereditary fitness.

At about the time that mortality began to decline there was renewed interest in the mother and child relationship. Child care became the major concern of the public and the state. In addition to the economics and statistics of diet, clothing and feeding, the quality of care came to be appreciated as the key issue in the maintaining of a healthy family life. Intense emotional yearning for children became a theme of naturalist and symbolist literature and art. Between 1903 and her death from childbirth in 1907, Paula Modersohn Becker painted hundreds of pictures of infants and mothers; often they were suckling, and on occasions bottle-feeding. She elevated the peasant mother into a Gauguin-like symbol of exotic paradise. Käthe Kollwitz's obsession with the themes of mother, death and child began from around 1903, which was the year when Gustav Mahler's *Kindertotenlieder* were first performed. Heinrich Zille's earthy pictures of poverty in Berlin show squalid rooms packed to bursting point with babies and children. These artists were responding to a widespread sense of public concern about the high rates of infant mortality. Through her husband, a doctor with a large sickness insurance practice, Kollwitz became aware of the tragedy and difficulties of proletarian

[127] A. Ploetz, 'Die Lebensdauer der Eltern und die Kindersterblichkeit', *ARGB*, vol. 6 (1909), 33–44.

[128] A. Bluhm, 'Stillunfähigkeit', in A. Grotjahn and I. Kaup (eds.), *Handwörterbuch der Sozialhygiene* (Jena, 1912), vol. 2, pp. 555–70; Bluhm, 'Stillhäufigkeit und Stilldauer', *Handwörterbuch der Sozialhygiene*, vol. 2, pp. 570–91.

[129] F. Prinzing, 'Die angebliche Wirkung hoher Kindersterblichkeit im Sinne Darwinscher Auslese', *Zentralblatt für öffentliche Gesundheitspflege*, vol. 22 (1903); H. Helbrich, 'Ist hohe Säuglingssterblichkeit eine Auslese im Darwinschen Sinne?', Diss. Greifswald, 1907.

[130] G.F. Still, *Common Disorders and Diseases of Childhood* (London, 1912), pp. 616–35.

[131] Spree, 'Sozialisationsnormen', p. 659.

life.[132] The dramatic entry of the Empress into the campaign to promote infant health was of great importance in raising the ideological temperature. She was the mother of seven children, and was a model wife in her sense of duty to her impulsive husband. She became a symbol of the caring mother. Her efforts were crucial in giving the infant health movement social prestige and moral ardour.

As public concern with infant health reached a high point in the early twentieth century, a number of pressure groups agitated for state action. Midwives and socialists demanded free midwifery and maternity benefits. Doctors urged welfare measures, improved artificial diets and breast feeding. For example, in 1893 Biedert began his tract on infant feeding with the observation that the state should promote infant health measures as a means of overcoming an individualistic struggle for survival. Social welfare measures could transfer the struggle for survival from a struggle between individuals to a struggle between societies that depended on overall levels of health. The state was urged to support children's hospitals, the training of paediatricians, and promotion of dietary improvements.[133] While most paediatricians rejected the view that high infant mortality was symptomatic of a healthy survival of the fittest, biologically based welfare measures resulted in a proliferation of infant welfare clinics and services.

Midwifery

Improved midwifery and encouragement of breast feeding were the two responses by the state to the problem of infant mortality. From 1900 Althoff presided over the Prussian Medical Advisory Committee.[134] He took keen interest in discussions of the provision of midwives, and infant nutrition, as well as in the problems of abortion and contraception. Taken with his efforts to initiate action on tuberculosis and VD, Althoff's plans amount to a covert population policy using the state's public health apparatus. He directed the attention of medical scientists and welfare organizations to critical issues affecting family health and the birth rate.[135]

In 1900 the German Association of Midwives petitioned the Reichstag to grant them a monopoly over attendance at birth. They envisaged that each midwife should have a district with between 80 and 120 births per year, and that they should have a guaranteed income of 1,200 marks.[136] In 1902 the question came before the Prussian Medical Advisory Committee. The administration was concerned with the high infant mortality rates in rural areas, where often only a small percentage of births were attended by a qualified midwife. In the East Prussian district of Königsberg, only 20 per cent of births had a midwife present. The committee recommended improved education, the support of midwives' professional

---

[132] Kollwitz, *Ich sah*, p. 274.
[133] P. Biedert, *Die Kinderernährung im Säuglingsalter* (Stuttgart, 1880), (2nd edn 1893).
[134] *Wissenschaftlicher Beirat für das Medizinalwesen.*
[135] ZSTA M Rep 76 VIII B Nr 37 Wissenschaftliche Deputation für das Medizinalwesen.
[136] ZSTA M Rep 76 VIII B Nr 37; GSTA Dahlem Rep 84a Nr 10994 Bl 190, Hebammen.

associations, raising income by guaranteeing an income of 500 marks for a district midwife, and sickness benefits. Specially dutiful and industrious midwives should be rewarded with the title of *Oberhebamme*. It was a prescription for state-sponsored professionalization of midwifery. Similar schemes were mooted in other states. The Saxon Ministry of the Interior rejected compulsory attendance of midwives as an infringement of individual liberty. Midwives protested that implicit in such liberalism was the fact that more prosperous families could afford to have safer births with a doctor in attendance, whereas no provision was to be made for the majority of the population.[137]

Between 1901 and 1914 maternal mortality wavered between 3.1 and 3.6 per 1,000 live births. There was less concern for the mother than for infants, but it was felt that here too was a human wastage that could be reduced. 10,000 mothers died a year, and about 4,000 from childbed fever, which was attributed to lack of cleanliness in the home and on the part of the midwife. Officials hoped that midwives would monitor maternal health and disseminate advice on child care and nutrition. In 1902 midwives were asked to measure the temperature of mothers with a thermometer until nine days after birth.[138] This extension of midwives' responsibilities was a result of pressure from innovative paediatricians against the more conservative obstetricians who taught midwives. It was suggested that midwives should have certificates from the police stating that they were of good character, and that their rights to choose where they practised should be limited so as to ensure that they were evenly distributed throughout rural areas. In return midwives' salaries, training and status should be improved. The Prussian Ministries of Finance and Justice doggedly opposed any reform of midwifery. They insisted on the liberal principle that it was not the state's role to intervene in family matters.[139] This was not the standpoint of the Prussian Medical Department. The Minister of the Interior in 1907 and 1908 issued edicts that midwives should be educated in matters of infant welfare. The official textbook of 1912 on midwifery was to include a section on the care and feeding of infants. In 1908 a reform of midwives' fees was achieved. The public health lobby had to be content with piecemeal reform rather than comprehensive reorganization of midwifery services.

Political pressures for midwifery to be treated as an issue of national importance began to mount. The liberal Reichstag representative of the *Fortschrittliche Volkspartei* (Progressive People's Party) Otto Mugdan, saw improved education of midwives as a means to reduce infant mortality. He demanded a national reform as the question seemed to lie beyond the capacities of individual state administrations. In the following year, the Centre Party took up the question of midwifery reform

---

[137] STA Dresden MdI Nr 15249 Bl 240–7, Hebammenwesen 1911–14.
[138] STA Dresden MdI Nr 15245 Bl 201 Hebammenwesen, *Allgemeine deutsche Hebammen Zeitung*, vol. 17 (1902).
[139] GSTA Dahlem Rep 84a Nr 10995, Hebammen 1905–21; ZSTA M Rep 151 I C Nr 9071 Bekämpfung der Säuglingssterblichkeit und des Geburtenrückganges 1904–1916.

in the light of the declining birth rate. It urged that the Reich assume responsibility for a strong and healthy future generation. It also wanted private training institutions to continue, whereas the midwives' association campaigned for state facilities. On 7 February 1914 socialists joined in the pressure for national regulation of midwifery. They considered that through reform of midwifery, 8,000 mothers could be saved each year from invalidity and death. Antiseptic births were attacked as a class privilege, because deaths from childbed fever were lower among the wealthy. Maternity homes were the way to prevent the poor from dying in aseptic conditions. State officials attributed the slight rise in childbed fever to criminal abortions.

In line with the official principle that medical affairs should be left to individual states, Bethmann Hollweg (the Prussian Minister of the Interior) rejected the demand that midwifery reform required national legislation. This would violate the rights of federal states. The Reich administration defended this view until 1918. The only solution was that the Imperial Health Office should liaise with each state over the introduction of legislation. The states defended their autonomy when they submitted details of their provisions for infant health, but the Office's director, Franz Bumm, concluded by 1912 that some co-ordination was desirable. Here one can see how professional expertise – in this case, of the directors of midwifery training institutions – curbed the liberal federalism. Leading figures such as Bumm continued to emphasize the important role of private charity in the welfare sphere. Yet a comprehensive reform of midwifery was delayed until the changed constitutional circumstances of the Weimar Republic, and was then achieved only with difficulty.[140]

Breast feeding and purer milk

Whereas officials from the Ministry of Finance prevented health officials from using their budget for such 'humanitarian' ends as subsidizing educational courses on infant welfare, medical officials supported the campaign to extend breast feeding.[141] Medical officials had reservations over artificial feeding, but breast feeding seemed to be an ideal solution. It meant encouraging personal responsibility and provided a medically acceptable solution to the problem of infant deaths.

Whatever the causes of infant mortality, there was a widespread conservative tendency to blame mothers for infant deaths. Failure to breast feed, ignorance and incompetence were major accusations. These were associated with criticisms of the growing participation of women in the industrial labour force – and in the SPD. The breast feeding campaign was launched on a nation-wide basis, but in reality feeding practices varied from region to region. In certain districts of Bavaria *not* to

---

[140] M. Stürzbecher, 'Die Bekämpfung des Geburtenrückganges und der Säuglingssterblichkeit im Spiegel der Reichstagsdebatten *1900–1930*. Ein Beitrag zur Geschichte der Bevölkerungspolitik', PhD Freie Universität Berlin, 1954, pp. 55–77.
[141] ZSTA M Rep 76 VIII B Nr 2764 Bl 63–4, in 1906.

breast feed was a tradition. Confronted by numerous diets based on milk, cereals, eggs, sugar and rice, doctors sought to reduce the confusion based on local customs to a single correct diet on a proven scientific basis. Liebig invented a 'soup for infants' based on analogies to mother's milk and physiological needs. Nestlé followed with a milk and cereal diet, and then physiologically trained paediatricians experimented with the aim of making cow's milk like mother's milk in its mineral and protein content. Urban expansion meant a decline in breast feeding, and much attention was given to milk hygiene in cities such as Berlin.[142] Medical science sought to restore a natural diet – or its artificial equivalent – to counter urban degeneration.

Infant feeding practices became the object of surveys and campaigns. In 1887 the Berlin statistician and patriotic ideologist, Boeckh, discovered that the mortality among those infants not breast fed was six times as great as among those who were. An unfortunate feature of the statistics on infant feeding practices was that they were not correlated with social class or mother's occupation.[143] Mothers – especially working mothers – were criticized for neglecting their children. Yet no statistics of the proportion of working women who were mothers were ever produced. Nor did the state correlate infant mortality statistics with feeding practices, class or maternal occupation. Some local surveys of infant feeding between 1905 and 1912 did ask for the mother's occupation. These showed that 5–15 per cent of mothers gave occupation as a cause of not breast feeding. That these surveys were compiled by crusaders for the mother's duty to breast feed meant that physiological reasons such as the cessation of milk or illness might be exaggerated.[144] Biases in the attitudes of compilers of these surveys should be taken into account since these can give the statistics the quality of ideological gauges of groups of concerned experts rather than accurate representations of child-rearing practices.[145] Among other accusations against mothers were a range of moral censures of the lapse of maternal duty for self-indulgent luxury. Not breast feeding was blamed on such fashions as the wearing of corsets.[146] The substantial proportion of women working was the object of much high-minded criticism. Here was a society unable to adapt to industrial working practices and to consumer demand. Official morality was itself a type of corset that sought to restrain the population from enjoying benefits of a consumer and market-oriented society. That such a high proportion of infant deaths was among the illegitimate reinforced the moral argument. Eugenicists blamed alcoholism, inherited incapacity and the physically degenerating urban environment as causes of not breast feeding.[147] The

[142] Kintner, 'Determinants', pp. 218–25; A. Peiper, *Chronik der Kinderheilkunde* (Leipzig, 1951), pp. 156–207.   [143] Spree, *Soziale Ungleichheit*, p. 66.   [144] Spree, *Soziale Ungleichheit*, p. 70.
[145] Spree, *Soziale Ungleichheit*, pp. 69–72.
[146] W. Artelt, 'Kleidungshygiene im 19. Jahrhundert', in Artelt, E. Heischkel, G. Mann and W. Rüegg (eds.), *Städte-, Wohnungs- und Kleidungshygiene des 19. Jahrhunderts in Deutschland* (Stuttgart, 1969), pp. 119–35.
[147] 14. A. Bluhm, 'Stillfähigkeit', in A. Grotjahn and I. Kaup (eds.), *Handwörterbuch der sozialen Hygiene* (Leipzig, 1912), II, pp. 555–70; Bluhm, 'Stillhäufigkeit und Stilldauer', in Grotjahn and Kaup, *Handwörterbuch der sozialen Hygiene*, pp. 570–91.

state sought to impose a nationalist ideology of motherhood by ignoring demands for purer milk while concentrating on breast feeding as a panacea for physical, moral and social ills.

At the turn of the century there was much public concern over the purity of milk. In the late 1890s certain bacteriologists, particularly Theobald Smith, an American, and Bernhard Bang, a Dane, emphasized that the best means to prevent TB would be its control in cattle. But in Germany, despite innovations in milk hygiene through measures such as pasteurization and sterilization, the state was reluctant to support efforts to provide purer milk. Scientific experts disagreed over the links between infected milk and infant deaths. At the International Tuberculosis Conferences in 1901 and 1908, Koch pronounced that human and bovine TB were totally distinct, and that no precautions were necessary to protect humans against infection with the bovine bacillus. He considered that the prevalence of unboiled milk showed the lack of infectiousness. Behring took the opposite view, believing that tuberculosis in humans was contracted in childhood by the drinking of infected milk. He developed an expensive bovovaccine for cattle herds. Later research rejected the extremes of Behring and Koch's views. American, British and German commissions (in 1907) supported the opinion of the transmissibility of TB from animals to humans, but considered that there were two distinct forms of human and bovine TB. The questions of virulence and incidence were left unanswered. The situation was further complicated by the opinions on the relations between the human, avian and bovine baccilli originating from a common stock but having evolved 'racial peculiarities' due to their different food, temperature and resistance in different animals. These opinions show how bacteriology was an extension of evolutionary biology.

Although some bacteriologists claimed that there were large numbers of tuberculosis bacilli in milk, their observations were shown to have confused harmless bacilli widely present in food with the tuberculosis bacillus. It was suggested that the human bacillus was more virulent than the bovine bacillus, and as a consequence adults were unaffected. In children, however, bovine TB was considered to cause a quarter of all cases of TB, resulting in alarming numbers of crippled children. The quality of milk became an emotive issue. Studies made of mortality relating to milk showed that this was greatly exaggerated as a carrier of diseases. Some researchers accused milk of containing a germ causing 'cholera infantum'. This was never substantiated. Milk was accused of harbouring infections such as diphtheria and scarlet fever, but epidemiological studies showed that milk might have been the carrier of the infection in only a few cases. Moreover, consumption of milk during epidemics was generally low. The issue of the infectiousness of milk was kept alive by the veterinary profession which made its professional reputation by 'saving' humanity from the dubious perils of infected cattle and contaminated milk.[148] As better transport, cooking and household

---

[148] P.G. Heinemann, *Milk* (Philadelphia and London, 1919).

handling of milk were introduced, the differential in mortality between breast fed and artificially fed infants began to disappear.

The provision of milk was bound up with the question of women's work. France had taken the lead in providing *consultations de maternité* in the early 1890s. Sterilized milk was supplied to mothers who could not breast feed, and babies were weighed and seen by a doctor. In 1892 the Paris doctor, Pierre Budin, organized *consultations de nourrissons*, and in 1894 Léon Dufour opened a dispensary at Fécamp called the *Gouttes de Lait*. He provided hygienically controlled milk for the babies of working mothers and for those mothers needing to supplement breast milk.[149] This developed into an international mass movement for infant feeding. But it did not win official German approval. The reports by the Paris consulate on the provision of cheap sterilized milk were disapproved of by medical officials.[150] Gottstein made a statistical study of the aetiology of TB in 1901. He concluded that the mortality from TB in children who were breast fed was half that of those nourished on cow's milk. The Imperial Health Office reported that breast feeding was to have a priority over milk provision.[151] The Prussian medical official, Eduard Dietrich, and the Prussian Medical Advisory Committee gave priority to breast feeding and to the moral strategy of raising the sense of maternal duty. In 1907 he reported that at the International Gouttes de Lait Congress, the French emphasis on artificial feeding was being replaced by the German methods of natural feeding and education.

Social Darwinists such as Röse, the Dresden expert on dental hygiene, argued that the inability to breast feed was a sign of the degeneration of the white race.[152] University professors and medical officials rejected the assertion that civilization caused degeneration. The Berlin paediatrician, Heubner, supported breast feeding as superior to any artificial method at the Prussian Medical Advisory Committee. In 1904 Prussian officials had decided that mothers should be educated on the dangers of artificial feeding and alcoholism, and on the need to breast feed. Special dispensaries (modelled on TB dispensaries) should supply welfare subsidies to breast feeding mothers. Antagonism to artificial feeding meant that in 1907 the Imperial Health Office declined to recommend a hygienic design of bottle. In contrast, in France a law regulating their design came into force in 1910. Only an especially hot summer and high mortality in 1911, caused the German authorities to consider action against bottles with long feeding tubes. A survey on their manufacture and use established that they were difficult to clean and that the milk

[149] D. Dwork, *War is Good for Babies and Other Young Children* (London and New York, 1987), pp. 94–102.
[150] ZSTA P 15.01 Nr 11989 Bekämpfung der Säuglingssterblichkeit in fremden Staaten Bl 1–2; ZSTA M Rep 76 VIII B Nr 2763 Bl 76, report of 20 July 1905.
[151] ZSTA M Rep 76 VIII B Nr 38 and 2765 Bl 31–5.
[152] C. Röse, 'Die Wichtigkeit der Mutterbrust für die körperliche und geistige Entwicklung des Menschen', *Deutsche Monatsschrift für Zahnheilkunde*, vol. 23 (1905), in ZSTA M Rep 76 VIII B Nr 2762 Bl. 353–76.

went cold.[153] In 1912 a baby's bottle law was prepared. The proposed law met with a stormy response in the Reichstag. It was asserted that most deaths were due to inherited diseases, so that such a law was unnecessary. Socialists opposed the legislation as too limited in scope, and conservatives emphasized that the state should not interfere in an area where private charity was the solution. The law did not reach the statute books.[154] Although it had been hoped that breast feeding would instil patriotic values into the family, the complexities of diverse infant feeding practices were politically divisive. Officials refused to recognize that artificial feeding under hygienic conditions could achieve a mortality rate as low as for breast feeding.

Entrepreneurs of infant health

Special hospital facilities for infants were a product of the enhanced sense of value attached to infant life and of the application of science to social problems. Arthur Schlossmann pioneered such hospitals as part of comprehensive schemes for social hygiene of infants. Schlossmann was born in 1867, and his father was a wealthy merchant. In 1891 he qualified in medicine and received training in child health in the Kaiser und Kaiserin Friedrich-Kinderkrankenhaus, a specialized children's hospital opened in 1890 in Berlin. It was supported by voluntary contributions, until it passed into municipal control in 1900. Schlossmann moved to Dresden in 1893 where he set up as a general practitioner in a working–class district. In March 1894 he opened a 'Policlinic for Infants and Children' in his practice. He organized a range of initiatives on infant health between coming to Dresden in 1893 and moving to Düsseldorf in 1906. These illustrate a distinctive blend of personal careerism, humanitarian zeal and academic specialization at a time when there was genuine hardship among recently qualified doctors.

Schlossmann offers insight into the combination of professional and social factors that produced an innovative type of social medicine – or social hygiene – in Germany around the turn of the century. Similar pursuit of welfare aims in medicine can be seen in several other young general practitioners during the 1890s. Gottstein, as general practitioner in Berlin during the 1890s, took on honorary responsibilities for child health in the municipality of Charlottenburg. He developed Charlottenburg into a model health and welfare administration with an exemplary range of infant and child health services such as breast feeding premiums and family allowances for officials. There were numerous examples of such career development from general practice to social hygiene during the 1890s and 1900s. The overcrowded university system produced excessive numbers of doctors, who applied their scientific expertise to develop hitherto marginal areas of medicine

---

[153] ZSTA M Rep 76 VIII B Nr 2789 Die Berichte der Ober- und Regierungspräsidenten auf den Runderlass von 21 Dezember 1911 betr. die Benutzung von Rohrsaugflaschen.

[154] M. Stürzbecher, 'Bekämpfung', pp. 138–147; M. Stürzbecher, 'Zur Geschichte der Kindersaugflaschen', *Forschungen und Fortschritte*, vol. 33 (1959), 78–83.

such as dermatology and child health. While an element of personal careerism underlay the rapid expansion of social medicine, these doctors responded to the social crisis of exceptionally rapid industrialization.

Saxony had one of the highest infant mortality rates in Germany: between 1890 and 1895 it stood at 28 per cent. Dresden, the capital of Saxony, was the fifth largest German city and rapidly growing. (Its population rose from 177,000 in 1870 to 548,000 in 1910.) A children's hospital had been founded in 1878, but infant care was still neglected. In 1896 Schlossmann established an association for infant and child health for the support of the *Kinderpoliklinik* in a Dresden suburb, the Johannstadt. His next step was to transform this policlinic into a specialized hospital for infant care.[155] In August 1898 he opened the first infant hospital (*Säuglingsheim*)[156] in Germany where nurses for infants were trained. It was initially on a small scale with ten beds. Schlossmann argued that infants required special nutrition and nursing. This shows the drive towards professionalism and specialization, resulting in a breaking away from general paediatrics, which had developed as a branch of general practice and was supported by middle-class philanthropic initiatives. He linked infant health to the development of specialized hospitals that required the training of infant nurses. Institutions provided the opportunity for research into scientific aspects of infant care. Schlossmann furthered his career with a habilitation thesis in 1898 on the differences between cow and human milk, and in 1902 he was granted the title of professor. He continued to undertake chemical and physiological researches on infant nutrition, which he regarded as the key to infant health. It was an approach that went with the demand for large-scale institutions and professionalization of infant care. He argued that panel and poor law doctors could cope with minor ailments among infants, whereas special institutional care was needed for the really sick. His infant hospital was a model for others which opened in Vienna, Heidelberg, Strasburg, Solingen, Berlin and Danzig by 1914.

Schlossmann cultivated the support of doctors and of academics at the Technical University. But most finance came from industrialists. From March 1896 he negotiated with Karl August Lingner of the Dresden Chemical Laboratories and manufacturer of the mouth wash Odol. The hospital was expanded with Lingner's support, the benefactions of other industrialists and the efforts of a women's committee chaired by the mayor's wife. By 1904 it could take fifty infants, and in 1907 it became a municipal institution. Schlossmann's social hygienic approach was based on stringent asepsis, natural methods and education. Where possible the infants were to be suckled by wet-nurses, who were provided with accommodation and could bring their own babies into the institution. Mothers were also encouraged to breast-feed their babies. There were farm facilities for the supply of cow and goat milk, so that this should be free of infections. The milk kitchen also

---

[155] P. Wunderlich, 'Arthur Schlossmann und seine Bemühungen um die Anerkennung der Kinderheilkunde in Dresden, 1893 bis 1906', *Beiträge zur Geschichte der Universität Erfurt*, vol. 12 (1965–66), 167–80.   [156] infant hospital.

supplied infants being cared for outside the institution, and mothers were to be educated as to the proper diets for their babies. The influence of the parallel campaign for public TB sanatoria was reflected in Schlossmann's enthusiasm for fresh air. His hospital was designed with balconies where infants could be kept during warmer months. A forest settlement provided a further ninety beds for convalescent children and for those with TB, rickets and anaemia aged up to three years, and a department for premature births. There was great concern for those infants with syphilis. The attached policlinic was used to distribute special meals and welfare supplements. The policlinic was carefully designed with facilities for prams, and there was a pharmacy, laboratory and gymnasium. Contact with general practitioners was maintained. It became a model institution of world renown.[157] Schlossmann attracted the attention of Althoff, who was keen to support the application of socially relevant advances in medical science. It was due to Althoff that in 1906 Schlossmann moved to the recently founded medical academy at Düsseldorf where he pioneered state-supported welfare facilities, linking the training of nursing specialists to state services. Schlossmann regarded the Ruhr as a challenge because of high concentration of industry. In contrast to Dresden he developed centralized welfare institutions and networks of midwives and health visitors with a combination of state and municipal support. He regarded integrated welfare services as making the difference between guerilla warfare and national mobilization to reduce infant mortality and to promote a strong and numerous *Volk*.[158]

Infant health was a key element of Lingner's plans to promote health education on a massive scale. In 1908 he produced a memorandum on the organization of infant and maternal health. This reflected the views of Schlossmann in its strong nutritional bias. He attributed over 60 per cent of infant deaths to poor nutrition. Lingner's aim was to have a complete national coverage of maternal clinics, crèches and milk depots. He demanded what he called *Säuglingsgrundbücher* – a type of infant register, which could then be correlated with health records of, for example, the school health services.[159] He continued to collaborate with Schlossmann in efforts to create national systems of surveillance for infant welfare. Lingner died in 1916 leaving a foundation with capital of ten million marks. This was to be used primarily for infant welfare, health education and school medical services in Saxony. One quarter of the foundation's income went towards boosting state measures in infant welfare in Saxony.[160] That this final bequest was designed to supplement state resources exemplifies the transition in infant care from philanthropy to state-supported measures.

[157] W. Haberling, *Arthur Schlossmann, sein Leben und Werk* (Düsseldorf, 1927).
[158] A. Schlossmann, 'Ueber die Organisation des Vereins für Säuglingsfürsorge im Regierungsbezirke Düsseldorf', *Concordia*, vol. 15 (1908), 239–49.
[159] K.A. Lingner, *Betrachtungen über die Säuglingsfrage mit einem Vorschlage für die Organisation einer Landeszentrale Säuglingspflege und Mutterschutz in Hessen*, (Dresden, 1908); Sächsischer Landesgesundheitsrat, *Einrichtungen auf dem Gebiete der Volksgesundheits- und Volkswohlfahrtspflege* (Dresden, 1922), p. 48.   [160] *Einrichtungen*, p. 110.

Imperialism and infant health

The infant welfare campaign rapidly left its basis of support in voluntary associations of individual philanthropists to become a national and imperialist movement in the decade before 1914. There emerged a 'national social' ideology of welfare, best articulated by the liberal Friedrich Naumann. He not only had links with a range of reforming groups ranging from feminists in the League of German Women (*Bund deutscher Frauen*) to the German *Werkbund* (an arts and crafts organization), but he also inspired initiatives in social hygiene. For example, his disciple Alfons Fischer developed the idea of maternity insurance as the central feature of a campaign for social hygiene on an educative model in Baden.[161] Naumann fostered the development of social work as a specifically female occupation to serve the nation. His journal, *Die Hilfe*, approved of feminism as part of a movement of patriotic social reform. He argued that a strong nation had to promote social welfare measures. Infant and child nursing followed the pattern of development from voluntary organizations into a state registered and secular profession. The movement influenced Schlossmann (a left-wing liberal) and a number of other infant welfare experts. It provided an ideological basis for state bureaucrats, professional experts, and church nursing organizations to co-operate in promoting the health of the German family.

The infant welfare movement developed with exceptional vigour after 1904. This coincided with the decline in infant mortality. Of all the various public health campaigns – such as for TB, VD and alcoholism – the infant welfare campaign developed the most centralized institutions. Bourgeois philanthropy was linked to imperialism through influential official patronage. The result was the founding of the Kaiserin Auguste Viktoria Haus (KAVH) for the Combating of Infant Mortality. Between 1906 and its opening in 1909 there was a massive campaign to mobilize public support as the KAVH assumed direction of infant health measures.[162] This model institution for infant care was the product of developments in the sphere of welfare policy, and professional specialization in medicine and nursing. That it was a specialized institution for infant care was in itself remarkable. Paediatricians were divided over the merits of separating infant care from child health. In Berlin they were overridden by a mixture of welfare concerns and socio-political motives. During 1904 the Prussian medical authorities debated with alarm the high infant mortality rates in Berlin, where over one-fifth of all infants died in their first year of life.[163] The success in Dresden in providing adequate hospital facilities for sick infants meant that other municipal and state authorities wished to emulate these.[164]

[161] K.-D. Thomann, *Alfons Fischer (1873–1936) und die Badische Gesellschaft für Sozialhygiene* (Cologne, 1980), p. 12.
[162] *Schriftenreihe zur Geschichte der Kinderheilkunde aus dem Archiv des Kaiserin Auguste Viktoria Hauses (KAVH) – Berlin*, vol. 1–4, (1986–7).
[163] ZSTA M Rep 76 VIII B Nr 2762 Bl 62, Die Sorge um die Erhaltung des Neugeborenen.
[164] 'Säuglingsschutz', *Berliner Tageblatt* (19 July 1904).

A precursor for the KAVH was the *Berliner Krippenverein* (Crèche Association), which provided crèches. This association typifies the transition from a liberal bourgeois philanthropic association (it was founded in 1877) to a specialized medical institution. In 1901 the Empress became its patron; officials such as Dietrich and Althoff and aristocrats such as Behr-Pinnow, a member of the personal retinue of the Empress, took over the managing committee. It supervized smaller crèches in industrial districts. Here, the wives of industrialists such as Rathenau were active. To mark the silver wedding of the Emperor and Empress in 1906, it built a day and night crèche with medical facilities. In association with the neighbouring Pestallozzi-Froebel Haus, it offered training in infant care and nursing. In 1908 Fritz Rott was appointed as its medical superintendent, and the professor of paediatrics and the state officials groomed him for duties in the Kaiserin Auguste Viktoria Haus, where he opened a department of social hygiene.[165] Rott along with the aristocrat Behr-Pinnow was instrumental in fusing eugenics with the movement for infant health.

State officials shared in the sense of alarm at high rates of infant mortality. They considered that it was the responsibility of the mother to care for her babies, and that artificial feeding was a sign of a lack of maternal duty. A distinct vision of the German mother began to take shape in the official mind. The Prussian medical official, Eduard Dietrich – of a pietistic and patriotic disposition – insisted that the caring German mother was not like the egotistic French mother; the German preferred 'natural' methods of care to bottle feeding her infant, and was prepared to devote herself to her family and country rather than to indulge herself with consumer luxuries. A new term gained currency, that of the 'child rich' family, which became a much-vaunted ideal for official welfare policies and for nationalist pressure groups. Social biology provided a rationale for such high-minded infant welfare. The infant health campaign contradicted the Social Darwinist theory that high infant mortality was a sign of a healthy process of selection. Lower infant mortality went with a lower child mortality. If the Darwinian theory was correct, high infant mortality would have been the precondition for improved child and adult mortality rates. French infant mortality rates were lower and the rates of survival to productive adulthood were higher.[166] Given that infant health experts were convinced that most deaths were due to bad diets and dirt, effective action could be taken. There was faith that environmental improvements would secure the health of future generations. Biology supported environmental and social reforms as vital for maintaining the long-term survival of the nation.

Although medical officials urged state intervention, they were limited by the liberal constitution that relegated family welfare to the private sphere of individual philanthropy. A way of circumventing this was to sponsor welfare organizations. In 1904 a Society for Combating Infant Deaths[167] was founded by Prussian officials and a number of dignitaries such as aristocrats, bankers and their wives. Its

[165] M. Stürzbecher, *100 Jahre Berliner Krippenverein* (Berlin, 1977).
[166] STA Dresden MdI Nr 15245 Das Hebammenwesen Bl 108.
[167] Gesellschaft zur Bekämpfung der Säuglingssterblichkeit.

propaganda was aimed not only at instructing mothers in domestic hygiene, but at broader targets. One was that of consumerism and personal luxury; another was the eugenic argument that industrialization had caused degeneration which made mothers physically unable to breast feed. In contrast, the Berlin paediatrician, Heubner, diagnosed the situation as a lack of will on the part of mothers. He endorsed the ideology that a healthy state was based on a strong family. These opinions were echoed by the Empress. In November 1904 the Empress preached the virtues of breast feeding and education in child care to the Patriotic Women's League. Auguste-Viktoria had taken a lead in building churches in industrial suburbs, and was renowned for her piety and dedication to charitable causes and to her family. She headed the League, which engaged in voluntary nursing. The Empress gave full support to the infant health campaign, and the need for state support was urged. The Empress' political outlook was highly conservative, and her intervention into infant health coincided with the growing influence of conservative philanthropists over social policy. Imperial power and infant health were intertwined.[168] In 1894 the Red Cross in association with the Patriotic Women's League established a section for infant care. Leading state officials like Althoff and Dietrich joined forces in establishing the Society to Combat Infant Mortality in 1904. They organized infant crèches and clinics (on the model of TB dispensaries) to advise mothers on infant care in Berlin. They wished to'encourage breast feeding and improve standards of maternal care by education. In 1904 the Prussian state granted funds for the first child welfare clinic. The Empress supported these campaigns and the Patriotic Women's League staffed the clinics. Premiums were paid for breast feeding. In 1909 the idea of a mother's milk bank was proposed.[169] By 1915 there were over one thousand infant clinics.

The political edge to the infant health campaign was clear, since it gathered force in reaction to the establishing of the League for the Protection of Mothers in 1905. This was a radical organization to promote the welfare of unmarried mothers and to campaign for social and sexual liberation for women. Its message was that the mother was the source of the *Volkskraft*. The League attracted the support of feminists, liberal industrialists, innovators in social medicine and eugenicists. In March 1905 its well-attended meetings were causing alarm among official circles and there were attempts to have it suppressed. Behr-Pinnow, a Privy Councillor and member of the Empress' personal staff, wrote to the Berlin Police President, Georg von Borries, that the Emperor and Empress were outraged by the League. The Police President replied that he could do little except under the public indecency laws, because the League was supported by the educated middle class. The League for Protection of Mothers campaigned for 'sexual reform', and it posed a radical challenge to official views on the role of women and the family for the next twenty-five years.

---

168 ZSTA M Rep 151 I C Nr 9071 (Finanz Ministerium) betr. die Bekämpfung der Säuglingssterblichkeit; I.V. Hull, *The Entourage of Kaiser Wilhelm II* (Cambridge, 1982), pp. 18–22.
169 ZSTA M Rep 77 Tit 662 Nr 44 Beiakten 9 Vereine zur Bekämpfung der Säuglingssterblichkeit.
170 ZSTA M Rep 77 Tit 662 Nr 123 Betr. den Bund für Mutterschutz.

Conservative philanthropists tried to wean the public away from the radicalism of the League for the Protection of Mothers. In October 1905 a committee on infant health began to meet in the Prussian Kultusministerium. It was chaired by Althoff, the education official. Again Behr-Pinnow was a key figure. In 1905 he circulated a manifesto among state officials denouncing Social Darwinist arguments on the selective value of high infant mortality. He urged that infant care committees be established throughout Germany and that there be a model central institution for infant care. In June 1906 the Chancellor announced to the Reichstag that there was to be a public campaign for an infant welfare institution. The organizing committee was itself managed from above with Althoff and Behr-Pinnow directing public health officials and child welfare specialists. Their efforts in co-ordinating municipal, state and voluntary bodies ensured that the infant welfare campaign had a 'national' aura. They drummed up public support with pamphlets, lectures, and exhibitions on infant care. The Municipality of Charlottenburg gave the site for building the infant hospital, and the Reich contributed 500,000 marks and Prussia 200,000 annually. Contributions from associations and individuals amounted to only a small proportion in comparison with funds from state sources. This was all the more remarkable at a time when there were few national medical institutions. The KAVH was called a *Reichsanstalt* (Reich institution) and was to serve the needs of all states, although it was independent from the Reich administration. It maintained the position of an independent but national organization, under the supervision of a highly conservative board of governors, until the Third Reich.[171]

The 'infant palace' had multiple functions, as it aimed to provide institutional and outpatient care through a policlinic and welfare centre. It had an obstetrics department, and a mothers' home. It cared for both healthy and sick infants. There was an institute for study of the physiology and social hygiene of infant development. Its kitchens prepared model diets. It acted as a centre for training of infant and children's nurses. The KAVH supported a policy of separate training for those who were to care for sick infants (the *Säuglingskrankenpflegerin*), and for those who would look after healthy infants, particularly in the context of a family (the *Säuglingspflegerin*). The English nursery nurse or nanny was the model, although a more scientific type of training was considered necessary. In any case, training was to be supervised by paediatricians. A comprehensive curriculum covering all aspects of infant care was formulated: diet, clothing, bedding, and accommodation were all part of this. For infant psychology, Friedrich Froebel was prescribed.[172] The KAVH imposed uniform standards on the forty welfare training establishments.[173] It compiled and distributed manuals in infant care which were given official status. It also had a public function as it launched a mass education

---

[171] ZSTA M Rep 151 I C Nr 9071; ZSTA P 15.01 11982 Errichtung einer Musteranstalt zur Bekämpfung der Säuglingssterblichkeit; 15.01 Nr 11983.
[172] ZSTA M Rep 76 VIII B Nr 27911.   [173] ZSTA P 15.01 Nr 11974 Bl 147.

programme for mothers and mothers-to-be by means of courses, pamphlets and lectures. It sought to dragoon the nation's babies into a regimented pattern of regular feeds and hygienic habits. In periods of high infant mortality during the summer months (as during 1911), it issued emergency mass publicity leaflets (*Hitze-Merkblätter*) on the care of infants.[174]

During its first decade, research was conducted on the physiology of child development and nutrition. In these areas the KAVH followed the dominant physiological model in medicine. This was the interest of its first director Arthur Keller. However, this post required a degree of diplomatic tact and a type of sanctimonious, moral nationalist outlook that Keller evidently did not possess. The board of governors, composed of high ranking aristocrats and ministerial officials, dismissed Keller in 1911.[175] He was succeeded by Leo Langstein, who was also interested in nutrition, but gave more emphasis to questions of social hygiene. Rott, the senior physician from 1911 and the co-director from 1922, blended infant care with nationalist ideology. He had made his mark at the *Krippenverein*, and continued to work in association with the ministerial official, Dietrich. As director of the department for social hygiene, Rott developed a comprehensive strategy of preventive care in infant and child health. He wrote on crèches, prams, mother-craft instruction, and the co-ordination of the work of midwives and infant nurses. He directed the Prussian central office for infant care[176] and was honorary secretary of the German Association for Infant Care[177] (founded in 1908).[178] The aim of the state was to co-ordinate the efforts of all local infant welfare associations. As with the TB clinics, their functions were those of education and the dispensing of welfare supplements. The central agency's chairman was Otto Krohne, the medical official responsible for investigating the declining birth rate.[179] Rott's approach illustrates the expansiveness of the infant care movement; he regarded all infants as at risk, and so requiring professional supervision. Furthermore, he considered that two-thirds of the new born required medical attention. The KAVH led the drive towards comprehensive supervision of parents and infants.[180]

The link between scientific and national concerns was exemplified by Behr-Pinnow, who took over the administration of the KAVH. He drew moralistic conclusions from infant mortality statistics, and wrote on the importance of combating the declining birth rate and on the value of improved welfare services. Rott and Behr-Pinnow inculcated a strongly moralistic and nationalist tone in

[174] E. Dietrich, 'Fürsorgewesen für Säuglinge', *Bericht über den XIV internationalen Kongress für Hygiene und Demographie. Berlin 23–29 September 1907* (Berlin, 1908), II, pp. 393–427.
[175] M. Stürzbecher, 'Zum 100. Geburtstag von Arthur Keller', *Medizinische Monatsschrift*, vol. 23 (1968), 544–9.   [176] *Centrale für Säuglingsschutz*.
[177] *Deutsche Vereinigung für Säuglingsschutz*.
[178] D. Tutzke, 'Die Habilitanden Alfred Grotjahns (1869–1931)', *Clio Medica*, vol. 3 (1968), 251–64.
[179] ZSTA M Rep 77 Tit 662 Nr 44 Beiakten 9.
[180] F. Rott, 'Das Problem der Erfassung fürsorgebedürftiger ehelicher Säuglinge', in L. Langstein (ed.), *Beiträge zur Physiologie, Pathologie und sozialen Hygiene des Kindesalters* (Berlin, 1919), pp. 603–39.

infant care associations. In September 1913 they emphasized that infant health was vital to Germany's position as a world power. Langstein criticized the eugenicists as underrating the extent to which paediatricians could remedy weakness at birth. But Behr-Pinnow and Rott accepted positive eugenics by the First World War.[181] At the same time Behr-Pinnow modified some of his moral outrage vented at the League for the Protection of Mothers when he conceded that special care was needed for babies born out of wedlock. Conservative morality was persuaded by medical considerations into accepting broader-based public welfare measures. During the 1920s Behr-Pinnow took a lead in eugenics organizations, and in 1933 came out in favour of sterilization, indicating the extent to which welfare campaigners acted in accordance with prevailing political powers.

The KAVH exemplifies how the idea of motherhood was appropriated by imperialist and national ideology. One of its most important functions was to shift the responsibility for family welfare from a private concern to the professions and the state. Moral and educational strategies, reinforced by scientific rationales, came to predominate in hygiene. If the early work of Schlossmann is compared with the later phase of the KAVH, an interesting contrast emerges. Schlossmann used considerable skills of entrepreneurship and tapped private reserves of bourgeois philanthropy for the support of the Dresden infant hospital. Once he moved to Düsseldorf he became influenced by Naumann's social imperialism. According to Bethmann Hollweg, the Prussian Minister of the Interior, Schlossmann's writings on child care merited the widest public distribution.[182] Schlossmann influenced the establishing of a network of infant and child welfare facilities in the administrative district of Düsseldorf with specially trained urban and rural social workers. Concern centred on the problems of 'child rich' but economically poor families. The imperialist atmosphere prior to the war resulted in a fusion of social interests. When the German Association for Infant Protection (*Deutscher Verein für Säuglingsschutz*) held its first conference in 1909, its committee consisted of Behr-Pinnow, Lingner and the ministerial official, Dietrich. This represented the fusion of the state, the imperial court and commerce. The Society for Child Health in 1911 rallied to imperialist aims by seeing children in the context of 'health, fitness, and military power'. The drive to develop specialized nursing cohorts showed that imperialism went with an impulse to further medical specialization. This was a two-edged process. On the one hand it expanded opportunities for training and specialized careers for male paediatricians. On the other, there were ancillary caring professions for which it was felt that women were especially suited.

The infant health movement illustrates a change in German liberal values during the crucial decade prior to the First World War. The state, and ruling elite, as well as professional specialists in infant care, came to dominate humanitarian

---

[181] M. Stürzbecher, 'Zum 100. Geburtstag von Fritz Rott', *Der Kinderarzt*, vol. 10 (1979), 601–3; ZSTA M Rep 151 IB IC Nr 9071.

[182] ZSTA P 15.01 11973 Bekämpfung der Säuglingssterblichkeit, Bl 159, dated 19. Jan. 1908; STA Dresden MdI Nr 17219.

philanthropic associations. The Empress' involvement imprinted the infant health campaign with a distinctive imperialist character. Once the ruling elite was removed in the wake of the First World War, maternal and infant health became symbols of national unity in their own right. Disparate interests in the infant welfare campaign sought a common basis for unity in promoting the health of the German family.

The struggle for school health

Officials responded to the public outcry over child health by supporting demands for school medical services and youth welfare. Child health was considered crucial to national renewal and future military fitness. Such health and welfare issues were a means of mobilizing nationalist sentiments among the public. Officials and medical officers sidestepped the constitutional restrictions that health and welfare were matters for private philanthropy and that federal states should be responsible only for the control of epidemics and infectious diseases. National child and youth welfare institutions and organizations were established. At the same time school health services became a state priority. The state fostered the development of approved youth organizations and promoted physical education.

Comparisons were made between rural and urban child health, and the health of military recruits from town and country. The assumption of greater inherent fitness of rural population stocks prompted a concern to promote fresh air, exercise and a reformed lifestyle as an antidote to the class room. In 1896 a German Schools Association to Combat Alcohol was founded by teachers and pupils. During the 1890s, at the same time as the authorities reversed their hostility to the natural sciences, such outdoor pursuits as school gymnastics and sports were introduced. Associations for playgrounds, sports facilities and holiday colonies grew in popularity. The youth hostel and *Wandervogel* movements began during the 1890s. From the turn of the century the spread of socialism stimulated the state to develop and centralize social facilities for youth so as to promote fitness and inculcate national values. Nationalists and radical reformers competed in the resort to natural values and outdoor activities.

School medical services became a national priority. They were initially demanded by liberal doctors and organized on a municipal basis, before being subject to state intervention at the turn of the century. When Virchow in 1869 complained that a school pathology was necessary, he wished for improved ventilation and heating to reduce the risks of foul air.[183] In 1864 a Breslau ophthalmologist, Hermann Cohn, discovered a high incidence of short-sightedness while undertaking pioneering medical inspections. In 1888 a Prussian decree on school health sounded a note of concern with the physical well-being of school

---

[183] R. Virchow, 'Ueber gewisse, die Gesundheit benachteiligende Einflüsse der Schulen,' *Archiv für pathologische Anatomie*, vol. 46 (1869), 447–70.

children. In 1887 a journal of school hygiene for teachers was launched by Ludwig Kotelmann in Hamburg, where there was a well-developed organization for philanthropic help for needy children.[184] In line with a physiological and environmental approach to hygiene, attention was initially given to physical growth, gymnastics, and the design of school buildings and their interiors. During the 1880s there was controversy on whether school children were overburdened by too much knowledge and deformed by long hours cramped up at badly designed desks in overcrowded class rooms. Public alarm was signalled by school-boy suicides that were attributed to academic overburdening. It was pointed out that concern for physical development was lacking, and a balance between mind, body and nature became the aim of educational and medical reformers.[185]

Municipal school medical services in Germany date from the 1880s. In 1883 Alexander Spiess was appointed *Stadtarzt* in Frankfurt-on-Main, his duty being to inspect schools. He measured the height and weight of 15,000 children, and improved the design of desks and buildings.[186] In 1895 the municipality of Wiesbaden took an important initiative by employing school doctors for regular medical examinations of all children. Their role was to screen for TB and for mental abnormalities like epilepsy and hysteria. These biological concerns opened the way to ideas of preventive medicine and marked a great advance over the quantitative anthropometric and building-design approach.[187] School doctors revealed an alarmingly high proportion of illness with a quarter of children having some disease, parasite or disability. In 1898 the Prussian state decreed that municipalities were free to employ school doctors. In 1899 medical officers were made responsible for buildings, sanitation and prevention of infectious diseases. Conservatives protested that school doctors meant unwarranted undermining of parental responsibility for children.[188] By 1900 there were twenty school doctors (although still part-time) in Berlin, and in 1913 there were 3,000 school doctors in Prussia. The first full-time school doctor was appointed in 1904. Conservative and state authorities reversed their hostility to school health services. In 1909 the Prussian *Kultusminister*, August Trott zu Solz, wrote to the Kaiser to the effect that Berlin children were weaker than average.[189] Paediatricians were asked to examine school health in relation to military needs. Erich Peiper, professor at Greifswald, conducted a survey of military fitness in 1910.[190] In January 1914 the

[184] A. Gräfin zu Castell-Rüdenhausen, 'Die Überwindung der Armenschulen, Schülerhygiene an den Hamburger öffentlichen Volksschulen im zweiten Kaiserreich', *Archiv für Sozialgeschichte*, vol. 22 (1982), 201–26.
[185] J.C. Albisetti, *Secondary School Reform in Imperial Germany* (Princeton and Guildford, 1983).
[186] K. Hartung, 'Einhundert Jahre schulärztlicher Dienst – ein beinahe vergessenes Jubiläum', *Öffentliches Gesundheitswesen*, vol. 45 (1983), 615–17.
[187] C. Schmid-Monnard, 'Die Aufgaben des Schularztes', *Politisch-Anthropologische Revue*, vol. 1 (1902/3), 201–4.
[188] ZSTA M Rep 76 VIII B Nr 2828 Bl 285; 'Der Schularzt', *Nationalzeitung*, (10 February 1899).
[189] 'Dienstordnung für die Schulärzte in Wiesbaden', *Centralblatt für die gesamte Unterrichtsverwaltung in Preussen* (18 May 1898), 390–7.
[190] ZSTA M Rep 76 VIII B Nr 1917 Bl 149, 200–7.

War Ministry intervened in order to make school health a national priority.[191] School medical services were subject to the shift from liberal sanitary hygiene to militarism.

School dental services expanded from the turn of the century after they were initiated in Strasburg in 1900. The founder of the Strasburg dental clinic and school dental service, Ernst Jessen, was inspired by Hueppe's emphasis on the importance of eating habits for dental health. Poor teeth were regarded as a mark of degeneration for they were considered foci for a range of infections. Jessen argued that education in dental health ought to be a priority. Other pioneering work was undertaken by Röse in Dresden between 1896 and 1902. Röse conducted surveys of dental caries in 70,000 children and military recruits. He attributed caries to environmental factors (especially the lack of mineral salts in drinking water), to life-style (for example, the lack of breast feeding) and to racial factors. Noting that caries was more frequent among the more prosperous, he argued that it was a sign of racial degeneration.[192] Germany was to take a *Führerrolle* in the hygiene of the teeth and mouth. The school medical services underwent the same process of centralization as other welfare services. A German Central Committee for School Dentistry was established in 1908 under state patronage. Local committees raised money for school dental clinics. These were financed by a mixture of municipal, state and voluntary contributions. The committees arranged public lectures and educational pamphlets on dental hygiene.[193] This was part of a movement obsessed with measuring, weighing and medically examining school children. Statistics on height, weight, short-sightedness and dental caries added material to the debate on degeneration of the race and the declining health of military recruits.

The concern was not only to establish the physical condition of school children but also to inculcate healthy habits and a sense of responsibility to future generations. Eugenicists took a lead in demanding a school curriculum with health education as a major feature. Academic education was deemed insufficient for girls: Gruber, the Munich professor, demanded that they be trained in mothercraft and domestic science.[194] The 'future generation' became a rallying cry, bringing together teachers, medical experts, the clergy and eugenicists. Health and fitness were to be an integral part of education. Municipalities were able to take pioneering initiatives beyond the capacity of state authorities. This is exemplified in certain municipalities such as Charlottenburg and Düsseldorf which achieved the reputation of providing model child welfare institutions. In Charlottenburg,

---

[191] ZSTA M Rep 76 VIII B Nr 2831; C. Schmid-Monnard, 'Soziale Fürsorge für Kinder im schulpflichtigen Alter', in T. Weyl (ed.), *Handbuch der Hygiene* (Jena, 1904), 4th suppl. vol., pp. 409–44.

[192] C.P. Heidel and G. Heidel, 'Zu Carl Röses wissenschaftlichen Verdiensten um die Kariesätiologie und die soziale Zahnheilkunde', *Stomatologie DDR*, vol. 34 (1984), 173–9.

[193] E. Jessen, *Die Aufklärung des Volkes über die Bedeutung der Zahnpflege für die Gesundheit* (Berlin, 1900); *Mitteilungen aus der Strassburger Poliklinik für Zahnkrankheiten* (Berlin, 1901); H. Kientopf, 'State of School Dentistry in German Schools in 1909', in *The School Dentists' Society* (London, 1910), pp. 34–6. [194] M. v. Gruber, *Mädchenerziehung und Rassenhygiene* (Munich, 1910).

Gottstein as medical officer pioneered a range of public health measures: school meals, open-air schooling for children suffering from TB, school health services and holiday colonies. School health was part of a broader concern with the family.[195]

Gottstein's work exemplifies the way in which the extension of public health opened the door to eugenics. His scepticism of bacteriology and advocacy of social hygiene went with a strong commitment to eugenic measures. Believing that politics was applied biology, he typified the positivistic attitude to social reform. The extension of school health meant a shift from the technical approach characterizing early initiatives to screening for hereditary abnormalities and diseases. The forms for the examination of children show that doctors were to look out for inherited TB, hereditary syphilis and a range of other inherited conditions.[196] In Saxony the investigations were extended to teachers, one quarter of whom were regarded as suffering from chronic nervous conditions. Konrad Biesalski, an orthopaedic specialist, carried out a national survey in 1906 of the number of crippled children, showing that there were 100,000 crippled children who required institutional care, therapy and education. Other health experts seized on the high numbers of mentally defective children. In 1912 there was a survey of 'mentally defective' children in primary schools and in 'special education' in Prussia. The state asked about *erbliche Belastung*, or hereditary traits of inherited TB, syphilis, alcoholism or criminality of parents, and about degenerate signs (*Entartungszeichen*) in physical development. Head and body measurements were made for comparison with 'normal children'. Hereditarian medicine was extending its domain.[197]

The struggle for youth

In 1900, as a result of anxieties over youth delinquency, Prussia imposed a reformed system of education for youth criminals. 'Physical and moral purification' was to be achieved by custodial detention followed by training in selected families. In the same year the German Central Association for Youth Welfare was established in Berlin under the patronage of the Kaiser,[198] with the aim of preventing youth crime and delinquency.[199] In 1908 – at the same time as the Kaiserin Auguste Viktoria Haus for infant care was opened – a *Zentrale für Jugendpflege* was established to co-ordinate youth welfare, continuing education and exercise to ensure physical fitness. Its basis was the *Zentralstelle für Volkswohlfahrt*, a charity

---

[195] M. Stürzbecher, 'Adolf Gottstein als Gesundheitspolitiker', *Medizinische Monatsschrift* (1959), 374–9; *Die gesundheitlichen Einrichtungen der königl. Residenzstadt Charlottenburg, Festschrift gewidmet dem 3. internationalen Kongress für Säuglingsschutz* (Berlin, 1911).
[196] ZSTA M Rep 76 VIII B Nr 2828 and Nr 2830 Bl 336–7 Die Hygiene in Schulen.
[197] ZSTA M Rep 76 VIII B Nr 2828 Bl. 343, 347–8; A. Uffenheimer, *Soziale Säuglings- und Jugendfürsorge* (Leipzig, 1912), pp. 123–43.   [198] *Deutscher Zentralverein für Jugendfürsorge.*
[199] O. Krohne, *Erziehungsanstalten für die verlassene, gefährdete und verwahrloste Jugend in Preussen* (Berlin, 1901).

organization society and a central committee for youth sports. Here, the eugenicist Kaup gave priority to improved diet, regular exercise, an annual holiday in the open air, and rural health.[200] Kaup deployed economic arguments and the statistics on the health of military recruits in a campaign for improved youth welfare services. He argued that these would result in financial savings for employers, sickness funds and municipalities, and that a healthy adolescent constitution was vital from a national biological point of view as here were the parents-to-be of future generations.[201] A survey of 1911 showed that only 10 per cent of youths took regular exercise. By 1914 two million youths were dragooned into the adult-directed youth organizations for sports, gymnastics and drill. The first boy scout groups were established in 1909 by two veterans of the South West Africa campaign, Major Maximilian Bayer and the medical officer, Alexander Lion. By 1910 military recruitment statistics and the declining birth rate gave urgency to improving youth health. A Prussian decree of 1911 encouraged a national network of youth organizations. Doctors were appointed to schools for continuing education, the first such appointment being in the Berlin municipality of Schöneberg. The racial hygienists Kaup and Gruber encouraged such medical supervision of youth. Doctors also took a prominent role as physical educators in the *Jungdeutschlandbund*, an organization for improving the health of country youth. It was intended that this *Bund* co-operate with rural welfare clinics.[202] By 1914 there were 80,000 boy scouts and about two million youths in the *Wandervogel* and in the officially approved and directed youth movement.[203]

In reaction to adult and official controls, the free youth movement took shape, growing to a membership of 25,000. Youthful idealists regarded nature as the basis for a reformed lifestyle. The movement itself attracted praise from eugenicists. The medical student Lenz exchanged ideas on biology and philosophy with leaders of the 'Free Students' at the University of Freiburg. He appreciated their enterprising vigour, and dedication to the pursuit of a free and healthy lifestyle.[204] Early in 1913 the racist-inclined *Deutsche Vortruppbund*[205] floated the idea of a mass youth-gathering. At the fabled mass rally on the Hoher Meissner hills during October 1913, the free youth movement achieved unity. It was seen as an occasion for releasing the potential for those eugenic ideals publicized by Hermann Popert of the *Vortruppbund*. Popert was the author of *Helmut Harringa*, an adventure story about a Nordic hero crusading for racial hygienic virtues of abstinence from

[200] M. v. Gruber, 'Fürsorge für die schulentlassene Jugend', *Bayerisches ärztliches Correspondenzblatt* vol. 13 (1910), 76–80; I. Kaup and T. Fürst, *Körperverfassung und Leistungskraft Jugendlicher* (Munich and Berlin, 1930).
[201] I. Kaup, 'Sozialhygienische Vorschläge zur Ertüchtigung unserer Jugendlichen', *Concordia*, vol. 18 (1911), 141–5, 163–9, 191–200.
[202] K. Saul, 'Der Kampf um die Jugend zwischen Volksschule und Kaserne', *Militärgeschichtliche Mitteilungen*, vol. 10 (1971), 97–143; *Der Arzt als Erzieher*, vol. 10 (1914), 86.
[203] P.D. Stachura, *The German Youth Movement* (London, 1981), p. 35.
[204] F. Lenz, 'Rassen-Hygiene', *Studentische Monatshefte vom Oberrhein*, no. 7 (1911), 8–11; no. 8 (1911), 3–9.   [205] Advance Crusade.

alcohol, health and superior morality.[206] Lenz praised the *Freischar* as embodying the racial hygienic values of fitness and a sense of national duty.[207] The meeting was approved of by such intellectual social reformers as Avenarius, Max Weber, Naumann and Gerhart Hauptmann. But the youth movement sought to create its own life forms. Freedom from alcohol and smoking went with demands for self-determination over mind, body and lifestyle. The movement unleashed a generation of radical *Lebensreformer* on to the terrain of health and welfare policy. Some, such as Friedrich Weber, became active in extreme right-wing circles and the *Freikorps*; but others veered to the left, such as the medical student Max Hodann, who later joined the communists and the radical sexual reformers, or Wilhelm Hagen, who in 1918 sought to convert the free youth movement to socialism and became a municipal medical officer. A qualitative change occurred as the movements conjured up by the state and establishment figures broke away to establish their own identities.[208]

CONSTITUTIONAL PATHOLOGY

Social hygiene

During the 1890s perceptions of the ill-effects of industrialization resulted in a shift from individualist to collectivist approaches to hygiene.[209] The democratic values of the medical reform tradition were superseded by professional, scientific and collective social values. The emphasis changed from hygienic improvements for individual benefit to the collective welfare of societies, cultures and races. Biology offered a means of formulating concepts of social cohesion and development, and medical science provided standards of fitness and health. The doctor became a demagogue, asserting authority as a 'Führer', organizing welfare institutions and ordering the nation to adopt a healthier and more orderly lifestyle. This went with a comprehensive programme for collecting data on how nutrition, income, occupation and housing affected health in everyday life.[210] The most important initiative was 'social hygiene'. This was a product of medical practice, corporate professionalism, eugenics and socio-political concerns. Hereditarian biology and social science gave the fledgling discipline academic aims and credentials. There was a shift of focus in medical theory away from individual disease processes to social causes, prevention, and to positive health-promoting efforts. Whereas earlier

[206] F. Lenz, review of *Helmut Harringa, Eine Geschichte aus unserer Zeit* (22 edn, 1913), in *ARGB*, vol. 11 (1914–15), 279–80; Mosse, *German Ideology*, pp. 104–6.

[207] F. Lenz, review of *Freideutsche Jugend. Festschrift zur Jahrhundertfeier auf dem Hohen Meissner* (Jena, 1913), in *ARGB*, vol. 10 (1913), 823–4.

[208] P.D. Stachura, *German Youth*, pp. 31–3; W. Lacqueur, *Young Germany* (New York, 1962), pp. 32–40.

[209] C.L.P. Trüb, *Die Terminologie und Definition Sozialmedizin und Sozialhygiene in den literarischen Sekundärquellen der Jahre 1900 bis 1960* (Opladen, 1964).

[210] E. Lesky (ed.), *Sozialmedizin. Entwicklung und Selbstverständnis* (Darmstadt, 1977); for Britain, see G. Jones, *Social Hygiene in Twentieth Century Britain* (London, 1986).

writers on social hygiene had argued merely for limited medical measures to control VD, now there were by the 1890s elaborate attempts to analyze in biological terms the effects of demographic and economic forces on the health of total populations.

The context of social medicine during most of the nineteenth century was legalistic. It was linked either to forensic medicine, or targeted at the destitute. Poor Law medicine was a means of segregating and controlling marginal groups.[211] During the 1890s a change occurred. The Poor Law was resented because it deprived recipients of welfare of their political rights and carried a social stigma, and sickness insurance was limited to the elite of the working class. Reforming schemes of social medicine were developed to take account of society as a whole. The initiative was taken by radical critics of prevailing medical systems. Zadek in Berlin and Ludwig Teleky in Vienna developed models of social medicine on a socialist basis.[212] Teleky's analysis was primarily in economic terms. Zadek analyzed social inequalities in health in a biological framework. His views on free medical care were adopted in the 1893 Erfurt programme of the SPD. A priority was the sweeping away of the Bismarckian sickness insurance system, and extension of the role of the state and municipalities in providing comprehensive and free medical care.[213] It was in reaction to these radical proposals that theories of social hygiene were formulated. These took account of the effects of demographic and economic change on the health and hereditary constitution of population groups.

Professional expertise

Social medicine was supported by a wide range of political and professional interests as a response to changing conditions in the organization and status of the medical profession. There resulted a comprehensive set of theories and institutions regulating relations between individuals and the family, populations, medical practitioners and the state. General practitioners were hard-pressed to make a living on the traditional form of consultations with patients on an individual basis. Mass urban society opened up opportunities for extending medical practice, career openings and supplementary income. It was necessary for doctors to specialize in such areas as neurology, paediatrics or dermatology. As there were few full-time posts, doctors avidly accumulated offices on a pluralist basis. For example, Moritz Fürst (a dermatologist with an insurance practice) was a Poor Law doctor, school doctor, and police doctor in Hamburg during the 1890s. Others took lucrative part-time positions as state medical officers (*Kreisärzte*), or with municipalities, railways, and factories. These responsibilities deepened doctors' academic understanding and stimulated socio-political activities. For example, the Frankfurt police

---

[211] Tennstedt, *Vom Proleten*, pp. 272–7.
[212] I. Zadek, *Die Arbeiterversicherung. Eine social-hygienische Kritik* (Jena, 1895).
[213] D.S. Nadav, *Julius Moses*, pp. 73–5.

doctor, Max Flesch, became interested in venereology, the regulation of prostitutes and in criminal anthropology. Grotjahn's work for sickness insurances aroused interest in occupational diseases, and Weinberg's experiences in obstetrics led to research in human genetics. Innovative schemes in social medicine and welfare resulted from this fusion of academic, professional and political interests.

The next steps were to integrate these diverse interests in a coherent theory of social hygiene, backed up by publications, societies and full-time professional appointments. Initially, opportunities for full-time work in public health were in municipal service as *Stadtarzt*. The first medical officers were appointed by Frankfurt-on-Main in 1883 and by Stuttgart in 1888. Rapid urbanization and associated health problems confronted these new municipal officials with a wide range of public health problems. They acquired responsibilities for co-ordinating state and voluntary spheres of health care. Enterprising medical officers took initiatives that linked many towns and cities with innovations in public health: examples were Wiesbaden for school medical services, Strasburg for school dental services, Halle for TB clinics, Leipzig for guardianship of foster children, Charlottenburg for infant welfare, and Hamburg for VD clinics. The special services set up to ameliorate urban living conditions were grouped into unified agencies for administering and dispensing health care. This process of the bureaucratic and central administration of health care resulted in the creating of a full-time *Stadtmedizinalrat*. The medical officer gained executive responsibilities in the municipal administration, rather than acting as a mere agent of municipal policies. The first appointment, in 1905, was of Peter Krautwig in Cologne, and was followed by the appointments of Johannes Rabnow in Berlin-Schöneberg in 1906, of Wilhelm von Drigalski in Halle in 1907, of Gottstein in Berlin-Charlottenburg in 1911, and of Friedrich August Weber in Berlin in 1913. These municipal officials pressed for the establishing of municipal health offices in order to co-ordinate all aspects of sanitation, disease prevention and health education.[214] Leading exponents of preventive medicine found these positions attractive career openings. Gottstein was not only highly innovative in Charlottenburg, but he also developed theoretical interests in the solution of public health problems. By 1914 he used the local hospital (Westend) as a location for lectures on social medicine. He intended to develop the hospital into a teaching centre.[215] Rabnow, appointed in Schöneberg, took a lead in the anti-TB campaign. Grotjahn received only twelve votes in the election for the Berlin post, which went to the bacteriologist, Weber, who polled eighty-two votes, having just excelled as general secretary of the Dresden hygiene exhibition.[216] Grotjahn was compensated in 1912 by a university

---

[214] W. Piechocki, 'Zur Geschichte des Stadtgesundheitsamtes Halle', in W. Kaiser and H. Hübner (eds.), *Theodor Brugsch (1878–1963)* (Halle, 1979), pp. 58–75.

[215] M. Stürzbecher, 'Aus der Geschichte des Charlottenburger Gesundheitswesens', *Bär von Berlin* (1980), 43–113.

[216] M. Stürzbecher, 'Von den Berliner Stadtmedizinalräten, Stadtmedizinaldirektoren und Senatsdirektoren für das Gesundheitswesen', *Berliner-Ärzteblatt*, vol. 94 (1981), 789–90.

teaching post in social hygiene, although he continued to support himself by medical practice until 1915 when he was appointed to head a department of social hygiene in the municipality of Berlin.

The state improved career opportunities and adopted ambitious public health policies, so that municipalities should not have a monopoly of innovation in public health services as this would have given socialist and liberal radicals power and prestige. In 1899 a Prussian law for district medical officers (*Kreisärzte*) made full-time appointments possible. Fifteen full-timers were appointed in 1901, and by 1908 the number had reached forty-three. At the same time there was a tendency to appoint professionally trained physicians from the ranks of the district medical officers to central administrative posts, so eroding the tradition of legally trained administrators. Scientific expertise replaced legalistic approaches to social problems. Professional examinations raised the requirements in hygiene based upon experimental biology, but limited forensic medicine. This had the dual effect of limiting access of part-timers to public health, and replacing a legally bound curriculum by one that was biologically based. State medical officials were generally staunch conservatives, but they retained strong allegiances and personal contacts with their professional colleagues in municipalities, universities or in insurance practice. They too acted on the premise of a coherent theory of social hygiene. In 1911 Kirchner, a high-ranking military medical officer who had trained with Koch, was appointed as the first medically trained *Ministerialdirektor* of the Prussian Medical Department. An administrative hierarchy based on centre-periphery contacts began to take shape. An outstanding example of the resulting type of career pattern was Otto Krohne. From 1891 he was a general practitioner in Thuringia, and also took on the functions of a miners' medical officer. Opportunities for an energetic medical officer lay not in industrial health, but in the public health administration and family welfare. In 1901 Krohne was appointed *Kreisarzt*, and in 1904 he entered the provincial administration in Düsseldorf, and he was promoted to the central administration in 1911. He took a lead on matters associated with the declining birth rate, and in 1922 he became President of the Racial Hygiene Society. This career pattern was to allow a number of nationalist-minded doctors to enter the central administration, but to maintain professional allegiances with doctors in academic, welfare and specialist organizations, and develop sympathies for eugenics.

The rallying of the medical profession to collectivist ideologies can be detected around 1900. Doctors' associations combined defence of corporate professional interests with a sense of social mission. The powerful association for the defence of the economic interests of the medical profession, the *Hartmannbund*, represented the conservative majority who resented the ability of insurance societies to dictate terms on which doctors were admitted to their lists. While they were politically antagonistic to Zadek and his socialist allies among sickness insurance administrators, common professional interests provided issues over which socialist and conservative doctors could unite. A broad political spectrum among doctors supported the efforts of a League to Combat Quackery, founded in 1904.[217] Left-wing doctors such as Zadek and Blaschko were here at one with conservatives in their opposition to nature therapy. The League allied with advocates of social medicine to attack quacks and nature therapists in a widely supported public campaign. The League to Combat Quackery and broadly-supported public health organizations for the prevention of TB and VD showed the shift that had occurred in the medical profession from liberal individualism to corporate monopolistic aspirations.

Politics

Left-wing politics was replaced by nationalist consensus and professionalization of social hygiene. There was a shift from a politicized concept of health, based on liberal and legalistic premises, to a technocratic model of professional medical expertise. Initiatives in social hygiene came from all parts of the political spectrum. Professional allegiances and common national assumptions unified the movement for an academic discipline of social hygiene. While some advocates of social hygiene had limited aims to reform systems of medical insurance, others were allied to a range of political groupings. Just as biology and concern with the birth rate had led radicals such as Kautsky to Marxism, there continued to be a vein of biological and medical socialists. Zadek, Hermann Weyl and Karl Freudenberg were SPD representatives. In Austria the first academic appointment in 'social medicine' went to Teleky, who had left-wing sympathies. Grotjahn, who was to take a leading position as a theoretician of social hygiene, had contacts with the reformist wing of the SPD in the 1890s, but regretted their lack of nationalism. Blaschko wavered between left liberalism and the revisionist socialist circles of the *Sozialistische Monatshefte*. The shift to corporatism could lead from liberalism to socialism: Julius Moses in Berlin supported the liberal *Freisinnige Vereinigung* of Barth, but he progressed to socialism by 1912.[218] Biological materialism and concepts of organic cohesion continued to channel doctors and scientists towards socialism.

Liberal doctors illustrate the shift from Virchow's democratic individualism to corporatist professional authority. The slogan of 'medical reform' stood for ideas of organic social integration, reinforced by organicist theories of social co-operation. Indeed, medical reform was the title of a journal edited from 1905 by the liberal TB expert, Rudolf Lennhoff, who also contributed to the liberal national daily paper, the *Vossische Zeitung*. An ideology of 'one nation' and moral leadership was given immense publicity by Naumann who endeavoured to fuse the science of Darwinism with the unifying spirit of Rousseau.[219] Fürst was a member of the liberal *Fortschrittlicher Volkspartei*. Lennhoff, one of the organizers of the society for

---

[217] ZSTA M Rep 76 VIII B Nr 1342 die Deutsche Gesellschaft zur Bekämpfung des Kurpfuschertums 1904–1928 Bl 1–6, 49, 57 for ministerial support.   [218] Nadav, *Julius Moses*, pp. 132–3.

[219] F. Naumann, 'Die psychologischen Naturbedingungen des Sozialismus', *Politisch-Anthropologische Revue*, vol. 1 (1902/3), 564–71.

social medicine in 1905, was a member of another liberal faction, the *Freisinniger Volkspartei* (Free Peoples' Party). The doctor Mugdan represented this party in the Reichstag between 1903 and 1911, and was vociferous on public health issues.[220] Other liberal experts in social medicine were Schlossmann, municipal health officials such as Wilhelm Hanauer in Frankfurt and the Berliners, Max Mosse and Gustav Tugendreich, who co-edited a eugenically oriented work on social medicine.[221]

Gottstein, the critic of bacteriology, was an outstanding example of an ardent liberal. During the 1890s he attended the Berlin Society for Political Economy.[222] His social views had a basis in biology rather than in politics: he justified free trade by reference to the theory of teleological mechanics advanced by the physiologist, Eduard Pflüger. He contributed articles to Theodor Barth's weekly, *Nation*, including discussions of racial hygiene.[223] He was a campaigner for the extension of municipal health services. He was to become one of the most powerful practitioners of social hygiene, and in 1919 took over directorship of health services in Prussia. He regarded public health measures in the field of infant and child health as strengthening the social organism. He was a persuasive advocate of the view that the doctor should use his authority and scientific expertise to guide the nation towards health and efficiency, rather than just entering general political life. His staunch liberalism was reinforced by authoritarian convictions. He typified the Führer ideology of liberal medical reformers.[224]

From 1900 there were moves to combine 'social' and professional commitments. From 1902, Alfons Fischer belonged to Naumann's 'national-social' movement. The ideal of the *Sozialstaat* influenced his programme of *Kulturhygiene*. He campaigned for the extension of state social welfare. His treatise, 'Outlines of Social Hygiene', was written not only for doctors but also for economists, administrators and social reformers, and was dedicated to the socialist welfare expert, Heinrich Braun, whose wife, Lily Braun, pioneered the concept of maternity insurance.[225] Fischer's reformist sympathies were in keeping with Naumann's ideal of centre-left coalition from 'Bassermann to Bebel'. Other sympathisers of nationalist aims underlying welfare reforms were Grotjahn, Krohne, the paediatrician Schlossmann and the hygiene professor Martin Hahn. Social biology and concepts of a healthy social organism provided a positive basis for social progress and the overcoming of class divisions.[226]

There was a medical and nationalist consensus that cut across party divisions, and linked socialist, Centre Party and conservative doctors around the themes of social

[220] E. Hamburger, *Juden im öffentlichen Leben Deutschlands* (Tübingen, 1968), p. 366.
[221] M. Hubenstorf, 'Sozialhygiene und industrielle Pathologie im späten Kaiserreich', R. Müller *et al.* (eds.), *Industrielle Pathologie in historischer Sicht* (Bremen, 1985), pp. 82–107.
[222] *Berliner Volkswirtschaftliche Gesellschaft.*   [223] *Die Nation*, (12 November 1904).
[224] Compare W. Mommsen, *Max Weber und die Deutsche Politik* (Tübingen, 1979).
[225] A. Fischer, *Grundriss der sozialen Hygiene für Mediziner, Nationalökonomen, Verwaltungsbeamte und Sozialreformer* (Berlin, 1913).
[226] M. Hahn, *Grenzen und Ziele der Sozialhygiene* (Freiburg, 1912).

and racial hygiene and population policy. Centre Party disciples among medical officers included Krautwig, and the Kreisarzt Jean Bornträger. The Centre Party, which was strong in the Rhineland and the densely populated Ruhr, was innovative in welfare schemes. The hygienist, Gruber, abandoned the radical commitments to reform as a Fabian in Vienna during the 1890s and after he had moved to Munich in 1902 he encouraged social hygiene from nationalist perspectives. He developed concepts of natural selection of vital factors (*natürliche Vitalauslese*) and of *National-Eugenik*. He appointed the nationalist advocate of rural regeneration, Kaup (a sometime sympathiser of the Austrian nationalist and anti-semitic politician, Georg von Schönerer) in 1912 as head of a department of social hygiene. Kaup inaugurated the concept of a *National-Biologie. Völkisch*-minded popularists of racial ideas had erratic and often strained relations with more academic and medical advocates of racial hygiene such as Ploetz, Kaup and Gruber. The right considered that social hygiene was part of *Volks-* or *Rassenhygiene.* Both Kaup and Gruber were prepared to co-operate with eugenicists, such as Grotjahn, who were further to the left and with whom they shared a common basis of hereditarian biology, public health and nationalist ideals. Ploetz conformed to the prevailing disdain for party politics by declaring racial hygiene to be without party political ties. He cultivated contacts with a broad range of experts in hygiene including Bornträger, Gottstein and Kaup, and lectured on racial hygiene to the German Society for Public Health in 1910.[227] Eugenicists regarded medicine and biology as offering a broadly based solution to social problems.

Theory

The term *Sozialhygiene* derived from reforming French initiatives in the 1840s and was introduced into German by Pettenkofer in 1882. It initially represented the liberal approach to hygiene as based on sanitary improvement and philanthropic welfare.[228] During the 1890s, the term was used in a limited sense to mean the implementation of public health legislation and the application of social welfare measures in areas such as housing, in order to reduce mortality. When Theodor Weyl, a *Privatdozent* at the Technical University Charlottenburg and author of several volumes on municipal health during the 1890s, published a volume on 'social hygiene' in 1904, he meant it in this limited sense of applied epidemiology. The term 'social medicine' was also current, with a restricted meaning of insurance medicine and related to administrative practice. After 1900 these terms acquired greater breadth.

Social hygiene was transformed around 1900 as criticisms arose of bacteriologi-cal and physiological approaches to hygiene. Instead of disease being attributed to pathogenic micro-organisms, social causes such as poverty, housing and occupa-

---

[227] Ploetz papers, diary, 4 and 14 February 1904, 23 June 1906, 25 October 1909.
[228] K. Georg, *Soziale Hygiene* (Berlin, 1890); A. Nossig, *Einführung in das Studium der sozialen Hygiene* (Stuttgart, 1894).

tion were held to be paramount. The liberal heritage of legal and economic concepts was rejected in favour of social concepts, which were heavily influenced by hereditary biology and biologistic sociology. Consequently, social hygiene represented a step forward in the technocratic direction. In the shaping of social hygiene as an academic discipline, a leading role was taken by Grotjahn who was primarily a theoretician. In 1904 he defined social hygiene as a descriptive science of the factors affecting the health of population groups, and as a normative science of the measures necessary to spread hygienic values among individuals and their offspring. At the same time he attacked the 'physical-biological' hygiene of the bacteriologists. His approach combined statistical social science with reproductive biology as the link between generations.

From 1896 Grotjahn took part in the evening discussions held by the revisionist socialist, Leo Arons, and was in contact with Heinrich Lux, Woltmann and Joseph Bloch. There were strongly nationalist sentiments among these bourgeois 'academic socialists'.[229] Grotjahn withdrew from left-wing politics in the summer of 1901, as he attempted to build up a professional pressure group for social medical reform. From 1902 he co-edited an annual bibliography of social hygiene. Grotjahn established a network of contacts with advocates of social medicine and with medical statisticians such as Prinzing and Roesle. Teleky and Schallmayer were also contributors to Grotjahn's journal, *Zeitschrift für Soziale Medizin*, the first number of which appeared in 1906. In 1912 Grotjahn joined forces with Kaup to edit a massive handbook of social hygiene. Grotjahn also published a volume on 'social pathology' that year, combining biology and social science as ways of combating physical degeneration and the declining birth rate. In 1905 Grotjahn and Lennhoff were prime movers in the founding of an Association for Social Medicine, Hygiene and Medical Statistics.[230] This challenged the established Berlin Society for Public Health.[231] The social hygenic reformers emphasized demographic and welfare issues such as infant and maternal health rather than bacteriology. The demographer, Paul Mayet, was elected president, and Gottstein and Dietrich were vice-presidents. Although they were cold-shouldered by bacteriologists of the Koch Institute and the Imperial Health Office, that both Mayet and Dietrich were in state service shows a rapprochement with the authorities. This is borne out by the fact that Zadek's socialist grouping refused to join Grotjahn's association, instead establishing an alternative Association of Socialist Doctors.[232] Grotjahn's abandoning of political activism meant that the main thrust of social hygiene was to be academic and administrative rather than party political.

Grotjahn's programme was supported by the social scientists Schmoller and Tönnies who were veterans of the Association for Social Policy.[233] The friendship

[229] D. Tutzke, 'Alfred Grotjahns Verhältnis zur Sozialdemokratie', *Zeitschrift für ärztliche Fortbildung*, vol. 54 (1960), 1183–7; Grotjahn, *Erlebtes*, pp. 63–5.
[230] *Verein für soziale Medizin, Hygiene und Medizinalstatistik in Berlin.*
[231] *Berliner Verein für öffentliche Gesundheitspflege.*   [232] Grotjahn, *Erlebtes*, pp. 132–4.
[233] *Verein für Sozialpolitik.*

with Tönnies dated from 1892, when Grotjahn turned to Tönnies for advice on topics such as national sentiments, about which he felt the party political literature was deficient. Grotjahn, however, complained that Tönnies' approach was overly deductive and should have been based more on natural science and statistics.[234] Schmoller and Tönnies encouraged Grotjahn in the plan of fusing hygiene and social science.[235] Grotjahn claimed to be the first medical *Kathedersozialist*. Due to a recommendation by Schmoller, *Ministerialdirektor* Althoff took an interest in Grotjahn's work and interviewed him in 1903.[236] In 1905 Schmoller attempted to persuade the Berlin medical faculty to appoint Grotjahn as *Privatdozent*, but this was blocked by Rubner, the professor of hygiene, who defended Pettenkofer's traditional approach according to which hygiene was applied physiology. Rubner dismissed social hygiene as an empty slogan, arguing that as all hygiene was social, the attempt to establish a separate discipline was unjustified. Between 1905 and 1907 the elitist faculty resisted pressure for professorships in socially relevant specialisms such as venereology, laryngology, otology and pulmonary diseases. The one concession was a teaching post in social medicine as a branch of forensic medicine in 1908.[237] Despite the opposition of the Berlin professor of hygiene, Rubner, others supported Grotjahn's social hygiene. They considered that it was a means of countering radical socialist criticisms of social conditions. In 1912, when Rubner was away in the United States, Grotjahn was appointed *Privatdozent* in social hygiene. Ministerial officials regarded Grotjahn's positivism as a means of suppressing politically more radical concepts of health. Grotjahn thus succeeded in his strategy of attaining academic recognition by withdrawing from left-wing political circles.[238]

Grotjahn's allegiance to social science encountered much criticism among his colleagues. Fischer preferred an approach to hygiene based on history, culture and education, rather than Grotjahn's analyses of family income and other socio-economic factors. Gottstein also criticized Grotjahn's programme. He considered that problems of health lay in the inter-relations of social groups, and in the relations of groups or their offspring to general social levels of health. He would have preferred the term *Gesellschaftshygiene* (social hygiene). He warned against ecological dangers which threatened the degeneration of total societies. Grotjahn's combination of social science and biology did not achieve the consensus that he desired. Some of the strongest criticisms of his approach came from the racial hygienists.

---

[234] Grotjahn, *Erlebtes*, pp. 56–7.
[235] Tönnies papers, Grotjahn to Tönnies, Sig C564: 56, 21 September 1895.
[236] ZSTA M Rep 72 Althoff A I Nr 37 Bl 195, Schmoller to Althoff, 30 October 1903.
[237] ZSTA M Rep 76 Va Sekt 2 Tit X Nr 176, Errichtung eines Seminars für soziale Medizin 1908–1909.
[238] ZSTA M Rep 76 Va Sekt 2 Tit 12 Nr 83 Bd 12 Bl 275, and Bd 13 Bl 5; D. Tutzke, *Alfred Grotjahn* (Leipzig, 1979), pp. 37–9.

Social hygiene and eugenics

Apart from Teleky's analysis based on socio-economic conditions, twentieth-century theories of social hygiene were located within a framework of social biology. As eugenics was a distinct form of social biology, relations of social hygiene with eugenics and racial hygiene involved many theoretical and personal differences of opinion. While racial and social hygiene shared common ground in biology and in human reproduction, social hygiene included a greater degree of social science and racial hygiene drew more on racial anthropology. The distinction was not clear cut, and there were many conflicting formulations of the relations between social and racial hygiene. While taking a deep interest in economic conditions as a major factor in differentials in health, Grotjahn saw 'reproductive hygiene' as central to social hygiene.[239] Heredity was a major factor. As a medical practitioner in Berlin from 1896, Grotjahn paid attention to the hereditary aspects of diseases and nervous states. On a visit to England in 1902 he observed how industrial conditions had produced a congenitally deformed caste. He defined social hygiene in a study of social statistics on degeneration, and he conceived of the discipline as *Entartungshygiene* (degenerative hygiene).[240] He was a friend of Woltmann, who turned from socialism to Aryan racism, and was well versed in the hereditarian theories of Schallmayer, Ploetz, Hegar and Haycraft. Grotjahn praised Ploetz as *geistreich*, but criticized him for ignoring the importance of descriptive social science and the analysis of social conditions. Grotjahn was irritated by Ploetz's use of the term 'race' on the grounds that racial hygiene and Aryanism were liable to be confused. Grotjahn deliberately avoided any mention of 'race'. Schallmayer congratulated Grotjahn on this in 1904, explaining that he preferred the term *Rassehygiene*, with race in the singular to denote the whole human race. He wished to dissociate his ideas from Aryan anthropologists and ideas of biological inequality between races. Instead he was concerned with biological inequalities between economic and other population groups.[241] To Ploetz, 'social' hygiene was merely a sub-category opposed to 'individual' hygiene. The overarching status ascribed by Grotjahn to society, Ploetz gave to the race. Indeed, Ploetz could present his definition of race as a breeding community in social terms. There was considerable overlap between Grotjahn and Ploetz, despite their contrasting priorities and different sets of academic and social allegiances.[242]

Grotjahn enjoyed far better relations with the eugenicist, Schallmayer, than with Ploetz, and here the difference between a single or a pluralistic concept of *Rasse-* or *Rassenhygiene* was significant. Whereas Ploetz pointed out the risks of

---

[239] Grotjahn, *Erlebtes*, p. 118.
[240] A. Grotjahn, 'Soziale Hygiene und Entartungshygiene', in T. Weyl (ed.), *Handbuch der Hygiene* (Jena, 1904), 4th Suppl. vol., pp. 727–89.
[241] Grotjahn papers, Schallmayer to Grotjahn, 20 November 1904.
[242] A. Elster, 'Die Abgrenzung der Begiffe: Rassen- und Gesellschaftshygiene (und -Biologie). Soziale Hygiene und Soziale Medizin', *ARGB*, vol. 4 (1907), 80–9.

hygenic improvements, as with anti-TB measures, by 1910 Schallmayer accepted the therapeutic benefits in hygiene.[243] Schallmayer confided that he had a low opinion of Ploetz as a scientist, but admired the intensity of his personal propaganda for racial hygiene.[244] Grotjahn's concept of *Fortpflanzungshygiene*,[245] introduced in 1912, was close to Schallmayer's understanding of eugenics and *Vererbungshygiene*.[246] They were both concerned with the statistics which showed a declining birth rate and indicated an increased level of physical degeneration among military recruits. Medicine took on the social function of maintaining the quality and quantity of the population, and preventing degeneration. Grotjahn praised Schallmayer's suggestion of marriage certificates. An academic discipline of 'sexual hygiene' was necessary to reconcile individual interests to the need to prevent disease by preventing the existence of weaker members of society or at least to improve conditions of antenatal care. This conclusion was similar to Ploetz's proposals for control of variation. In a study of municipal hospitals in 1908, Grotjahn initiated the suggestion that TB sanatoria, mental hospitals and medical institutions should detain the weak so as to 'humanely' prevent their procreating.[247]

Ploetz had to defer to Grotjahn while planning the *Archiv für Rassen- und Gesellschaftsbiologie* in 1903. He wrote to Grotjahn that the journal was to have a social science orientation because of the need to secure financial backing from his brother-in-law Nordenholz. They had originally thought of including the term *Sozialhygiene* in the title. But so as to avoid a collision with Grotjahn's journal, *Jahresberichte für Sozialhygiene*, they suggested the term *Gesellschaftshygiene*. They stressed that this was narrower in scope than Grotjahn's enterprise. Although there might be some overlap between the two publications, Ploetz hoped that they could co-exist amicably, and be as two powers marching forward side by side.[248] The polite exchanges between Grotjahn and Ploetz concealed rivalry and conflicting opinions on racial issues. Ploetz made considerable efforts to win converts among the social hygienists. From 1905 he cultivated contacts with experts in hygiene. Rubner rebuffed Ploetz just as he resisted Grotjahn.[249] Ploetz approached Theodor Weyl, the editor of a major handbook on hygiene, but condemned him as a philistine and materialist. Ploetz dismissed Kriegel as *den Trabanten Grotjahns*[250] because he co-edited the rival *Jahresberichte*. Ploetz and Bluhm were present at the founding of the Society for Social Medicine, Hygiene and Medical Statistics on 16 February 1905.[251] Ploetz noted that Grotjahn was the leading light, and that three-quarters attending this 'boring meeting' were Jews. Ploetz was actively planning to found the Racial Hygiene Society, discussing the matter with Rüdin soon

---

[243] Grotjahn papers, Schallmayer to Grotjahn, 3 June 1910.   [244] Grotjahn papers, 30 April 1910.
[245] reproductive hygiene.   [246] hereditary hygiene. Trüb, *Terminologie*, pp. 27–8, 56.
[247] A. Grotjahn, *Krankenhauswesen und Heilstättenbewegung im Lichte der sozialen Hygiene* (Leipzig, 1908).   [248] Grotjahn papers, Ploetz to Grotjahn, 1903. Ploetz papers, Grotjahn to Ploetz 26 January 1901.
[249] MPG Rubner papers, Ploetz to Rubner. 1 March 1910, Gruber to Rubner 14 March 1910.
[250] Grotjahn's minstrel.   [251] Ploetz papers, diary, also 4 Feb 1905.

afterwards on 18 February 1905. Ploetz and his supporters resented what they perceived as a materialist and Jewish predominance in social hygiene. Despite a common core of biological theories, racial hygiene and social hygiene were destined to be rivals. That Schallmayer praised Grotjahn for having spread the gospel of eugenics in those circles interested in social hygiene indicates how social hygiene extended the appeal of eugenics.[252]

Welfare, social hygiene and racial hygiene were united when the Central Office for Welfare[253] appointed the eugenicist Kaup in February 1907. This was a state-subsidized organization, but the initiative for its establishment came from Graf Hugo Sholto Douglas, an industrialist and free conservative who from the 1880s devoted his life to philanthropy and anti-alcohol campaigns. The Central Office was developed out of a socialist welfare organization founded in 1891, which was transformed as a result of Douglas's scheme for a national anti-alcohol organization in 1902.[254] Kaup must be regarded as one of the first racial hygienists to have received official funds, albeit indirectly.[255] From 1908 he directed the hygiene department and obtained a post teaching occupational hygiene at the Technical University in Berlin-Charlottenburg. Kaup was concerned with the degenerative effects of toxic poisons in the workplace. He saw the solution to degeneration to lie in improving conditions for the peasantry. He demanded *Lebensraum* for the peasantry to better their socio-economic conditions, so as to ensure the survival of the race.

The first university to recognize social medicine was Vienna. Teleky applied for a teaching post in 'social hygiene' in 1907. As in Grotjahn's case in Berlin, the professor of hygiene defended the unity of his discipline; it was agreed that the appointment could be made under the rubric of 'social medicine'. Teleky linked social hygiene not only to welfare work (he was secretary of the Austrian committee for combating tuberculosis) but also to the application of medicine for the purposes of socialist political agitation with studies of industrial diseases.[256] In 1912 social hygiene won recognition as an academic discipline with the establishment of academic posts in Munich and Berlin. The process as seen in Munich suggests how far responses to a left-wing political movement opened opportunities for *völkisch* eugenics. Longstanding left-wing agitation for the development of social and occupational medicine came to a head during 1906. But when instituted, social hygiene was developed on a positive scientific rather than on a politically reformist basis. Lectures on these topics were given by Hahn from 1907 to 1911 who enraged Gruber by receiving special state grants for a laboratory of occupational hygiene. He was appointed professor of hygiene at Königsberg and

---

[252] Grotjahn papers, Schallmayer to Grotjahn, 14 July 1914.
[253] *Zentralstelle für Volkswohlfahrt.*
[254] 'Graf Douglas', *Concordia*, vol. 19 (1912), 191–4.
[255] ZSTA M Rep 76 VIII B Nr 2023, Die Schaffung eines Volkswohlfahrtsamts, 1904–1906.
[256] L. Teleky, 'Geschichtliches, Biographisches, Autobiographisches', in Lesky, *Sozialmedizin*, pp. 355–70.

then at Freiburg, where he insisted that hygiene was a unified academic discipline with social hygiene as an integral part. His successor, Kaup, was appointed in 1912 as lecturer in social hygiene in Gruber's Munich Hygiene Institute.[257] The appointment of Kaup meant that racial hygiene became substituted for occupational hygiene. As dean of the medical faculty, Gruber argued that occupational hygiene was too narrow, and that a precondition for understanding the social basis of health and disease were investigations of their natural biological basis. Only this would guarantee against the abuse of an academic discipline for hidden party political ends. Gruber recommended Kaup's abilities in bacteriological and physiological research, as well as his dedication, independent of party politics, to research on social policy.

This triumph of social hygiene was simultaneously a victory for racial hygiene. This can be seen in a survey of the major textbooks and monographs published around 1912. Gruber and Kaup steered social hygiene in a racial biological direction. Gruber introduced a substantial *Handbook of Hygiene* in 1911 with the definition that hygiene was to maintain the health of the germplasm; the decisive criterion of health was the breeding of healthy and numerous offspring.[258] Alfons Fischer gave a lengthy exposition of Schallmayer's 'national eugenics', and concluded that social hygiene and eugenics complemented each other.[259] The compendium on social medicine edited by Mosse and Tugendreich included much discussion of racial and eugenic issues, as in a contribution by Schallmayer. It was published by the *völkisch* Munich publisher, Lehmann.[260] Grotjahn's *Soziale Pathologie* of 1912 intensified discussions of eugenic issues. In the climate of heightened nationalism and concern with the birth rate, racial hygiene won over converts among advocates of hygiene and social hygiene. By December 1913 Ploetz's Racial Hygiene Society included many experts in hygiene: among the Berlin Racial Hygiene Society were Blaschko, Flügge (the professor of hygiene), Grotjahn, Kisskalt and Korff-Petersen, an assistant at the Hygiene Institute. Grotjahn chaired the Berlin branch of the Racial Hygiene Society, Kisskalt was vice-chairman and Korff-Petersen was secretary: Gruber presided over activities in Munich. That 'progressive', left-wing intellectuals were prepared to join forces with racial hygienists was revealing of the authoritarian and elitist dynamic within social medicine. The democratic potential of social medicine was fading fast. The reformulation of medicine in terms of racial biology was under way.

Mass Education

The wave of concern with social hygiene and heredity led to innovative schemes for promoting the health of families. Although these represented the culmination

---

[257] University of Munich archives, Hygienisches Institut IH 37.144; Gewerbehygiene, Medizinische Statistik und Gesundheitspflege I Gen 26 Ser, Gruber, 27 July 1912.

[258] M. v. Gruber, 'Einleitung', M. Rubner, M. v. Gruber and P.M. Ficker (eds.), *Handbuch der Hygiene* (Leipzig, 1911), I, pp. 1–16.   [259] Fischer, *Grundriss*, p. 166.

[260] W. Schallmayer, 'Soziale Massnahmen der Verbesserung der Fortpflanzungsauslese', in M. Mosse and G. Tugendreich (eds.), *Krankheit und soziale Lage* (Munich, 1913), pp. 841–59.

of the shift from individualism to corporatism in medicine, there were competing state-socialist and commercially sponsored ventures. The state's attempts to improve positive health were based on the dispensaries for TB and infant health and on home visiting, which ushered in a concern with domestic hygiene. Hygienic advice regulated contact between members of a family: between the parents, and between parents and children, between the sick and the healthy, and between those intending to marry. Nose-blowing, spitting, coughing, cooking, washing, clothing, and sleeping arrangements were all objects of hygienic advice literature. Prescriptions for one handkerchief, one set of cutlery, and one bed per person were the order of the day. Whereas in the 1890s moral advice characterized hygienic campaigns, after 1900 hereditary biology had an impact. School doctors and military doctors collected material on family background and heredity. Their data supported studies of hereditary diseases and the inherited constitution. An important commitment of social hygienists was to the popularization of hygienic culture.

The science of hygiene formed the basis of the campaigns for an orderly, sober and clean home environment. Health education was a priority in the movement to combat disease. Around 1900 there were, however, marked divisions between socialist schemes for workers' education, nationalist propaganda for *Volkshygiene* and commercially sponsored health education. The socialist *Arbeiter-Sanitäts-Kommission* (ASK) supported initiatives in health education, public lectures and a workers' health library. Doctors lectured to workers' emergency first-aid groups, as 'samaritan brigades' proliferated in Berlin during the 1890s.[261] ASK pamphlets projected a strictly scientific view of medicine, while dealing with topics like the care of hair, skin and teeth, domestic hygiene and clothing. Several pamphlets were eugenic in tone. Zadek emphasized a hereditary disposition to TB. Julian Marcuse (once Ploetz's Breslau comrade) dealt with sex education in the family. The revisionist socialist, Eduard Bernstein, produced a pamphlet on sexual instincts. He prescribed socialism, fresh air, exercise and vegetarianism as antidotes against alcoholism and depraved and unhealthy sexual indulgence, resulting from lack of self-control, particularly among youth.[262] Approval of the latest medical discoveries reinforced the image of socialism as modern and scientific in its analysis of social problems. At the same time it moderated demands for fundamental socio-economic revolution, by making workers responsible for adopting a hygienic life-style. Scientism was a feature of revisionist trends in the SPD.

There was concern that socialists should not have the initiative in health education. There was a conservative strategy of *Volkshygiene*, which aimed to inculcate nationalist values and moral conduct. Exercise, sports and fresh air were officially sanctioned. Gymnastics, for many years regarded as subversive, was

---

261 A. Labisch, 'Selbsthilfe zwischen Auflehnung und Anpassung: Arbeiter-Sanitätskommission und Arbeiter-Samariterbund', *Argument-Sonderband*, no. 77 (1983), 11–26; Labisch, 'The Work-ingmen's Samaritan Federation. Arbeiter-Samariter-Bund 1888-1933,' *Journal of Contemporary History*, vol. 13 (1978), 297–322.
262 E. Bernstein, *Der Geschlechtstrieb* (Berlin, 1910).

introduced into school timetables. Hueppe and Kaup advised on the medical value of exercise and praised the virtues of fresh air and of peasant life. Scientific hygiene was defended by the Society for National Health[263] which was founded in 1900. Its educational approach was encouraged by Althoff and had backing from *Reichskanzler* Bülow.[264] State officials were requested to distribute its journal and booklets in schools, prisons and other institutions. Professors of hygiene such as Rubner and Buchner took a lead in the society.[265] The first chairman was Graf Hugo Sholto Douglas who had co-operated with Rubner in public lectures since 1894.[266] The Society's aim was to restore public confidence in the science of hygiene, and to use this to prescribe a healthy lifestyle. Health propaganda was aimed at 'educated' craftsmen and workers. It attempted to arouse popular appreciation for hygiene as a science, and to emphasize the moral responsibilities of citizens of leading a healthy and hygienic life in obedience to the laws of hygiene. It reinforced the idea of the physician as educator of the *Volk*. Provincial officials distributed the society's journal, and pamphlets were written by leading scientists on alcoholism, TB, VD, infant care and nutrition.[267] These presented a simplified view of scientific facts. Special courses directed at workers were not a success. The Leipzig branch reported that for years they had been lecturing to empty benches, but when courses were run in conjunction with the sickness insurances the attendances were good.[268] Only broad-based public organizations could effectively spread the gospel of hygiene. There was to be co-ordination of the efforts of conservatives to solve 'the social problem', and those of socialist insurance officials and medical experts in social hygiene.

The hygiene eye

There were conflicting strategies of health education. Some believed that the public should be given the facilities to learn for itself. Others held that experts should dictate what was right. Lingner, the *Odol* mouthwash manufacturer, was outstanding in his efforts to make the facts of biology, medicine and statistics publicly accessible. His idea was to have attractive displays that could capture the attention of the onlooker. He sponsored a centre for dental hygiene[269] which opened in Dresden during 1898, where Carl Röse carried out pioneering research on the causes of dental caries as a symptom of racial degeneration. Lingner subsidized Schlossmann's infant hospital. He switched from the sewing machine business to manufacturing mouth water, called *Odol*, and the shampoo *Pixavon*. These products had bactericidal properties, as well as fulfilling consumer demands for cosmetics and personal hygiene. In 1903 at a municipal exhibition in Dresden,

[263] *Gesellschaft für Volkshygiene.*
[264] ZSTA M Rep 92 Althoff B Nr 8, B1 120–122, correspondence of Althoff and Beerwald.
[265] Staatsarchiv Munich, Pol Dir Mü Nr 5601 Verein f. Volkshygiene in München.
[266] ZSTA M Rep 77 Tit 662 Nr 44 Beiakten 5, Deutsche Verein für Volkshygiene; GSTA Dahlem Rep 84a 5585 Volkswohlfahrt 1902–1932; MPG Rubner papers, Douglas correspondence.
[267] *Blätter für Volksgesundheitspflege*, vol. 1–33 1900–1933.
[268] Tennstedt, *Vom Proleten*, pp. 555–72.   [269] *Zentralstelle für Zahnhygiene.*

he impressed the public with a display of epidemiological statistics. In 1908 he developed his hygienic theories with plans for an infant welfare organization in Hessen.[270] Already brilliant at advertizing campaigns for *Odol*, for which he employed outstanding artists, Lingner sought to use these commercial techniques in a massive hygiene exhibition.

Hygiene exhibitions had been imported from England. They were initially displays of sanitary technology, and were little more than trade exhibitions. Galton, ever inventive, had taken advantage of the International Health Exhibition held in London to organize a public laboratory for anthropometry. The first hygiene exhibition was held in Berlin in 1883, and went on permanent display at the university's hygiene institute.[271] However, when Rubner succeeded Koch, he disliked the public in his institute and ran the exhibition down. A change came when Lingner financed a hygiene exhibition in Munich in 1905, after which he attempted to establish a permanent home for the collection. He considered that there was great popular interest in learning about disease but that academic experts in hygiene spoiled the displays that he wished to show.[272] A more ambitious hygiene exhibition was held in Berlin to coincide with the international congress of hygiene and demography of 1907. This had sections for infant and child care, for TB prevention, and a display on the evils of quackery. Lingner turned the exhibition into a mass spectacle.[273]

The authorities distrusted Lingner for his *amerikanischen Smartness*. Having excelled in *make-money*, he wished to impress with a giant undertaking. Lingner declared that the nation's health amounted to capital, which if well tended could be made to increase. Poor hygiene led to popular discontent. He termed his strategy of mass education 'social hygiene'.[274] Whereas the authorities thought that such an exhibition would interest only experts, Lingner was convinced that it would have mass appeal.[275] There was so little support from officials that he postponed plans for an exhibition in 1906. With much persistence he overcame official reluctance in promoting his venture – reluctance shown, for example, when the Reich Ministry of the Interior refused to sanction the request that the Kaiser be patron.

Lingner's brilliance lay in his ability to recruit talented experts, and in his grasp of how to mount a striking spectacle. He engaged outstanding artists and scientists to mount the displays. The experts included the medical statistician Emil Eugen Roesle, the paediatrician Schlossmann, and the bacteriologist Weber, who became the general secretary of the Hygiene Exhibition.[276] The symbol of the exhibition

270 H. Brose, *40 Jahre Lingner Werke* (nd, Dresden).
271 STA Dresden MdI 3579 Die Errichtung eines Gesundheitsmuseums zu Dresden.
272 BHSTA Mk 11167 Bekämpfung der Volkskrankheiten. Sammlung und Ausstellung (Lingner'sche Stiftung) in München.
273 A. Fischer, 'Zur Geschichte der Hygiene-Ausstellungen', *DMW*, vol. 61 (1935), 165–7; H. Horn and W. Mattjäi, 'Die erste Deutsche Hygiene-Ausstellung', *Zeitschrift für die gesamte Hygiene*, vol. 9 (1963), 563–76. 274 STA Dresden Kreishauptmannschaft Dresden Nr 535.
275 STA Dresden MdI Nr 3572 Internationale Hygiene Ausstellung Dresden.
276 E. Roesle, 'K.A. Lingner†', *Archiv für Soziale Hygiene und Demographie*, vol. 11 no. 4 (1916), 459–61.

was the 'hygiene eye' – a striking adaptation of the all-seeing eye of God. It was created by Franz von Stuck, the Munich secessionist artist. Lingner retained a bias towards conventional scientifically based hygiene. There were displays by the Social Medicine Society, and by state public health administrations. An anti-alcohol exhibition was mounted by Gruber and Grotjahn, and Lingner was among the audience when Gruber lectured.[277] From 1910 the circulars mention the *Sondergruppe Rassenhygiene*, which staged a successful display, as well as lectures and meetings on racial hygiene. But there was friction with both the League for the Protection of Mothers and the campaigners for nature therapy. The most significant group to be excluded was the trade union movement which wished to organize a section on domestic labour. A cartoon of slum life had a child asking, 'Mother, what is hygiene?'.[278]

Millions of onlookers flocked to the International Hygiene Exhibition, when it opened in Dresden during 1911. The theme was *Der Mensch*. The high spot was a model of the 'Visible Man'. This used a special technique for see-through anatomical models, making the interior organs visible.[279] These models by Professor Spalteholz, an anatomist, were a public sensation, and Lingner established a lucrative company (called *Natura Docet*) to supply a world-wide demand for these transparent models. Lingner planned a national hygiene museum on the model of the Deutsches Museum in Munich. There was to be a travelling exhibition for schools.[280] The museum was to be an academy where all could learn visually, with the aim of a reform in lifestyle, as well as satisfy a popular interest in hygiene. The museum was to have sections on the human body, history and ethnology. It constituted a popular anthropology of health and physical culture. That Lingner admired the Jews for their hygienic lifestyle that ensured their survival suggests that this popularized medical anthropology was not anti-semitic. Lingner was able to marry the science of hygiene with popular consumerism and love of spectacle. He took hygiene in a popular direction that contrasted to the rigid scientificity of the state-sponsored *Volkshygiene* movement or to the elitism and the professionalism of racial hygiene. His 'hygiene eye' – which became a trade-mark of the health educators – was indeed far-seeing, as the movement that he initiated drew together scientists, radical reformers and the public.

Genealogy and Mendelism

Biological studies of the family and heredity, led to demands for national institutions for screening the health of total populations. Widespread public interest in heredity supported the scientific movement for studies of human

---

277 STA Dresden MdI Nr 3573; Ploetz papers, diary 3 August 1911.
278 G. Pässler, *Die Geschichte des Deutschen Hygiene-Museums Dresden bis 1945* (nd, np), p. 9.
279 H. Spalteholz, *Ueber das Durchsichtigmachen von menschlichen und tierischen Präparaten* (Leipzig, 1914).
280 K.A. Lingner, *Denkschrift zur Errichtung eines National-Hygienischen Museums in Dresden* (Dresden, 1912).

biology. During the 1890s genealogy gained in popularity, particularly in conservative circles. Medieval styles and ideas became fashionable among the middle class and aristocracy. This 'feudalization' found an expression in the eugenic creed of a revitalized order of chivalry, in the Gobineau Society, and in a variety of cultural forms such as neo-Gothic architecture and Wagner's Germanic operas. Societies for genealogy flourished. These represented far more than just nostalgia for pre-industrial forms of authority. There was a professionalism and scientific approach to the pursuits of genealogy. A number of genealogists, including the royal genealogist, Bernhard Koerner, joined the Racial Hygiene Society and in Leipzig a central office for the study of genealogy was sympathetic to eugenics. Collecting coats of arms or the names of family descendants was condemned by scientific genealogists as dilettantism. Historians, physicians and scientists envisaged that genealogy would form the basis of national schemes for the scientific study of families on aspects including physique and diseases.[281]

This programme was realized between 1900 and 1914. Politics and professionalism underlay the rise of hereditarian ideas in medicine. The controversy on the declining birth rate generated interest in social biology and hereditary pathology. Human genetics arose as part of a broader public movement of hereditarian ideas, as well as being a scientific response to Mendelian theories of biological inheritance. During the 1890s historians developing genealogy as a science were influenceed by positivism. Darwinism, which had drawn so much from historical theories of national progress, was looked to as a basis for a scientific history. In 1898, the Jena historian, Ottokar Lorenz, published an innovative textbook on genealogy which related it to sociology and science. He replaced the traditional family tree or *Stammbaum* with its single lines of only male ancestry, suggesting that an ancestral table or *Ahnentafel* should be constructed. This took account of male and female ancestries. He related his approach to Weismann's biological concept of the ancestral germplasm.[282]

Lorenz's innovations were welcomed by medical researchers with an interest in heredity. They appreciated that genealogy had immense potential for human biology and medicine. The biologists Oscar Hertwig and Hermann Poll considered that it created the possibility for evaluating the female contribution to inheritance.[283] The clinician, Martius, recommended that patients' families be comprehensively reconstructed. Carriers of diseases could be located, and their ratio of incidence could be established. The physician Julius Grober urged the compilation of patients' genealogies.[284] Lorenz's programme pre-dated the

---

[281] R. Sommer, *Familienforschung und Vererbungslehre* (Leipzig, 1911).

[282] O. Lorenz, *Lehrbuch der gesammten wissenschaftlichen Genealogie. Stammbaum und Ahnentafel in ihrer geschichtlichen, sociologischen und naturwissenschaftlichen Bedeutung* (Berlin, 1898).

[283] O. Hertwig, 'Das genealogische Netzwerk und seine Bedeutung für die Frage der monophyletischen oder der polyphyletischen Abstammungshypothese', *Archiv für mikroskopische Anatomie*, vol. 89 part 2 (1917), 227–42.

[284] J. Grober 'Die Bedeutung der Ahnentafel für die biologische Erblichkeitsforschung', *ARGB*, vol. 1 (1904), 665.

development of Mendelism in Germany from 1900. The wider hereditarian movement encompassed historical and social concerns as well as an interest in natural laws of heredity. Few German biologists were orthodox Mendelians, and their studies of inheritance were conducted on a broader intellectual basis than on strictly Mendelian lines. The 're-discovery' of Mendel's laws of inheritance reformulated hereditarian convictions in terms of the hereditary mechanisms of the cell nucleus and chromosomes. German biologists, notably Carl Correns the botanist, took a lead in 1900 in postulating that units of inheritance followed regular ratios of inheritance. Mendelians showed that parental traits could be isolated, and were inherited according to a 3:1 ratio, and that some traits were dominant and others recessive. These discoveries gave an immense boost to studies of hereditary properties in families.[285]

Inherent in Mendelism was a combined administrative and research programme for the collection and analysis of genealogies. By this means scientists and eugenically trained doctors could establish how congenital defects were inherited and locate the carriers of pathological genes. Darwinian concepts of blending inheritance were liberal in that male and female contributed equally to the formation of a new individual. The implications of Mendelism were that traits were immutable or persisted over generations. The medical status of Mendelism increased with the research of the physician Archibald Garrod who, in 1902, pointed out that a rare inborn error of metabolism known as alkaptonuria could be attributed to Mendelian recessive genes as a result of consanguinity of parents who were cousins. He considered that there was an inborn incapacity of the body to carry out normal chemical processes.[286] Garrod entered into correspondence with German doctors on hereditary diseases. Mendelism had institutional ramifications. In 1904 the US biologist, Charles B. Davenport, established the Eugenic Record Office at Cold Spring Harbor.[287] This acted as a vast collection centre for details of diseases, mental traits and vital statistics.[288] The demand arose in Germany for a national institute for the study of human heredity, where scientists could oversee the collation of legal, administrative and medical records. In Germany the re-discovery of the Mendelian ratios of inheritance cemented links between biologists, clinicians, genealogists and statisticians. Mendelism offered a way of understanding the biology of inherited diseases. It shifted the emphasis in biology to study of reproduction and of the inheritance of constant traits. This contrasted with the continuous evolutionary process emphasized by Darwinians. Mendelian study of hybridization offered an empirical approach to the problems of inheritance. Medical scientists such as Martius, Aschoff and Abderhalden gave attention to

[285] O. Meijer, 'Hugo de Vries No Mendelian', *Annals of Science*, vol. 42 (1985), 189–232.
[286] A.G. Bearn and E.D. Miller, 'Archibald Garrod and the Development of the Concept of Inborn Errors of Metabolism', *Bulletin of the History of Medicine*, vol. 53 (1979), 315–27.
[287] D.J. Kevles, *In the Name of Eugenics* (Harmondsworth, 1986), pp. 40–6.
[288] G.E. Allen, 'The Eugenics Record Office at Cold Spring Harbor, 1910–1940: An Essay in Institutional History', *Osiris*, 2nd series vol. 2, (1986), 225–64.

heredity as a predisposing factor in disease. Studies began to be made of patients' genealogies. For example, when Grotjahn held patient consultations he asked about ancestry – how many suicides, criminals and bankruptcies there had been in a family. Indeed Grotjahn diagnosed himself as having been the neurotic child of a father who had been a morphine addict. Underlying the medical concern with heredity and disease was the sense of personal and economic insecurity.[289]

At the meeting of German Physicians and Naturalists held in 1898, the clinician Martius proclaimed a programme for research on hereditary diseases. This was based on the constitutional theories of inherited predisposition to disease as formulated by Gottstein and Hueppe, who argued in general epidemiological terms that infecting agents should have a variable rather than constant statistical value. Martius formulated constitutional theories from the point of view of a specialist in internal medicine, and suggested that infections depended not only on bacteria, but on the variable condition of the infected organism. Since 1889 he had been observing individual cases such as heart disease and jaundice, for which inherited disposition seemed the best explanation. In 1901 he combined these views with the genealogical method of Lorenz to produce a theory of 'constitutional medicine'.[290] He believed that since Ibsen's *Ghosts* the public had been in the grips of a 'pandemic' fear of degeneration. While he praised Ploetz for his scientific analysis of degeneration, he considered that Ploetz's demands for public controls of reproduction still lacked a feasible scientific basis. The restrictions on marriage of the sick and criminal urged by the psychiatrists Näcke and Gebhardt were also premature. But he considered that Lorenz could provide the basis for an exact scientific analysis of these problems.[291] Between 1899 and 1909 he published a comprehensive account of heredity and disease, based on study of patients' genealogies. He criticized the experimental approach as isolating individual instances from their context in population biology. Psychological studies on heredity, such as those by Ribot, were condemned as anecdotal due to their lack of systematic observation. Martius regarded the genealogical approach as a means of synthesizing scientific research with the clinical observations of the practising physician.[292] He used what he called 'the historical concept of a constitution' to explain disease processes. It meant that infectious diseases such as TB had to be understood in terms of the defence systems and the constitutional condition of a body. He agreed with Gottstein that there was a variable relationship between the cause of the disease and the constitution.[293] He developed concepts of the 'family disease' by combining clinical observations with hereditary biology.[294]

Martius suggested that Lorenz's historical approach had a counterpart in

---

[289] Weindling, 'Medical Practice', p. 406.
[290] F. Martius, 'Das Vererbungsproblem in der Pathologie', *Berliner klinische Wochenschrift*, vol. 38 (1901), 781–3, 814–18.   [291] Martius, 'Das Vererbungsproblem', pp. 781–3, 814–18.
[292] F. Martius, *Die Pathogenese Innerer Krankheiten* (Leipzig and Vienna, 1899), pp. iii–v.
[293] Martius, *Pathogenese*, pp. 158–63.
[294] 'F. Martius' in L.R. Grote (ed.), *Die Medizin der Gegenwart in Selbstdarstellungen* (Leipzig, 1923), I, pp. 105–40.

chromosomal studies of inheritance. He drew on H.E. Ziegler's concept of the chromosome as containing all the hereditary qualities of its ancestors and the hereditary mass out of which the new individual would be formed. He agreed with Ziegler that every human carried chromosomes containing the disposition to diseases such as cancer, mental illness and TB. Martius recommended that in the choice of a partner in marriage a good general constitution was desirable; the intended spouse should also be without the accumulation of specific disease determinants. It was necessary not to marry relations such as cousins, as this would cause a loss of accumulated diversity. Thus Wilhelm II had only 162 of a possible 512 'individual ancestors' when traced back to the ninth generation.[295] The social overtones of such examples of inbreeding in the discussion of 'constitutional diseases' suggest that biologists were claiming to be in a position superior to the privileged aristocratic elite, and that the population would be healthier if biologists were in a position of power.

In 1902 the distinguished clinician, Wilhelm Ebstein, criticized the concept of 'constitutional diseases'. He argued that every disease had an element of a constitutional cause.[296] He attributed diseases such as jaundice, obesity and diabetes to anomalies in the protoplasm resulting from inherited factors. Martius replied that it was necessary to establish why these diseases did not occur in every generation, and why the form that the diseases took was liable to alter. He considered this was necessary as a basis for a preventive medicine that could protect the human species in the 'coming generation'. He quoted Rüdin's opinion on the need to prevent marriage between persons with diseases such as epilepsy and diabetes. He considered that preventive medicine administered by doctors offered the middle way between the anarchy of political individualism and a system of public health that amounted to a police state.[297] To Ploetz's delight, Martius publicly supported racial hygiene at the Congress for Internal Medicine in April 1905. He affirmed a holy duty towards the coming generation. He envisaged a state registry office that would record all sickness and other anomalies.[298]

The idea of a 'constitutional pathology' came to permeate other branches of medicine. In 1904 the Jena psychiatrist, Wilhelm Strohmeyer, announced a research programme for psychopathology based on statistical genealogy.[299] Hereditary disposition and the defence systems of the body came to characterize many branches of pathology. The Bonn pathologist, Hugo Ribbert, emphasized the role of hereditary and racial immunity in addition to the cellular factors detected by Behring.[300] The Berlin professor of pathology, Johannes Orth,

[295] Martius, *Pathogenese*, pp. 380–4; Martius, 'Der Familienbegriff und die genealogische Vererbungs-lehre', in C.H. Noorden and S. Kaminer (eds.), *Krankheit und Ehe* (Leipzig, 1914); see also H. Senator, S. Kaminer and R. Fischer (eds.), *Krankheiten und Ehe. Volks-ausgabe*, (Berlin nd).
[296] W. Ebstein, *Vererbbare celluläre Stoffwechselkrankheiten* (Stuttgart, 1902).
[297] Martius, *Pathogenese*, pp. 234, 424–6.   [298] Ploetz papers, diary, 12 April 1905.
[299] W. Strohmeyer, 'Ziele und Wege der Erblichkeitsforschung in der Neuro- und Psychopathologie', *Allgemeine Zeitschrift für Psychiatrie und psych-ger. Medizin*, vol. 111 (1904), 355.
[300] H. Ribbert, *Ueber Vererbung* (Marburg, 1902); Ribbert, 'Die Vererbung der Krankheiten', *Politisch-anthropologische Revue*, vol. 3 (1904), 85–101.

stressed the importance of heredity to pathology in 1906, and joined the Racial Hygiene Society.[301] The standard textbook on pathological anatomy, edited by the Freiburg pathologist Aschoff, was introduced by a chapter on heredity. Genealogies of the inheritance of colour blindness and haemophilia were not yet Mendelian, but Mendelism was given prominence. There was emphasis on the hereditary predisposition of pathological conditions. The author of the introductory chapter, E. Albrecht, declared that the Mendelian laws should enable the location of pathogenic substances in the chromosomes. Their elimination was necessary to improve the health of races and families through control of marriage and child rearing.[302]

Whereas the anthropological surveys of eyes, hair and skin conducted during the 1870s had aimed to map the geographical distribution of external variations, the concern now shifted to the prevalence of degenerative traits in all parts of the body. The ophthalmologist Arthur Crzellitzer studied eye diseases. From 1900 until 1912 he reconstructed genealogies of 104 families of his patients. He carried out a large survey of 786 families in a working class area of Berlin.[303] He dismissed as useless observations that a father and son were suffering from the same disease, since they gave no idea of the incidence of the diseases in other members of a family. He investigated such conditions as short-sightedness, long-sightedness, squinting, astigmatism, cataract and nystagmus. Like earlier researchers he emphasized the role of incest in causing blindness and other eye diseases. In the 1880s Alexis Magnus had examined 374 marriages resulting in blind children. Crzellitzer used Mendelian ratios to show latent inheritance over three generations. He studied diseases in relation to birth order and family size. As with Pearson's studies of TB and criminality, he pointed out that the first born was at greater risk. Crzellitzer elaborated the concept of the discipline of 'family research'.[304] Heredity was acknowledged as essential in the social hygienic aim of maintaining the health of families.

Mendelian racial hygiene

The fusing of racial hygiene and Mendelism was rapid. In the first volume of Ploetz's *Archiv* the re-discoverer of the Mendelian laws, the botanist Correns, contributed an essay on experimental Mendelian research. Erich von Tschermak, who also claimed (with less justice) to have rediscovered the laws, published in the

[301] J. Orth, *Aufgaben, Zweck und Ziele der Gesundheitspflege* (Stuttgart, 1904).
[302] L. Aschoff (ed.), *Pathologische Anatomie* (Jena, 1909), pp. 18, 22.
[303] A. Crzellitzer, 'Die Berliner städtischen Familienstammbücher und ihre Ausgestaltung für die Zwecke der Vererbungsforschung und der sozialen Hygiene', *Medizinischer Reform*, vol. 19 no. 11 (1911).
[304] A. Crzellitzer, 'Methoden der Familienforschung', *Zeitschrift für Ethnologie*, vol. 41 (1909), 182–98; Crzellitzer, 'Familienforschung', in A. Grotjahn and I. Kaup (eds.), *Handwörterbuch der sozialen Hygiene* (Leipzig, 1912), I, pp. 326–36; Crzellitzer, 'Die Vererbung von Augenleiden', *Berliner Klinishe Wochenschrift*, no. 44 (1912), 2,070–4; Crzellitzer, 'Die Aufgaben der Rassenhygiene', *Deutsche Medizinische Wochenschrift*, vol. 38 (1912), 1,651–3.

Archiv on Mendelism and Galton's theory of ancestral heredity (translated as *Ahnenerbe* – a term later to be used by the SS).[305] The zoologist, Plate, who was a close friend of Ploetz and became Haeckel's successor in Jena, published on the need for an institute for experimental zoology, and on the inheritance of human diseases.[306] The *Archiv* became a home for genealogical studies of local populations and families. Mendelian researchers, such as Weinberg in Stuttgart and Fischer in Freiburg, organized branches of the racial hygiene society; Baur and Rüdin were dedicated Mendelian researchers while campaigning for racial hygiene.

Eugenicists became major exponents of the application of mathematics to reproductive patterns and diseases. A lead was taken by the Stuttgart general practitioner and Poor Law doctor, Weinberg. In the course of his practice he attended 3,500 births including over 120 twin births. In 1901 he published on the physiology and pathology of multiple births. He developed a method for determining the proportion of identical twins deriving from one fertilized egg or fraternal twins from two eggs. He used the principle of probability that single eggs always give rise to unisexual pairs, whereas two eggs give rise to randomly determined sexual combinations. He proceeded to discover differences between the two classes of twins in their life expectancy, diseases and fertility in terms of an inheritance of the tendency to have twins.[307] He became interested in pathological inheritance and genealogical statistics in 1903.[308] In 1905 after a lecture from Ziegler (the instigator of the 'Krupp' Prize) on hereditary biology, Weinberg quickly recognized the possibilities of Mendelism for statistical research on inheritance. In 1908 he published on the validity of the Mendelian ratios for humans. He discovered the equilibrium law for successive generations of monohybrid populations. He showed a recurrent balance of dominant and recessive genes in successive generations. He calculated the frequency with which genotypes occurred in populations breeding at random. These results were published in 1908[309] but Weinberg's work did not find international recognition because of his criticisms of Karl Pearson. He argued in 1909 against Pearson and Yule's assertion that the Mendelian laws could not be applied to human populations.[310]

Weinberg greatly refined statistical methods of investigation. In 1909 he showed that studies on the reproductive fitness of selected individuals was nothing but a mathematical consequence of the fact that selection of children favours selection of

---

[305] E. v. Tschermak, 'Der moderne Stand des Vererbungsproblems', *ARGB*, vol. 2 (1905), 663.
[306] L. Plate, 'Ueber Vererbung und die Notwendigkeit der Gründung einer Versuchsanstalt für Vererbungs- und Züchtungskunde', *ARGB*, vol. 5 (1908), 67; Plate, 'Ein Versuch zur Erklärung der gynephoren Vererbung menschlicher Erkrankungen', *ARGB*, vol. 8 (1911), 164.
[307] C. Stern, 'Wilhelm Weinberg 1862–1937', *Genetics*, vol. 47 (1962), 1–5.
[308] W. Weinberg, 'Pathologische Vererbung und genealogische Statistik', *Archiv für klinische Medizin*, vol. 78 (1903), 521–40.
[309] It was not until 1943 that he was given joint credit for this discovery with the British statistician G.H. Hardy.
[310] For later discussions of Weinberg's statistics see correspondence in R.A. Fisher papers, Adelaide.

the more highly fertile parents. This should be compensated for by examining the fertility of the siblings of these parents. In 1912 he focused on the problem of incomplete selection of human material. For example, in the case of albinism, only families with albinos were located whereas those without any escaped attention. This resulted in too high a proportion of the relation of albinos to the normal in such families. Weinberg invented the 'sib', 'proband' and 'a priori' methods for correcting for this. These innovations provided a scientific rationale for comprehensive screening of total populations.[311]

The classic text book on heredity, published in 1911 by the Berlin botanist Baur extended the Mendelian discoveries to man. He compared the German Empire to an *Antirrhinum-Volk* – a nation of snap dragons. Its composition was equivalent to the population resulting from crossing three to four varieties of snap dragons. Drawing on the observations of the eugenicists Grotjahn and Schallmayer, Baur warned that the declining birth rate was counter-selective. The *führenden Elemente* in the population were in danger of dying out and could never be replaced. Negative selection was the main problem, whereas the burden of the degenerate was only a secondary issue. He considered that the North American laws for castration of criminals and mental patients would achieve little as the capacity for modifications of the hereditary characters resulting in these defects was so large that they could never all be located.[312] Baur indicated the need for more comprehensive means of weeding out degenerate population stocks.

In 1911 Fischer, the Freiburg anthropologist, consolidated the biological method in his researches on the Rehoboth in German South-West Africa. The Rehoboth arose from inter-breeding between white settlers and natives. Fischer's aim was to investigate the inheritance not so much of pathological characteristics but of the normal. He tested the conclusions of other researchers, such as the Davenports, for hair and eye colour. He claimed to show Mendelian patterns of inheritance as for the height of the forehead. He saw a constant recurrence of individual characteristics. Fischer praised this 'mixed race' as 'healthy, strong and fertile'; they were ideally adapted for military service and industry in this region. His study stimulated research on the biological anthropology of families in general.[313]

Another model of practical relevance was produced by Hermann Lundborg, a lecturer in psychiatry at the University of Uppsala. The title of his giant-sized book was, *Medico-biological Family Researches on a Strain of 2,232 Swedish Peasants*. This ambitious study of inherited diseases was published in Germany in 1913 with the support of the Swedish state and the Swedish Racial Hygiene Society. Swedish household books and the high quality of local population registers enabled research

[311] W. Weinberg, 'Ueber Methoden der Vererbungsforschung beim Menschen', *Berliner Klinische Wochenschrift* vol. 49 (1912), 646–9, 697–701.

[312] E. Baur, *Einführung in die experimentelle Vererbungslehre* (Berlin, 1911).

[313] E. Fischer, *Die Rehobother Bastards und das Bastardierungsproblem beim Menschen* (Jena, 1913).

[314] H. Lundborg, *Medizinisch-biologische Familienforschungen innerhalb eines 2232 köpfigen Bauernge-schlechtes in Schweden (Provinz Blekinge)* (Jena, 1913).

on a total population in any locality rather than just those actually in a clinic or visiting a doctor. This permitted study of latent carriers of a disease. Lundborg showed how certain nervous diseases such as epilepsy, and schizophrenia were passed on from generation to generation. Each disease had a different incidence and pattern of heredity although there were common causes such as incest.[314] The introduction to Lundborg's study was written by Gruber as chairman of the Racial Hygiene Society. Gruber considered that inherited constitution was the major factor determining health. The best hygienic conditions were impotent against inherited genetic defects. Inequality was a result of different biological capacity. The only way to improve the condition of the nation was to allow those with superior hereditary qualities to reproduce. He considered that this study pointed to the need for a state institute for heredity and state-established health passports.[315]

The medical lobby for more systematic population registration and correlation of demographic and medical data became vociferous after 1900. Weinberg benefited from family registers, which were kept in Württemberg and parts of Baden. He recommended that the statistics of school doctors, recruitment authorities, criminal records and suicides be correlated. There was already an index of cancer, TB and multiple births kept for over two centuries in Stuttgart.[316] Crzellitzer demanded compulsory family registers, and other researchers into hereditary diseases urged that population registration be as comprehensive as possible.[317] Following Lundborg's model, Rüdin researched the problem of the inheritance of schizophrenia. His attention had been drawn to schizophrenia by Kraepelin in Munich. Kraepelin had analyzed this as a degenerative disease beginning in youth, and as a result named the disease *dementia praecox*. By contrast with Kraepelin's clinical approach, Rüdin researched on the family background to the disease. He was convinced that as mental diseases had an organic basis, the characteristics of such diseases must be inherited in the same way as Mendelian factors in plants and animals. Rüdin claimed to show that the disease caused a recessive pattern of inheritance with a 1:16 ratio. Rüdin, like Lundborg, stressed the need to research on total populations rather than on just the individual sick.[318]

A generation of medical students was exposed to hereditarian medicine. In Freiburg Lenz was impressed by the lectures of Fischer. Lenz studied the human genetics of pioneers such as Baur, Bateson, Boveri, Morgan, Garrod and Weinberg. In 1912 he completed his dissertation on sex determination and inherited disease. He then worked in Gruber's hygiene institute in Munich. He fused social and racial hygiene on a Mendelian basis.[319] These developments

[315] M. Gruber, 'Vorrede', foreword to Lundborg, *Familienforschungen*.

[316] W. Weinberg, 'Aufgabe und Methode der Familienstatistik bei medizinisch-biologischen Problemen', *Zeitschrift für soziale Medizin*, vol 3 (1907), 4–26.

[317] *Medizinische Reform* (1911), 218.

[318] E. Rüdin, 'Einige Wege und Ziele der Familienforschung mit Rücksicht auf die Psychiatrie', *Zeitschrift für die gesamte Neurologie und Psychiatrie*, vol. 7 (1911), 487–585; Rüdin, *Zur Vererbung und Neuentstehung geistiger Störungen* (Berlin, 1916).

[319] F. Lenz, *Ueber die krankhaften Erbanlagen des Mannes und die Bestimmung des Geschlechtes beim Menschen* (Jena, 1912).

suggest that from about 1911 there was a far greater acceptance of racial hygiene in academic medicine. This can be seen in the gynaecological lectures and academic orations by the Strasburg professor Heinrich Bayer to the Strasburg Medical and Scientific Society.[320] Medical expertise fuelled a growing movement for genealogical research. Courses on genealogy were organized by the psychologist, Robert Sommer, at Giessen in 1908 and 1912. The first course was on 'inherited feeble mindedness', and criminal psychology was the major concern. The second course combined genealogists, lawyers and experts in hygiene such as Kaup, Crzellitzer and Weinberg. Sommer added an historical dimension to hereditarian research, using monuments, coins, coats of arms and pictures to reconstruct genealogies stretching back into the Middle Ages. The course was supported by the Prussian state as suitable for the training of medical officers, psychiatrists, pathologists, prison doctors and lawyers.[321] The problem of degeneration led to a reorientation of attitudes to welfare institutions and politics. As psychiatrists discovered a growing mass of degenerates, confidence was shaken in whether it was right and economically feasible to provide therapeutic institutions. In 1911 the weekly, *Die Umschau*, held a competition for answers as to the costs to state and society in supporting inferior elements. The winner was an asylum official, Ludwig Jens, who emphasized the high costs of welfare provision.[322] The eugenicist Kaup called for radical measures to isolate the congenitally degenerate.[323]

A national institute

The popularity and prestige of biology was shown when national research institutes were planned from 1907. It was hoped to harness the might of industrial capital to support a national institute for biological research. There were fears that Germany was losing its world leadership in biological research. When the Kaiser Wilhelm Gesellschaft (KWG) was planning the foundation of research institutes there was much support for institutes for biological heredity, anthropology and medical research. Eugenicists urged that these schemes be extended to human heredity, as well as to anthropology and sociology. The idea of a national eugenics institute was a long-standing aim of supporters of racial hygiene. Gruber outlined a scheme for an institute for human heredity.[324] Kraepelin lobbied for a psychiatric institute which should contain a department for genealogical studies of inheritance.

---

320 H. Bayer, *Über Vererbung und Rassenhygiene*, (Jena, 1912); also W. Oettinger, *Die Rassenhygiene und ihre wissenschaftlichen Grundlagen* (Berlin, 1914).
321 R. Sommer, *Bericht über den II. Kurs mit Kongress für Familienforschung, Vererbungs- und Regenerationslehre* (Halle, 1912).
322 L. Jens, 'Was kosten die schlechten Rassenelemente dem Staat und der Gesellschaft?', *Archiv für Soziale Hygiene*, vol. 8 (1913), 213–37, 265–322.
323 I. Kaup, 'Was kosten die minderwertigen Elemente dem Staat und der Gesellschaft?', *ARGB*, vol. 10 (1913), 723–47; J. Noakes, 'Nazism and Eugenics', in R.J. Bullen *et al.* (eds.), *Ideas into Politics* (London, 1984), pp. 75–94.
324 G. Wendel, *Die Kaiser-Wilhelm-Gesellschaft 1911–1914* (Berlin 1975), pp. 116–22; M. v. Gruber, 'Organisation der Forschung und Sammlung von Materialien über die Entartungsfrage', *Concordia*, vol. 17 (1910), 225–8.

This demand was supported by his Munich colleagues, Alzheimer and Rüdin. They envisaged either the Imperial Health Office or the recently founded KWG as the home for a national department for *Familienforschung* (family research). This should co-ordinate official statistics and registration procedures with scientific research.[325]

Human heredity was also an aim of some of the wealthier patrons of the KWG. They had many links to biology through family and friends as in the cases of Boveri (the brother of an engineer), Goldschmidt (supported by Frankfurt commercial interests) and Wassermann (the son of the banker). The industrialist, August Ludowici (himself an amateur biologist), wanted an appointment for the environmental biological theorist, von Uexküll. His priority was research on inheritance. This was also the opinion of Paul Mankiewitz, the director of the Deutsche Bank. He considered research on human heredity would have especial significance for medicine.[326] Similar opinions were heard among the general public. The psychologist, Sommer, advocated a Reich Institute for Family Research, Heredity and Regeneration.[327] In April 1914 Géza von Hofmann, the Hungarian consul in Berlin and author of a study of US sterilization laws, wrote to Adolf von Harnack (the church historian and secretary of the KWG) of the need for a national institute of racial biology.[328] The demand for a national eugenics institute remained a major aim.

Although the elite of academics in Imperial Germany were staunch nationalists, they abhored biological racism as unscientific and a violation of personal liberty. This was seen when Woltmann petitioned the Prussian Academy of Sciences for funds for support for a research programme on the racial lines established by Gobineau and Chamberlain. The academy secretary, Hermann Diels, rejected the application as 'a raw dilettantism'. When the Kaiser himself supported an application by the Gobineau Society for an edition to be edited by Schemann, the Academy condemned the enterprise as of no scientific value, amateurish and confused.[329] Harnack blocked proposals for racial research. When leading university professors were asked for their ideas for biological institutes, the plans elicited were couched in positivistic and cautious terms. After a conference in 1912 Harnack decided to support biological research on heredity, bacteriology, brain research and experimental physiology. These were conservative choices, still very much in line with the positivistic approach to research. Harnack recognized that racial hygiene had been one of the aims of medical research since 1900, but he did not allow this to become part of the KWG's programmes. Medical research was restricted to protozoa research, and thus in line with bacteriology. Research on

[325] Rüdin, 'Wege und Ziele', pp. 570–2.
[326] Wendel, *Kaiser-Wilhelm-Gesellschaft*, pp. 175–8.
[327] R. Sommer, 'Organisation und Aufgaben eines Reichsinstitutes für Familienforschung und Vererbungslehre', *Deutsche Medizinische Wochenschrift*, vol. 46 (1914), 708–11.
[328] MPG Arbeitsphysiologie Gen II 8 Bd II (1911–1918) Bl 80, 81; BAK R 86 Nr 2371 Bd 1 Bl 108.
[329] *Die Berliner Akademie in der Zeit des Imperialismus* (Berlin, 1975), pp. 89–91, *ein blutiger Dilettantismus*.

heredity was to be carried out on animals and plants, with an eye at most to agricultural improvement.[330]

The Kaiser Wilhelm Gesellschaft was a bastion of scientific positivism. The older generation of professors and administrators was resistant to racial ideas. Its positivism accepted only empirical research on heredity as scientific, and condemned the transfer to the human and social spheres as beyond the pale. The initial proposals show that leading industrialists and the public had great interest in biology and its application to human heredity and society. The rising tide of patriotism from 1914 meant that the divisions between patriotism and positivism would be swept away.

THE DECLINING BIRTH RATE

The human economy

The synthesis of biology and hygiene, and the concern with the deterioration in health of future generations made reproductive hygiene a central issue, and gave medicine the major task of improving the quality of the population and maintaining its quantity. Advocates of social hygiene made common cause with feminists who were demanding improved welfare for mothers and babies. Such social hygiene was a response to the declining birth rate, which was regarded as precipitating a disrupting shift to 'modern', 'rational' values. Large families with many births but a high infant mortality were typical of Germany until the 1890s. Small families with a low birth rate and a low infant mortality then became the norm. With hindsight this decline has been regarded as a normal consequence of industrialization. But at the time it was condemned as a sign of degeneration, as morally and physically pathological, and as an alarming threat to the military and economic power of the nation. From 1900 there was concern among conservatives and religious groups such as the Centre Party over the decline, which was perceived as a moral decline resulting from a materialistic attitude to life. National values of health and maternal duty were deemed necessary to maintain the will to have families with more than three children. A slogan in popular moral and medical tracts was that of the 'scream for the child'. Medical reformers joined in the agitation, because reduction of high rates of infant mortality would reduce the burden of childbirth on mothers. Child health became a common rallying cry of feminists, doctors, welfare experts, social scientists and eugenicists. The remainder of this chapter describes how debate was carried out at a variety of levels – the political, official, academic – as well as among feminists and social reformers. The 'scream for a child' was to pierce the sinews of social life and, harmonizing with both radical and nationalist ideals, to prompt a chorus of propaganda for more babies of better quality.

During the nineteenth century Germany was regarded as over-populated.

[330] MPG archives, KWI für Biologie. Biologische Institute im Allgemeinen, Gen 4 Bd I.

Malthusian opposition to population increase outstripping economic resources underwent a change from absolutist authoritarianism in the 1820s to liberalism. Early German Malthusians advocated that moral restraint be reinforced by state coercion, and in a notorious case, by mass infibulation as a means of preventing the poor and chronic invalids from reproducing. Laws on marriage restrictions were a short-lived Malthusian experiment between the 1820s and 1860s. During the economic crises of the 1920s these authoritarian precedents were cited to legitimize medical remedies for the problem of the surplus population.[331]

Liberal economists remained Malthusians, convinced that there was a lack of natural resources. Although liberalism had the effect of removing restrictions on marriage (in 1868) and migration, liberal social theorists continued to be preoccupied by the problem of over-population as a cause of poverty. In 1881 Gustav Rümelin published on the problem of over-population, suggesting that the growth of the proletariat should be curbed by marriage restriction. The influential 'academic socialists' – the economists Lujo Brentano, Schmoller and Adolf Wagner – pointed out that the population was increasing faster than the means of subsistence. The poor had too high a rate of reproduction whereas the higher social classes could support their families. As liberal, 'Manchester' economics became outmoded at the turn of the century, economists transferred their attention to social and demographic questions. There was a shift away from political economy to what was termed the 'human economy'. Biological standards of wealth were suggested, expressed by the terms 'child poor' to denote small families, and 'child rich' to denote larger families. There was an interest in fiscal and taxation measures to boost the production of children. Although the population was continuing to grow, a declining birth rate was discovered. The earlier view that Germany was over-populated gave way to fears that the nation would not be able to sustain its military and industrial might.[332]

Demands were made that the state should stimulate a rise in the birth rate. A number of groups began to campaign for a quantitative increase in the birth rate, and for state subsidies for 'child rich' families. The neo-Malthusian advocates of birth control shifted their ground. They no longer said that fertility should be curbed to prevent over-population; instead, birth control should be used to prevent VD and to raise the quality of future generations. The issues of quantitative pro-natalism and qualitative eugenics caused much controversy among concerned groups of public health experts and social scientists. The discovery of the declining birth rate prompted economists to investigate how social conditions determined reproductive behaviour. A major preoccupation was the explanation of fertility change, and of the 'rational' values resulting in smaller families. Just prior to the German studies on the problem came analyses of differential fertility in Britain and

---

[331] D.V. Glass, *Introduction to Malthus* (London, 1953), pp. 38–47.
[332] Dietzel, 'Der Streit um Malthus' Lehre', *Festgabe für Adolf Wagner* (Leipzig, 1905); L. von Bortkiewicx, 'Die Bevölkerungstheorien', *Festschrift Schmoller. Die Entwicklung der deutschen Volkswirtschaftslehre im 19. Jahrhundert* (Leipzig, 1905).

France. In 1899 Jacques Bertillon published a study of fertility among women aged between fifteen and thirty living in Paris, Berlin, Vienna and London. He correlated very high birth rates with poverty, and opened up the disturbing possibility of a class differential in the birth rate which would result in the higher classes becoming swamped by the more fertile but less capable masses. In 1907 Sidney Webb published a Fabian pamphlet on *The Decline in the Birth Rate*: he observed that not only were the prosperous and thrifty sectors of society practising birth control, but skilled workers were also limiting family size; immigrant families of Irish and Jews had larger than average families. In 1910 the *École des Hautes Études Sociales* organized a conference on 'demographic' problems such as abortion and neo-Malthusianism. In 1911 the *Académie des Sciences* offered a prize for a treatise on population which was won by the pro-natalist statistician, Bertillon. The attention of the international community of demographers and welfare experts was thus firmly fixed on the birth rate.

These concerns with differential fertility were taken up by German economists, who pursued a variety of psychological and social biological analyses in attacks on the false psychological premisses of Malthus. In 1907 Paul Mombert (a student of Brentano) suggested that when there was an improved standard of living, further expectations of improved welfare were achieved by saving on the costs of having children. He analysed savings bank statistics in order to prove that those who saved more had fewer children. Fertility decreased with increasing prosperity and high birth rates remained a feature of poverty. He argued that the same psychological motive underlay saving and reproduction – a concern with personal well-being and securing the future of one's family. Prosperity meant a greater calculation of future economic circumstances. There occurred a decline in the instinct to reproduce – in contrast to a decline of reproductive potential or of sexuality.[333]

The economist Brentano analysed the situation from a Malthusian perspective. He denied the existence of a reproductive instinct to maintain the race. In 'lower' societies and classes children were conceived to satisfy personal sexual instincts. In 'higher' civilized societies and classes children were an expression of the love between parents. He argued that prosperity freed parents from animal instincts and allowed them rationally to calculate and choose their family size. Decreased fertility was caused by VD incurred as a result of postponing marriage, and mental stress due to the strains of urban civilization, but the main cause was a voluntary decision not to reproduce.[334]

Contrasting with the consumer theories of Mombert and Brentano were theories of collectivist-minded economists. In 1911 Goldscheid argued that the production of children was related to the production of economic goods. His study on the 'evolution of the human economy' suggested that the weakening of the

---

[333] P. Mombert, *Studien zur Bevölkerungsbewegung in Deutschland in den letzten Dezennien* (Karlsruhe, 1907).
[334] L. Brentano, 'The Doctrine of Malthus and the Increase of Population During the Last Decades', *The Economic Journal*, vol. 20 (1910), 371–91.

reproductive instinct was not to be understood in individualist terms. Similarly, manufacturing had to be explained not in terms of the individual entrepreneur but by reference to the technical and economic reproductive sector of the nation. Until now the masses brought up children at their own cost, but for the benefit of the state. As the masses became more educated, the realization had dawned that it was in one's personal interest to have less children. The state had a choice: either to allow immigration by foreign racial elements, or to subsidize the rearing of children. He argued that the state must invest in the human economy as in other productive sectors like agriculture or industry. He called for comprehensive research into the family.[335]

The falling birth rate prompted many different studies of its cause. There were two strategies of analysis. One was to conduct empirical demographic analyses of the affected sectors of society. Karl Oldenberg, an opponent of over-industrialization, suggested that migration from the countryside due to urbanization was the basic cause of the declining birth rate. He criticized Brentano's explanation based on neo-Malthusian responses to poverty. The poor living conditions in cramped urban conditions forced a limitation of fertility.[336] Another approach to the problem was to consider the underlying psychology of family limitation. Attention was fixed on the problem of 'rationalization' as linking economics, religion and demographic issues. In 1909 Sombart spoke of 'a rationalization of life style'. In 1911 the economist, Julius Wolf, employed the concept of rationalization to produce one of the most eloquent and influential analyses of the declining birth rate. Wolf illustrates the transition from fiscal studies to broader nationalist and welfare-oriented approaches. His arguments for a strong German-dominated Central European economy led to an interest in racial and demographic movements.[337] He analysed the decline in the birth rate as a 'rationalization of sexual life', due to feminism and social democracy. He argued that the birth rate was lower in electoral districts voting socialist, and higher in conservative areas. Wolf introduced the term, 'the two child system', to stigmatize the tendency to have smaller families. He regarded the religious commandment that birth control was a sin as far too weak. For he suggested that a major change had taken place in the psychic structure of the masses between 1895 and 1910 with a collapse of religious faith. This was the major single cause of infertility.[338] Wolf's analysis was taken up by churchmen such as the Berlin theologian, Reinhold Seeberg, and medical experts such as Gruber and the Catholic medical officer Bornträger.[339]

[335] G. Heinson, R. Knieper, and O. Steiger, *Menschenproduktion. Allgemeine Bevölkerungslehre der Neuzeit* (Frankfurt-on-Main, 1979), pp. 194–6.
[336] K. Oldenberg, 'Ueber den Rückgang der Geburten- und Sterbeziffer', *Archiv für Sozialwissenschaft*, vol. 32, (1911), 319–77; vol. 33 (1911), 401–99.
[337] J. Wolf, *Materialien betreffend den Mitteleuropäischen Wirtschaftsverein* (Berlin, 1904); Wolf, 'Das Rassenproblem in der Weltwirtschaft', *Zeitschrift für Sozialwissenschaft*, vol. 6 (1903), 30–42.
[338] J. Wolf, *Der Geburtenrückgang* (Jena, 1912).
[339] J. Bornträger, *Bewirkt die Geburtenbeschränkung eine Rassenverbesserung?* (Düsseldorf, 1913); R. Seeberg, *Der Geburtenrückgang in Deutschland, eine sozialethische Studie* (Leipzig, 1913).

The decline was a type of 'psychic infection'. Wolf's analysis cemented an alliance of the churches, eugenicists and welfare experts, marking the end of the antagonism between Social Darwinists and the churches. There followed studies correlating the decline in fertility to occupation and social status. The concept of rationalization was employed more to describe the mentality resulting from economic progress rather than, as in Wolf's pejorative sense, the dissolution of higher ethical and national ideals.

The concern with differential fertility reflected the sense of insecurity of the educated elite. The fear of the demise of the nation's elite led to debate on the fertility of Jews. The statistician, Felix Aaron Theilhaber, published in 1911 a treatise on 'The Decline of the German Jews. An Economic Study'. He argued that West European Jews had voluntarily decided to limit their fertility to such a great extent that they were on the verge of extinction. The Jews were a prototype of Germany's educated and commercial classes who would inevitably share the same fate. A major cause was the turning away from religion to secular values.[340] His work bore similarities to that of Sombart's studies on the Jewish origins of capitalism, and on luxury and capitalism. *Sterile Berlin* was the sensationalist title of Theilhaber's economic study of demographic trends in Berlin. Part of this had been used as an entry in the competition on the declining birth rate organized by the Racial Hygiene Society.[341] He argued that economic causes were a major factor in the limiting of fertility. Berlin could not replenish itself with its own low fertility. Unless immigration from the countryside was maintained, its schools and university, and its commercial and manufacturing institutions would stand empty. He pointed out that the ending of child labour removed an important rationale for large 'child rich' families. He suggested that the 'child poor' be taxed to benefit the 'child rich'. It was a problem not only limited to Berlin, but also affecting the whole of Germany. Theilhaber typified a shift in attitudes among social scientists away from commercial and fiscal problems and towards the problem that the 'human economy' determined the reproduction and quality of future generations.[342]

Medical diagnoses

There was a convergence of interest between economic and medical studies focusing on the motives behind the limiting of fertility. Studies by a number of Berlin doctors, combining clinical experience with sociological observation, came to dominate the debate. They sought to determine the medical causes for the decline in fertility. They were obsessed by the spread of chronic diseases such as VD and TB, and the possible effects of toxic substances at work on heredity. The social pathology of abortion, prostitution and contraception were major concerns.

---

[340] F.A. Theilhaber, *Der Untergang der deutschen Juden: eine volkswirtschaftliche Studie* (Munich, 1911).
[341] F.A. Theilhaber, 'Die Schädigung der Rasse durch soziales und wirtschaftliches Aufsteigen bewiesen an der Berliner Juden', *ARGB*, vol. 10 (1913), 68–92.
[342] F.A. Theilhaber, *Das sterile Berlin. Eine volkswirtschaftliche Studie* (Berlin, 1913).

Doctors praised the healthy virtues of early marriage, and were critical of economic factors causing postponement of marriage and childbirth.

There was intense propaganda against VD and alcoholism as racial poisons. The eugenic arguments of Ploetz and Rüdin that these conditions brought on a whole range of pathological characteristics as nervous diseases and damaged the quality of the nation's hereditary stock became accepted. Chronic and inherited diseases – whether short-sightedness, diabetes or neurological complaints – indicated a decline in the quality of of the population.[343] The eugenicists entered into the fray over neo-Malthusianism. Schallmayer attacked a Dutch neo-Malthusian tract to which the feminist Marie Stritt had written an introduction. Whereas the author, J. Ruttgers, believed that neo-Malthusianism was eugenic, Schallmayer warned of the cultural, political and biological dangers of contraception.[344] Gruber was outraged by feminist and neo-Malthusian lectures at the Dresden Hygiene Exhibition of 1911, and pressurized Ploetz to take a stand against the sexual reformers.[345] Ploetz addressed the International Eugenics Congress of 1912 on this topic, outlining his view that contraception was only justified for eugenic purposes. He conceded that neo-Malthusianism was beneficial to the parents and that those children born might be healthier; but it was harmful to the middle and upper classes (among whom contraception was widely practiced). Birth control was damaging to the social position of 'the highly endowed Nordic (Teutonic or Germanic) race', and more generally to 'the white race', as it interfered with the operation of natural selection.[346]

The medical debate became more sociological with analysis of the social distribution of chronic diseases, of their economic costs, and of the psychology of the modern, rational lifestyles. The expert in social hygiene, Kaup, stressed the degenerative effects of urban life. He emphasized occupational hazards such as lead and zinc poisoning. He argued that as women entered the labour market they risked exposure to hazards which caused congenital weakness and malformations. Urban industrial life thus resulted in physical degeneration.[347] The other side to Kaup's diagnosis was that the countryside was positively healthier than the cities. The nation's future depended on maintaining a fit and fertile peasantry. He was concerned that nutritional standards were declining. The mechanization of dairies resulted in less nutritious centrifuged milk. The healthy rural diet was losing its quality. Malnutrition led to degeneration, increased incidence of diseases, inability to breast-feed, and a decline in the fitness of military recruits.[348] There reached a point when it was felt that the argument that physical degeneration was the cause of

---

[343] O. Bumke, *Über Nervöse Entartung* (Berlin, 1912).

[344] J. Ruttgers, *Rassenverbesserung, Malthusianismus und Neo-malthusianismus* (Dresden and Leipzig, 1908); Weiss, 'Schallmayer', pp. 269–76.

[345] Ploetz papers, Ploetz to Gruber, 19 November 1911.

[346] A. Ploetz, 'Neo-Malthusianism and Race Hygiene', in *First International Eugenics Congress*, pp. 183–9.   [347] I. Kaup, *Frauenarbeit und Rassenhygiene* (Hamburg, 1914).

[348] I. Kaup, *Ernährung und Lebenskraft der ländlichen Bevölkerung*, (Berlin, 1910) = Zentralstelle für Volkswohlfahrt, Heft 6.

declining fertility had to be investigated. Berlin gynaecologists pioneered research on the social conditions affecting reproduction.

Max Marcuse and Max Hirsch were two leading medical analysts of the social causes of abortion. Marcuse regarded the decline in births as due to lower marital fertility because the numbers of illegitimate births remained high. He agreed with Mombert that rising prosperity resulted in savings made by having fewer children. Women's work was a further factor. He suggested that psychological preconditions of the declining fertility were due to a combination of technical and economic factors. In an effort to discover the social reality behind the public rhetoric on the birth rate, Marcuse carried out a survey of one hundred patients in his insurance-based practice. Women coming to his surgery for dermatological or gynaecological problems were asked how often they had had an abortion. Marcuse addressed them in colloquial terms – how often had they 'spilt' (gekippt)? How else had they prevented pregnancy? The hundred patients had experienced seventy-six abortions. One conception in four ended in abortion. He found that the most common method of contraception was coitus interruptus, followed by post-coital douching.[349] By way of contrast Hirsch considered that abortion was the birth control of the poor, whereas contraceptives were the methods of the prosperous. It was impossible to estimate the extent of abortions, but he was convinced that these were on the increase and that spontaneous abortion was rare. Poverty, inadequate housing, and economic inflation caused women to have abortions. The situation was worsened by working women being physiologically especially at risk. Abortion was condemned as a major cause of sterility, and laws to prevent abortion were seen as a fiasco. It simply could not be outlawed. After all, one could not ban all sorts of douches, sprays and implements such as hair and knitting needles, spindles, wires or glass rods. Hirsch's solution was to advocate medically administered abortion on eugenic grounds.[350]

Doctors became critics of industrialization as damaging to morals, health and family life. They offered compelling medical reasons for extension of welfare benefits to include such items as family allowances. A shift occurred in the categories of debate as the concept of 'child riches' was introduced. Liberal economists had equated small families with economic prosperity. The debate stressed the need for a revised scale of social values associated with national duty and a sense of maintaining the vigour and numbers of the population. This was to combat the modernized, rational lifestyle of small families and consumer luxuries. In 1912 Grotjahn used the concept of the 'rationalization of sexual life' in his social pathology.[351] The demand for a reorienting of priorities away from liberal

349 M. Marcuse, Der Eheliche Präventivverkehr. Seine Verbreitung, Verursachung und Methodik. Dargestellt und beleuchtet an 300 Ehen (Stuttgart, 1917); R.P. Neuman, 'Working Class Birth Control in Wilhelmine Germany', Comparative Studies in Social History, vol. 20 (1975), 408–28.

350 M. Hirsch, 'Der Kampf gegen die kriminelle Abtreibung', Zentralblatt für Gynäkologie, vol. 36 (1912), 995–7; Hirsch, Fruchtabtreibung und Präventivverkehr im Zusammenhang mit dem Geburtenrückgang (Würzburg, 1914).

351 A. Grotjahn, Soziale Pathologie (Berlin, 1912); Grotjahn, Geburtenrückgang und Geburtenregelung im Lichte der individuellen und sozialen Hygiene (Berlin, 1914).

capitalism meant that medical and psychological categories gained in importance. They reinforced the nationalist campaign for better health, as a means to secure a fitter and more fertile population. The second major development was that doctors took a leading role in the debate. There were two camps. One sought to ally itself with the state in order to stamp out all quacks and to extend the responsibilities of the medical profession over a range of population questions. The other argued that all state action was futile: that sexuality and reproduction were primarily medical problems, best dealt with in the inviolable privacy of a medical consultation. The best way to solve these questions was to make the doctor responsible for abortion and contraceptive advice. Both camps of medical reformers argued for greater professional powers of intervention in family life.

The birth strike

Eugenicists took a leading role in the debate on medical aspects of the declining birth rate. Marginal groups of socially concerned gynaecologists, dermatologists and public health experts found that the birth rate gave their work a sense of national importance. They used the opportunity of state and public concern to promote ambitious plans to extend professional responsibilities and improve medical facilities. These plans for reform of 'reproductive hygiene' drew on eugenics. Although contraception represented a vice if practised merely for the sake of personal convenience, it had ethical and medical potential as a form of negative eugenics. Birth control could be regarded as a means of sexual selection, and of improving maternal health and the quality of offspring. Professional reformers did not have a monopoly of eugenics: regeneration of the race was a repeated neo-Malthusian aim in addition to preventing disease and poverty by reducing the population size.

During the nineteenth century the neo-Malthusian movement for birth control in Germany was small and sporadic. There were a few isolated propagandists and innovators in contraceptive techniques. The Neo-Malthusian League, established in London in 1877, found an echo in Kautsky's widely disseminated writings on birth control, surplus population and the socializing of the means of production in 1880, that so influenced the Ploetz circle.[352] W. Mensinga, a doctor in Schleswig Holstein, pioneered the occlusive pessary, and published on contraception as the responsibility of the medical profession. From case histories he argued that medically administered contraception would prevent a wide range of inherited diseases such as female hysteria and tuberculosis, as well as premature invalidity through excessive numbers of pregnancies. Medically prescribed contraception was a means of preventing degeneration.[353] From 1910 Ernst Gräfenberg, a

---

[352] K. Kautsky, *Der Einfluss der Volksvermehrung auf den Fortschritt der Gesellschaft* (Vienna, 1880). Kausky, *Erinnerungen*, pp. 389–94.

[353] W.P.J. Mensinga, *Facultative Sterilität* (Berlin and Neuwied, 1888); Mensinga, 'Zuchtwahl und Mutterschaft', *Politisch-Anthropologische Revue*, vol. 2 (1903/4), 630–9.

gynaecologist in the Schöneberg district of Berlin which had one of the lowest birth rates, began to experiment on a contraceptive method that led to the pioneering of his eponymous ring. It was one of a number of technical innovations that led to the availability of a greater variety of contraceptives.[354] There were substantial ideological distinctions between personal choice in contraception, medical counselling, and public advocacy of contraception as general principle. The methods and moral implications of birth control were rarely discussed in public. Medical commentators wrote only for professional colleagues. This was to change around 1910. Birth control became an explosive political issue. Eugenicists were the first to advocate birth control from the point of view of improving the quality of health of offspring and the mother. But rival groups simultaneously seized on the ideology of birth control as a means of promoting personal liberation and fulfilment.[355]

From 1900 there was an international renaissance of neo-Malthusian propaganda. The debate on the birth strike had its origins in French anarchist agitation for *la grève des ventres* in 1908. Concepts of 'forced birth' and of resistance by a strike were rapidly disseminated. There were popular festivities when balloons carrying neo-Malthusian slogans were released. Successful songs had refrains such as 'Don't make us have any more children', or 'mothers strike'. Dramas by Eugène Brieux such as *Blanchette* and *Maternité* justified abortion.[356] Contraception was regarded as a political weapon to deny the state and the ruling class workers for factories and soldiers as cannon fodder. These ideas were popularized in Germany where there was already a lively debate on the family and welfare among the socialists.[357]

The conflict of personal fulfilment and consciousness of racial duty resulted in diverse syntheses of eugenics, reproductive biology and feminism. Marie Stopes was the first woman to gain a doctorate in science – in her case, palaeobotany – from the University of Munich in 1904, where she met a number of biologists who were concerned with the social aspects of reproduction and heredity. She underwent a turbulent transition from biologist to campaigner for birth control as a means of fulfilling motherhood. Stopes merits comparison with Helene Stöcker of the League for the Protection of Mothers and for Sexual Reform. Stöcker was more radical in her emphasis on personal fulfilment and support for the unmarried mother. She declared that neo-Malthusianism was one of the most effective means of solving the woman question and the social question.[358] Racial improvement and health were the themes of the third general conference of the League for the Protection of Mothers in 1911. Eduard David, the SPD representative, argued that

---

[354] K. Engel, 'Der Gräfenberg Ring. Zu seiner Vorgeschichte, Entwicklung und frühen Rezeption', med. Diss. Erlangen-Nürnberg, 1979; M.C. Stopes, 'Zur Geschichte der vaginalen Kontrazeption', *Zentralblatt für Gynäkologie*, vol. 55 (1931), 2,549–51.

[355] F. Ronsin, 'Liberté – natalité. Réaction et répression anti-malthusiennes avant 1920', in L. Murard and P. Zylberman (eds.), *L'Haleine des Faubourgs* (Fontenay-sur-bois, 1977), pp. 365–93; Ronsin, *La grève des ventres* (Paris, 1978). [356] Fernand Kolney, *La grève des ventres* (Paris, 1908).

[357] J. Donzelot, *The Policing of Families* (London, 1980), p. 177.

[358] R.J. Evans, *The Feminist Movement in Germany 1894–1933* (London and Beverly Hills, 1976), p. 132.

birth control was not harmful but beneficial to the race. It would prevent the physically and mentally degenerate from being conceived. Society should have the right to prevent those with hereditary diseases from having children. The positive aspect of racial hygiene was the selection of an appropriate mate. Such a choice was possible only if appropriate economic support was there. The social and racial questions were thus indistinguishable.[359]

There occurred a constant struggle between neo-Malthusians and moral purists. In France the statistician Bertillon headed an *Alliance nationale pour l'accroissement de la population française*. It sought to outlaw neo-Malthusian propaganda, and mounted its own propaganda to prevent the disappearance of the French race. For example, at the election of 1914, over one million pro-natalist leaflets were distributed. Michelin, the tyre manufacturer, supported the campaign with such slogans as 'large families can travel economically on Michelin tyres'.[360] In Germany the moral purity movement grew in fervour. From 1898 the Centre Party supported a massive campaign against prostitution, and immoral art and literature. This found favour among a range of clerical, conservative and medical interests. Lingner, the manufacturer of the mouthwash *Odol*, employed a number of medical experts examining the physical causes of degeneration, such as the dental expert Röse, or Roesle, who analysed the statistics of the declining birth rate. By contrast with the moral purity crusade, radical feminists demanded the removal of state controls from all private moral spheres, and argued that prostitutes were the victims of a male-dominated society. The disagreement between the moral crusaders and the radical feminists was extended to include the issue of contraception.

The radical sexual reformers were influential advocates of eugenically based moral codes. On 30 September 1911 a German Neo-Malthusian Committee and an International Society for Protection of Mothers and Sexual Reform were founded. Their manifesto stressed the need for racial improvement and sexual selection to ensure human progress. Members of the International Society represented an alliance of literary authors such as Carl Hauptmann and Wedekind, artists such as Kollwitz, politicians such as Bernstein, Potthoff and Eduard David, feminists like Stöcker, biologists such as Haeckel, and sexologists such as Bloch, Forel and Freud. The eugenicist Schallmayer gave support.[361] The society participated in conferences of the Monist League, the Society for the Prevention of VD, the International Order of Ethics and Culture, and the Sociological Society. They proclaimed the need for an 'organic-spiritual' culture that could bring about a nobler, happier lifestyle. This was to be achieved by racial health and selective breeding. It represented a more liberal form of eugenics than the International Society for Racial Hygiene.

[359] B. Nowacki, *Der Bund für Mutterschutz (1905–1933)* (Husum, 1983), pp. 73–4.
[360] W. Schneider, 'Towards the Improvement of the Human Race: The History of Eugenics in France', *Journal of Modern History*, vol. 54 (1982), 268–91.
[361] *Internationale Vereinigung für Mutterschutz und Sexualreform. Aufruf an Männer und Frauen aller Kulturländer*, (nd, np).

During 1912 a major controversy flared up among the feminists and sexual reformers. The moderate feminists of the *Bund deutscher Frauen* (BDF) proposed as alternatives to contraception a range of measures such as marriage certificates to screen for VD and mental disease. In contrast to the radical feminists of the League for the Protection of Mothers, the BDF resolutely condemned abortion. It appealed to the patriotism and racial conscience of women to bear more children.[362] Sexual politics cut across party lines. The BDF received support among more enlightened establishment circles. The SPD became deeply divided on the issue of birth control.[363] Two doctors, Alfred Bernstein and Julius Moses, took the lead in a campaign for the birth strike.[364] From 1912 they began to speak on women's right for self-determination over their own bodies. On 25 November 1912 the Berlin police president limited attendance at their lectures and those of Hirschfeld exclusively to adult males. Bernstein and Moses were not deterred. In March 1913 they proclaimed the birth strike as a 'weapon of the proletariat'. They were supported by the leading socialists, Kautsky and Luise Zietz. But in July and August 1913 Clara Zetkin criticized birth control as individualist and not part of a class strategy. If there would be fewer soldiers, contraception would also result in fewer revolutionaries. Her view was endorsed by Rosa Luxemburg, and this became the official party line. The socialist newspaper, *Vorwärts*, declared that the declining birth rate was a sign of the degeneration of capitalism. A meeting was held by the SPD on 22 August 1913 to condemn the birth strike as 'bourgeois reactionary quackery'. Over 4,000 attended. Moses replied that the birth strike was already a reality, and had disturbed Junkers and pastors. In a working-class family, too, a large number of children bring nothing but poverty and misery. Birth control meant improved health. At another rally Bernstein echoed the eugenicists by stating that the quality rather than the quantity of the population was important. Zetkin insisted on quantity. But other women SPD leaders did not follow Zetkin's line, and newspapers commented on the unpopularity of her view.[365] Moses organized further public meetings. On 15 October 1913 at a rally on 'The Declining Birth Rate – a Cultural Change', he announced the need to maintain quality of the population, and that the declining birth rate was the result of capitalism. Industrial work was making women infertile. Newspapers articles and even poems in satirical journals such as *Simplicissimus* began to appear. Moses proclaimed that the birth strike showed the impotence of the state in the area of fertility and the family. The state might be seeking to isolate its causes, to implement legislation banning contraceptives and quacks, or to recruit the clergy to preach against the decline – but all this was in vain. On 8 January 1914 Moses

---

[362] Evans, *Feminist Movement*, p. 158.
[363] U. Linse, 'Arbeiterschaft und Geburtenkontrolle im Deutschen Kaiserreich von 1891 bis 1914', *Archiv für Sozialgeschichte*, vol. 12 (1972), 205–71.
[364] K. Nemitz, 'Julius Moses und die Gebärstreik-Debatte 1913', *Jahrbuch des Instituts für Deutsche Geschichte*, vol. 2 (1978), 321–35.
[365] A. Bergmann, 'Frauen, Männer, Sexualität und Geburtenkontrolle. Zur Gebärstreik-Debatte der SPD 1913', in K. Hausen (ed.), *Frauen suchen ihre Geschichte* (Munich, 1983), pp. 81–108.

was censured by the Berlin *Ärztekammer* as having brought the profession into disrepute.[366]

Moses combined medical expertise with politics. There were other lay propagandists for birth control. Alma Wartenburg (from Hamburg) toured Germany giving popular lectures on women's diseases, contraception and pregnancy. She insisted on a woman's right of self determination over her body in defiance of the state. She was imprisoned for lecturing on contraception. Yet in whatever way the declining birth rate was politically conceptualized, it was a fact of life among many workers irrespective of party politics. Of one hundred interviews conducted by Max Marcuse only three couples justified birth control on political grounds. One said, 'We workers are no longer so stupid so as to provide children for the rich and for the state'.[367] But the concern with pro-natalism was paramount in the minds of state public health administrators who firmly linked the declining birth rate to socialism.

The cult of motherhood

The state's attitude to the declining birth rate was essentially pro-natalist. The eugenicists' commitment to the quality of the population meant that they were divided over the extent to which the quality of future generations would be jeopardized by quantitative population increase. Some of the more radical reformers argued that the health of mothers should be given greater priority; they demanded smaller families, and that single mothers and their children be given positive support. The *Bund für Mutterschutz*, the League for the Protection of Mothers, was an explosive alliance of feminists and social hygienists. The League campaigned for removing the moral stigma from being an unmarried mother, and argued that emancipation of women was a prerequisite for improving the health of mothers and their children. Its brazen demands for a new morality provoked a division of opinion among eugenicists and sexual reformers.

The founder of the League was Elisabeth Bouness, a teacher who composed poetry under the pseudonym of Ruth Bré. Her pamphlets pleaded for improved legal status for mothers, and for the protection of women by health certificates prior to marriage. On 12 November 1904 she founded the League with the utopian socialist doctor, Friedrich Landmann, who was at that time in Eisenach, and Heinrich Meyer, a Munich novelist who wrote on prehistoric themes. These associates show the influence of *völkisch* and medical ideas on Bré. Landmann was a friend of Woltmann, the editor of the *Political Anthropological Review* which was also published in Eisenach.[368] Bré also had contact with Willibald Hentschel, the

---

[366] K. Nemitz, 'Gebärstreik-Debatte', p. 323; Bergmann, 'Frauen', pp. 97–103.

[367] M. Marcuse, *Der Eheliche Präventivverkehr. Seine Verbreitung, Verursachung und Methodik. Dargestellt und beleuchtet an 300 Ehen* (Stuttgart, 1917); R.P. Neuman, 'Working Class Birth Control in Wilhelmine Germany', *Comparative Studies in Social History*, vol. 20 (1975), 408–28.

[368] For Landmann see: F. Tennstedt, 'Sozialismus, Lebensreform und Krankenkassenbewegung. Friedrich Landmann und Raphael Friedeberg als Ratgeber der Krankenkassen', *Soziale Sicherheit*, vol. 26 (1977), 210–4, 306–10, 332–6.

Aryan nationalist and anti-semite, the author of the Mittgart plan for selective breeding colonies.[369] Hentschel proposed to settle mothers on his estates.[370] These contacts and plans for utopian mother colonies arose from a distinctive blend of *völkisch* racism and feminism.

The aims of the League were: 'to protect motherhood in all its forms, as the mother was the source of the *Volkskraft*'; the 'improvement of the race and of national welfare by breeding of the healthy'; to establish rural settlements as an antidote to urban degeneration; and to secure paternal responsibility for offspring. The statutes declared in favour of racial hygiene so that the sick should not be a burden on the healthy and consume national strength and wealth. It was a mistake to take the sick and 'weak elements' into municipal maternity homes. Instead mothers should re-populate the countryside. Bré hoped for a mother's home in the rural East, so as to 'infuse German blood into the Ostmark'.[371] Bré's ideas were explicitly *völkisch*.

Bré contacted a progressive group of Berlin feminists and doctors. They transplanted the League for Protection of Mothers to Berlin on 5 January 1905. In March of 1905 the steering committee of the League was remarkably diverse. There were extreme *völkisch* eugenicists like von Ehrenfels, who advocated polygamy, Hegar, the gynaecologist and theorist of racial degeneration, the Aryan enthusiasts Wilser and Woltmann, and radical medical reformers such as Blaschko. Owing to the intervention of a liberal, Walter Borgius, the League became a broad coalition of reformers. Borgius was secretary of the Trade Treaty Union[372] an association of left-wing liberals, merchants and representatives of light industry. They opposed the tariffs advocated by heavy industry and agrarian interests. Borgius was interested in founding an association for sexual reform. He offered to set up a branch of the League for the Protection of Mothers in Berlin. This was joined by a varied collection of reformers who changed the tone of the League from being *völkisch* and utopian, to being urban, professional, scientific – leading the campaign for the liberating of restrictive moral codes. The league embraced neo-Malthusian advocates of contraception such as Mensinga and Max Marcuse; a racial hygiene lobby opposed to contraception led by Agnes Bluhm and Ploetz; distinguished neurologists and dermatologists such as Blaschko and Iwan Bloch (the secretary of the League during 1907), Erb of Heidelberg, Flechsig, Forel. Julian Marcuse, Willy Hellpach, Moll, and Neisser, and three more women doctors: Agnes Hacker, Moestra and Lydia Rabinowitsch-Kempner. Politically, the League was a coalition of reformers, including the Christian social liberal Naumann, Potthoff (a member of the Trade Treaty Union with an interest in eugenics), Hugo Boettger (a Social Democrat), and sociologists such as Oppen-

---

[369] This aspect of Hentschel is omitted from D. Löwenberg, 'Willibald Hentschel (1858–1947), Seine Pläne zur Menschenzüchtung, seine Biologismus und Antisemitismus', med. Diss. University of Mainz, 1978.

[370] R. Bré, *Das erste Jahr des 'Ersten deutschen Bundes für Mutterschutz'*, in ZSTA M Rep 77 Tit 662 Nr 123.

[371] ZSTA Merseburg Rep 77 Tit 662 Nr 123 betr den Bund für Mutterschutz; B. Nowacki, *Der Bund für Mutterschutz. (1905–1933)* (Husum, 1983), pp. 20–4.   [372] *Handelsvertragsverein.*

heimer (the theorist of rural settlements), Sombart and Max Weber. In 1905 there were overtures to socialists such as Eugen Simonowski and Bebel. Affiliation to the Monist League was contemplated. Maternal health was the focus of a wide range of interests.

The League continued to advocate racial improvement and a sense of responsibility to future generations. Yet the tone changed from Bré's lyrical Aryan utopian ideology to a plea for ethical values based on biological and social science. The League campaigned for maternity insurance, economic self-sufficiency for mothers, and improved legal status for single mothers. There emerged a major challenge from Stöcker, an author, teacher and monist. Stöcker venerated Nietzsche as a symbol of the freeing of creative, individual powers. She had a brief love affair with Tille, the advocate of a fusion of Darwinism with Nietzschean philosophy. Stöcker urged the fulfilment of women by having children and professional careers. The affair with Tille prompted Stöcker to reconsider her attitudes to marriage, which she began to see as a constraint on women living their lives to the full. Marriage caused the growth of prostitution and the stigmatization of the illegitimate. She rejected the view that woman was naturally chaste, believing that sexual love was the basis of partnership. From 1901 she took a leading role in the abolitionist movement in Berlin for repeal of laws regulating prostitution. Her radical views on sexuality caused dissension among the Berlin abolitionists. The founding of the League thus presented Stöcker with an ideal organization of which to assume control.[373]

The League was taken over by an alliance of abolitionist feminists (led by Stöcker) with Max Marcuse, the sexologist, and Borgius. Bré was persuaded to resign, in favour of Stöcker as president and Marcuse as secretary. The League concentrated on propaganda for a reform of sexual ethics, and practical aims. Bré was outraged that the League was supporting the inferior elements of society. She accused Stöcker of having stolen her brain-child, and seceded to form a rival but unsuccessful 'First League for German Mothers'.[374]

The League caused considerable alarm among the official establishment. Bré publicized the League by asking for Prussian state support. This was declined on 24 February 1905.[375] She also petitioned the commissioner for settlements in Posen.[376] It was in March 1905 when Behr-Pinnow wrote to the Berlin Police President, von Borries, about the Emperor and Empress's moral indignation against the League, and the chain of events leading to the founding of the Kaiserin Auguste Viktoria Haus was set in motion. The Police President replied that hundreds from educated higher social classes supported the League. Suppression of the League would be difficult, and possible only if the law on public morality was contravened.[377] Stöcker's presidency steered the League into a radical course of

---

[373] H. Stöcker, *Die Liebe und die Frauen* (Minden, 1906); R.J. Evans, *The Feminist Movement in Germany 1894–1933* (London and Beverly Hills, 1976) pp. 116–20.   [374] Nowacki, *Bund*, p. 24.
[375] ZSTA M Rep 76 VIII B Nr 2762, Bl 288–304, 285–6, letter from Bré, dated Hermsdorf, 11 February 1905.   [376] ZSTA M Rep 76 VIII B Nr 2763 Bl 62–3.
[377] ZSTA Merseburg, Rep 77 Tit 662 Nr 123 betr. den Bund für Mutterschutz.

sexual reform. She proclaimed a morality based on 'modern, individualist, scientific moral teaching'. Sexual activity was a 'natural and self-evident right'. Marriage should be a free contract between equals. The League compaigned for an extension of municipal welfare to unmarried mothers, for sex education in schools, and more generally for reformed sexual values in order to prevent prostitution, venereal disease and sexual crimes. Stöcker espoused the neo-Malthusian belief in contraception, and protested against the abortion laws as based on the state regarding the unborn child as its property.

Stöcker's radicalism was opposed by advocates of racial hygiene. Ploetz and Stöcker were initially on cordial terms until 1908.[378] Borgius and Sombart were keen that Ploetz join the committee of the League in 1905.[379] Ploetz was instrumental in deposing Ruth Bré. At a committee meeting of the League on 15 May 1905 Ploetz complained that Bré had added his name without his permission to a leaflet. Hegar made a similar complaint. There followed a discussion of the 'racial hygienic duties' of the League, especially with regard to Bré's opinion that the League should only support healthy mothers and their infants, while the degenerate should be left unassisted.[380] Ploetz's racial interpretation of the League's function was evident in early manifestos. The League was portrayed as a solution to the problem of degeneracy, since from the illegitimate were recruited the armies of criminals, prostitutes and vagrants. The state could reduce infant mortality and compensate for the declining birth rate by measures to support the health of the 'illegitimate'. Certain early supporters such as Bruno Meyer (an art critic) disapproved of the use of health as a criteria of racial selection.[381] Stöcker solicited a contribution from Ploetz on racial hygiene and motherhood for her journal, *Mutterschutz*.[382] Ploetz and Stöcker had antagonistic views on contraception, and Ploetz was vociferous in denouncing medical advocates of contraception such as Marcuse.[383] The most extreme critic of individualism was Agnes Bluhm, who maintained close contact with Ploetz. Bluhm opposed Stöcker's sexual individualism on eugenic grounds. At a meeting of the Berlin abolitionists in 1905, she proposed that no one be allowed to marry unless they had a certificate of good health. The abortion issue caused a split between the *Bund deutscher Frauen* (BDF) and the radical *Mutterschutz* group. A consequence was that physicians such as Blaschko, Bloch, Forel and Kromayer resigned from the League for the Protection of Mothers.[384] Bäumer assumed a leading role in the BDF. She rejected Stöcker's notion of sexual equality, arguing that woman was fulfilled not in sensuality but in the soul – in 'a deep alive Germanic racial instinct'.[385] Abortion was opposed as causing a dangerous drop in the birth rate. There was an increasing penetration of

---

378 Ploetz papers, diary, 20 March 1908, on visit of Stöcker.
379 Ploetz papers, Borgius to Ploetz, 6 January 1905; A. Ploetz, 'Bund für Mutterschutz', *ARGB*, vol. 2 (1905), 164.   380 Ploetz papers, Bund für Mutterschutz, Protokoll, 15 May 1905.
381 Ploetz papers, Bruno Meyer to Ploetz, 26 May 1905.
382 Ploetz papers, Stöcker to Ploetz, 10 August 1905 and 30 April 1906; also 13 March 1908 and 18 September 1910.   383 Ploetz papers, diary, 13 January 1907.
384 Evans, *Feminist Movement*, pp. 135–6.   385 Evans, *Feminist Movement*, p. 156.

Social Darwinism into German feminism, and an insistence on the need to defend the institutions of marriage and the family.[386]

Until February 1906 the doctor Max Marcuse directed the League, but from 1 April 1906 the radical feminists Marie Lischnewska and Stöcker were in control.[387] They opened an advice centre for mothers and provided welfare for mothers and mothers-to-be who were often adrift in Berlin having come from the provinces. The more radical position of the League still included racial priorities. Lischnewska continued to emphasize Germanic rural settlements as a state-social measure.[388] Her interest in racial hygiene was shown by her request to Ploetz to prepare a paper on the need for good quality, healthy mothers.[389] The League took up the campaign for maternity insurance, and a system of crèches and welfare facilities for women workers, which had first been proposed by the socialist Lily Braun in 1897.[390] From 1907 this was a major object of debate. Although in 1903 certain benefits were conceded these were only for insured women workers, and payment for the attendance by doctors and midwives was left to the discretion of individual sickness insurance funds. The economist and leading expert on sickness insurance statistics, Mayet, presented detailed costings for maternity benefits and breast feeding premiums. He regarded maternity insurance as a rational weapon in the struggle for survival, necessary to maintain progress and the higher developmental instincts. From 1907 the League favoured maternity insurance on the grounds that this would remedy the problem of racial degeneration at its root by improving the economic status of mothers and their offspring and petitioned the Reichstag.[391] The League's exposure of the inadequacy of the sickness insurance system was a substantial and valid criticism of the liberal individualist premises of insurance that only the insured worker and not the family dependants received benefits. The demand for maternity insurance and postnatal care became widespread. It was taken up by welfare oriented eugenicists; Grotjahn developed the concept of 'parental insurance' in order to guarantee the three children necessary to stem the declining birth rate. It was to be financed by a bachelor tax.[392]

The League focused on the lack of a healthy reproductive environment. Midwifery reform was a priority of 'practical Mutterschutz'. The paediatrician Heinrich Finkelstein said that this was a matter of national urgency, but one that posed a good many difficulties.[393] There were demands for outpatient clinics, convalescent homes and maternity hospitals. Bré and Stöcker agitated against what

---

[386] Evans, *Feminist Movement*, pp. 158–70.
[387] Marcuse left the league on 30 November 1907.   [388] Nowacki, *Bund*, p. 53.
[389] BAK Nachlass Schreiber Nr 25 Bl. 519, 15 May 1905.
[390] L. Braun, review of L. Frank, Keiffer and L. Maingie, *L'Assurance Maternelle* (Paris, 1897), in *Archiv für soziale Gesetzgebung und Statistik*, vol. 11 (1897), 543–8; Braun, *Mutterschaftsversicherung und Krankenkassen* (Berlin, 1906).
[391] Nowacki, *Bund*, pp. 43–4; BHSTA Mk 11166 Kinderheilkunde; Mayet lecture to the Verein für Mutterschutz München, 13 January 1908.
[392] Alfons Fischer, *Die Mutterschaftsversicherung in den europäischen Ländern* (Leipzig, 1911).
[393] BAK Nachlass Schreiber Nr 25 Bl. 504.

they considered to be harsh treatment of single mothers by Berlin gynaecological clinics in 1908. They were prosecuted by doctors whom they had criticized. In November 1909 the League attempted to establish its own gynaecological clinic. The dermatologist Kromayer secured the services of Wilhelm Liepmann, who provided free beds for single mothers. The plan encountered personal and financial difficulties.[394] The agitation against lack of hygienic antenatal and postnatal care continued. The League looked to radically minded doctors to provide such care, and thus remained dependent on professional expertise.[395]

The science of woman

Among gynaecologists the reforming spirit resulted in a movement for 'social gynaecology'. The lead was taken by the Berlin practitioners, Max Hirsch, Liepmann and Paul Strassmann. They diverted the movement of sexual reform into one for professional reform. In 1912 the Medical Society for Sexology and Eugenics[396] was established in Berlin. This was a forum for physicians interested in sexual questions, such as the venereologist Bloch, the campaigner for homosexual rights, Hirschfeld, and eugenicists such as Grotjahn.[397] The society was for medical reformers for whom the League for the Protection of Motherhood was too radical. Its transactions were published in a journal established by Hirsch, the *Archiv für Frauenkunde*. Hirsch coined the term *Eugenetik* as sounding more scientific than either *Eugenik* or *Rassenhygiene*. He recruited a scientifically distinguished group to support the journal. It included sexual reformers such as Havelock Ellis, eugenicists such as Grotjahn, Hegar and Schallmayer, and social scientists such as Goldscheid and Tönnies. Max Weber declined Hirsch's invitation as did a number of leading feminists who suggested that a journal for 'male studies' might be of greater interest than dissecting woman from scientific, social and cultural points of view.[398]

Hirsch proclaimed *Frauenkunde* as an inter-disciplinary study combining the expertise of biologists, medical scientists and social scientists. But physicians and especially gynaecologists were meant to have the major responsibility in this enterprise, for they supervised all aspects of life from the cradle to old age. Only physicians could judge the effect of paid labour on reproductive capacity. It was to provide answers to the 'Woman Question', which had been raised by feminism. Hirsch's programme greatly extended the scope of gynaecology. Instead of merely attending to women's diseases, the gynaecologist should evaluate all aspects of a woman's life, the repercussions for the declining birth rate and 'last but not least auf die Lebenskraft der kommenden Generation'. He viewed woman in terms of the 'human economy' as the reproducer of the 'most valuable of all goods'; the future

---

[394] Nowacki, *Bund*, pp. 59, 61; V.C. Grabke, 'Wilhelm Liepman als Sozialer Gynäkologe', med. Diss., Freie Universität Berlin, 1980.   [395] BAK Nachlass Schreiber Nr 25 fol 1, Bl 217–224.
[396] *Aerztliche Gesellschaft für Sexualwissenschaft und Eugenik*.   [397] Grotjahn, *Erlebtes*, p. 134.
[398] Hirsch papers, Staatsbibliothek Preussischer Kulturbesitz Berlin; M. Lennig, 'Max Hirsch: Sozialgynäkologie und Frauenkunde', med. Diss., Freie Universität Berlin, 1977.

of the human race depended on women's health. Eugenics was thus central to Hirsch's programme.[399] Grotjahn underlined this view by stating that the 'hygiene of reproduction'[400] should end the laisser faire in sexual affairs that resulted in degeneration.[401] Schallmayer regarded *Frauenkunde* as a means of awakening the racial conscience of women of superior moral and physical quality to their *Rassedienstpflicht* of having healthy families.[402] Their views typified the collectivist attitude towards childbirth.

This broadened vision of the 'social gynaecologists' displaced the feminist demand for social rights and improved status, by a view of women's health centred on social biology and eugenics. This was the outcome of a professionalism that gave priority to scientific research rather than to political campaigns. The scientifically based movement for sexual reform established itself as an independent entity. Eugenicists disassociated maternal health from the radical political strategies of the campaigners for sexual rights. It meant that there was a readiness among eugenicists to advise and guide the state on health and population questions.

Rural health: the last bastion

Theories of degeneration prompted investigation of declining birth rates. Officials in a number of European countries monitored birth rates as barometers of national health. The first country officially to consider the birth rate as a national problem was France which established a Commission on Depopulation in 1902. The German embassy reported on this and subsequent political debates in terms of how demographic weakness sapped the French desire for a war to avenge the defeat of 1870.[403] In Britain the Inter-Departmental Committee on Physical Deterioration of 1904 was followed by a Fertility of Marriage Census in 1911. There was an unofficial National Birth Rate Commission in 1913 and 1914 instigated by the National Commission for Public Morals.[404] In Germany there was a slower response to the decline in the birth rate. The first state to take the initiative of considering its effects was Prussia. The differential between the rural and urban birth rate meant that whereas the urban birth rate had been falling since the 1890s, the rural birth rate continued to rise. Only when the rural birth rate began to fall in the early twentieth century did the state become alarmed.[405] Reorganization of

[399] M. Hirsch, 'Ueber Ziele und Wege frauenkundlicher Forschung', *Archiv für Frauenkunde*, vol. 1 (1914), 1–13.   [400] 'Hygiene der Fortpflanzung'.

[401] A. Grotjahn, 'Die Eugenik als Hygiene der Fortpflanzung', *Archiv für Frauenkunde*, vol. 1 (1914), 15–18.

[402] W. Schallmayer, 'Eugenik, ihre Grundlagen und Beziehungen zur kulturellen Hebung der Frau', *Archiv für Frauenkunde*, vol. 1 (1914), 271–91.

[403] M.S. Teitelbaum and J.M. Winter, *The Fear of Population Decline* (New York, 1985); S.J. Holmes, *A Bibliography of Eugenics* (Berkeley, 1924).

[404] J. Lewis, *The Politics of Motherhood* (London, 1980), pp. 201, 203.

[405] ZSTA M Rep 76 VIII B Nr 4364 die Geburts- und Sterblichkeitsverhältnisse in den grösseren Städten Deutschlands 1906–1911.

the Prussian Medical Department in 1911 finally permitted substantial analysis of the problem.

Concern over the birth rate arose from the preoccupation with rural health. During the 1890s a number of authors, such as the racial anthropologist Ammon, discussed the health of rural military recruits. In 1895 – the same year as the Anti-TB League was founded – a Committee for Rural Welfare was established.[406] It observed that despite the annual surplus of births the rural population was declining. The association received backing from such notables as the Baden and Saxon Ministers of the Interior, the Prussian Minister of Agriculture, and the Minister of State, von Gossler. They instructed provincial officials to support local initiatives. The secretary was Heinrich Sohnrey, who was a follower of the left liberal politician, Naumann. Their ideal was a fit and fertile rural population. Sohnrey described various plans for rural health care. Drawing on the voluntary initiatives of the Patriotic Women's League, state officials were to oversee the provision of cottage hospitals and rural welfare workers. Other concerns were rural depopulation, settlement, and alcoholism. This organization conceived of the idea of *Kreisfürsorgestellen* – rural welfare centres which co-ordinated a variety of functions such as TB prevention and infant care. Rural welfare workers were to oversee the health aspects of housing, clothing and nutrition.[407]

The priority of rural health prompted the state to focus on improving midwifery, especially the securing of an even distribution of midwives in rural areas. The concern with rural health conditions meant that from the mid-1890s there was an informal population policy shown by the state's support of voluntary rural welfare organizations. In March 1905 and June 1907 officials considering the problem of rural health observed that rural mortality was significantly lower than urban mortality.[408] In 1907 the declining birth rate was placed on the agenda of the Prussian Medical Advisory Committee but time did not permit its discussion. As the debates among eugenicists, doctors and lay reformers intensified, the birth rate continued to attract officials' and politicians' attention. In 1909 Chancellor Bülow commented on a decline in the nation's physical vitality.[409] But there was no action on this issue until 1911.

Re-structuring the medical administration

From 1899 there were fundamental changes in the structure of the Prussian Medical Department. Contacts increased with the medical profession, members of whom

---

[406] This became the German Association for Rural Welfare, *Deutscher Verein für ländliche Wohlfahrts- und Heimatpflege*.

[407] Heinrich Sohnrey, *Wegweiser für ländliche Wohlfahrts- und Heimatpflege* (Berlin: Deutscher Dorfschriftenverlag, 1900); Hauser and A. Duttmann-Oldenburg, *Die Kranken- und Hauspflege auf dem Lande* (Leipzig, 1899). J. Grassl, *Blut und Brot. Der Zusammenhang zwischen Biologie und Volkswirtschaft bei der Bayerischen Bevölkerung im 19. Jahrhundert*, (München, 1905).

[408] ZSTA M Rep 76 VIII B Nr 1916 Bl 62; Die Hygiene auf dem platten Lande 1904–8.

were offered opportunities to advise on policy. Medically trained officials were promoted, and opportunities for service as state medical officers were enlarged with the reform of public health in 1899. The Medical Advisory Committee[410] was extended to include delegates of the doctors' representative chambers. Provincial doctors were consulted. The first such consultation was about the abuse of hypnosis in 1901, when doctors expressed concern about the prevalence of 'quacks'.[411] Medically qualified rather than legally qualified officials were appointed in the central administration. Medically trained officials were more susceptible to the influence of their professional colleagues. Legally educated officials were neutral on issues such as the practice of nature therapists, whereas medical officials stigmatized 'quackery' as a major cause of the declining birth rate.[412] The state steered an erratic course over the suppression of contraceptives, unlicensed practitioners and abortions. The medical profession used the issue of population policy to press for control of unlicensed practitioners, who were stigmatized as abortionists, and for ineffective 'quack' treatment of VD. Legally educated officials defended the right of all to practise medicine. In 1910 a draft law 'Against Abuses in Medical Practice' planned controls on unqualified practitioners, but it was quickly withdrawn. This attempt to suppress unlicensed practice was motivated by a combination of professional and demographic concerns.[413]

Whereas the Reich Health Office was directed by a legally trained official, Franz Bumm, medical officials gained increasing influence in Prussia. Dietrich exemplified the growing power of medically trained officials. He was responsible for infant welfare and took a leading role in voluntary organizations for infant and child care. The Department was joined in 1911 by the innovative and strong-minded Krohne, whose life's work became the implementation of population policy. His initial responsibility was midwifery but he rapidly developed plans for a comprehensive population policy. Professionalization was fortified in 1911 with the appointment of a medically qualified administrator as Ministerial Director. Kirchner who was a military doctor and bacteriologist had since 1900 been prominent in welfare organizations such as the Societies to Combat TB and VD.[414]

The year 1911 was a turning point for the Prussian Medical Department in that it was transferred from the Ministry of Religious Affairs and Education[415] to the Ministry of the Interior. Until the death of the education official Althoff in 1907 the Medical Department had a powerful ally in this mastermind of university expansion. Indeed, Althoff had pioneered dispensary clinics for TB, and in his role

409 ZSTA M Rep 120 Abt XV, Nr 63, Bd 1 B1–5.
410 *Wissenschaftliche Deputation für das Medizinalwesen.*
411 GSTA Dahlem Rep 84a Nr 10992 Hypnose und Suggestion 1897–1931.
412 GSTA Dahlem Rep 84a Nr 2326–2328 Reform der Medizinalbehörden 1896–1910.
413 GSTA Dahlem Rep 84a Nr 1241 Kurpfuscherei 1910–1933.
414 *25 Jahre preussische Medizinalverwaltung seit Erlass des Kreisarztgesetzes, 1901–1926,* (Berlin, 1927); P.J. Weindling, 'Die preussische Medizinalverwaltung und die "Rassenhygiene" 1905 bis 1933', in A. Thom and H. Spaar (eds.), *Medizin im Faschismus* (Berlin, 1983), pp. 23–35.
415 'Kultusministerium'.

as chairman of the Medical Advisory Committee from 1900 had encouraged intervention in welfare issues such as TB, VD and infant and school health.[416] The move of the Medical Department in 1911 to the Ministry of Interior was prompted by the feeling that the Department was more appropriately located alongside policing authorities. It marked a shift from a moral and educative view of health, as well as a return to the old idea of medical police; but controls were exerted in a modernized form in that the medical profession was to take a decisive role in formulating and implementing policies. The reorganization explains why the state did not tackle the issue of degeneration and the declining birth rate until 1911. But when it did so, the Medical Department had powerful allies in the Minister of the Interior and in the belligerent medical profession. Medical officials became intermediaries between the state and profession.

Public controversies over the birth rate had erupted. The varying interpretations were linked to political divisions, with socialists using the decline to denounce poverty and lack of housing, and conservatives attributed it to socialist materialism, immorality, and feminism. Between these extremes, medical commentators argued over the causes, some attributing the decline to contraception, and others to racial degeneration. There was incontrovertible evidence that the birth rate had fallen from 40.9 births per thousand inhabitants in 1890 to 28.2 in 1911. The Prussian medical administration felt compelled to establish the causes. It was concerned as to whether there were medical indications that the decline in mortality rates in Germany resulted from a physiological incapacity to reproduce.

Racial hygienists took a lead in exerting pressure on the state. In 1910 the Munich professor of hygiene, Gruber, argued that the *Zentralstelle für Volkswohlfahrt* ought to collect statistics on physique and on the quality of health of families. The office should become a national institute for racial hygiene and co-ordinate the issuing of health passports by school doctors. Genealogical data should also be collected so that the question of national degeneration could be thoroughly investigated.[417] A positive inspiration was that in 1910 the *Zentralstelle* held a meeting on rural health, when Kaup emphasized that peasants were a potential source of urban regeneration. He took up the demand for a network of state rural welfare centres.[418] From 1910 the Catholic Centre Party strengthened its agitation against contraception. When a law was proposed to suppress quackery, the Centre and conservatives demanded a clause that contraceptives be outlawed. The declining birth rate was consequently debated in the Reichstag. Conservatives attributed the decline to the corruptions of luxury, and socialists to poverty.[419]

Neo-Malthusianism was a spur to state intervention. Over 24–27 September 1911 the Fourth International Malthusian Congress was held at Dresden. On 25 October, the declining birth rate was discussed at the Prussian Medical Advisory

---

[416] ZSTA M Rep 92A Althoff AI 263 Wissenschaftliche Deputation.
[417] M. v. Gruber, 'Organisation der Forschung und Sammlung von Materialien über die Entartungsfrage', *Concordia*, vol. 17 (1910) 225–228.
[418] ZSTA M Rep 76 VIII B Nr 1917 Bl. 186.   [419] Stürzbecher, *Bekämpfung*, pp 148–58.

Committee. Moritz Pistor, a retired medical official, and Dietrich, the official responsible for infant welfare, reviewed the issue. The Committee consisted of eleven leading medical professors. Representatives of provincial doctors were admitted to their discussions. It was a means by which the German medical profession could influence state policy. That two of the professors, Flügge (a bacteriologist) and Orth (a pathologist), were members of the Racial Hygiene Society indicated that racial degeneration would be regarded as a real possibility. Pistor was aware of the eugenic theories of Schallmayer and Grotjahn.[420] He considered that there was no reason to believe that the advance of material prosperity limited sexual instincts. He observed that widespread use of contraceptives could be attributed either to poverty resulting from inflation or to material luxury. There was a sharpening of the economic struggle for survival. He recommended an increase of social welfare benefits in such areas as housing and travel, and that the price of food be prevented from rising. Such measures should benefit large families. Dietrich considered whether malnutrition and the general weakening of the constitution diminished the physiological capacity to reproduce. He prescribed breast feeding of infants, sport for youth and education of women in the performing of household duties.[421]

Otto von Schjerning, the chief military medical officer, rejected the view that recruitment statistics showed a deterioration in health and physique. Others on the Committee agreed that there was no evidence for racial degeneration, but further research was necessary. They concluded that the decline in fertility was primarily an urban phenomenon. There was a worsening struggle for survival in towns. Poor living conditions brought about alcoholism, occupational poisons and malnutrition. The cost of living was rising. They attributed the decline not to physiological degeneration but to a voluntary decision to have less children. The decline was occurring primarily among the married. They accepted that the eugenicists Gruber and Kaup were right to demand a government investigation into the causes of degeneration. Local surveys of degeneration were necessary. Committee members urged the state to consider measures as to how this evil could be combated.[422] The advice of medical experts was difficult for more traditional sections of the state to stomach. The Prussian Ministers of Agriculture and Trade were outraged by Pistor's conclusions that the current state policies were primarily in the agrarian interest.[423] In defence the Medical Department said that Pistor was speaking as a representative of the medical profession. Although it was agreed that the report should only have limited circulation, the Medical Department contrived to use the issue to mobilize leaders of public opinion.[424]

---

[420] Grotjahn papers, Schallmayer to Grotjahn, 3 June 1910.
[421] ZSTA M Rep 76 VIII B Nr 1998 Bl 1–21.
[422] ZSTA M Rep 76 VIII B Nr 1998 betr den Geburtenrückgang.
[423] ZSTA M Rep 76 VIII B Nr 1998, Bl 95–6.
[424] ZSTA M Rep 76 VIII B Nr 1998, Bl 105–6.

The survey

On 1 April 1912 the Minister of the Interior sent the minutes of the advisory committee to provincial officials. They were asked to report on the declining birth rate in their region and to seek the opinions of mayors, subordinate officials, medical officers, school inspectors, factory inspectors, medical chambers or *Ärztekammer* and provincial medical assemblies. 2,699 copies of the report were distributed, thereby bringing the issue of the declining birth rate to the attention of a large group of officials.[425] The replies to the questionnaire reveal the extent that the theory of racial degeneration was accepted by officials and the medical profession. The process of information-gathering relied primarily on medical officers, and was supplemented by consultation with other professional bodies. For example, the medical chamber of Breslau asked 1,900 doctors for their opinions. The medical press contained accounts of local discussions and general reviews by experts such as the economist Julius Wolf and the medical statistician Prinzing.

Officials were asked to reply to the following questions: 1. What evidence was there for a limitation of the capacity to conceive and bear children? 2. Was the decline in births restricted to certain sectors of the population, and was there physical degeneration due to occupational conditions? 3. Was the decline in births due to voluntary family limitation? – among which social groups? – and was this due to neo-Malthusian propaganda or to traders in contraceptives? Most officials considered that there was no racial degeneration. They saw the decline as emanating from the higher social classes, and as a spread of corrupting urban values of self-indulgent luxury to the countryside. Only a minority of officials attributed the decline to inflation or to poor urban housing. Other differentiating social factors were held to be the decline of religious observance and in moral standards. Smaller families were correlated in eleven cases to socialist voting, thus following the analysis of Wolf whose analysis reached the medical profession when the topic was being considered late in 1912 and early in 1913. In December 1912 Wolf published his idealistic analysis in the leading professional journal *Berliner Klinische Wochenschrift*.[426] He argued that the process of 'rationalization of sexual life' could be offset by reaffirming moral values of procreating many children. (See table 5 for a regional analysis of the replies.)[427] The decline in births was overwhelmingly diagnosed as due to voluntary limitation of fertility in marriage. It was agreed that the use of contraceptives was becoming widespread. Yet only occasionally did officials consider this to be due to neo-Malthusian propaganda. In Schleswig the officials objected to the presence of the neo-Malthusian pioneer of the occlusive

---

[425] ZSTA M Rep 76 VIII B Nr 1998, Bl. 84.
[426] J. Wolf, 'Der Geburtenrückgang und seine Bekämpfung', *Berliner Klinische Wochenschrift*, vol. 49 (1912), 2297–301, 2351–354.
[427] *Denkschrift über die Ursachen des Geburtenrückgangs und die zur Bekämpfung desselbes etwa in Betracht zu ziehenden Massnahmen* (Berlin, 1912).

pessary, Mensinga, as the first German physician to write that it was the duty of the doctor to advise on contraception.[428] Officials observed that contraceptives were being sold on a large scale by travelling salesmen, and by shops selling 'sanitary articles'. Commercialism and consumer demand rather than neo-Malthusian ideology were more important in the decision to control fertility.

The questionnaire tested the eugenic hypothesis of a decline in reproductive powers. VD and alcoholism were regarded as major causes of sterility. Exposure to toxic substances such as lead and zinc were held to result in infertility and congenital malformations. Nature therapists were singled out as contributing to the spread of VD through ineffective treatments, and of undertaking abortions. Officials varied in their opinions as to whether there was an increase in chronic diseases. There was most concern with VD, because it was regarded as a major cause of sterility. Alcoholism, nervous diseases, and lead and zinc poisoning prompted comment in a number of reports but they were not major objects of interest. A large number of reports saw nature therapists as a threat because of their supposed role as abortionists and their treatments of VD. Whatever the opinion on medical factors, the reports generally rejected the concept of racial degeneration. Instead they considered that the causes of the decline were primarily moral. The decline was correlated with a decline in religious values and the rise of socialism. Overall, the replies showed considerable uniformity of perceptions, despite the very diverse social conditions.

Among the few reports to argue categorically for racial degeneration as the cause was that compiled by the *Ärztekammer* of Berlin Brandenburg. This medical chamber attributed the increase in female infertility to abortions and VD. Male infertility was caused by neurasthenia in the higher classes, and was accompanied by the weakening of sexual powers. Late employment caused delay in marriage and prior sexual debauchery had consequences for a decline in fertility. Women were regarded as succumbing to neo-Malthusian sexual morality which was condemned as over-individualistic. Other Berlin authorities were also critical of modern morality. The municipality of Berlin observed that there was rising sexual neurasthenia and hysteria as a result of the struggle for survival. The Police President regarded such signs as women speaking too loudly on trams as evidence for the new shamelessness. He condemned the display of contraceptives in shops selling 'sanitary articles'.[429]

Certain medical experts spoke in racial terms. The Medical College of Breslau referred to the selling of contraceptives as 'racial suicide'. One local medical officer, Wilke, was well versed in the theory of degeneration. He rehearsed the arguments of the eugenicists Schallmayer, Grotjahn and Crzellitzer regarding how civilization restricted the workings of natural selection. While Grotjahn had suggested that a third of the population was degenerate, he regarded the matter as an open

---

[428] W. Mensinga, (pseudonym, C. Hasse), *Über facultative Sterilität* (Neuwied, 1885).
[429] ZSTA M Rep 76 VIII B Nr 2006 Bl. 194.

question, but recommended measures such as improved midwifery, restricted sales of contraceptives, maternal health insurance, a bachelor tax and anti-alcoholism. These were consistent with a programme of racial hygiene.[430] He convened a special meeting of medical officials. They concluded that there was no hope of preventing a decline in births, and that it would be better to improve hygienic conditions.[431] It was necessary to support campaigns against alcoholism, TB and VD, and against women working in factories, and on the positive side to promote breast feeding, school health, and youth social work. These measures would improve the quality of offspring and prevent the bad racial elements which cost immense sums to state and society.[432]

Many experts emphasized that 'child rich' families should be supported. If the birth rate fell this would be a threat to the political power of the Reich.[433] A gynaecologist complained about a devaluation of all moral values by the ideas of free love and female emancipation. Strong state measures were demanded to ban all contraceptives and to support the 'child rich'. There was a popular misconception that many births were unhealthy. It was necessary to dispel this with improved facilities for large families. Reports on contraceptives estimated sales and catalogued the different types. The police reports emphasized the difficulties in taking effective action against their spread. Prosecution against contraceptive displays could be undertaken only on the grounds of the laws on public decency. The Gynaecological Societies of the Lower Rhine-Westphalia, Berlin and Breslau condemned certain types of douches which caused internal damage resulting in sterility. There was much concern over abortion, and voices were raised against midwives as illegal abortionists. There was comparatively little interest in maternal mortality.[434] Most reports highlighted the growth of neo-Malthusianism in a commercial rather than ideological sense. Only a minority spoke of neo-Malthusian birth control propaganda; in general, officials were alarmed at the rise in commercial sales of contraceptives. This fitted the anti-commercial and nationalist tone of the reports.

The evidence used regional statistics on the birth rate, but was on the whole impressionistic, preferring qualitative to quantitative evidence. The inquiry contrasted with the British Fertility of Marriage Census which, with its eight occupational categories, correlated fertility with social status. The German survey lacked this class differential. The Prussian Statistical Office responded to Krohne's survey by stating that no firm conclusions could be drawn from the evidence. It warned against international comparisons as data-collecting procedures differed so widely. The varying explanations advanced for the declining birth rate were monocausal and statistically unfounded. Statisticians demanded an extension of the census to take account of health conditions and to improve data on infant mortality. The problem of population decline was used to extend medical and demographic expertise.[435]

Abortion

The debate on the birth rate prompted officials to review the abortion question. Prevention of abortion was a means of raising the birth rate. The authorities wished to find out the frequency and causes of abortion. Moreover, they feared medical and moral justifications of abortion. The sexual reformer Hirsch had written in favour of eugenic abortion. Similar to Kaup's attribution of degeneration to industrial causes, Hirsch challenged the state in linking abortions to urban poverty. Hirsch denied that it was possible to have a precise idea of the extent of abortions or for the state to take effective action. But in July 1913 the Ministry of the Interior requested additional information with regard to premature births and the incidence of induced abortions.[436]

Out of 11,700 doctors who were asked to provide information on abortions only 2,515 replied. Rural doctors participated more readily than their urban colleagues. Urban practitioners were more frequently faced with demands for abortions, and there was a sense of resentment that the state was prying into an area where its interference was unwelcome. As many as 40 per cent of doctors replied from rural Schleswig-Holstein (where the incidence of abortion was low), but only 3.2 per cent from urban Berlin-Brandenburg (where abortion rates were high). The statistics suggested a rise in premature births between 1910 and 1912. Nearly half the replies suspected that criminal abortions were a factor, and the remainder left the question unanswered. Estimates of the number of premature births being criminal abortions varied between 10 per cent and 100 per cent. More evidence was submitted to the effect that midwives, especially in towns, undertook criminal abortions. Mass-circulated nature therapists' writings such as Bilz's 'New Cures'[437] were attacked for publicising methods of inducing abortion. The tone of some replies was sensationalist. A police doctor from Dortmund declared that the state was an organism which now was sickening, infected by epidemics of abortion, socialism and luxury.[438]

As with the fertility survey, racial hygiene came under attack. In his evidence the gynaecologist Ernst Bumm criticized the illegality of eugenic abortion. He accepted the necessity of abortion in such cases as maternal blindness and pulmonary TB. But he warned that however noble the ideal of racial improvement, neither eugenic sterilization nor abortion was practicable. Other evidence criticized the arguments of Hirsch and Marcuse in favour of eugenic and social abortion. The uncertainties of medical science regarding the inheritance of diseases, as well as ethical considerations, supported arguments against eugenic

---

[435] ZSTA M Rep 76 VIII B Nr 1998 Bl. 243–6.
[436] ZSTA M Rep 76 VIII B Nr 1998 Bl. 242, 255.
[437] *Das Neue Heilverfahren.*   [438] ZSTA M Rep 76 VIII B Nr 39; *Bericht* (1915), p. 68.

abortion.[439] The results of the survey were placed before the Prussian Medical Advisory Committee on April 1914. The committee had the impression that there was rising pressure by patients on doctors to undertake abortions. The committee was aware of the justification for abortions on social and eugenic grounds. These progressive ideas were condemned as irreconcilable with the law that abortion could be induced only in cases of severe threats to the health or life of the mother.[440]

Krohne reported on the swelling tide of demand for abortion and voluntary sterilization. If a patient was denied an abortion by their family doctor, they could then find a practitioner in one of the larger cities, who carried out abortions as a lucrative fringe activity. Diagnoses such as 'latent TB' could suffice. A director of a maternity clinic reported that medical indications were coming to include eugenic items such as 'hereditary damage to health', as in the case of women diagnosed as suffering from 'nervous excitement' or 'depression' due to menstruation.[441] Krohne regarded abortions as posing a serious threat to the nation. He pronounced that the state had a prime interest in maintaining life not only of the newly born but also in the womb. He condemned abortion on grounds of social and racial hygiene. He considered that surrendering to demands for abortion on such grounds as poverty would mean that nothing would stop doctors from giving morphine to an incurable case of TB when the person was too poor to pay for treatment. For the same reasons the killing of the incurably mentally ill should not be allowed. Eugenic indications were inadmissible.[442] This statement by a leading medical official shows how the authoritarianism of Wilhelmine doctors stopped short of compulsory euthanasia and endorsed racial hygiene only when consistent with conservative moral convictions of the ruling elite.

The Medical Department was cautious in its reactions to the mass of evidence. Krohne was alarmed by the medical and official evidence that he had collected, showing the extent of the problems, and by the heated debates in newspapers about the social repercussions of the decline. His verdict was that there was a serious problem with the 'loss' of two million births per year. Taking venereal diseases as a symptom of racial degeneration, he admitted that although no statistics were available there was probably a moderate decrease in its incidence. Neither VD nor alcoholism could explain the loss of two million births. Although certain experts in occupational hygiene (such as Kaup) had attributed declining fertility to women performing physically hard work, only the Schleswig Holstein report considered women working to be a cause of racial degeneration. Nutrition had improved and sport was building up the physical qualities of youth. The most important evidence against racial degeneration was the increase in life expectancy.

With regard to the social sectors among which the decline in fertility was occurring, Krohne concluded that the greatest decline was among the Berlin

---

[439] ZSTA M Rep 76 VIII B Nr 2006 Bl. 43–4, 48.
[440] ZSTA M Rep 76 VIII B Nr 39.   [441] ZSTA M Rep 76 VIII B Nr 2006 Bl. 48–9.
[442] ZSTA M Rep 76 VIII B Nr 2006 Bl. 51–2.

working classes, while the least was in rural areas. Increased prosperity was a major factor, although he acknowledged that there were economic pressures on women to work. Certain craftsmen and middle-class professions were also facing economic difficulties, as shown by rising rents. Krohne censured excessive civilization – *Ueberkultur* – as causing the decline. Marriage and the family had to be maintained as the essence of the German national character. Moral purity and not racial purity had won the first round of the debate on the birth rate.

State solutions

The debates on the birth rate resulted in a combination of demands for tighter state controls, and for a renewed purity of morals campaign. There were demands for the registration of all 'quacks' or nature therapists. The police was urged to be more severe in the suppression of contraceptive sales, and they began to compile dossiers on offending shops and newspaper advertisers. A directive of 25 November 1912, controlled newspaper advertisements and announcements of births and marriages for the Ministry of the Interior suspected that these announcements were used by contraceptive sellers to locate potential clients. There was a difference of opinion on contraception: some officials favoured police intervention; others like the Magdeburg medical officers considered that no special harm was caused by contraceptives and that the trade should remain unregulated.[443]

In 1913 laws were proposed in the Reichstag to suppress abortifacients and contraceptives, and in February 1914 the Centre Party, the Economic Union and the Conservatives all gave support for such laws. These measures were not successful. There was division among state administrators with regard to the extent that the state could interfere in such matters. Whereas the Medical Department in the Ministry of the Interior favoured strong police action, the Prussian Ministry of Justice urged caution. The legislation did not go beyond the committee stages. There was more enthusiasm for informal methods of public propaganda. It was observed that while the Catholic church had official means of enforcing its doctrines, the Protestant church should develop a pastoral and educative strategy against the declining birth rate. In 1913 Seeberg, the Berlin professor of theology, began a campaign to reinstill women with a sense of their maternal duties. Medical officials approached the Protestant church in March 1914 asking that sermons be preached on the birth rate and against contraception. There was a need to build up religious and moral 'counter forces' against the socialist-inspired trend to have smaller families. The church was expected to provide courses on motherhood and to distribute pamphlets to newly weds condemning contraception. A circular was sent to all pastors warning them that contraceptives were spreading like a poison.[444]

---

[443] ZSTA M Rep 76 VIII B Nr 1998 Bl. 200–9, 260–3, 352.
[444] ZSTA M Rep 76 VIII B Nr 1998 Bl. 390–3.

Public pressure began to mount. The declining birth rate was debated by the Prussian Assembly in 1913.[445] Yet official and scientific experts had greater influence than elected representatives in the formulation of population policy. Wolf proposed a Society for Population Policy early in 1914 but was persuaded by the Imperial Health Office to withdraw the suggestion.[446] Instead health officials began to assume a greater public profile. In January 1914 Krohne addressed a meeting of German students on the hygienic and moral effects of the declining birth rate, calling for internal colonization. However, his demands did not stop here. He foresaw a struggle for new territory in which the population could expand.[447]

The agitation for population policy cemented the alliance between the medical profession, a group of reforming state administrators and clerics arguing for moral purity. These groups sought to redefine and extend the responsibilities of the state regarding health and welfare questions. Naumann's social liberalism linking welfare reformers to moral and national issues set the tone. The birth rate survey provides insight into the quality of provincial administration, and into the specific issue of the extent that the theory of racial degeneration permeated the state before 1914. The state was not an impersonal and detached monolith, but susceptible to influences such as professionalization and highly reactive to issues such as the birth strike. Concern with national fitness has to be understood as part of the mobilization of the public for war. A fit and fertile population was the precondition for military power. Krohne's report on the survey became the basic document in plans to impose national welfare legislation.

---

[445] ZSTA M Rep 169 C17 Nr 22 Bl. 1 betr. Bevölkerungsfragen 12 Juni 1913–9 November 1918. Haus der Abgeordneten, Sitzung 7 Februar 1913.
[446] BAK R 86 2375 18 February 1914, Bumm to Schjerning.
[447] O. Krohne, *Die Beurteilung des Geburtenrückganges vom volkshygienischen, sittlichen und nationalen Standpunkt* (Leipzig, 1914).

Table 5. *The Prussian survey of the declining birth rate of 1912: summary of provincial reports*

1 Factors causing declining fertility

Reporting authority	Increased abortion	Increased contraception	Voluntary causes	Neo-Malthusianism	Women's work
East Prussia:					
OP	yes	yes	yes	yes	no
Medkoll	yes	yes	yes	yes	yes
Ärztek	yes	yes		yes	yes
Gumbinnen RP		yes		no	
Allenstein RP	yes	yes	yes	no	
Königsberg RP	yes	yes		yes	
West Prussia:					
OP	yes	yes	yes	yes	no
Ärztek	yes	yes	yes	yes	
Medkoll	yes	yes	yes	no	
Danzig RP	yes	yes	yes	no	no
Marienwerder RP	yes	yes	yes	yes	
Brandenburg:					
OP	yes	yes	yes		yes
Potsdam RP	yes	yes			yes
Berlin Medkoll	yes	yes	yes	no	yes
Berlin Ärztek	yes	yes	yes	yes	
Berlin Magistrat		yes	yes	no	
Berlin Polpräs	yes	yes	yes	yes	
Frankfurt/O RP	yes	yes	yes	no	yes
Pomerania:					
OP	yes	yes	yes	no	no
Köslin RP	no	yes	yes	no	yes

Stralsund RP	yes		yes	no	yes
Stettin Medkoll	yes	yes	yes	no	no
Stettin Ärztek		yes	yes	no	no
Posen:					
Posen RP	yes	yes	yes	no	
Posen Medkoll	yes	yes	yes	no	
Posen Ärztek		yes	yes	no	
Bromberg RP	no	yes	yes	no	
Silesia:					
OP	yes	yes	yes	no	yes
Breslau RP	yes	yes	yes	no	no
Breslau Medkoll	yes	yes		no	yes
Breslau Ärztek	yes	yes	yes	no	no
Liegnitz RP	yes	yes	yes	no	
Oppeln RP	yes	yes	yes	yes	no
Priests/teachers	yes	yes	yes		
Saxony:					
OP	yes	yes	yes	yes	no
Magdeburg RP		yes	yes	yes	yes
Magdeburg Magistrat		yes	yes	yes	yes
Magdeburg Kreisärzte		yes	yes	no	
Magdeburg Ärztek	yes	yes	yes	yes	
Magdeburg Medkoll	yes	yes	yes	yes	yes
Merseburg RP	yes	yes	yes	yes	
Erfurt RP		yes	yes	no	no
Schleswig-Holstein:					
OP	yes	yes		yes	
Schleswig RP	yes	yes	yes	yes	yes
Schleswig Medkoll		yes			
Schleswig Ärztek		yes			yes

Table 5 (cont.)

Reporting authority	Increased abortion	Increased contraception	Voluntary causes	Neo-Malthusianism	Women's work
Hanover:					
OP	yes	yes			
Hanover RP	yes	yes	yes	no	no
Hanover Medkoll		yes			
Hanover Ärztek		yes			
Hildesheim RP	yes	yes	yes	yes	yes
Lüneburg RP	yes	yes	yes	yes	no
Stade RP	yes	yes	yes	yes	no
Aurich RP	yes	yes	yes	yes	no
Osnabrück RP	yes	yes		yes	
Westphalia:					
OP	yes				
Münster RP		yes		yes	
Gynaecological Society of Lower Rhine–Westphalia					
Arnsberg RP		yes			
Minden RP		yes			
Hessen-Nassau					
Cassel RP	yes	yes		yes	yes
Wiesbaden RP		yes	yes	yes	
Wiesbaden Ärztek		yes			yes
Rhine Province:					
OP	yes	yes			no
Trier RP					
Trier Medkoll					

	Racial degeneration	VD	Nervous disease	Alcoholism	Lead/zinc poisoning	Nature therapy
Trier Ärztek						
Koblenz RP						
Cologne RP						
Düsseldorf RP			yes			
Aachen RP	yes	yes	yes	yes		yes
Essen-Ruhr Ärztever	yes	yes	yes	yes		yes
Sigmaringen RP[a]						

2 Medical causes of declining fertility

Reporting authority	Racial degeneration	VD	Nervous disease	Alcoholism	Lead/zinc poisoning	Nature therapy
East Prussia:						
OP	no	no	no	yes	no	yes
East Prussia Medkoll	no	yes				
East Prussia Ärztek	no					
Gumbinnen RP	no	no	no			
Allenstein RP	no	no	no			
Königsberg RP	no	no	no	no		
West Prussia:						
OP	no	no			no	
West Prussia Ärztek	no	no		no		yes
West Prussia Medkoll		no				
Danzig RP	no					
Marienwerder RP	no					
Brandenburg:						
OP	no	no		no	no	
Potsdam RP	no	yes		yes		yes

Table 5 (*cont.*)

Reporting authority	Racial degeneration	VD	Nervous disease	Alcoholism	Lead/zinc poisoning	Nature therapy
Berlin Medkoll	no	yes		yes		
Berlin Ärztek	no	no	yes	no		
Berlin Magistrat	no	no	no	no		
Berlin Polpräs			yes			
Frankfurt/O. RP	no	no	yes	no		yes
Pomerania:						
OP	no					no
Köslin RP						yes
Stralsund RP	no					
Stettin Medkoll	no	no				
Stettin Ärztek	no					
Posen:						
OP						
Posen RP	no	no		no		
Posen Medkoll	no			yes	yes	
Posen Ärztek	no	yes				
Bromberg RP	no	no		yes		
Silesia:						
OP	no	yes				yes
Breslau RP	no			no		yes
Breslau Medkoll	no					
Breslau Ärztek	no				no	
Liegnitz RP	no			no		
Oppeln RP	no					yes
Priests/teachers		yes		yes		yes

Saxony:

	1	2	3	4	5
OP	no				yes
Magdeburg RP	no				yes
Magdeburg Magistrat	no		no		no
Magdeburg Kreisärzte	yes				no
Magdeburg Medkoll	no		yes		
Magdeburg Ärztek	no		yes		
Merseburg	no	yes	yes		
Erfurt RP	no	no	no		

Schleswig-Holstein:

	1	2	3	4	5
OP				yes	yes
Schleswig RP	yes	yes	yes		yes
Schleswig Medkoll	no	no	no		yes
Schleswig Ärztek	no				yes

Hanover:

	1	2	3	4	5
OP	no		no		
Hanover RP					
Hanover Medkoll					
Hanover Ärztek					
Hildesheim RP	no		no		
Lüneburg RP	no	no	no		
Stade RP	no	no	no		yes
Aurich RP	no		no		
Osnabrück RP	no				

Westphalia:

	1	2	3	4	5
OP	no		no		
Münster RP	no				
Gynaecological Society of Lower Rhine–Westphalia					
Arnsberg RP	yes				
Minden RP	no				

Table 5 (cont.)

Reporting authority	Racial degeneration	VD	Nervous disease	Alcoholism	Lead/zinc poisoning	Nature therapy
Hessen-Nassau:						
OP						
Cassel RP	no	no				
Wiesbaden RP	no					
Wiesbaden Ärztever	no	yes				
Rhine Province:						
OP	no	no				
Trier RP		yes				
Trier Medkoll		yes				
Trier Ärztek		yes				
Koblenz RP		no				
Cologne RP	no					
Düsseldorf RP	no					
Aachen RP	no	yes				
Essen–Ruhr Ärztever	no	no				
Sigmaringen RP[a]						

3 Social causes of declining fertility

Reporting authority	Imitation of higher classes	Migration	Excess of luxury	Economic Inflation	Rise of socialism	Housing shortage	Religious/ moral decline
East Prussia:							
OP	yes	yes	yes				

	C1	C2	C3	C4	C5	C6	C7
East Prussia Medkoll							
East Prussia Ärztek							yes
Gumbinnen RP	yes	yes	yes				
Allenstein RP	yes	yes	yes				
Königsberg RP	yes	yes	yes				yes
West Prussia:							
OP	yes	yes	yes				
Danzig Ärztek	yes		yes		yes		
Danzig Medkoll	yes		yes				yes
Danzig RP	yes	yes		yes			yes
Marienwerder RP	yes						
Brandenburg:							
OP	yes	yes	yes	yes			
Potsdam RP	yes		yes	yes	yes		
Berlin Medkoll			yes				
Berlin Ärztek	yes	yes	yes				
Berlin Magistrat				yes	yes		
Berlin Polizeipräs				yes			
Frankfurt/O RP	no		yes	yes			yes
Pomerania:							
OP	yes	yes	yes				
Köslin RP	yes		yes				
Stralsund RP	yes		yes	yes		yes	
Stettin Medkoll	yes		yes	yes			
Stettin Ärztek	yes		yes				
Posen:							
OP	yes[b]		yes			yes	
Posen RP	yes[b]		yes			yes	
Posen Medkoll	yes		yes			yes	
Posen Ärztek			yes	yes			
Bromberg RP	yes		yes	yes	yes		

Table 5 (cont.)

Reporting authority	Imitation of higher classes	Migration	Excess of luxury	Economic Inflation	Rise of socialism	Housing shortage	Religious/ moral decline
Silesia:							
OP	yes	yes	yes				no
Breslau RP		yes	yes				no
Breslau Medkoll							
Breslau Ärztek	no						
Liegnitz RP	yes		yes			yes	yes[c]
Oppeln RP	yes	yes	yes				yes
Priests/teachers	yes						
Saxony:							
Magdeburg RP	yes		yes		yes	yes	yes
Magdeburg Magistrat	yes		yes		yes	yes	
Magdeburg Kreisärzte		yes	yes				
Magdeburg Medkoll	yes		yes				
Magdeburg Ärztek		no				yes	
Merseburg RP	no		yes	yes			
Erfurt RP			yes	yes			yes
Schleswig-Holstein:							
OP							
Schleswig RP	yes		yes			yes	
Schleswig Medkoll							
Schleswig Ärztek							
Hanover:							
OP							
Hanover RP	yes		yes			yes	yes

Hanover Medkoll						
Hanover Ärztek						
Hildesheim RP		yes		yes		
Lüneburg RP	yes	yes				
Stade RP	yes[b]				yes	yes
Aurich RP						
Osnabrück RP						yes[c]
Westphalia:						
OP						
Münster RP				yes		
Gynaecological Society of Lower Rhine–Westfalia						
Arnsberg RP						
Minden RP	no					
Hessen-Nassau:						
OP						
Cassel RP	yes			yes		
Wiesbaden RP	yes			yes	yes	
Wiesbaden Ärztever				yes	yes	
Rhine Province:						
OP	yes			yes	yes	
Trier RP						
Trier Medkoll						
Trier Ärztek						
Koblenz RP						
Cologne RP						
Düsseldorf RP			yes			
Aachen RP						yes
Essen-Ruhr Ärztever	yes					

Table 5 (*cont.*)

Notes:

This survey was compiled from reports submitted by provincial officials, some with the advice of local medical and professional authorities. OP = Oberpräsident (chief regional official), RP = Regierungspräsident (chief provincial official), Medkoll = Medizinalkollegium (State Medical Assembly), Ärztek = Ärztekammer (Medical Chambers), Ärztever = Ärzteverein (Medical Society), Polpräs = Polizeipräsident (police chief).

[a] no analysis as only slight decline in births
[b] higher Polish fertility attributed
[c] occurring among Catholics.

4

Struggle for survival, the 1914–1918 war

Medical mobilization

During the war, informal state control over welfare was centralized. The hitherto covert and fragmented population policy, supported by health officials and public health reform associations, became an explicit part of the planning for post-war reconstruction. Social hygiene supplied a rationale for unifying the diverse initiatives of national welfare associations, municipalities and sickness insurance funds, and for ensuring the co-operation of the medical profession. Official recognition for social hygiene meant that certain eugenic demands were incorporated in welfare legislation. What had been an outrage to official morality before the war, became recognized as intrinsic to the national interest: demands of the League for the Protection of Mothers for better conditions for single mothers and their children, contraception and certificates of good health prior to marriage found support among officials. That eugenics had gained influence in organizations to combat VD and TB meant that eugenic views came to permeate the state, which relied on welfare organizations to solve problems of civilian health. The state's population policy promoted the importance of social hygiene. Welfare-oriented eugenics was victorious by 1918.

The prestige of social hygiene rose in the context of the war-time crisis over civilian health. Added to those killed in combat, there was an alarming increase in adult civilian mortality. Food shortages resulted in severe ill-health. Among the worst hit groups were school children. Their low mortality concealed high rates of disease and severe starvation. That the birth rate continued to fall, and could no longer be offset by increased life expectancy, meant that policies to improve family health became urgent. Family health took priority over food rations and welfare for the mentally ill and other long-term hospital patients, who suffered high mortality rates. Health officials hoped that opposition within other ministries to family-oriented policies could be overcome, and that the strikes and boycotts of militant doctors against the sickness insurance funds would cease in a conciliatory spirit of the 'peace in the citadel', which political parties supported.

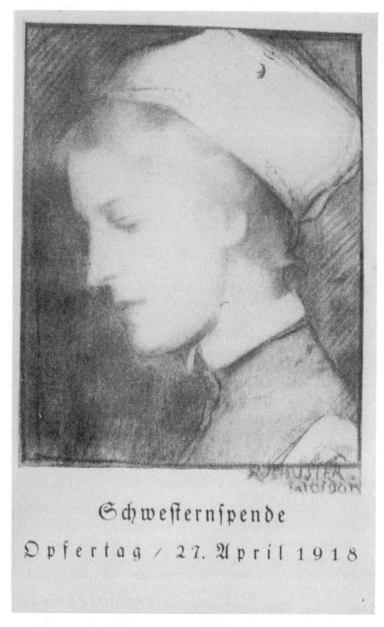

Schwesternspende

Opfertag / 27. April 1918

4 Nursing Flag Day, 27 April 1918. Postcard designed by R. Schuster, and printed by Pass und Garleb Gmbh, Berlin. The War saw the rapid development of nurse training as many female volunteers gained professional qualifications. This is exemplified by the emergence of children's nursing as a specialization.

Initially, there was confidence in the superiority of German science, medicine and civilized values. The nationalist pride in scientific achievements inspired the faith that these would contribute to a swift military triumph. The experience of mobilization of August 1914 became crucial to German history. It represented an ideal of unity aimed for by imperialists and conservatives in the Kaiserreich. Thereafter, its memory was immortalized by nationalists who tried to revive its spirit as a permanent condition. The nation was idealized as a highly integrated community or *Volksgemeinschaft*. An important element of these patriotic 'ideals of 1914' concerned the notion of a healthier society.[1] The expectation was not of a Social Darwinist survival of the fittest, but of a primarily moral and nationalist regeneration of the family and *Volk*. The materialist culture of France and Britain was synonymous with the worst features of industrial and urban Germany. France was condemned as the embodiment of the two-child system, and as ravaged by alcoholism, nervous diseases and by the *morbus gallicus* on a scale far worse than Germany. War was an opportunity for the nation to purge itself of the materialism that brought on these diseases. The war could provide an antidote to the threat of Germans being demographically swamped by the larger Slav families in the East, with the conquest of territories for the settlement of large German families.[2]

Measures imposed during mobilization expressed this medical optimism. Consumption of alcohol and tobacco was placed under strict control, as threatening military efficiency.[3] Active military service was glorified as healthier than urban life. The fresh air and exercise of the front meant that it could be a vast open air sanatorium. Another indicator of health was the fall in the number of mental patients, and a decrease of suicides.[4] Even food shortages were regarded as beneficial, as declining rates of diabetes, obesity and jaundice were recorded.[5] The medical profession mobilized with enthusiasm. About 24,000 out of 33,000 male doctors served. Leading university professors, who often were reserve officers, set an example by quickly reporting for duty. Months and years elapsed before the army realized that gynaecologists and obstetricians were more useful in a university clinic than at the front.[6] Experts in social hygiene and eugenicists signed manifestos

---

[1] T.W. Mason, *Sozialpolitik im Dritten Reich* (Opladen, 1977), p. 26. On the medical profession in the 1914–18 war see: W. Hoffmann, *Die deutschen Ärzte im Weltkriege* (Berlin, 1920); W. His, *Die Front der Ärzte* (Bielefeld and Leipzig, 1931); M. Kirchner, *Ärztliche Kriegs- und Friedensgedanken* (Berlin, 1918); G. Jeschal, *Politik und Wissenschaft deutscher Ärzte im ersten Weltkrieg* (Pattensen, 1978). On health conditions see: F. Bumm, *Deutschlands Gesundheitsverhältnisse unter d. Einfluss d. Weltkrieges* (Stuttgart, 1928). For the demographic context see J. Knodel, *The Decline of Fertility in Germany* (Princeton, 1974); P. Marschalck, *Bevölkerungsgeschichte Deutschlands im 19. und 20. Jahrhundert* (Frankfurt-on-Main, 1984); P.J. Weindling, 'The Medical Profession, Social Hygiene and the Birth Rate in Germany, 1914–1918', in R. Wall and J. Winter (eds.), *The Upheaval of War. Family, Work and Welfare in Europe 1914–1918* (Cambridge, 1988) pp. 417–37.

[2] O. Krohne, *Die Beurteilung des Geburtenrückgangs vom volkshygienischen, sittlichen und nationalen Standpunkt* (Leipzig, 1914).

[3] On the health benefits of war see: Bumm, *Gesundheitsverhältnisse*, I, pp. 58–60.

[4] ZSTA M Rep 76 VIII B Nr 1951 Bekämpfung der Truncksucht 1913–1922.

[5] ZSTA M Rep 76 VIII B Nr 1960 Bl. 77; Hoffmann, *Ärzte im Weltkrieg*, pp. 60, 64.

[6] W. Stoeckel, *Erinnerungen eines Frauenarztes* (Leipzig, 1980), pp. 86–7.

on German war aims. Pan-Germanist annexation of territories was supported by Gruber, the Munich professor of hygiene, the paediatrician Schlossmann, the venereologist Neisser, and the professor of hygiene, Rudolf Abel (who until 1915 was a Prussian medical official).[7] More moderate social hygenists such as Grotjahn favoured a peace settlement without annexations. That the majority of doctors saw active service meant that the profession was inculcated with military and authoritarian values.

. The priorities were medical examination of recruits, the organization of field hospitals, and the prevention of epidemics at the front. Hygenic regulations concerning, for example, the provision of latrines were to be strictly observed. Confidence in the recent German bacteriological triumphs over epidemic diseases was unbounded. Typhus was controlled by de-lousing. Dysentery and typhoid that could be spread by inadequate sanitation were kept in check. Cholera – spilling over from Russia – was contained. Tetanus immunization for the wounded was a remarkable medical innovation. Advances in antiseptics meant that a relatively low rate of 3 per cent mortality occurred among the 10 million field hospital patients. The warning of medical demographers that epidemics resulting from wars could cause greater loss of life than military action was well heeded.[8]

Civilian welfare

As the war proceeded, fears arose regarding the deteriorating health of soldiers' families. State medical authorities defended the health of families with methods of social hygiene: welfare clinics, health propaganda, and family income supplements reinforced civilian health. Military medical authorities communicated their concerns to the High Command and the Prussian War Ministry. As VD constituted the highest incidence of all infections that afflicted the army, this posed a threat to the family as well as to military efficiency. Medical officials sought to convince other ministries of the need for a population policy. The army pressed for action from civilian authorities with regard to maternity allowances for soldiers' wives, the control of VD, and improving school medical services. By 1916 the army supported the demand for a comprehensive population policy.[9] Given that eugenics had established itself in various specialisms dealing with chronic diseases such as VD and TB, the state accepted certain eugenic remedies. Family allowances, VD prevention, measures to improve midwifery and school health became part of a strategy for a comprehensive social welfare and population policy.

Campaigners for financial subsidies for families won a swift victory in December 1914 with maternity benefits being granted to soldiers' wives. Whereas in the Imperial Insurance Code (*Reichsversicherungsordnung*) of 1911 maternity

[7] *Berliner klinische Wochenschrift*, vol. 52 (1915), 1383.
[8] F. Prinzing, *Epidemics Resulting from Wars* (Oxford, 1916); His, *Die Front*, p. 13.
[9] ZSTA P 15.01 Nr 9345 Massregeln gegen den Geburtenrückgang Bl. 141.

benefits were discretionary, mandatory maternity benefits marked a stage in the advance to family insurance for a worker's dependants. The benefits were extended during the war to single-parent families.[10] It was a move towards the realization of the demands of the League for the Protection of Mothers for improving the conditions of the unmarried mothers and their children. Progressive sickness insurance funds, which were controlled by socialists and disciples of Naumann's social liberalism, were keen to promote preventive medicine. The state insurance offices, which had contributed towards the costs of dispensaries, were sympathetic to sickness insurance funds providing additional family benefits, despite falling insurance contributions during the war.[11] But the Prussian Finance Ministry resisted plans for altering taxation to benefit large families, and so checked the advance of social hygiene into the realm of state finance.

Military pressure was effective on public health issues such as VD prevention. The state had first discussed clinics at the Reich Health Council in 1908. Only in 1911 did VD become a statutory obligation of sickness funds. In January 1914 the first advisory clinic financed by a provincial insurance office was opened in Hamburg. During the war a national system of VD clinics was established to provide free consultation on the model of TB dispensaries. Treatment by doctors in a private practice was to be paid for by an insurance office.[12] The Governor General of the occupied territories in Belgium, von Bissing, brought it to the attention of the Reich Insurance Office that the incidence of VD was far higher in troops not at the Front.[13] On 14 June 1915 the Prussian War Ministry decreed that all soldiers leaving the army were to have a health examination; those with VD were to be placed under the supervision of a welfare centre. The Chancellor, Bethmann Hollweg, showed that more than just military efficiency was at stake when in March 1915 he called for vigorous state intervention to defend the health and numbers of future generations.[14]

An alliance was established between military authorities and medical reformers on the basis of efficiency and social need. In December 1915 two conferences on VD prevention were held by the authorities in Belgium and by the Prussian Ministry of the Interior. Experts in social hygiene such as Blaschko and Neisser were summoned to these conferences. That Blaschko was secretary and Neisser president of the Society for the Prevention of Venereal Diseases exemplifies how the policies of a reforming pressure group achieved influence. The state and army distributed the propaganda of the anti-VD society. Social hygienists impressed on the military the fact that VD accounted for a loss of 60 births per 100 marriages, and 100,000

[10] Stürzbecher, 'Bekämpfung', 45.
[11] ZSTA M Rep 151 I C Nr 9073 Bl. 280; ZSTA M Rep 76 VIII B Nr 4197 Bekämpfung der Geschlechtskrankheiten Bl. 320.
[12] ZSTA P 15.01 Nr 11869 Massregeln gegen Geschlechtskrankheiten Bl. 31, 84–96.
[13] On VD see: H.C. Fischer and E.X. Dubois, *Sexual Life During the World War*, (London, 1937), pp. 357–398; M. Hirschfeld (ed.), *Sittengeschichte des Weltkriegs* (Leipzig and Vienna, nd), I, pp. 219–48.
[14] ZSTA P 15.01 Nr 11868 Bl. 68.

babies each year had congenital syphilis.[15] Venereologists successfully defended the value of condoms as prophylactics against VD. The medical advisors demanded that VD control be primarily a medical rather than a police responsibility, and that there be compulsory medical treatment of soldiers and prostitutes. Doctors' demands were realized in the emergency decree for VD prevention of 11 December 1918, which was a step towards achieving a monopoly of treatment for VD.[16] The medical profession's powers represented a victory over nature therapists as well as an erosion of the voluntaristic principles of health care that had prevailed in Imperial Germany. VD prevention exemplifies the state centralization of hygienic measures that occurred during the war.[17]

Concern to protect the family motivated state intervention in infant and child health. By 1916 it was calculated that Germany had 'lost' 680,000 births in the course of the war on the basis of the pre-war high, albeit falling, birth rate. By 1917 the Prussian Statistical Office reckoned that Germany 'lost' 1.5 million births. It feared that by 1936 only 235,000 infants would survive the first year of life in comparison with 620,000 in 1914.[18] Lowering the infant mortality rate was to compensate for the decline in births. Remedies were the improvement of midwifery and infant feeding practices, and the training of children's nurses. The state regarded midwifery reform as the best means of raising standards of infant care. Plans for reform, which had foundered because of opposition from the Finance Ministry in 1902 and 1908, re-surfaced. Midwives enthusiastically supported state plans. Conflict erupted when doctors continued to criticise midwives for their ignorance, and to accuse them of performing criminal abortions.[19]

The remedy suggested by the Association of German Midwives was to raise their professional status. They demanded improved training, higher income, recognition as state officials rather than as *nicht beamtete Medizinalpersonen* (non-official medical personnel), and legislation for their compulsory attendance at all births. Midwives interpreted lack of state support for the final demand as implying a preference for doctors to attend births, especially in prosperous families.[20] Otherwise, medical officials supported their demands but planned to restrict where midwives could practise. Supervision by police and medical officers would ensure

---

[15] *Massnahmen zur Bekämpfung der Geschlechtskrankheiten* (Brussels, 1915); ZSTA P 15.01 Nr 11868 Bl 195–234, Nr 11869 Bl. 390. F. Tennstedt, 'Alfred Blaschko – das wissenschaftliche und sozialpolitische Wirken eines menschenfreundlichen Sozialhygienikers im Deutschen Reich', *Zeitschrift für Sozialreform*, vol. 25 (1979), 513–23, 600–13, 646–67; ZSTA M Rep 77 Tit 662 Nr 44 Beiakten 4 Deutsche Gesellschaft für Bekämpfung der Geschlechtskrankheiten.

[16] ZSTA P 15.01 Nr 11881.

[17] S. Schmitz, *Adolf Neisser* (Düsseldorf, 1968), p. 57; P. Kaufmann, *Krieg, Geschlechtskrankheiten und Arbeiterversicherung* (Berlin, 1916).

[18] ZSTA M Rep 151 I C Nr 9071 Bl 327, 329; *Denkschrift des Ministers des Innern über die Ergebnisse der Beratungen der Ministerialkommission für die Geburtenrückgangsfrage* (Berlin, 1917), pp. 5, 7, 50.

[19] ZSTA M Rep 76 VIII B Nr 2766 Sorge um die Erhaltung der Neugeborenen Bl. 103.

[20] Staatsarchiv Dresden, Ministerium des Innern Nr 15249 Das Hebammenwesen Bl. 88–92.

that midwives were of good character and would prevent illegal abortions.[21] An even distribution of midwives would remedy the considerable regional variations in infant mortality.[22]

In order to improve hospital clinics the state carried out surveys of obstetric facilities in 1914, 1915 and 1918. Despite recognition of a growing public preference for hospital births, the Prussian Ministry of the Interior favoured home births supervised by a midwife over births in district maternity hospitals.[23] At the Inter-ministerial Committee on the Birth Rate in February 1916, the Finance Ministry opposed midwifery reform. But the Agriculture Ministry championed the cause of midwifery to improve rural health. In July 1916 a survey of midwifery ascertained whether a district midwife was necessary.[24] Grants were made to each province to educate midwives so that they could train mothers in methods of infant care. Midwives were to be alerted to the nation's economic and military need for healthier babies, and to their own patriotic responsibilities in working to offset the declining birth rate.[25] The Association of German Midwives in 1917 requested state subsidies for courses on social science and hygiene, so that midwives could contribute to the population policy.[26] Medical officials were confident that midwives could reduce numbers of still births and the maternal mortality rate of 65,000 deaths a year.[27] But when a law for the reform of midwifery was drawn up in 1917, it encountered the same opposition to state regulation and subsidies from the Ministry of Finance as it had in 1908. The Ministry of the Interior was forced to continue with its policies of re-educating midwives and extending supervision by medical officers.[28]

The centralization of resources to combat infant mortality found expression in the state's reliance on the Kaiserin Auguste Viktoria-Haus (KAVH). It exerted influence through a widespread network of infant care clinics, milk depots and local associations for maternal welfare.[29] Behr-Pinnow continued to mediate between the Emperor and Empress, ministerial officials and paediatricians. He condemned ignorant mothers as responsible for 200,000 infant deaths a year. He recommended that all districts should have an integrated system of clinics under control of the medical officer and that the state should educate girls for motherhood.[30] Health officials took up his demand that all districts with over 30,000 inhabitants should have infant care and maternal advice clinics. The Finance

[21] Staatsarchiv Dresden, Ministerium des Innern Nr 15248 Bl. 78–79.

[22] GSTA Dahlem Rep 84a Nr 10995 Bl. 111.

[23] ZSTA M Rep 76 VIII B Nr 1734 Schaffung von Entbindungsanstalten. Nr 1735 Bl. 90, 100.

[24] ZSTA M Rep 151 I C Nr 8892; Rep 76 VIII B Nr 2766 Bl. 118; Rep 76 VIII B Nr 1443 Bl. 82.

[25] ZSTA M Rep 76 VIII B Nr 1415 Bl. 106, 152.

[26] ZSTA M Rep 76 VIII B Nr 1415 Bl. 220.   [27] GSTA Dahlem Rep 84a Nr 865 Bl. 67.

[28] ZSTA M Rep 76 VIII B Nr 1416 Decree of 5.i.1918; Nr 1443 Bl. 158–61; Rep 151 I C Nr 9071 Bl. 233; Denkschrift über die Ursachen des Geburtenrückganges und die dagegen vorgeschlagenen Massnahmen. Bearbeitet im Ministerium des Innern (Berlin, 1915), p. 47; M. v. Gruber, Hygiene des Geschlechtslebens (Stuttgart, 1917).   [29] A. Peiper, Chronik der Kinderheilkunde (Leipzig, 1951), p. 109.

[30] ZSTA M Rep 76 VIII B Nr 2766 Sorge um die Erhaltung der Neugeborenen Bl. 164, 194–198.

Ministry objected as its policy was to oppose all areas of social hygiene, which it was proposed to administer or directly subsidize by the state. The Finance Ministry considered infant health a charitable issue which was beyond the needs of a war economy and thus beyond the competence of the state. The most that was achieved was an increase in subsidies to infant welfare organizations.[31] The power of the Finance Ministry demonstrates how a conservative administrative structure was maintained even at a time of rapid expansion of welfare services.

The KAVH contributed to the transition from voluntary work to a professional ethos. It raised standards in training infant nurses by instigating a professional exam in May 1917.[32] The KAVH prepared the official textbook based on the principles of social hygiene, outlining the responsibility of nurses to supervise not only a child's physical condition, but also character and sexuality.[33] Officials regarded child nursing as a suitable occupation for women from 'better families' to develop their experience in war nursing as a career.[34] The Bund deutscher Frauenvereine (BDF) protested on 19 August 1917 that the child nursing regulations confused domestic infant care, public service, and the nursing of sick children. Women doctors were excluded from the examining commission, as indeed they were from most doctors' war services. The criticisms revealed the hierarchy of control envisaged with medical officers in charge of nurses recruited from the ranks of the Vaterländische Frauenvereine.[35] Marie Baum of the BDF objected that the motive for combining nursing care of sick and healthy children in the domestic and public spheres was to incorporate these functions in the district welfare centres that were the state's main aim. These would undermine the independence of voluntary organizations. At the Inter-ministerial Committee on the Birth Rate, Anna von Gierke emphasized the need to give women social workers administrative training so that they could have the status of officials rather than remain as ancillaries.[36]

The war ushered in a more compassionate attitude to the problems of single mothers. When the Kaiser recognized the urgent need for a population policy on 14 October 1916, he stressed that measures should be devised to improve the chances of survival of illegitimate babies. It was recommended that medical officers supervise and teach foster parents in methods of infant care.[37] Health officials relaxed their animosity against artificial feeding and became concerned with the unhygienic design of babies' bottles and with the quality of the milk supply.[38]

School health was a major component of population policy. Children were

---

[31] ZSTA M Rep 76 VIII B Nr 2803 Bl. 2–5.

[32] ZSTA M Rep 76 VIII B Nr 2791 Ausbildung von Säuglingspflegerinnen Bl 53–55, 117, 144; 2.2.1 Nr 24546 Bl. 3; STA Dresden Ministerium des Innern Nr 15221 Ausbildung von Säuglingspfleger-innen Bl 328; ZSTA P 15.01 Nr 1 1974 Bl.147.

[33] ZSTA M Rep 76 VIII B Nr 2791 Bl. 203–5.   [34] ZSTA M Rep 76 VIII B Nr 2791 Bl. 198.

[35] ZSTA M Rep 76 VIII Bl. 136–9; Rep 76 VIII B Nr 1704 Bl. 167–8.

[36] M. Baum, 'Die Staatliche Anerkennung von Säuglingspflegerinnen. Bemerkungen zu dem Erlass des Ministeriums des Inneren von 31.iii.1917', *DMW*, (1917), 913–15, concerning 27 September 1916, Ministerialkommission zur Geburtenrückgangsfrage.

[37] 8 April 1916, Ministerialkommission zur Geburtenrückgangsfrage.

[38] ZSTA M Rep 76 VIII B Nr 2789; Nr 2051 Volksgesundheitliche Fragen während des Krieges.

among the worst-off of social groups because of the catastrophic food shortages. The extension of medical supervision of school children became urgent. Malnutrition resulted in an increase in rickets, stomach and intestinal disorders, and hunger oedema. Whereas the demands of population policy meant that children and young women were a high priority social group, others were neglected. Patients in mental hospitals and in homes for the elderly and infirm suffered an exceptionally high death rate.[39] (This experience of unco-ordinated neglect was used as a justification for systematic medical killing in the Second World War.)

The winters of 1916 and 1917 brought widespread starvation. Yet the state continued to be optimistic. It relied on nutritionists, who took a quantitative and physiological approach to food values, ignoring the quality of diet or overall social conditions. The physiologist Rubner, who had introduced the concept of calories, preached the virtues of a high fat and high protein diet. Medical officers were censured for having undertaken surveys of the extent of hunger among children. Officials rejected the validity of asking children to list the diet of one day when meat was eaten and one day without meat, as the children had concluded that they were continually hungry. Personal experience was too impressionistic for the scientific stance of the state. But socialists produced devastating criticisms of health and nutritional conditions by using sickness insurance and factory inspectorate statistics.[40] The state administration pressed for central controls over the food supply. Health officials and physiologists such as Rubner took an optimistic view that the nation could withstand short-term food shortages, despite the rise in mortality from infectious diseases. The physical powers of resistance to infections weakened. TB rose to the level found twenty-five years previously.[41]

As the military situation worsened, officials urged implementation of population policies. The diverse areas of reform such as VD control and infant health measures required a co-ordinated strategy of social reform, accompanied by a growth of the powers of doctors and public health officials. The debate intensified in nationalistic fervour with the glorification of Germanic family life. Such a heightening of phraseology can be seen in the reports on the birth rate drafted by the Prussian Medical Department in 1912, 1915 and 1917. They were reinforced by a military report in spring 1918, advising that ethical, material and *völkisch* reserves be mobilized for a comprehensive population policy. The Chief of Staff in 1918 made urgent recommendations regarding infant health, and suggested that dermatology and paediatrics should be incorporated in medical education.[42] It

---

[39] ZSTA M Rep 76 VIII B Nr 2051 Bl. 16.

[40] ZSTA M Rep 76 VIII B Nr 2051 Bl. 208–396; M. Kirchner, 'Kriegsernährung und Volksgesundheit', *Berliner Lokalanzeiger*, (6 Nov. 1916); ZSTA M Rep 76 VIII B Nr 2079 Bl. 30–4.

[41] *Denkschrift* (Berlin, 1917), pp. 32–3; *Stenographischer Bericht der Verhandlungen des Reichstags* (10 June 1918), 5364.

[42] *Denkschrift über die Ursachen des Geburtenrückgangs und die zur Bekämpfung desselbes etwa in Betracht zu ziehenden Massnahmen* (Berlin, 1912); *Denkschrift über die Ursachen des Geburtenrückganges und die dagegen vorgeschlagenen Massnahmen. Bearbeitet im Ministerium des Innern* (Berlin, 1915); *Denkschrift des Ministers des Innern über die Ergebnisse der Beratungen der Ministerialkommission für die Geburtenrückgangsfrage* (Berlin, 1917).

marked the high point of official support for a population policy based on social hygiene.

The Inter-ministerial Committee on the Birth Rate held fifteen sessions between 13 October 1915 and 3 February 1917. Because rural health (the topic of the first session) was a major priority, other ministries gave support; for in 1912 the Prussian Ministers for Finance and Trade had objected that the state survey on the birth rate implied criticisms of government neglect of urban living conditions. Rural areas had high infant and adult mortality rates (higher than in many cities). This differential provided the Prussian Medical Department with reasons for its programme of state centralization, it being consistent with powerful landed interests. The number of full-time medical officers was to be increased, as 86 per cent of the 520 officers were part-time appointments. District health and welfare centres – *Kreisfürsorgeämter* – were established in Cologne, Düsseldorf and Potsdam, and it was hoped that these could provide the basis of a social hygienic solution to the declining birth rate. It was important that these were under the auspices of central government rather than of municipalities. *Ministerialdirektor* Kirchner disliked the municipal health departments (as much as socialists favoured these), although certain state medical officers had dual appointments with municipalities.[43] The planning of health centres was a sign that an innovative era of central state welfare planning had dawned, and that the aims were to reinforce state power and a conservative social structure.

Despite the support of the Kaiser and *Staatsministerium*, the main means for achieving a population policy, that of subsidies for large families, was successfully blocked by the Finance Ministry. On the committee discussing the birth rate were several economists invited by the Prussian Medical Department. Their expertise was to be used on a sub-committee for taxation reforms introducing fiscal benefits for the 'child rich'. Each time such proposals were raised, they were quashed by the Finance Ministry, which insisted on its exclusive prerogative over fiscal matters. Finance and Justice officials defended the vestiges of the non-interventionist state. The medical department's report on the birth rate of 1917 was unable to discuss taxation reform other than in the most general terms. The Ministry of Justice had consistent reservations over any extension of doctors and midwives' responsibilities. Entrenched positions of those opposed to population policy meant that the hoped-for advances in welfare legislation became bogged down. The medical authorities were fighting on two fronts: they had to contend with the traditional legal barriers to state welfare and with the radicalism among the eugenicists, who urged population policy oriented to selective quality rather than quantity of births.

[43] ZSTA M Rep 76 VIII B Nr 1998 Der Geburtenrückgang Bl. 87; *Denkschrift* (1917), pp. 28–31.

ORGANICIST IDEOLOGY AND RACIAL HYGIENE

Defenders of the family

Links between the medical profession, eugenicists and the state became closer. They shared a distinctive organicist ideology which showed how social hygiene, eugenics and nationalism had become intertwined. Medical and demographic conditions were regarded as barometers of national patriotism. Statistics and commentaries on health were more ideological constructs than reflections of actual conditions. By focusing attention on the declining birth rate, state medical authorities shifted debate away from the extent to which the war had exacerbated the social causes of ill-health. Germany's enemies were blamed for social deprivation. Dietary deficiencies could be attributed to the enemy blockade. 'Child rich' families were by definition healthy families. These were threatened by 'epidemics' of abortions, harmful contraceptives and VD. Official statistics of these immeasurable phenomena revealed the ideological commitments of their compilers. Organicist theories of the state were popularized. The state was conceptualized as an organism, the family as an elemental cell, and the decreasing family size as cancer or cellular degeneration. This implied that the professional expert and state medical officer had a patriotic duty to intervene in issues of family health. The hostility to small families indicated consensus on pro-natalism, which was shared by the various family welfare organizations and public health officials. The war gave rise to a holistic ideology of *Ganzheit*, that brought about state centralization of the Red Cross, medical and welfare organizations, and a rise of professionalism.[44] This ideology lay behind the concept of the welfare state.

Theories of social hygiene were based on eclectic combinations of medical, biological, social and ethical theories. The tone was set by the 'one nation' ideology of Naumann. He had long been urging welfare measures as necessary to strengthen military prowess. He considered that the birth rate was an index of national vitality, the *Lebensbejahung des Volkes*. Krohne, the official responsible for organizing population policy, approved of Naumann's views on the birth rate and on the responsibility of officials to have more children.[45] Naumann's moral priorities influenced officials. They were unsympathetic to attributing the decline in births to increasing poverty, apart from recognizing the economic difficulties of the

[44] D.V. Glass, *Population Policies and Movements in Europe* (Oxford, 1940), pp. 270–3; A. Mendelssohn-Bartholdy, *The War and German Society, The Testament of a Liberal* (New Haven, 1937), pp. 135, 139.

[45] ZSTA P 15.01 Nr 11982 Musteranstalt zur Bekämpfung der Säuglingssterblichkeit; T. Heuss, *Friedrich Naumann* (Stuttgart and Tübingen, 1949), pp. 206, 314; A. Fischer, 'Der Frauenüberschuss. Eine sozialhygienische Betrachtung Naumannscher Aufsätze', *Hilfe*, vol. 17 no. 31, 32 (1911), 484–5, 499–500; K.-D. Thomann, *Alfons Fischer [1873–1936] und die Badische Gesellschaft für soziale Hygiene* (Cologne, 1980); P.J. Weindling, 'Soziale Hygiene, Eugenik und medizinische Praxis', *Argument – Sonderband*, no. 119 (1984), 6–20.

Mittelstand. Instead, a diagnosis was made in moral terms: that of *Überkultur*, of egoism and personal indulgence, of materialist socialism, and disregard for the higher interests of the nation. A moral diagnosis of the nation's ills underlay organicist analogies in war propaganda. The rationalism of the 'two-child system' was identified as an enemy characteristic. The antidote was pro-natalist propaganda to strengthen the woman's *Wille zum Kind*. Naumann took an active interest in population policy, and addressed the opening meeting of the Society for Population Policy in 1915.

Naumann's emphasis on social integration was used to counter theories based on conflict, whether class struggle or Darwinian survival of the fittest. This can be seen in the views of leading university professors, who were self-elected spokesmen for the medical profession. They condemned eugenics and Social Darwinism. Bumm, the Berlin professor of gynaecology, criticized eugenic theories in his speech as rector in 1916. The professor of anatomy, Oscar Hertwig, attacked the biological premises of eugenicists but favoured an ethical and Christian view of the social organism in terms reminiscent of Naumann's belief in the need to fuse Darwin with Rousseau. The public debate on eugenics occurred simultaneously with a debate on eugenics within the state. The official memorandum on the birth rate drafted by Krohne rejected the theory that smaller families would improve the race. If the eugenic theory that one in six of the population was of a higher quality was correct, then large numbers of children were necessary.[46] Naumann preached that officials should have larger families. Such remedies to the declining birth rate were to strengthen the existing social structure. '

Racial hygiene and social hygiene overlapped through their common focus on reproduction. But only those eugenic solutions conforming to the moral precepts of Naumann's Christian nationalism were officially acceptable. The eugenicists were divided by bitter disagreements over issues such as the admissability of Aryan racial categories, and the value of abortion and sterilization on racial hygienic grounds. Proposals regarding matters such as marriage certificates provoked disagreements over their effectiveness. State advisers with affiliations with eugenic organizations, such as Blaschko, Behr-Pinnow and Rott, favoured positive eugenics but were cautious about negative eugenic measures. Rott advised intensification of measures against hereditary diseases and glorification of family life as a means of improving the race.[47] Ploetz and Schallmayer enjoyed a degree of influence in Bavaria where a medical commission for population policy was convened. But they were decisively rejected as too radical by Prussian medical officials such as Dietrich, Kirchner and Krohne, who also determined the tone of

---

[46] P.J. Weindling, 'Theories of the Cell State in Imperial Germany', in C. Webster (ed.), *Biology, Medicine and Society 1840–1940* (Cambridge, 1981), pp. 99–155; E. Bumm, *Ueber das deutsche Bevölkerungsproblem. Rede zum Antritt des Rektorats . . .* (Berlin, 1916); P.J. Weindling, 'Cell Biology and Darwinism in Imperial Germany: the Contribution of Oscar Hertwig', PhD dissertation, University of London, 1982.

[47] Rott papers, FU Berlin, Leitsätze 24 März Fachkommissionssitzung; ZSTA M Rep 76 Va Sekt 2 Tit 12 Nr 83 Bd 12 Bl. 275, Bd 13 Bl. 5.

Reich policies. The Munich Racial Hygiene Society developed connections with the Pan-German League. They demanded conquered territories for re-settlement of families. This was a further reason for official distrust, as the bellicose League clashed with government policy. The nationalist publisher Julius Lehmann was censured for alarmist propaganda on venereal disease and attacks on Bethmann Hollweg. Extremes of medicine and politics were linked.

The defeat of negative eugenics occurred over official discussions of induced abortion and of marriage certificates. Leading gynaecologists and state officials allied against eugenics. In April 1914 the Prussian Scientific Committee for Medical Affairs demanded a tightening of controls on induced abortion, and in May 1917 the Ministry of Justice reiterated that induced abortion on racial or social grounds was illegal. That doctors could undertake abortions when there was a 'severe threat' to the health of the mother, was a vestige of state reliance on professional autonomy. The laxity with which a 'severe threat' could be interpreted came to be regarded as a loop-hole in the law. Medical officials hoped to secure registration for all abortions with permission given by a minimum of two doctors. Prosecutions, such as that of the Jena professor of gynaecology, Max Henkel, showed how efforts were made to impose more stringent standards on the profession. Since 1914 he had carried out abortions on thirty-three patients with TB, nine with heart disease, and six with mental illness. He was reported by two assistants to the authorities, and in the autumn of 1917 there was a widespread debate among medical circles and politicians as to Henkel's guilt. Leading psychiatrists and gynaecologists, including Bonhoeffer and Bumm, condemned Henkel for these abortions. However, they accepted that eugenic abortions for such mental illnesses as hysteria were justified. Henkel incurred the wrath of both conservatives and the Evangelical League for having harmed the future of the race. Socialists such as Haenisch commented that Henkel was a victim of changing moral and medical standards. Eugenicists were divided over the issue of eugenic sterilization. A minority praised the American sterilization legislation, and argued that male vasectomy at least was a straightforward operation. The majority regarded sterilization as unrealistic and an unsuitable topic for public discussion. Sterilization on eugenic or social grounds was also condemned by health and legal officials.[48]

Serious consideration was given to renewed demands for marriage certificates as a means of preventing hereditary diseases. Certificates were a long-standing demand of the League for the Protection of Mothers, of the Monist League which had petitioned the Reichstag in 1912, of the Society to combat VD, and of eugenicists. In 1915 the League to Increase and Sustain the German National Vitality[49] demanded specially trained doctors for marriage advice. Blaschko (who combined his secretaryship of the VD Prevention Society with membership of the committee of the Racial Hygiene Society) had shown that most cases of VD

---

[48] ZSTA P 15.01 Nr 9346 Bl. 220–230, 282–3, Nr 9345 Bl. 30–59.
[49] *Bund zur Erhaltung und Mehrung der Deutschen Volkskraft.*

among the married had been contracted before marriage. His finding influenced the Berlin Racial Hygiene Society to petition for marriage certificates from September 1916. The Berlin eugenicists invited representatives from welfare organizations concerned with VD and alcoholism, a representative of the Society for Population Policy, experts in municipal health such as Gottstein, and the Berlin Police President. The eugenicists regarded health examinations as a means of achieving their aim of 'as many high-value and as few useless offspring as possible'. In contrast to compulsory laws in the USA, the German eugenicists argued that although the examinations were to be carried out by a medical official, the decision to marry should remain voluntary. The certificate was thus to have educational value. Eugenics could be effective only if there was a popular understanding of its aims. But Blaschko spoke against the proposal because of the difficulties of certifying positive health prior to marriage. Even the lack of symptoms of infection was an unreliable indicator of VD. The VD clinics had often encountered popular opposition. Compulsory registration of VD had not worked. Instead he urged that all those marrying should be given a health education pamphlet. Gottstein prescribed regular health examinations for all those insured, just as school children were regularly inspected.[50]

In February 1917 the Berlin Racial Hygiene Society organized a further meeting with welfare organizations to publicize certificates as an educative measure.[51] At the suggestion of the anatomist, Gustav Schwalbe, it was agreed that a leaflet, recommending a health examination, be distributed by the clergy and registry officials. The Berlin eugenicists decided to petition the *Bundesrat* for the appointment of a special doctor for each district to monitor for inherited diseases, mental diseases, drug addiction, alcoholism and VD. A booklet on the subject was prepared by the Berlin eugenicists and was published by Lehmann.[52] Diagnostic difficulties persuaded the Reich Health Office to reject the proposal in December 1917. It preferred increased health education, and special advisory clinics. In February 1918 the Ministry of the Interior pronounced that such certificates were premature, given the lack of understanding of eugenics among the population. The Ministry was concerned that the certificates represented an intrusion into personal freedom.[53] Certificates were suitable only as a measure of positive health education, not as a compulsory negative eugenic measure.

The emphasis on pro-natalism rather than eugenics, meant that the state favoured associations for family welfare. Shortly before the war, there were moves to subsidize large families by groups such as Wilhelm Polligkeit's Office for 'Child

---

[50] Rott papers, Vorberatung über die Frage des Austausches von Gesundheitszeugnissen vor der Eheschliessung, 23 September 1916.

[51] *Korrespondenz für Bevölkerungspolitik*, no. 43 (3 February 1917), and no. 44 (10 February 1917).

[52] *Ueber den gesetzlichen Austausch von Gesundheitszeugnissen vor der Eheschliessung und rassenhygienische Eheverbote* (Munich, 1917).

[53] ZSTA P 15.01 Nr 9379; *Berliner klinische Wochenschrift*, no. 1 (1918); ZSTA M 2.2.1. Nr 24546 Bl. 101–105.

Rich' Families[54] in Frankfurt-on-Main. The concept of 'child riches' was a product of the fusion of biological and economic ideas. During the war the numbers of such societies increased, and these coalesced after the war into the powerful Reich League for Child Rich Families[55]. The state supported societies with a local basis. The Düsseldorf medical officer, Bornträger, encouraged the formation of the Association for Family Welfare[56], which subsidized large families of more than seven children. After a number of towns had followed this example, the Association of Child Rich Families and Widows[57] was established in the Rhineland. Other regions followed this pattern.[58]

A remarkable number of biologists and medical scientists were active in these associations. Halle provides a classic example with its League to Increase National Vitality[59] which was organized by the physiologist, Abderhalden. His long-standing concerns with abstinence from alcohol and nutrition, dating from his studies in Basel, were extended into the reproductive realm. He recruited other university biologists such as the geneticist Valentin Haecker to the pro-natalist campaign. The League for the German Family and National Vitality[60] founded in April 1917 included a number of scientists and administrators. The organizer was a school doctor, Hermann Paull. With distinct echoes of Naumann, the League campaigned against materialism and for the nation to become a 'great and mighty organism'.[61]

Population policy triumphant

National associations were more problematic than local organizations for distributing welfare. Coinciding with the start of the Inter-ministerial Committee on the Birth Rate, the Society for Population Policy was called into being on 19 October 1915. The charity organization agency, the Zentralstelle für Volkswohlfahrt, held a major conference on the Increase and Raising of National Vitality[62] on 26–28 October 1915. The programme was initially meant to include speeches by Ploetz and Gruber on racial regeneration and the need to prevent degenerative diseases. Gruber proposed to speak on marriage certificates as a means of preventing the degenerate from reproducing. Other participants such as Behr-Pinnow, Gottstein, Rott and Kaup shared similar eugenic convictions. There was official dissatisfaction at these initiatives, however, and at the emphasis the Zentralstelle placed on eugenics. The eugenic settlement policies initiated by Kaup were continued by his successor, Max Christian. Officials initially distrusted the Society for Population Policy, although it attracted prominent politicians to its

---

[54] *Zentrale für kinderreiche Familien.* [55] *Reichsbund für kinderreiche Familien.*
[56] *Vereinigung für Familienwohl.* [57] *Vereinigung kinderreicher Familien und Witwen.*
[58] ZSTA P 15.01 Nr 26234 Bl. 11 Entwicklung des Reichsbundes für Kinderreiche.
[59] *Bund zur Vermehrung der Volkskraft.* [60] *Bund für deutsche Familie und Volkskraft.*
[61] Bund für deutsche Familie und Volkskraft, *Mitteilungen*, no. 1 (1918).
[62] *Die Mehrung und Hebung der Volkskraft.*

meetings. Its president was the economist Wolf, who analyzed the declining birth rate in terms of increasing rationalization of personal values, and the secretary was the Berlin sexologist Moll. They were unable to convince state officials that the society merited support. Behr-Pinnow wrote to the Prussian Minister of the Interior denouncing the society, as he felt it had compromised too much with radical women's leaders such as Käthe Schirmacher who favoured birth control. The medical officials Krohne and Roesle criticized Wolf as a dilettante and the society as unproductive. A reversal occurred in February 1916 when the Berlin theologian Reinhold Seeberg was appointed chairman. He campaigned for a moral approach to the population question such as was favoured both by the state and churches. At the same time as the society was distancing itself from the eugenicists, it was granted an official subsidy.[63]

Conferences were a means of co-ordinating voluntary and professional efforts. Doctors' organizations formed an alliance with the organizations for population policy. Hugo Dippe of the Association to Defend Economic Interests of the Medical Profession (*Hartmannbund*) organized a conference on the family doctor and population policy[64] in 1916. The Darmstadt conference on the reconstruction of the German family life after the war[65] was an important meeting of different organizations. In Dresden the Hygiene Museum organized travelling exhibitions on child health.[66] In Munich medical societies favoured eugenic demands for marriage certificates and in 1917 promoted a commission for 'maintaining and increasing national vitality'.[67] The eugenicists Gruber, Ploetz and Schallmayer took leading roles in lobbying among public health officials, policing authorities and professional bodies. They aimed to introduce positive eugenic measures. Gruber outlined plans for rural settlements of selected families of sound hereditary health with at least three children and formulated a law for welfare benefits for the child rich. Ploetz recommended early marriage as a means of rejuvenating the *Volk* in the wake of war. He pointed out that intellectuals married too late in life. Child allowances should be granted on the basis of academic qualifications. It amounted to a campaign for social dominance by an intellectual meritocracy.[68] The nationalism of the medical profession served professional ends by establishing the need to extend infant and family health measures.

The war strengthened the ideology of the *Volksgemeinschaft* and enhanced professional and state power over the family. Doctors and midwives were allotted

[63] ZSTA M Rep 76 VIII B Nr 2002 Bl. 3; Rep 169 C 17 Nr 26 Bl. 2; ZSTA P 15.01 Nr 9344 Bl. 51–52; BAK R 86 Nr 2376 Wolf on 27 May 1915, and condemnation by Roesle; ZSTA P 15.01 Nr 9350 Bl. 90; ZSTA M Rep 76 VIII B Nr 4388 Ausstellungen.
[64] *Hausarzt und Bevölkerungspolitik.*
[65] *Der Neuaufbau des deutschen Familienlebens nach dem Kriege.*
[66] ZSTA M Rep 76 VIII B Nr 2002 Bl. 199 re. Hausarzt und Bevölkerungspolitik conference.
[67] *Kommission zur Beratung von Fragen der Erhaltung und Mehrung der Volkskraft.*
[68] M. v. Gruber and D. Pesl, *Rassenhygienische Bevölkerungspolitik auf dem Gebiete des Wohungs- und Siedlungswesens* (Munich, 1918); A. Ploetz, 'Die Bedeutung der Frühehe für die Volkserneuerung nach dem Kriege', *MMW*, vol. 65 (1918), 452–5.

additional responsibilities by a state anxious to promote welfare measures as an antidote to political discontent. A shift occurred away from moral to racial precepts. Demographic and medical statistics could be taken as indicators that the German nation might no longer survive. Deaths alarmingly outstripped births. A shift occurred from Naumann's Christian humanitarianism, suiting a voluntary system of welfare, to biological values that expressed the ethos of scientifically trained professionals. Welfare measures meant a strengthening of the eugenic lobby. Eugenic theories were introduced into the prescribed training courses for doctors, nurses and social workers. Social hygiene was a central feature of policies for pro-natalism and positive eugenics designed to promote family health. Policies were determined by medically educated administrators. Social hygiene went with a reorientation of interests within the state; a new technocracy, drawn from the medical profession, midwives, nurses and social workers, gained considerable professional advantages. War-time population policies provided the opportunity for co-ordinating and centralizing health measures dealing with diverse social sectors: rural and urban, infants, school children and mothers. They could all be placed in a co-ordinated scheme that was to strengthen the social order by extending medical and welfare facilities.[69]

Despite all the propaganda and support, the welfare policies made many enemies. One line of criticism came from socialist feminists. The socialist newspaper, Vorwärts, published an article in October 1915 condemning 'the absolutely male character' of the demands for population policy. The woman was allotted a passive role, and was only the object of social policies.[70] The war-time policy was only a partial success owing to the entrenched opposition of other ministries. A diversity of interests and policies became apparent in the state. Ironically, population policy that aimed to reinforce the existing social order could not remove other fundamental features of that order. Obstacles included the right of self-determination in the choice of medical practitioner and in matters concerning the family and marriage. Well-defined administrative divisions obstructed state intervention in welfare, or prevented a ministry from using a medical rationale to institute family allowances.

The clash of interests within the state was symptomatic of how social hygiene was part of a broader process of socio-political change. It pointed the way towards a

---

[69] On socialist health strategies see: E. Hansen et al., Seit über einem Jahrhundert . . . Verschüttete Alternativen in der Sozialpolitik, (Cologne, 1981); P.J. Weindling, 'Shattered Alternatives in Medicine. [Essay Review of the Verschütteten Alternativen Project]', History Workshop Journal, issue 16 (1983), 152–6; A. Labisch, 'Die gesundheitspolitischen Vorstellungen der deutschen Sozialdemokratie von ihrer Gründung bis zur Parteispaltung (1863–1917)', Archiv für Sozialgeschichte, vol. 16 (1976), 325–70; D.S. Nadav, Julius Moses und die Politik der Sozialhygiene in Deutschland (Gerlingen, 1985); on public health and eugenics see: P.J. Weindling, 'Die Preussische Medizinalverwaltung und die "Rassenhygiene"', 1905–1933', Zeitschrift für Sozialreform, vol. 30 (1984), 675–687; A. Labisch and F. Tennstedt, Der Weg zum "Gesetz über die Vereinheitlichung des Gesundheitswesens" (Düsseldorf, 1985).

[70] Paula Müller in Vorwärts, no. 290 (20 October 1915); on war and women's social work, see C. Sachsse, Mütterlichkeit als Beruf (Frankfurt-on-Main, 1986), pp. 162–73.

redefinition of the state and a realignment of social interests with greater symbiosis between the state and professional and welfare organizations. There was acceptance of the primacy of the family in social policy. Professional interests gained a technocratic hold on government as advisers and policy makers. Public health officials and the medical profession extended their authority over issues of welfare and family size. The fusion of professional, state and military interests supported a socialized programme for public health and for the extension of welfare benefits. The welfare state, conceived amidst the destruction of war, was set to embark on ambitious policies of social reconstruction.

MILITANT EUGENICS

War transformed racial hygiene. At the outbreak of the war, the Racial Hygiene Society was primarily concerned with the health of elite social groups. By the end of the war a polarization brought the rift between welfare technocrats and racist ideologues into the open. One wing of the Racial Hygiene Society became committed to a welfare-oriented population policy, and looked to the state for support. The other wing was allied with *völkisch* and national organizations. It saw racial hygiene as a means of national salvation, justifying territorial conquests, and it sought to co-operate with Austrian and Hungarian groupings on the ultra-right. Racial hygiene thus became politicized.

During the build-up to war, the Racial Hygiene Society had enthusiastically joined the patriotic crusade to raise the birth rate. In June of 1914 it issued a declaration against the trend to have smaller families.[71] It demanded a rural settlement policy.[72] This agitation on population matters continued during the war with various recommendations being produced on welfare and settlement issues. War aroused much concern among eugenicists because of the mass slaughter of the 'fittest'. Population policy was meant to compensate, and gave eugenics relevance to plans for post-war reconstruction. Racial hygienists were faced with a contradiction between their patriotic hopes for a German victory, and the demographic costs of the loss of the nation's elite.

The Racial Hygiene Society was not only internally divided but it also had to compete with several new organizations. It stressed the differences between pro-natalism and its own distinctive emphasis on the quality of future generations. There was a need to separate the allies from enemies among the other associations. Thus a Society for Inner Colonization instigated by Kaup was supported, as were demands by other groups for marriage certificates. The Racial Hygiene Society condemned the irresponsibility of those organizations like the Society for Population Policy advocating quantitative population increase.[73] But whereas the Society for Population Policy had official support, the Racial Hygiene Society

---

[71] *Deutsche Tageszeitung* (25 June 1914).   [72] *ARGB*, vol. 11 (1914–15), 707–9.
[73] Lenz papers, MS Minutes, p. 25.

remained a small grouping. The situation was similar in Austria, where in 1917 a Society for Population Policy was founded with prestigious medical and political backing. This included the welfare experts and eugenicists Kaup, Goldscheid, Tandler and Hainisch, and the theoretician of social medicine, Teleky. As in Germany the society provided a means for academics and state officials to interact.[74]

In 1914 the Racial Hygiene Society's statutes expressed its aims as the advance of the science of racial and social hygiene, and of racial and social biology. Popularization of the results of scientific researches was required. That the aims gave priority to scientific activities was indicated by a clause that the society could be dissolved if a German academy or institute for racial hygiene and biology were established. The scientific emphasis was important in distinguishing the society from Aryan enthusiasts, and for winning the support of medical experts. The intensification of racial values was apparent among many eugenicists. Ploetz's 'Bow' – his Nordic sporting group – continued to thrive. It had twenty-seven members during the war.[75] The Racial Hygiene Society was transformed from an international to a national society. On 22 and 23 July 1916 the committee of the German Racial Hygiene Society met formally to reconstitute the society. The committee was thoroughly Munich-dominated with Gruber, Ploetz, Lehmann, Lenz, Spatz and Rüdin; Weinberg came from Stuttgart, and the Berlin society was represented by von Hoffmann and Patz. The Berliners continued the attempt to fuse the society with the new associations for population policy. Official registration of the society fitted in with their efforts to secure greater recognition. All agreed that the internationalism of the society hampered recruitment. Constitutions were drafted up by Gruber and by the Berliners, and it was necessary to compromise between the more expansive plans of the Berliners, who were aiming at a broader membership and the use of propaganda, and the more selectionist and nationalist position of the Munich racial hygienists. The upshot was a tense situation between the two factions that continued for the duration of the war.[76]

Propaganda campaigns

The priority of the Racial Hygiene Society was the use of eugenic propaganda to arouse a sense of responsibility in the *Volk* towards future generations. The aim was to promote both the quantity and the quality of the race by public and private means. Petitions to official authorities, and the instituting of health examinations prior to marriage were envisaged. A stream of pro-natalist propaganda poured from the society which had Lehmann's publishing machinery at its disposal. The society urged that the health of the population be defended and the birth rate be sustained; for in a few decades it predicted a war of revenge. Such a war could be

---

[74] *Mitteilungen der Österreichischen Gesellschaft für Bevölkerungspolitik*, vol. 1 no. 1 (July 1918), 1–40.
[75] Ploetz papers, 'Münchener Bogenklub. Anschriften von Mitgliedern'.
[76] Ploetz papers, Christian to Ploetz, 27 February 1918.

prevented if the nation was so highly populated that no-one would dare attack.[77] From July 1916 the Racial Hygiene Society underwent reorganization to equip itself for the circumstances of the war. A category of membership was added for those aged between eighteen and twenty-five. Previously, membership was confined to unblemished or *unbescholtene* members of the white race, in line with the idea of a breeding elite. The society was now prepared to admit as members official bodies, associations and institutions. More attention was given to the relations between the national and the constituent local societies, as well as to laying down guidelines for expansion.[78] The society was registered in Munich on 7 April 1917.[79]

The society found difficulties in reconciling its desire for a large-scale impact with its elitist pretensions. At a delegates' meeting in October 1917, the problem of local groups admitting 'undesirable elements' was aired. The Munich eugenicists pressed for stronger controls from the centre, whereas the Berliners wished for greater autonomy, given that the German Racial Hygiene Society was Munich-dominated.[80] The aim of popularization led to plans for a popular racial hygiene journal. This was advocated by Berlin. There was a critical response from Lehmann, the Munich publisher, who represented a *völkisch* commitment to racial hygiene. It was agreed that a sixteen-page, illustrated journal, costing twenty pfennigs, should be published from 1 January 1917. Preparations were to be made by Patz, treasurer of the Berlin group, and Christian was appointed editor. Lehmann was more nationalist than the welfare-oriented Berliners, and he wished to have such a journal under his control. The financing of these activities required additional sources of money. It was agreed that industrialists, especially from heavy industry, should be approached, as the war had boosted their profits. The economic benefits of racial hygiene were to be emphasized. The inadequacies of the quantitative approach of the Society for Population Policy and the need for a qualitative approach were to be pointed out. In October 1917 a Berlin memorandum on publicity was accepted as the basis for a large-scale effort at popularization. The Berlin Society recruited members and drummed up funds. The Berlin Racial Hygiene Society produced detailed costings of a journal that was to spearhead a large expansion. It was hoped that by 1919 there would be 500 new members, ten member societies and an income of 60,000 marks from affiliated state and municipal bodies. The Berlin group did manage to raise three donations adding up to 23,000 marks for a racial hygiene journal with a paid administrator.[81]

On 29 July 1917 Berlin's efforts were again derided by Lehmann. He argued that all money collected belonged to the German rather than Berlin Society and that it would be better spent on a large-scale project such as a racial hygiene museum.[82]

[77] *Aufruf der Deutschen Gesellschaft für Rassenhygiene.*
[78] Lenz papers, MS Minutes pp. 1–18, 'Sitzung des Ausschusses der Deutschen Gesellschaft für Rassenhygiene'.
[79] *Satzung der Deutschen Gesellschaft für Rassenhygiene e.V.*, (10 April 1917).
[80] Lenz papers, MS Minutes, p. 23.   [81] Lenz papers, Freiburg Kostenvoranschlag.
[82] Lenz papers, MS Minutes, pp. 26–7.

The museum was to include an exhibition, a racial archive, and a library; it was also meant to produce a journal.[83] In March 1918 the Berliners expressed frustration that the advance of effective racial hygiene was hampered by lack of financial resources.[84] By October 1918 the committee agreed that the political situation prevented any further development of the museum scheme.[85]

The dispute over the journal indicated the divisions between the welfare-oriented Berlin approach, and the more nationalistic Munich group. Hoffmann, the Hungarian consul, who had been secretary of the society, was recalled to Budapest to advise the Hungarian government on the setting up of a welfare ministry. He used the opportunity to institutionalize racial hygienic ideals, and to organize a Hungarian Racial Hygiene Society. Berlin elected a committee which intensified propaganda activities from June 1917. The impetus came from the geneticist, Baur, who became chairman; the deputy chairman was the pathologist Westenhöfer; the third chairman was the infant welfare expert Behr-Pinnow. That the left-wing venereologist, Blaschko, was on the committee also emphasized the medical and welfare orientation of the group. The group's programme of lectures and outings during 1917 showed its concern to infuse eugenic ideas into the discussion of the declining birth rate. Popularization and degeneration were the topics of a lecture by Claassen (a publicist of the Land Owners' League). Another was on Grotjahn's views of the need to direct the inevitable rationalization of sexual life among women into eugenic channels. Christian reviewed theories of the declining birth rate, and appropriate state measures such as family allowances for officials. The society issued a news bulletin, and a series of widely disseminated pamphlets. Baur contributed a pamphlet on population policy and racial hygiene. Comparing Germany with a field of oats where the bad seed was being replanted, he argued that there should be greater selectivity.[86] He was convinced that there should be a national eugenics institute. He emphasized that American philanthropists were spending millions of dollars on eugenic research at Cold Spring Harbor, and a pamphlet was issued on the achievements of the Americans in Racial Hygiene. Baur urged that there should be legislation on settlement, taxation and contraception. His case exemplifies how a biologist's experience of war intensified nationalist and eugenic convictions.

Racial values

There was an even more extreme nationalism in Munich. Lehmann and his cousin Spatz became influential in fusing Pan-Germanic demands for conquered territory for German settlement with eugenics. Lehmann's wilder dreams of an overseas empire became fixated on settlement policy. Annexationist demands were

[83] Lenz papers, MS Minutes, Meeting of 10 August 1917, p. 29.
[84] Ploetz papers, Christian to Ploetz, 20 March 1918.
[85] Lenz papers, MS Minutes, Meeting of 16 October 1918, pp. 30–1.
[86] E. Baur, 'Bevölkerungspolitik und Rassenhygiene' in BAK R86 Nr 2371 Bd I Bl. 106–7.

contrary to official policy, and meant that Lehmann had a running battle with the censor. Kaup and Gruber also took a lead in plans for settlements to regenerate the peasantry. Lehmann advocated depopulation of the inferior Slavs to make way for German settlers. He was ferociously anti-Jewish. In 1915 Ploetz had to calm Lehmann down in a dispute with the editor of a medical journal (Sarason of the *Zeitschrift für ärztliche Fortbildung*), when Lehmann attacked 'the international Jewish world conspiracy'.[87] In April 1917 – just when the Berlin eugenicists were proposing a journal – Lehmann launched a Pan-German journal, *Deutschlands Erneuerung*, calling for national regeneration and territorial acquisitions. It accused the establishment of cultural decadence and with allowing alien and inferior racial elements to sap the vigour of the nation. Such nationalist and racist ideologues as Houston Stewart Chamberlain and the Pan-Germanist Heinrich Class were joined by Gruber on the editorial board. Lenz was an enthusiastic supporter of the venture. Lehmann's influence grew among the Munich racial hygienists. He donated 3,000 marks to the Anthropological and Racial Hygiene Societies for a picture collection of pure German types.[88]

Lenz illustrates how the war reinforced a sense of race as a fundamental value on which could be based a socially active and racially-oriented eugenics. Lehmann encouraged Lenz while on active service to publish on topics such as the German settlement of the Ukraine.[89] Lehmann published Lenz's tract on 'Race as a Principle of Value' in 1917, as well as an article on the renewal of ethical values.[90] Temperamentally, Lenz's outlook was pessimistic, and he sought solace in the darker beliefs of Schopenhauer that all life was a struggle. Racial hygiene was a means of giving this struggle a cosmic significance. He contributed three rousing articles to *Deutschlands Erneuerung*, and formulated a eugenic version of the ten commandments. He combined admiration for classical aesthetic values of physical prowess with biological, moral and nationalist convictions. He was acutely concerned over the long-term social and spiritual effects of the war. His writings on eugenic ethics fitted the need for a nationalist moral code. Racial history was a value that lay beyond science. Blood and race were natural and historical entities which had a primacy over such transient artefacts of civil society as the nation, politics, science, culture, education, and, indeed, individual life. Of these only race had a moral significance as an archetypal value. Race was to form the basis for a 'new German Weltanschauung'. Socialism was to be replaced by an 'organic-social' type of racial socialism. He believed that eugenics needed to be a racial religion if it was to succeed. He cited Gobineau to the effect that the German race was faced by alternatives of extermination or reaching great heights. The German

---

[87] Lehmann papers, Box 3 Zur Judenfrage, Ploetz to J.F. Lehmann, 5 April 1915.

[88] G.D. Stark, *Entrepreneurs of Ideology. Neoconservative Publishers in Germany, 1890–1933* (Chapel Hill, 1981), pp. 127–30.

[89] Lenz to Lehmann 25 December 1915 in M. Lehmann, *Verleger J.F. Lehmann. Ein Leben im Kampf für Deutschland* (Munich, 1935), pp. 64–6.

[90] F. Lenz, 'Die Judenfrage und das Problem des Rassenwertes', *Freideutsche Jugend* (1916), 289–99.

nation was the last carrier of the supreme Nordic racial values that had taken centuries to evolve. Lenz felt that Germany was at a crucial turning-point. He systematically rejected the values of civil society, including hallowed German institutions such as culture and the state. Racial hygiene was showing a heightened radicalism in the non-socialist critique of Imperial institutions. As the sense of crisis deepened, racial hygienists claimed that they were offering a creed of practical and spiritual relevance to their nation's struggle.[91]

Politicization of the racial hygienists, who had hitherto prided themselves as being above party politics, occurred when in September 1917 the ultra-nationalist Fatherland Party (*Vaterlandspartei*) was founded. This mass patriotic party provided popular support for generals such as Erich Ludendorff, who was opposed to any peace plans. By July 1918 its membership exceeded that of the SPD. Professors and students led the agitation for strengthening the will to victory. In Munich the local party organization was dominated by racial hygienists. Lehmann and Gruber took a lead in organizing a Bavarian section. Other Munich racial hygienists such as Richard von Hertwig, Ploetz and Kraepelin were fervent supporters.[92] The *Vaterlandspartei* opened the way to a political stance among the Munich eugenicists, fusing eugenics with right-wing nationalism.

The war saw a renewed effort to realize racial hygienic ideals. There were a number of promising developments: population and social welfare policies in the domestic sphere, and on the international front foreign conquests and the Central European ideal of *Mitteleuropa* could be reinforced and manipulated by racial hygienists. The internationalism of the pre-war eugenics movement was replaced by a triple alliance between German, Austrian and Hungarian eugenicists. This worked through informal contacts between eugenicists and sympathetic politicians made possible by such intermediaries as Hoffmann, the Hungarian consul. Munich eugenicists such as Gruber and Ploetz continued to cultivate Austrian contacts. Gruber's colleague, Kaup, was able to return to Austria in order to take part in establishing a welfare ministry. There were also more formal initiatives made possible by Ploetz's long-standing friendship with the Hungarian politician Teleki, who was in charge of civilian rationing. On 23 September 1918 the first German-Austrian-Hungarian conference was to be convened. The Hungarian Society for Racial Hygiene and Population Policy was to host the conference in conjunction with the 'Medical Department of the Fraternal Military Association'. The speakers were to include Gruber, the geneticist Weinberg, Wilhelm Hecke (on Austrian population policy) and Teleki (on Hungarian population and racial policies). The congress was cancelled at the last minute.

Eugenicists did not find the unity they had hoped for. Underlying the disputes, such as that over the control of the journal, were pronounced differences over

[91] F. Lenz, 'Zur Erneuerung der Ethik', *Deutschlands Erneuerung*, vol. 1 (1917), 35–56; Lenz, 'Gedanken zur Erneuerung des deutschen Volkes', *Deutschlands Erneuerung*, vol. 2 (1918), 765–75.
[92] Ploetz papers, *Landesverein Bayern der Deutschen Vaterlandspartei*, 'Bayerische Landesleute!' (pamphlet); W. Albrecht, *Landtag und Regierung in Bayern* (Berlin, 1968).

völkisch racism between Berlin and Munich. The Berlin group with its welfare orientation won the support of influential welfare organizers such as Behr-Pinnow and public health experts such as Krohne. The Munich group became inclined to Pan-Germanism and sympathetic to Nordic racial ideals. Polarization between racial selectionists and pro-natalist welfare eugenicists occurred. But during the final months of crisis, racial hygienists renewed their institutional and ideological onslaught. Their strength was that they pursued objectives that were not wholly dependent on military victories. In the shock of defeat they were able to rally support and continue to use racial hygiene as a value by which to judge measures in the spheres of politics and civil society. At the same time the war's legacy of legislation, plans for population conquering and ideals of unity lingered on in the memories of those campaigning for eugenic policies.

5

Revolution and racial reconstruction

RACIAL TERRORS

For some Germans the war was never to end. The fervent patriots of the *Vaterlandspartei* continued to support annexation of territories and opposed peace even after the armistice. There were the Eastern frontiers to be protected against the incursions of the fledgling Soviet Union and Poland, and in the West the allied occupation was resisted. Above all, the Versailles Treaty became a focus of opposition: the allies were accused of continuing their 'hunger blockade' of Germany by draining away scarce economic resources. There were enemies within German society. Alien socialist, democratic and racial elements had to be purged so that a truly Germanic social order could be realized. This was the mentality of the *Freikorps* and the nationalist right. The 'birth of a new Germany' had a different, but no less apocalyptic significance to the left. It was the long awaited opportunity for constructing a democratic and economically just social order. Planning and professionalism would replace the coarse authoritarianism of the army and aristocracy. Brave new plans of social reform and social reconstruction were drawn up. Restrictions were to be lifted on artistic expression, there was to be equality between men and women, and a freedom of choice of lifestyle which included family planning. Eugenics was caught between these two entrenched extremes.

The threats to national survival gave rise to a sense of alarm at impending racial extermination. The foreboding of racial extermination was given reality by mass starvation, and epidemics. Hunger meant widespread dependence on soup kitchens and other forms of public welfare. A ferocious influenza epidemic reached a high point late in 1918. Mortality from diseases such as TB continued to rise. The fear of an epidemic of VD arose with the breakdown of military controls on demobilized troops. The apparent political and economic chaos suggested that the nation's mental health was under immense strain. These concerns with health moved to the forefront of daily perceptions. The breakdown of social order gave the family a renewed importance as the basic life-sustaining element of society. Demobilized soldiers returned to their families and homes, and there was a post-war increase in

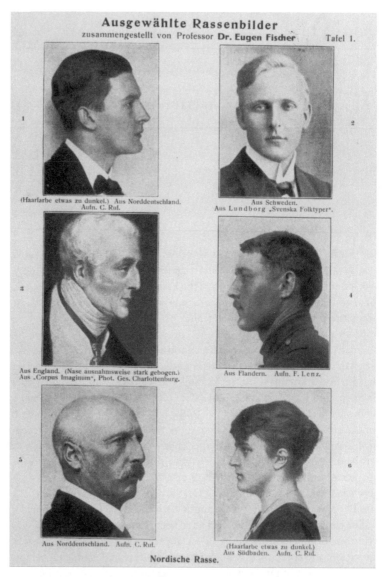

Ausgewählte Rassenbilder
zusammengestellt von Professor **Dr. Eugen Fischer**   Tafel 1.

(Haarfarbe etwas zu dunkel.) Aus Norddeutschland.
Aufn. C. Ruf.

Aus Schweden.
Aus Lundborg „Svenska Folktyper".

Aus England. (Nase ausnahmsweise stark gebogen.)
Aus „Corpus Imaginum", Phot. Ges. Charlottenburg.

Aus Flandern. Aufn. F. Lenz.

Aus Norddeutschland. Aufn. C. Ruf.

(Haarfarbe etwas zu dunkel.)
Aus Südbaden. Aufn. C. Ruf.

Nordische Rasse.

5 'The Nordic Race'. Reproduced from E. Baur, E. Fischer and F. Lenz, *Menschliche Erblichkeitslehre*, 2nd edn (Munich, 1923). The photographs were from the collection of Eugen Fischer, and included some by Fritz Lenz. The book established the scientific status of the concept of a Nordic race, which had been publicized by Hans Günther. The two-volume work was published by the Lehmann Verlag, which had originally planned a *Handbook of Racial Hygiene* prior to the War. Its publication was delayed until 1921. It became a standard textbook of eugenics, and was reissued in an extended and revised fifth edition in 1940.

marriage and a brief baby boom. The difficulties of material day-to-day existence meant that there was a popular sense of a struggle for survival. A feeling arose that it was necessary to reconstruct society on the basis of fundamental biological values. There was an outburst of theorizing on the social organism and of interest in eugenic social policies. At the same time mass poverty, political polarization, and the shift towards socialization were all signs of that at the very time that democracy became reality, liberal and democratic values were in jeopardy. The defeat gave eugenics relevance with regards to national reconstruction. Virtually every aspect of eugenic thought and practice – from 'euthanasia' of the unfit and compulsory sterilization to positive welfare – was developed during the turmoil of the crucial years between 1918 and 1924.

Revolution and counter-revolution

During 1917, leading racial hygienists in Munich – Gruber, Richard von Hertwig, Kraepelin, Lehmann and Ploetz – had moved to an alliance with the political right. Gruber was secretary of the Bavarian section of the *Vaterlandspartei* and in October 1917 issued a manifesto calling for the Bavarians to support Admiral von Tirpitz's demands for a peace based on foreign conquests so as to replace Germany's 'lost blood'. Early in 1918 the *Vaterlandspartei* swayed the Kaiser against a peace settlement. Annexationist aims were satisfied by the Treaty of Brest Litovsk; Germany imposed massive territorial losses on the Soviet Union in the expectation that it could dominate these Eastern territories in a Central European federation. These successes redoubled the demands of eugenicists for a population policy. In July 1918 Gruber, Kraepelin, Lenz, Ploetz and Schallmayer met at the Munich police headquarters to urge the imposition of a population policy. At meetings of the Pan-German League, Ploetz heard of the worsening morale of the troops. Socialist initiatives in Munich prompted counter-revolutionary impulses. Lehmann, the publisher, took a leading role in organizing the forces of the right by instigating popular *völkisch* radicalism with the recruitment of future Nazis such as the railway worker Anton Drexler. On 24 October 1918, he called a meeting of the Munich branch of the Pan-German League of which he was chairman, and of the anti-semitic Thule Society. They organized a Committee of National Defence.[1] Kurt Eisner's socialist *coup* in Munich on 7 November stole the initiative from Lehmann and the nationalists. From November 1918 isolated strikes and demonstrations became a revolutionary mass movement. Councils of soldiers, workers and peasants were established. These took charge of food distribution. Eisner's seizure of power prompted the liberal Chancellor, Prince Max of Baden, to transfer power to the SPD. The regime declared a Republic. Lehmann responded by taking a lead in turning the *völkisch* national front into an armed organization

---

[1] J. Petzold, 'Die Entstehung der Naziideologie', in D. Eichholtz and K. Grossweiler (eds.), *Faschismusforschung* (Berlin, 1980), pp. 261–78.

with the belligerent Nordic name of *Kampfbund Thule*. This allied with another national fighting unit called the *Bund Oberland*, in which Lehmann's son-in-law, Friedrich Weber (a veterinary surgeon), was active. They planned to overthrow Eisner's Soviet. Weapons were supplied by the army and were stored on Lehmann's premises. Ploetz noted in his diary on Christmas Eve 1918 that Lehmann was 'very busy'. Shortly afterwards, the plot was discovered, and Lehmann was imprisoned until February 1919. Bavarian society was becoming militarized with the conflict of socialist and *völkisch* forces.[2]

On his release, Lehmann participated in organizing a League for the Defence of German Honour and Ethics, called the *Deutsch-völkische Schutz- und Trutz-Bund*. This mobilized the public on anti-semitic and ultra-nationalist lines. Lehmann put the resources of his publishing house at the League's disposal.[3] In March 1919 he tried to persuade Ploetz to contribute to a series of anti-semitic publications.[4] He blamed the defeat of 1918 on alien Jewish elements, and the League was banned for a period in 1922. When an associate of the Thule group assassinated Eisner on 21 February 1919, Lehmann was again arrested. As the Munich government passed from being a democratic council to a communist soviet, there was an intensification of the counter-revolutionary forces. The right launched anti-semitic propaganda against intellectuals such as Ernst Niekisch, Ernst Toller, Gustav Landauer and the poet Erich Mühsam who dominated the Munich *Räterepublik* of 6–13 April 1919 and the ensuing soviet republic. Lehmann escaped and joined the *Freikorps* of General Epp in neighbouring Württemberg, and took a lead in the reconquest of Munich from 30 April to 2 May 1919. He was proud of his role in persuading reluctant troops to follow his lead. There were six hundred deaths in the 'liberation' of Bavaria, as a brutal white terror was unleashed.[5]

The *Freikorps* nurtured a generation of racial crusaders. They feared that Germany was succumbing to waves of decadent bolshevism and materialism. Rudolf Hoess is a notorious example of a Nazi racist. A First World War hero, he moved through association with the *Freikorps*, political terrorism and rural settlement with the racist Artamanen League from 1928, to become *Kommandant* of Auschwitz. The militaristic racist nationalism of the *Freikorps* bred a future generation of Nazi leaders. Yet there was a medical dimension to the *Freikorps'* nationalist crusade: they imagined horrifying epidemics of VD, diseases resulting in hereditary degeneration and corruption of the German blood; that the world's most civilized and cultured nation was in the grip of psychopathic disorders; and that the rising tide of sexual immorality was ending in epidemics of abortions. These male fantasies strengthened their resolve to defend the nation. They idealized a patriarchal family, and the sisterly care of the nurse.[6]

[2] G.D. Stark, *Entrepreneurs of Ideology. Neoconservative Publishers in Germany, 1890–1933* (Chapel Hill, 1981), pp. 158–9.
[3] U. Lohalm, *Völkischer Radikalismus. Die Geschichte des deutschvölkischen Schutz- und Trutz-Bundes 1919–1923* (Hamburg, 1970).
[4] Ploetz papers, Lehmann to Ploetz, 24 March 1919, concerning a Pan-Aryan League.
[5] O. Spatz, 'J.F. Lehmann zum hundertsten Geburtstag', MS, p. 6.
[6] K. Theweleit, *Männerphantasien* (Reinbek bei Hamburg, 1980).

Youthful medical students and biologists joined in the vicious reign of terror. They became the future leaders of Nazi science and medicine. Karl Astel exemplifies how the spirit of armed aggression infused medical ideals. As a boy he had been a *Wandervogel* and enjoyed breeding animals. After military service, he returned to be a medical student at Würzburg. He joined a *Freikorps* unit so as to free Würzburg from the bolsheviks. Then he saw action with the *Freikorps* Epp in Thuringia, and participated in student leagues and in the *Schutz- und Trutz-Bund* in Schweinfurt where he first met his life-long ally, Fritz Sauckel. In 1920 he was active in the *Bund Oberland*. He qualified in medicine and at the Bavarian Gymnastics School, and from March 1926 was employed as a sports doctor in Munich. In 1933 he headed a model health and racial hygiene administration in Thuringia.

Adolf Bartels is another example of the link between militant attitudes and medical ideals. He was active in the anti-Red *Hodlerbund* from the summer of 1919, assumed political leadership of a student fraternity called Cimbria, and joined the NSDAP in February 1920 and the anti-semitic *Eiserne Faust*. He saw action with the *Freikorps* Oberland in Silesia in 1921. From 1922 he began a career as a doctor in welfare clinics while maintaining nationalist contacts with Hugo Stinnes and the DNVP (*Deutschnationale Volkspartei*). He linked ideas of health and hereditary fitness, and was interested in industrial health. After quarrelling with a socialist superior in Dortmund, he moved to Eisenach, where he carried out research in occupational medicine at the BMW car factory. He took a lead in industrial health in the Third Reich, and became deputy Reichsärzteführer. The future Nazi Reichsärzteführer, Gerhard Wagner, was active in the *Freikorps* Epp and Oberland, before settling down to medical practice in Munich from 1924.

The profile of wartime experience at the front, activism in the *Freikorps* and then a few years of medical practice typified those future Nazi doctors, who were highly ideologically motivated in employing medicine as a weapon for racial purity. Other examples were Gregor Ebner and Max Sollmann of the SS's *Lebensborn* welfare institutions, who both served in the *Freikorps*. A substantial proportion of those involved in the medical killing of victims of hereditary diseases were conditioned by experiences in the *Freikorps*. Examples were the Austrian psychiatrist, Max de Crinis, and Werner Heyde who had participated in the Kapp Putsch. The war for national survival and then against bolshevism was subsumed into medical studies and practice.[7]

A remarkable example of the link between *Freikorps* terror and eugenics is provided by Otmar von Verschuer. He belonged to the lethal Marburg student *Freikorps*, and was active in the Kapp Putsch. He moved to the University of Tübingen, and was adjutant to Bogeslav von Selchow in a campaign against socialists in Thuringia. When he returned to Tübingen racial priorities prompted research on medical genetics.[8] It was as if the aim of the *Freikorps* in exterminating

[7] R.J. Lifton, *The Nazi Doctors. Medical Killing and the Psychology of Genocide* (New York, 1986),pp. 120–1, 126–9.
[8] B. Müller-Hill, *Tödliche Wissenschaft* (Reinbek bei Hamburg, 1984), p. 160.

the bolsheviks was transposed to locating and eradicating the genes of hereditary diseases. Geneticists wrote in militarist terms, comparing chromosomes to military units carrying out manoeuvres, and genes were seen as machine gun bullets. During the Second World War, Verschuer reflected that his military experience helped him to conduct research under adverse conditions.[9]

Despite the virulence of right-wing extremism among students, there were the germs of a socialist student movement. In Munich the free youth leader, and medical student, Wilhelm Hagen, turned to socialism. He was commissioned by the socialist politician Landauer to act in the cause of university reform. The student *Freischar* invited the racial hygienist Lenz to explain his genetic research. Lenz maintained that revolutionaries were dark, round-headed types. A rapid survey of those present showed that the majority of the socialists were pronounced Nordic types. Lenz took umbrage at this behaviour, and abandoned his attempt to unite the socialist and *völkisch* free youth.[10] Hagen exemplifies a transition from free youth leader to becoming an expert on public health. Despite his socialist convictions, he was a convinced eugenicist and retained the friendship of such right-wing extremists as Friedrich Weber.

The earliest membership list of the NSDAP shows that between 1919 (when the party was still the DAP) and autumn 1922, 72 out of 3,214 members were doctors or dentists. They represented 22.5 per cent of the academic professionals who were members.[11] Doctors were useful to the embryonic movement for tending the wounded SA members and, indeed, Hitler when he was wounded during the Putsch of 1923. Doctors provided money, prestigious contacts and, like Dr J. Dingfelder, could speak with authority on racial questions.[12] Some doctors fell by the wayside. Early enthusiasts, such as the *Oberland* and NSDAP member Dr G. Sondermann, withdrew by the time of the Third Reich. The path to Nazi racism even for the Nazis was tortuous.

Nordic regeneration

The medical publisher, Lehmann, continued to provide a link between nationalist propaganda, political terrorism and medicine. Racial hygiene was the ideal fusion of these spheres. He supported the *Feme* murders of politicians such as Walther Rathenau, claiming them to be the administration of *völkisch* justice. Vehemently nationalist publications poured from his presses, on issues such as the Versailles Treaty and the French occupation of the Rhineland. He attacked the Weimar Republic as a compromise of Jewish capitalism with Catholic and masonic internationalism. A culmination to his activities came in 1923 when there was a

[9] O. v. Verschuer, 'Rasse', *Deutsche Politik, ein völkisches Handbuch* (Frankfurt-on-Main, 1924), part 1; Verschuer, 'Rassenhygiene', *Deutsche Politik* (1925), part 15; Verschuer, *Leitfäden*, (Leipzig 1941), p. 6.   [10] IfZ ED66 Wilhelm Hagen papers, vol. 4, MS autobiography.
[11] F. Kudlien (ed.) *Ärzte im Nationalsozialismus* (Cologne, 1985), pp. 19–20.
[12] Kudlien, *Ärzte*, pp. 18–19.

proliferation of such nationalistic racist associations as the *Wikingbund* and *Bund Oberland* in reaction to a revival of the left. In order to stabilize the situation, a General State Commissioner was appointed. This was Gustav von Kahr, a monarchist with ties to the Pan-German League. Kahr used connections to the army and police to organize an anti-republican movement. The Bavarian government threatened to suppress growing communist influence in Saxony, and to initiate a nationalist movement, beginning with a march on Berlin from Munich. Lehmann gave his support, but was also at the Bürgerbräu beer hall when Hitler proclaimed his seizure of power on 8 November 1923. Members of Kahr's government were imprisoned at Lehmann's villa (of a remarkable Germanic architecture at Grosshesselohe). When the Putsch failed on the next day, Lehmann – forever keen to heal rifts on the right – persuaded the Nazi guards to flee rather than to execute the hostages. When Hitler was in prison, Lehmann campaigned on his behalf, and gave mass distribution to Hitler's writings.[13] During the mid-1920s Lehmann continued to support ultra-nationalist groups and secret armaments factories.[14]

Lehmann was a gifted racial propagandist. He wished to publish a racial geography of Europe so as to remind readers that the many ethnic German groups in the East justified the vision of a Greater Germany. His academic model was William Ripley's *The Races of Europe*, which was based on divisions between Teutonic, Alpine and Mediterranean racial groups. The superiority of the Nordic race had been popularized by Madison Grant's *The Passing of the Great Race*, which praised the Nordic type for its mental qualities of independence and tenacity. These works provided the geographical, historical and scientific basis for studies of national psychology, that were biased towards ideas of Nordic superiority.[15] Lehmann had personal contact with Grant and Lothrop Stoddard, and hoped that the geneticist Lenz could undertake his projected racial study.[16] Lenz declined. His interests lay more in the direction of research on inherited diseases, and in applying Mendelism to racial hygiene. He did not wish to compromise his scientific reputation with a popular racial anthropology. The Munich anthropologist Rudolf Martin also refused Lehmann's invitation because he considered that the scientific material was incomplete.[17] In 1920 a Freiburg-educated philologist and school teacher, Hans F.K. Günther, submitted a manuscript called 'Knight, Death and the Devil. An Account of the Nordic Man'.[18] This used Albrecht Dürer's engraving as the basis for a chivalrous romance about a knight who vowed to fight

13 Stark, *Entrepreneurs*, pp. 159–71, 207–11.   14 Lehmann papers, Box 3 Politik.
15 W.Z. Ripley, *The Races of Europe: A Sociological Study* (New York, 1899); M. Grant, *The Passing of the Great Race, or the Racial Basis of European History* (New York, 1916).
16 M. Grant, *Der Untergang der grossen Rasse* (München, 1925); L. Stoddard, *The Revolt against Civilization* (New York, 1920), translated as *Der Kulturumsturz*, (Munich, 1925).
17 K. Saller, *Die Rassenlehre des Nationalsozialismus in Wissenschaft und Propaganda* (Darmstadt, 1961), p. 26.
18 H.F.K. Günther, *Ritter, Tod und Teufel. Eine Darstellung der Wesensart des nordischen Menschen* (Munich, 1920).

for national ideals. Lehmann recruited Günther to his nationalist campaign. Lehmann invited Günther to join him on an Alpine walk, when on a high mountain ridge they surveyed the issues determining the fate of Germany. Lehmann transformed Günther from a heroic and chivalrous-spirited nationalist into a biological racist. This metamorphosis encapsulated the transition to a new type of scientific racism. Lehmann persuaded Günther to write a piece on racial biological identity. He arranged for Günther to visit Lenz and Ploetz. Günther made revisions armed with an article by Lenz on 'The Nordic Race and the Blood-mixture of our Eastern Neighbours'.[19] Lenz, Ploetz and Lehmann all approved of the resulting work, and Lehmann invited Günther to write a racial study of the Germans. Lehmann supported Günther's research with money and such scientific materials as photographs of racial types, and encouraged him to acquire the skills of a practising anthropologist. In the autumn of 1922 Günther's 'Racial Lore of the German Volk' appeared.[20] It was an instant popular success. Lehmann was convinced that it placed the racial question on the popular political agenda. By 1932, over 30,000 copies were sold.

Not all the racial hygienists shared Lehmann's enthusiasm for Günther's work. The Munich professor of hygiene, Gruber, sent a critical commentary, emphasizing its scientific inadequacies. Gruber rejected the distinction between high value and low value racial types, when based on such racial features as blond hair and blue eyes. He stressed that Germans were of mixed races.[21] Lehmann replied in a lengthy anti-semitic diatribe, defending Günther as one who had persuaded Germans of the need to recover consciousness of their Nordic racial blood and spirit. Although very few Germans had pure Nordic blood, Lehmann argued the Nordic had a superior right to leadership of the nation, and drew anti-semitic and anti-democratic conclusions from the book.[22] Lehmann went on to publish a steady stream of Günther's books. These defined the Nordic race on the basis of Gobineau's classification, and established a stereotype of the Jewish race. Fischer, the Freiburg anthropologist gave Günther's works enthusiastic reviews in academic journals.[23] Günther and Lehmann did much to fuse racial hygiene with racist nationalism and anti-semitism.

Ploetz and Gruber (by 1921 a member of the *Deutschnationalen Partei*) were politically less extreme than Lehmann. They continued to uphold the scientific standards of eugenics, while blending these with Nordic racism. But they did not whip up popular anti-semitism or *völkisch* racism. Their Nordic ideals were more refined and their scientific priorities made them more elitist than Lehmann's

---

[19] F. Lenz, 'Die nordische Rasse in der Blutmischung unserer östlichen Nachbaren', *Osteuropäische Zukunft*, cited as offprint.

[20] H.F.K. Günther, *Rassenkunde des deutschen Volkes* (Munich, 1922).

[21] Munich university archives, Gruber file containing 'Geheimrat von Gruber gegen die deutsche Rasse', *Völkischer Beobachter*, no. 25 (8 January 1926).

[22] Lehmann papers, Lehmann to Gruber, 1 February 1923.

[23] E. Fischer, review of Günther, *Rassenkunde* in *Zeitschrift für Morphologie und Anthropologie*, vol. 25 (1926), 160–3.

populist vision of a broad front. Depressed by the worsening situation in October 1918, Ploetz found consolation in Nordic ideals. He kept closely in touch with Lehmann and Gruber, with whom he intensively discussed the Nordic race. On 9 November 1918 he reacted to the armistice with the decision to form an armed militia against 'plunderers'. He retreated to his country house, Schloss Ried, at Herrsching on the Ammersee. He fortified this with machine guns and armed a local militia. He lived in terror expecting the Munich Soviet to storm his nationalist enclave. On a visit to Munich, Ploetz narrowly escaped arrest by hiding in the mental hospital of the psychiatrist Kraepelin.[24]

Ploetz's Nordic Archery Club survived the war. Its twenty-five members included Lehmann and Lenz. On 22 December 1918, just at the time that Lehmann was plotting a *coup*, Ploetz and Arthur Wollny, a doctor, transformed the Archery Club into a Nordic group called the *Widar Bund*. This was called after Widar the Strong who fought to restore the realm of light. Members met to hear Icelandic sagas, and to discuss politics, biology and race. Lehmann lectured on how the crippling wound of the Versailles Treaty meant Germany was bleeding to death. At Christmas he distributed his nationalist publications to members. Lenz lectured to the *Bund* on the races of Eastern Europe in July 1919, and Gruber lectured on national regeneration. In 1920 Lenz and Ploetz concentrated on racial hygiene, presenting a comprehensive course of lectures on degeneration and natural selection. Wollny, Lenz, Ploetz and Pauline Ploetz-Rüdin planned a medical clinic for racial hygienic advice on family matters and for eugenic examinations according to the procedures of the Racial Hygiene Society. An economic department was opened to recruit support among craftsmen and businessmen.[25] The *Bund* distributed groceries, prams and walking frames.

The *Widar Bund* was a substitute for the Racial Hygiene Society. At a time of social and moral crisis, the *Bund's* fellowship and Nordic ideology offered more hope than a purely scientific eugenics. During 1920 its organization was formalized.[26] In 1921 Ploetz became chairman and Lenz became vice-chairman. A meeting on the 'German Man' in November 1920 was attended by sixty members and their guests. Christmas and midsummer were specially celebrated. A pamphlet issued on 3 March 1919 declared that Germany had sacrificed two million of its best sons, and that the population was degenerating into a criminal, malingering and feeble-minded mass. Most Germans were to be valued neither as citizens nor humans. It was necessary to restore hereditary fitness to the nation, and to provide a healthy environment in which the people could recuperate. This contrasted with the political necessities of the moment, when there was a duty to take positive action. While it was possible to have a state which could provide a basis for regeneration, this was in itself not enough. It was necessary for family, friends and

---

[24] Ploetz papers, diary, 1, 16, 21 and 30 October, 9, 18, 26, 29 and 30 November 1918.
[25] *Widar Blätter*, no. 2 (February 1920).
[26] The chairman, secretary and vice-secretary were all architects; the treasurer was Lenz, and the vice-treasurer was Wollny; the 'Ordner' was Ploetz.

patriots to band together in order to resurrect the old organic forms of blood relationships. Their movement should regenerate national qualities, and restore a natural aristocracy to its pristine vigour. The statutes affirmed that as the *Bund* was to further the health, social welfare and prosperity of families, it stood above party politics. The *Widar Bund* registered with the authorities on 9 February 1923, and an inner group registered as the *Widar Ring* on 23 March 1923.[27]

Ploetz continued to cultivate relations with a small group of enthusiasts. These included the medical student, Verschuer, who while active in the *Freikorps* found occasional refuge in Ploetz's mansion.[28] Although regarded by such as Verschuer and Lenz as their *Geistiger Führer* Ploetz withdrew more and more to his estate. Here he concentrated on scientific research. Benefiting from Swiss nationality and investments, he sank his resources in an ambitious programme of scientific research. He bought expensive microscopic equipment and organized a team of assistants to help him. He investigated the effects of alcohol on heredity in mice and rabbits. His old friend, Bluhm, who became a respected geneticist in her own right, continued to supply encouragement and advice on Ploetz's grandiose schemes for genetic research. He was motivated by a concern with the loss in the war of two million of the nation's best breeding stock. For Ploetz considered that only 10 per cent of the nation were free from signs of degeneracy. He decided to study the effects of alcohol as a cause of degeneracy. By 1927 he had used nearly 5,000 rabbits in examining the effects of alcohol on vitality, growth and on the organs of dead animals. However, he found that alcohol was not as great a cause as might have been expected.[29] He hoped to solve the question of how pathological hereditary factors could be eliminated. This was to supply the empirical basis needed for legislation on racial hygiene. Ploetz was as devoted as an alchemist in his pursuit of genetics research, searching for a biological panacea to end all social ills.

Ploetz retreated from the Racial Hygiene Society, and became obsessed by his scientific quest. He secured complete control of the eugenic journal, *Archiv für Rassen- und Gesellschaftsbiologie*, and bought out his partners. On the 11 October 1918 Ploetz acquired Nordenholz's share for 100,000 marks. Thurnwald on 22 November 1919 sold his share for 20,000 marks.[30] The *Archiv* was transferred to Lehmann's publishing house. It continued to publish scientific papers, and avoided popularization. The post-war situation drove Ploetz into isolation. He was ignored by those eugenicists who saw opportunities for implementing eugenics in the welfare state. He kept aloof from Lehmann's Nordic radicalism, despite his personal sympathies for Nordic physical culture. He was anxious to maintain scientific standards, yet lacked the capacity to make any contribution to genetics. Ploetz's stance was an indication of how scientists who assumed responsibility as

---

[27] STA München Polizei Direction München 5453, 5454; *Satzung des Deutschen Widar-Bundes e.V.* and *Was will der Deutsche Widar-Bund?*

[28] O. v. Verschuer, 'Alfred Ploetz', *Der Erbarzt*, vol. 8 (1940), 69–72.

[29] Ploetz papers, MS 'Die Aufgaben der Tierzucht-Anlage des Dr Alfred Ploetz in Herrsching – Rezensried'.   [30] Ploetz papers, 22 September 1919, Thurnwald to Ploetz.

guardians of national and racial values were frustrated by adverse social and economic circumstances.

The revival of racial hygiene

During the post-war crisis the Racial Hygiene Society was virtually defunct. The core members of the original society, Ploetz and Gruber, preferred the Nordic idealism of the *Widar Bund*. By way of contrast, supporters of welfare-oriented eugenics captured influential positions within the state. By 1922 they began to salvage the remnants of the Racial Hygiene Society, which was revived as a scientific forum and as a means of infusing eugenics into welfare measures. The Society for Population Policy[31] wished to join forces with the eugenicists. It had grown faster than the Racial Hygiene Society. By 1918 it had a membership of 1,337 individuals and 188 corporations. Given that this society had semi-official status, it offered the prospect of state subsidies. The Prussian health official, Krohne, was an active supporter. The Prussian Welfare Ministry paid a 1,000 marks subsidy in 1920, and supported the idea of a combination of societies.[32] The warrior theologian, Seeberg, converted the eugenically minded scientists Baur, Gruber and Fischer to the idea of a broad eugenic front. They planned a popular eugenic journal, called 'The Coming Generation' which first appeared in November 1920.[33] Concern with future generations was to be a keynote of Weimar eugenics. The journal was sponsored by the Society for Population Policy, and later supported by the Association for Family Welfare.[34] This was a Rhineland-based organization for social welfare and had a large element of Centre Party support. It was indicative of the extent to which modern scientific approaches were to replace sentimental philanthropy in social welfare.[35] The negotiations did not proceed smoothly. The Berlin Racial Hygiene Society resented the journal, because it was to be edited by the Jesuit expert on family welfare, Hermann Muckermann. Ploetz was asked to withdraw from the editorial board although the medical official Krohne remained a member along with Seeberg, Francis Kruse and the Centre Party welfare expert Martin Fassbender. The Berliners continued their campaign for a popular journal. They wished the committee of the Racial Hygiene Society to withdraw from Muckermann's journal, and suggested a new journal to be called *Nordische Rasse*. There should be local groups established throughout the Reich, a national museum and a library.[36]

The first plenary meeting of the German Society for Racial Hygiene since the war was held on 14 and 15 October 1922 in Munich. Gruber reported that the Racial Hygiene Society had been virtually defunct since the end of 1918. He

---

[31] *Deutsche Gesellschaft für Bevölkerungspolitik.*
[32] ZSTA M Rep 76 VIII B Nr 2003 Bl. 188, 195.   [33] *Das kommende Geschlecht.*
[34] *Verein für Familienwohl.*
[35] Lenz papers, Fischer to Seeberg, 2 April 1919, 17 April 1919.
[36] The Racial Hygiene Society reconsidered the matter on 23 June 1922.

moved that the society should be transferred to Berlin. Given all the energies that the Munich group had given to extreme right-wing organizations and the *Widar Bund*, it was not surprising that the Racial Hygiene Society had been dormant. The chairmen were to be Krohne, the Prussian medical official, and the lawyer, E. Schubart, who took the lead in the campaign for marriage certificates. It meant that the society's links with the sympathetic administration in Berlin could be strengthened. Krohne moved that Gruber and Ploetz be elected honorary presidents of the society. These veterans of racial hygiene were thus promoted into retirement. The new direction was underlined when the Jesuit Muckermann joined the committee of the society. He was a force combining scientific welfare with religious zeal. That his election was twenty-one votes in favour and one against was an indication of the deep and lasting rift with Muckermann as there was intransigent opposition from the rabidly anti-Catholic Lehmann.

The move to Berlin revived the Racial Hygiene Society. A forty-one point programme was agreed in 1922. This was a social programme of remedial measures against degeneration, ranging from voluntary sterilization to eugenic education. The quality rather than the quantity of the race was stressed. Links to the state meant that subsidies for eugenics became available when Krohne took over the direction of the society. In June 1923 the Berlin Racial Hygiene Society received 50,000 marks. Yearly subsidies of between 1,500 and 2,500 marks were then granted to the society in 1927.[37] In December 1924 the society requested state funds for carrying out genealogical studies of criminals. The society continued to provide a forum for discussion of social aspects of heredity. Public lectures were designed to popularize eugenic legislation, such as that concerning marriage certificates from 1924. In September 1923 the society was admitted to the International Commission of Eugenics, signifying a step towards the rehabilitation of German eugenics.[38]

Local groups were founded. In 1922 Philaletes Kuhn, the bacteriologist, established a Dresden group. The secretary was a talented young eugenicist and doctor, Rainer Fetscher. Whereas Kuhn represented a racial approach to health, Fetscher was primarily interested in social welfare questions. He organized eugenic counselling, reinforcing welfare-oriented eugenics which later had state support. In 1923 there were groups established in Bremen and Kiel. At Kiel the impetus came primarily from university experts in hygiene and medicine, and links were established with the Schleswig Holstein Scientific Society. Lectures were held on standard topics such as family health, the laws of heredity and health certificates. The Bremen group was dominated by public health experts, and the group founded in Tübingen in 1925 also had a medical nucleus. The professor of hygiene, Kurt Wolf, was chairman. Wilhelm Weitz, the clinician and brother-in-law of Lenz, was vice-chairman, and the secretary was Wolf's pupil, Verschuer. They organized a clinic for 'scientific family advice in racial hygienic, marital and

---

[37] ZSTA M Rep 76 VIII B Nr 2073 Bl. 90, 106, 448.
[38] Ploetz papers, Leonard Darwin to Ploetz, 27 September 1923. The commission was later called the International Federation of Eugenics Organizations.

occupational matters'. The group was proud of the support from the churches.[39] Church, welfare organizations and medical men found common ground in eugenics.

The social composition of the societies show that they remained comparatively small academic groupings. In Freiburg there were thirty members in the 1920s (compared with fifty-nine before 1914). The decline in numbers reflected a defeatist spirit. In December 1918 Fischer, the anthropologist, declared that he believed in the ideal of defending the German race, but so far nothing had been achieved by the Racial Hygiene Society. His verdict was that the ideals were excellent, but the environment was hostile. Yet the society soldiered on.[40] As twenty-one of its members were medically qualified, it remained a scientific elite. A substantial number were leading scientists such as Aschoff, the pathologist. Others were socially prominent such as Hermann Paull of the *Bund der Kinderreichen*, and the ministerial official, Römer. Against the medical dominance should be set the membership of the Gobineau apostle, Schemann. The overwhelmingly medical character persisted throughout the Weimar period. In Munich in 1933 there were 119 members (compared with ninety-three in 1913). Of these, fifty-six were doctors, besides which there were others from related professions such as Plate, the biologist. The Marburg Hygiene Institute and the Bavarian associations of registry officials and for family studies were corporate members. Only eight of the doctors were members (although some carried considerable weight) of the Nazi Doctors League in Munich. There were eighteen women members. The society retained its overwhelmingly medical character.[41]

Berlin–Munich tensions

Although it was denied that there was a Munich–Berlin split, when the first general meeting was held in 1922 disagreements indicated deep tensions within the Racial Hygiene Society.[42] The rift that opened was between scientificity and social welfare on the one side, and racial ideology and authoritarian politics on the other. A welfare-oriented eugenics meant working within the political parameters of voluntarism and of the Weimar welfare state, whereas racial elitism meant opposition to republican institutions as alien constructs. The public health orientation of the Berlin society was indicated by its regular meetings in the Prussian Welfare Ministry from November 1920. These were on welfare-oriented topics such as education and heredity in February 1923. The Munich Racial Hygiene Society remained dominated by Gruber who was chairman until his death in 1927. The next professor of hygiene, Karl Kisskalt, took over as chairman of the society. Rüdin was vice-chairman from 1921 until 1933, except for his brief period in Basel. Lenz and Lehmann served terms as secretaries, and Lehmann's cousin,

---

[39] *ARGB*, vol. 17 (1925), 177–8. [40] Ploetz papers, Fischer to Ploetz, 25 December 1918.
[41] Rüdin papers, MS list. [42] *ARGB*, vol. 14 (1922), 371–5.

Bernhard Spatz, and then the latter's son, Otto Spatz, were treasurers. Ploetz was a conspicuous absentee.

The Racial Hygiene Society showed a glimmer of life when on 15 September 1921 its statutes were registered. Membership was below pre-war levels. Meetings were infrequent, money was short, and attendances were low at meetings to elect officers.

Date	Attendance
25 January 1923	7
7 January 1924	15
13 October 1924	8
19 January 1925	11
28 July 1926	12
2 January 1927	?
19 January 1928	10
31 January 1929	21

From January 1923 the Munich Racial Hygiene Society joined the *Widar Bund* in the opening of a Clinic for Biological Family Research at the Anthropological Institute. The clinic was planned by Lenz and Astel. There were also occasional lectures such as those by Rüdin on mental health and by Gruber on the 'Racial Hygienic Ideal'.[43]

The tensions of racial versus welfare eugenics surfaced in Austria. There were racial hygiene societies founded at Linz in 1923, and in Graz and Vienna (established by the anthropologist and blood group expert, Otto Reche) in 1924. The Allied measures to control nationalism meant that these societies could not affiliate to the German Racial Hygiene Society. But they adopted the statutes of the German Society, and, after combining as the *Verband der Oesterreichischen Gesellschaften für Rassenhygiene*, published news in Ploetz's *Archiv*. The nationalist racial hygienists continued to clash with socialist-oriented welfare experts. In 1919 the anatomist and socialist, Julius Tandler, disagreed with the eugenicist Kaup from the Austrian Ministry of Health over the issue of the socialization of health services. Kaup supported nationalist and Christian social policies. Tandler energetically pursued measures to improve the biological condition of the race and to restore the vigour of the 'body politic' by youth welfare and anti-tuberculosis measures. He campaigned for marriage certificates, and established a clinic for hereditary counselling with Karl Kautsky jun. in 1922.[44] But gradually, the welfare-oriented group of doctors lost ground in the state and university to racial hygiene and the right. Teleky, a pioneer of a social medicine based on economics rather than eugenics, left for Düsseldorf. His lectures on social medicine were replaced by those of the racial hygienist, Heinrich Reichel who combined with the anthropologist Otto Reche to stress race as central to public health. From 1923 the state authorities

---

[43] STA München, AG 33204 Registraturakten des Amtsgerichts München, Münchener Gesellschaft für Rassenhygiene.

[44] K. Sablik, *Julius Tandler. Mediziner und Sozialreformer* (Vienna, 1983), pp. 159–69, 275–80.

adopted the terminology of 'racial hygiene and population policy'. Vienna remained an enclave of pioneering social medicine on eugenic lines with model child health and genetic advice clinics.[45]

Of the other branches, the Bremen society was a microcosm of the tensions between the social welfare approach of health officials, and racially oriented eugenicists. The city medical officer, Hermann Tjaden, was active in pro-natalist organizations, and had been an early member of the Racial Hygiene Society. He supported the founding of the Bremen Society for Racial Hygiene in 1923, which became dominated by right-wing doctors. In 1925 a politically conservative gynaecologist, Friedrich Kirstein, had become active, and he used the society as a propaganda organization. Negative eugenics was stressed. Meetings were advertized in the Bremen medical journal on such topics as 'the extermination of western civilized races' and on the declining birth rate. Officials of the Bremen Senate declined invitations to such lectures. In February 1929 Verschuer lectured to the Medical Society on constitutional research and heredity. The links with the medical establishment were tightened when in May 1931 it became a Society for Heredity and Hereditary Welfare of the Bremen Scientific Society, having forty members. Kirstein hoped that doctors and scientists would lead a mass eugenic movement.[46]

During the 1920s the German Racial Hygiene Society and its constituent groups survived as a medical forum with nationalist tendencies. The societies continued to recruit among professionals such as doctors, scientists and teachers, but membership generally slumped below the pre-war level. It suggests that Ploetz's ideal of racial hygiene as producing a biological aristocracy had failed. The racial hygiene movement split between state-supported eugenic research institutes and welfare schemes, and Nordic racism.

Confronted by the first flare-up of Nazism and popular racism in 1919, Munich medical professors adopted a distinctive stance: *völkisch* but detached from popular politics. Figures such as Gruber, the surgeon Ferdinand Sauerbruch, the psychiatrist Kraepelin and the clinician Friedrich von Müller were very much part of the conservative circles, who were the first to be patrons of Hitler. Although the racial hygienists recognized Hitler's abilities as a potential Führer, they did not identify with his movement. Sauerbruch had a firm conviction that Germany's greatness and strength had to be defended. Early in 1919 he lectured to students on Germany's need to regain its position as world leader, and participated in *völkisch*-nationalist meetings against the Versailles Treaty. He moved in the circles of the Nazi writer Dietrich Eckart; he was acquainted with close associates of Hitler such as the rich and respected Ernst Hansfstaengel, and he met Hitler. He knew of the coming Putsch in 1923 and tended the wounded in his clinic. Yet at the time of the

---

[45] M. Hubenstorf, 'Sozialmedizin, Menschenökonomie und Volksgesundheit', in F. Kadruosk (ed.), *Aufbruch und Untergang, österreichische Kultur zwischen 1918 und 1938* (Vienna, 1981), pp. 247–66.

[46] H. Riggelsen, 'Bremer Ärzte auf dem Wege zum Nationalsozialismus. Die Problematik der Rassenhygiene und Eugenik', Diplomarbeit, Bremen, 1982.

Putsch he participated in student meetings, where it was argued that although Hitler had worthy nationalist aims, it was necessary to remain moderate. His verdict on Hitler was that he was a half-educated psychopath.[47]

Gruber took up a similar position – *völkisch*, eugenic but critical of Hitler. He suffered a mental collapse when Germany was defeated. Without an army, he believed that 'Germany was ripe for extermination'.[48] In spring 1919 when Hitler was assigned by the army to educational duties, lecturing to the troops (as well as spying on political parties), Gruber lectured to soldiers on racial hygiene as the most important aspect of *völkisch* domestic policy. His denial of a pure Germanic racial type enraged the *Völkischer Beobachter*.[49] Gruber observed Hitler as a popular lecturer at the Circus Krone in January 1923. He found Hitler's message acceptable regarding national issues such as the Versailles Treaty, and that he was an effective speaker. But he also recognized an unrealistic delusory quality in Hitler's demands about removing the yoke of foreign economic oppression. Gruber's admiration was far greater for Erich von Ludendorff, regretting his participation in the Hitler Putsch. Gruber condemned Hitler as a psychopath, and as an impure *rassischen Mischling*. This detachment was indicative of a deep distrust among the scientifically oriented racial hygienists who saw Hitler as a popular demagogue.[50] The old guard among the eugenicists were in danger of becoming isolated because of their scientific elitism. They had to choose between Weimar welfare or national opposition in order to regain a position of influence.

BIOLOGICAL POLITICS

The collapse of the imperial order created the need for enduring values and social foundations on which to reconstruct the nation. There was an outburst of visionary social philosophies. *Völkisch* prophets of doom such as Chamberlain and Spengler predicted a decline in Western civilization unless Germans drew on their cultural reserves to inspire a national rebirth. Cultures were organisms subject to natural cycles of birth, maturity, and decay, and German culture was diagnosed as in its death-throes unless it could be rejuvenated. Progressives such as Walther Rathenau, the industrialist, economic planner and politician, pointed to the need to blend industrial progress with organic national values.[51] From the left came renewed impulses for a socialist and pacifist democracy. A common element to the diverse visions was the faith in science as providing objective laws for social planning, economic prosperity and health. Yet many scientists harboured animosity towards the Republic and had visions of reviving the imperial state that

---

[47] F. Kudlien and C. Andree, 'Sauerbruch und der Nationalsozialismus', *Medizinhistorisches Journal*, vol. 15 (1980), 201–20.   [48] Lehmann papers, Lehmann to Gruber, 1 February 1923.
[49] U. Stolzing, 'Geheimrat von Gruber gegen die deutsche Rasse', *Völkischer Beobachter*, no. 25 (31 January 1926).
[50] F. Kudlien, 'Max von Gruber und die frühe Hitler-Bewegung', *Medizinhistorisches Journal*, vol. 17 (1982), 373–89.
[51] J. Herf, *Reactionary Modernism, Technology, Culture and Politics in Weimar and the Third Reich* (Cambridge, 1984), pp. 109–29.

had done so much to support science. While regaining lost territories and colonies was only a faint hope, there was an overwhelming sense that intensive cultivation of German culture and science could provide the means for improving social conditions and regenerating the nation's will to survive.

The natural sciences claimed objective authority over politics, whether left or right wing. Scientists argued for a 'human economy' that placed national welfare above profits. A rational socio-biological economy was to be introduced with improved nutrition and welfare services. Professional expertise justified scientists in instructing civil servants, politicians and the public as to what policies ought to be pursued. Scientists made bids for leading positions on expert state committees; they demanded funding for their disciplines and engaged in the popularization of nationalist forms of science. While many academics condemned socialism as culturally sterile, a few innovative scientists forged alliances with socialists. Scientists, advising on social policy, argued for state support for socially relevant research, and formulated social philosophies for a scientifically planned society. Scientists joined corporate organizations to secure funding and status. The 1920s marked the beginnings of a national science policy.

Biology and eugenics were central to this scientific movement for social reform and modernization. Biology captured the imagination of a wide variety of social groups. Ideas of the social organism were given biological rigour. Organicist social thought was modernized on the basis of Mendelian research and of other advances in human biology. Demography, medicine, plant and animal breeding and nutritional science were reformulated in line with social biology. Biologistic social philosophies appealed to critics of mechanistic rationalism and of liberal economic progress. Biology offered an opportunity of humanizing industrial society, and restoring natural values by improving the urban environment and reviving rural society. Many aspects of social thought bore imprints of biology and of organicist concepts of national unity as the antidote to class and political conflicts.

Mystic irrationalism, occultism and theosophy, which were much in vogue, could come to terms more readily with biology than with the rationalism of the physical sciences. Radical changes also occurred in the physical sciences. There was an attack on narrowly restrictive positivism. The funeral of the poet Carl Hauptmann in 1921 provided an occasion for criticism of exact natural sciences which Hauptmann in league with Ploetz had once sought to promote. The educationalist, Rudolf Steiner, accused science of being impersonal and materialist, and *Lebensphilosophie* continued to mesmerize many who were discontented with the harshness of life in defeated Germany. Physicists of progressive social views and modern literary interests were inspired by organicism, in contrast to conservatives such as Philipp Lenard and Johannes Stark who insisted on the concept of causality. Albert Einstein's theory of relativity undermined the rigid certainties of mechanistic physics and deterministic causality.[52] Biologists found that eugenics

---

[52] P. Forman, 'Weimar Culture, Causality and Quantum Theory, 1918–1927', *Historical Studies in the Physical Sciences*, vol. 3 (1971), 1–111.

offered a readily available means of extending their competence to all aspects of social and personal life. The immortality that biologists once saw as confined to the germplasm was transposed to the nation and race. Religious thinkers such as Paul Tillich saw biology as a redemptive creed starting with observation and experiment, and ending with healing and salvation. Biology became a creed of national salvation.

Defeat profoundly shocked nationalist-minded biologists. Richard Semon, the Lamarckian biologist, shot himself wrapped in the imperial flag. As Semon's ideas of inherited memory had impressed a wide range of intellectuals, his dramatic act symbolized the sense that all cultural life was on the verge of extinction. Biologists and doctors banded together in corporate associations to lobby for improved status and to mobilize support against the Treaty of Versailles. The Berlin professors Rubner and His, and the medical officer Krautwig mobilized the medical profession against the Treaty as 'causing many thousands of deaths in the German Volk'.[53] Universities were hot-beds of reaction. Faculties resisted the appointment of 'revolutionary professors'. By defending their corporate privileges, universities expressed their hostility to the Republic. Institutes flew the monarchist flag and university rectors, senates and faculties mobilized against republicanism and socialism. They turned a blind eye to the violence of right-wing students.[54]

The universities were filled with demobbed students. Still 95 per cent middle class, students polarized between a minority on the left and a vociferous right, who were anti-semitic and in favour of racial hygiene. They often remained in military uniform and relished the chance to attack the left. Their desperate extremism was heightened because students were impoverished and without career prospects. From 1922 the eugenicists Lenz in Munich, and Lothar Loeffler, Verschuer and Weitz in Tübingen organized student health services and racial surveys to cope with the disease and malnutrition of this hard-pressed *Führerschicht*.[55] Students readily banded together in corporate nationalist associations, and resisted women, Jews, Poles and socialists in university life. More extreme students took to political violence. Student volunteers in the *Freikorps* could be excessively brutal. In the wake of the Kapp Putsch in 1920, a student militia from Marburg seized fifteen workers who were beaten and shot. The rector and senate declared solidarity with the killers. Progressive intellectuals risked being beaten up or assassinated.

The fragility of the reformers' position was well shown by the case of Friedrich Nicolai, the cardiologist, who during the war had been demoted to being a nursing orderly for lecturing and writing on the *Biology of War*. This Darwinian pacifist returned to Germany and took a lead in pacifist organizations such as the *Bund*

[53] MPG, Rubner papers, Hartwich to Rubner, 12 December 1922.
[54] K. Töpner, *Gelehrte Politiker und politisierende Gelehrte. Die Revolution von 1918 im Urteil deutscher Hochschullehrer* (Göttingen, 1970).
[55] L. Loeffler, 'Allgemeine ärztliche Studentenuntersuchungen', *Mitteilungen der Gesellschaft Deutscher Naturforscher und Ärzte*, vol. 3 (1926), 35–6; Loeffler, *Ueber den Gesundheitszustand der deutschen Studentenschaft* (Göttingen, nd); O. v. Verschuer, 'Zur Frage Körperbau und Rasse', *Zeitschrift für Konstitutionslehre*, vol. 11 (1925), 754–61.

Neues Vaterland. The campaign for peace and international reconciliation had the support of only a few university professors such as Einstein, the sociologist Alfred Weber, the mathematician David Hilbert, the embryologist Driesch, and the biochemist Otto Meyerhof. Musicians, artists and writers were more enthusiastic. Nicolai's organicist social theory justified pacificism on biological grounds. When Nicolai tried to resume his post as university professor and clinician at the *Charité* hospital, he was opposed by the military authorities overseeing the *Charité* and by right-wing students. His opening lecture in January 1920 on 'Brain and Soul' occurred amidst a confrontation between the Socialist Students' Union who occupied the lecture hall, and a riotous mob of right-wing students, who claimed that the 'deserter-professor' was unfit to lecture and should not defile a German clinic. Nicolai was forced to suspend his lectures. The ultra-conservative university rector, the historian Eduard Meyer, and the senate supported the accusation that Nicolai was unworthy to be a university teacher because he had acted contrary to 'the ideal of the community as a binding social contract'. Although Nicolai protested that his opposition to the war had arisen from moral and patriotic reasons, the senate judged that he was unworthy of the rank of professor. The students were elated by their success, and finally forced Nicolai to emigrate. One of the ringleaders was the medical student, Leonardo Conti, who was to become the *Reichsgesundheitsführer* in 1939.[56]

The SPD educational policy was less radical than imagined by conservatives. The socialist, Konrad Haenisch, who was Prussian Education Minister, appealed to German students to resist the 'floods of bolshevism'. His concern for maintaining order meant that he was forced to tolerate the Marburg students' violence. He tried hard to reinstate Nicolai, but was blocked by the conservativism of the university's senate. Haenisch attempted to promote academics who would stabilize the Republic against the extremes of both left and right. Eugenicists such as Grotjahn were favoured because they were deeply hostile to left-wing socialism, and, while promising to help to improve social conditions, promoted social order with their stress on biology and family.

The ability of the sciences to salvage their prestige from the national crisis was shown by the founding of the Emergency Fund for German Science on 30 October 1920. The chemist, Fritz Haber, proclaimed that 'our existence as a nation depends on the scientific great power status, which is inseparable from our scientific organization and activities'. The president of the Fund, Schmidt-Ott, the last *Kultusminister* of Imperial Prussia, was a conservative. The Fund aimed to mobilize belligerent scientific nationalism by co-ordinating the nation's intellectual and economic resources. It served the needs of universities, academies of science, and learned societies such as the German Society of Doctors and Naturalists. It was supported by an association of industrialists and by the Reich government. Such a

---

[56] W. Zuelzer, *The Nicolai Case* (Detroit, 1982); ZSTA M Rep 76 vf Lit N Acta betr den ausserordentlichen Professor in Berlin Dr Georg Nicolai 1915–1932.

co-operative scientific organization was unprecedented. The competition between academic institutions that had prevailed in Imperial Germany was replaced by the new spirit of national co-ordination. Scientists gained the upper hand over state officials, and as a result the Emergency Fund feuded with the Prussian *Kultusministerium*. Academics were far better off with the Fund. Hitherto they had been subject to the interventionism of civil servants such as Althoff. Now they controlled specialist committees, which gave grants to individual scientists. It marked the beginning of the modern system of 'peer group review'. The committees included several for medicine and biology, and for eugenic topics like racial studies, ethnopathology and criminal biology, and (with echoes of Lehmann's Ripley scheme) for an atlas of German ethnology. Eugenics thus gained a place in the pantheon of German sciences.[57]

The geneticist Baur pressed for a national science policy. He was impressed by the agricultural research of Nilsson-Ehle in Sweden, and by Soviet and US funding of applied genetics. War work for the Navy Office had made him depressed at manpower shortages and hostile to pro-industrialist economic policies. He wished to revive German agriculture and improve conditions for the rural population. Post-war starvation hardened his resolve to apply genetics to make Germany economically and agriculturally self-sufficient. Agricultural improvements as in the production of vegetable oils and crops would augment the natural resources, and would help to raise the birth rate and prepare Germany for the next war. He typified the trend towards a planned science policy so as to make the most rational use of the nation's human and economic resources. As adviser to the Emergency Fund for German Science, he enlisted the help of the liberal-minded industrialist, Carl Bosch, and of the embryologist, Spemann, to urge the appointment of a national organizer, or Führer, to co-ordinate all scientific activity. Baur hoped such a national policy would provide remedies to the declining birth rate, food shortages, and improve agriculture. He established links with agriculturalists and his assistant, Hans Nachtsheim, who underwent a similar nationalist conversion, took a lead in public associations for breeding domestic animals such as rabbits. Hereditarian biology thus established links with the people as well as with government. Science could help Germany attain self-sufficiency, regain national self-respect and resist cosmopolitanism and mass culture.

The Rockefeller Foundation intervened from 1922 to save German medical sciences. American scientists, many of whom had trained in Germany, regarded German medicine as being of world significance. Leading scientists argued that the German universities had an international role in training researchers from all over the world. For their part the Germans pointed out that destruction of middle-class wealth and the lack of state finance meant that German science was fighting for survival. Schmidt-Ott of the Emergency Fund reported on 24 July 1922 that 'Lack

[57] B. Schroeder-Gudehus, 'The Argument for the Self-Government and Public Support of Science in Weimar Germany', *Minerva*, vol. 10 (1972), 537–70.

of courage to devote oneself to scientific pursuits is so great that workers are lacking for important scientific undertakings in every field. You will recognize that this will necessarily result in the destruction of the scientific life in Germany.' Admirers of the past glories of German *Kultur*, such as Abraham Flexner, reported that German science was on the brink of extermination. Abderhalden, the physiologist, warned Flexner that 'If the scientific activity of Germany collapses, if it fails in the matter of succession, then a perceptible regression over the whole world is bound to take place.'[58] Lenz was among those who gave evidence that the younger generation of German researchers was not only being deprived of research materials, but was literally starving. But the Foundation's New York office profoundly distrusted the universities. It argued that universities had nurtured the nationalism that had caused the war, and that the German economy had over-invested in science and learning. They decided to set up a committee of outstanding medical scientists to promote research rather than to subsidize the universities as institutions. The aim was to ensure the survival of the next generation of research workers by providing fellowships for gifted young scholars. Its secretary was the eugenicist, Heinrich Poll. He sought to divert the funds to genetics and to the neglected fringe medical specialisms. It was ironic that many in the younger generation were even more nationalistic than the older generation of liberal monarchist professors.[59]

Regenerationist biology

Biology inspired national values during a crisis when the state seemed to have lost its direction. Leading biologists reaffirmed the commitment of their science to German culture.[60] On a personal level professors had lost sons in combat, and family wealth was eroded in the inflation. Professors and their students were starving, and their institutes were starved of resources. At a time when Spengler's categories of organic destiny gripped the imagination of the scientific community, biologists offered creeds of national regeneration, combining the scientific with resonating categories of nature, life and the race. The organicist philosophy of the Berlin professor of anatomy, Oscar Hertwig, typified the sense that biologists should continue to publicize fundamental principles of social organization and development. In 1922 Hertwig depicted the state as an altruistic and humane social organism. It was a swan-song to the humane Christian welfare creed of Naumannism. Whereas during the war Hertwig argued against ultra-nationalist and selectionist Social Darwinism, now he turned on Marxism and socialism as the

---

[58] RAC 1.1/717/8/46, Schmidt-Ott to Pearce, 24 July 1922, Abderhalden to Flexner, 8 July 1922, Flexner to Vincent, 22 July 1922.
[59] P.J. Weindling, 'The Rockefeller Foundation and German Biomedical Sciences 1920–1940: From Educational Philanthropy to International Science Policy', in N. Rupke (ed.), *Science, Politics and the Public Good. Essays in Honour of Margaret Gowing* (Basingstoke, 1988), pp. 119–40.
[60] M. Verworn, *Biologische Richtlinien der staatlichen Organisation* (Bonn, 1917); Verworn, *Aphorismen* (Jena, 1922); Weindling, 'Theories of the Cell State', pp. 135–55.

enemies of national unity. He conceded that the republic needed a socialized work ethic in order to overcome industrial conflicts. The greater the division of labour, the more co-ordination by a centralized state was necessary. The state was a moral force that should combine socialism with Christian ethics. He suggested that Whitsun be transformed into a celebration of the unity of interests between employers and workers. Christmas should become a festival of love of fellow citizens. There should be a shortened working day and more hygienic working conditions. In the work-oriented *Berufsstaat*, knowledge must serve the needs of the 'human economy'. Politically, Germany should be governed by leaders who could act in the interests of the nation's general will. Such organicist utopias were a typical expression of the corporate spirit in German politics. Science provided national symbols to express social cohesion that matched the veneration of monuments of national culture, processions, festivals, and demands for charismatic leadership.[61]

The call to infuse science with the needs of the corporate state did not go unheeded. 1921 saw a momentous discovery by Spemann, the embryologist. He located the region in the embryo which, he claimed, controlled all organic form, and called this 'the Organizer'. This was a vitalistic and organicist concept, based on the idea that a particular region was endowed with superior controlling force. This is the only discovery in embryology ever to have earned a Nobel Prize. Spemann's research instigated a holistic phase of experimental embryology. Whereas Hertwig had concentrated on the formative role of individual cells, Spemann analyzed the formative role of whole regions in terms of controlling forces. A further discovery was how the eye lens was induced to form – a process described by Spemann as 'the dictatorship' of the optic cup over the lens. Spemann's work was inspired by a sense that nature was hierarchical, and form required controlling regions. At a time of national collapse, Spemann's research expressed a longing for order. Spemann was deeply nationalistic. As rector of the University of Freiburg in 1923 he led the professors in a *cortège* of homage to the coffin of Leo Schlageter, the Rhineland national resistance fighter.[62]

The organicist theories of Hertwig and Spemann had symbolic value, as they projected biology as a basis for national unity. They typified the older generation's continuing aloofness from politics. But there were others among the younger generation who sought to harness science to more direct political participation. In Tübingen, Ernst Lehmann, the botanist, was demoralized by the return of the defeated troops and he felt the Treaty of Versailles as a bitter blow. His patriotic ardour was rekindled by a march of Tübingen students to the Bismarck Tower during 1919. He joined the *Schutz- und Trutz-Bund*, the Pan-German League, and attended meetings of the embryonic Nazi Party. He praised the patriotism of full professors in the Association of German Universities.[63] As a lecturer, he was

---

[61] O. Hertwig, *Zur Abwehr des ethischen, des sozialen und des politischen Darwinismus* (Jena, 1918); Hertwig, *Der Staat als Organismus* (Jena, 1922).

[62] T. Horder and P.J. Weindling, 'Hans Spemann and the organizer', in Horder, J. Witkowski and C. Wylie (eds.), *A History of Embryology* (Cambridge, 1986), pp. 183–241.

[63] *Verband der deutschen Hochschulen.*

impressed by Julius Schaxel's manifesto to non-professors: that biology had a mission to solve the problems of public and private life. Lehmann felt that a nationalist response was needed to attempts to formulate a socialist biology. Schaxel attempted to bridge the rift between academic and popular science by modernizing Bebel's Lamarckism in a radical Trotskyist biology.[64] The Marxist threat provoked a massive campaign to rekindle nationalist values in science.

Lehmann considered that it was necessary to re-establish contact with amateur naturalists and to launch a popular movement of nationalist biology and national history. Between 1919 and 1925 a circle of academics from all faculties met to discuss the general significance of biology. This group included Edmund Mezger (a lawyer), Ernst Kretschmer (a psychiatrist whose categories on physique and character became standard), Theodor Haering (a philosopher), Heinrich Prell (a biologist specializing in forestry), Philaletes Kuhn (the hygienist), and Kolbenheyer (the zoologist, author and Paracelsian researcher). They were unified by an enthusiasm for popularizing a nationally oriented biology. They formed the nucleus for Lehmann's *Biologenverband*, and for a popular journal.[65]

The politicization of Haeckel's monistic legacy can be illustrated by conflicts at the university of Jena. Haeckel's successor, Plate, (who was a founder member of the Racial Hygiene Society) was active in the Pan-German League and conservative politics. He became the leader of a monarchist political faction. Schaxel, although especially close to Haeckel in his final years, joined the SPD in 1918. Plate and the professor of hygiene, Abel, organized counter-revolutionary demonstrations in 1919, and the Mendelian botanist Otto Renner was another vociferous conservative. From a podium draped with the monarchist black, white and red flag, they gave anti-socialist and anti-semitic speeches. They supported the Kapp Putsch in 1920, and Plate was taken into protective custody.[66]

Schaxel plunged into socialist politics as he pioneered a Marxist biology. Although he had been a pupil of the nationalists, Haeckel, Richard Hertwig and Plate, he harnessed developmental biology to dialectical materialism. In 1918 he established an Institute for Experimental Biology for research into the causal determinants of animal form, by such means as transplant experiments. Schaxel campaigned for a democratic university which was to infuse a socialist spirit into society and create a socialist-minded people. He formed the 'Coalition of Republican Professors' after the assassination of Rathenau in 1922. At the time of the socialist and communist coalition in Thuringia, between 1922–24, he took a leading political role in the government which initiated such radical schemes as sponsorship of *Bauhaus* architecture.[67] When the left lost power, he supported in 1924 the *Urania* organization for proletarian science. This challenged the right-wing *Kosmos* movement for popularizing science, and arose from Schaxel's

---

[64] L. Poliakov and J. Wulf, *Das Dritte Reich und seine Denker* (Frankfurt-on-Main, 1983), pp. 421–4.
[65] BDC Lehmann file, Lecture on Heimatbiologie 1944.
[66] M. Steinmetz, *Geschichte der Universität Jena* (Jena, 1958), vol. 1, pp. 542–5.
[67] B. Miller Lane, *Architecture and Politics in Germany 1918–1940* (Cambridge, 1968), pp. 69–76.

involvement in free thought organizations. He established a popular science journal, and lectured to publicize socialist science and biology. The local KPD Secretary, Walter Ulbricht, retained a lasting affection for monist biology. From 1925 Schaxel cultivated contacts with the USSR. Schaxel sought to establish a theory of development based on successive acts of historical formation when ontogenetic and environmental forces interacted. Far from a naive reductionist, Schaxel tried to combine the psychology of individual perception with a materialist philosophy of life. There was a continual process of historical change in nature. Heredity meant the production of ever-new combinations of genetic material. He was among the few biologists who were critics of racial science, and condemned *völkisch* demands for racial purity.[68]

There was only a minority camp of liberal democrats among university professors prepared to support the Republic. While hostile to *völkisch* racism, they still perceived the social order in organicist terms. Noted exponents of organicism were Willy Hellpach, the Baden DDP leader and psychologist, and the eugenicists Robert Gaupp and Abderhalden. Others such as Eugen Fischer fluctuated between acceptance and rejection of the Republic.[69] The liberal tradition of organicism lived on in the work of Driesch, the embryologist and philosopher. He was the leading advocate of vitalist organism and of holistic theories, and was an enthusiastic liberal-democrat and pacifist. He rejected racism and imperialism, and believed in the necessity of a world state. The year 1919 was a turning-point for Driesch as he enthusiastically entered into public life, and lectured incessantly on human rights issues. He rallied to the defence of other liberal professors such as the philosopher Theodor Lessing, who was under attack from right-wing students. He rejected force and dictatorship as immoral and culturally damaging. Driesch justified democratic ethics on the basis of holistic vitalism. He argued that there was an ethical imperative to combat nationalism, racism and anti-semitism.[70]

Geneticists became preoccupied with the shortage of funds, and the distressed condition of Germany. This can be seen in the tone of their work and in their research aims. Many geneticists distanced themselves from the Amercian concern with the chromosomes as the carriers of Mendelian genes. This sort of work represented a modern type of rational and mechanistic science of which there was a profound distrust. Instead, German geneticists examined the cytoplasm surrounding the nucleus, and several continued to investigate Lamarckian environmentalism. The scornful attitude to chromosomes was shown by their characterization of this as a *Kernmonopol* (nuclear monopoly) theory. This term echoed academic dislike of US capitalist trusts. Some compared the cell to an army, the plasma to the mass of soldiers and the genom to the general staff. Correns compared hereditary units to machine gun bullets. Other geneticists were concerned with how the natural vigour of populations in the wild was sustained.

[68] J. Schaxel, *Entwicklung der Wissenschaft vom Leben* (Jena, 1924).
[69] H. Döring, *Der Weimarer Kreis* (Meisenheim on Glan, 1975).
[70] R. Mocek, *Wilhelm Roux – Hans Driesch* (Jena, 1974), pp. 131–9.

This was very different from US laboratory confined·research.[71] German geneticists wished to know more about the active physiological role of genes in development. German genetics of the 1920s can thus be seen as shaped by a distinctive set of nationalist and scientific values in a search for a dynamic morphology.

Geneticists remained committed to a broader philosophical biology. Many were inspired by Max Hartmann's search for a rigorous philosophy that would reveal the formative powers among organisms; an example was the law of bi-sexual polarity.[72] Demands for greater social outlets for their work were frustrated by lack of resources. The only institute for pure genetic research was the Kaiser Wilhelm Institute for Biology. Its geneticists, Correns and Goldschmidt, had to share facilities with embryologists, biochemists such as Otto Warburg and protozoa specialists such as Hartmann. Other geneticists such as Baur and Haecker worked in agricultural training colleges. After the war, geneticists made a determined effort to improve their working conditions, and in 1920 founded a Society for Hereditary Science, obtaining support in the Prussian state and *Landtag*. Baur established an agricultural research station at Müncheberg in 1923, and Haecker obtained a university post at Halle, although many geneticists remained in 'applied' settings such as medical or agricultural institutions. Genetics fitted the criteria of being an exact science. Rapid US and Soviet advances convinced the Germans that there was an especial need to nurture this novel science of immense practical relevance. Nationalist preoccupations meant that there was a strong bond between eugenicists and genetics so that in many cases the two spheres were indistinguishable. Leading geneticists such as Baur, Haecker, Goldschmidt, Nachtsheim and Poll were sympathetic to eugenics. They cultivated links with eugenicists, as can be seen in the membership of the German Society for Hereditary Science.[73] Its members included Behr-Pinnow, Bluhm, Crzellitzer, Fetscher, Fischer, Lenz, Muckermann, Plate, Ploetz and Rüdin, as well as radical reformers such as Hirschfeld and Schaxel. The links between genetics and eugenics were apparent when Richard von Hertwig, Germany's most eminent zoologist and the mentor of many geneticists, contributed a foreword to the Festschrift for his 'dear friend' Ploetz.[74]

Geneticists were preoccupied with the pathological effects of war. They debated whether its physical and psychological effects could be inherited, causing lasting

[71] J. Harwood, 'The Reception of Morgan's Chromosome Theory in Germany: Inter-War Debate over Cytoplasmic Inheritance', *Medizinhistorisches Journal*, vol. 19 (1984), 3–32; Harwood, 'Geneticists and the Evolutionary Synthesis in Inter-War Germany', *Annals of Science*, vol. 42 (1985), 279–301; J. Harwood, 'National Styles in Science: Genetics in Germany and the United States between the World Wars', *Isis*, vol. 78 (1987), 390–414.

[72] H. Nachtsheim, 'Max Hartmann†', *Sitzungsberichte der Gesellschaft Naturforschender Freunde zu Berlin*, n.s. vol. 3 (1962), 14–20.

[73] 'Deutsche Gesellschaft für Vererbungswissenschaft', *Bericht über die sechste Jahresversammlung in Hamburg* (Leipzig, 1929), pp. 108–18.

[74] R. von Hertwig, 'Sympathiebrief', *ARGB*, vol. 24 (1930), xvi–xvii.

damage to the hereditary germplasm. Lenz argued that the effects of war were environmental and could never be inherited. Lamarckism raised the question of the inheritance of such defects. But the Lamarckian geneticist, Haecker, pointed to botanical examples of species which had shown the capacity for regeneration. While domestication could have degenerative effects, Haecker believed in spontaneous regeneration. He implied that nature was a regulatory force which could maintain and rejuvenate the nation.[75] Baur was more pessimistic. In 1920 he addressed the Prussian Racial Hygiene Committee of the Welfare Ministry on the problem of emigration. He considered the nation's regenerative powers were limited. Each permanent loss caused by underfertility and mass emigration, lessened the capacity of the *Volk* to produce natural leaders. The emigrant represented the fit, healthy and enterprising type, whereas the weak and chronically ill remained at home.[76] Geneticists were convinced of the importance of their work for rebuilding the damaged biological fabric of the German race, and frequently lectured on eugenics. For example, in 1923 Haecker lectured on human racial and family research. His lectures on agriculture were attended by Walther Darré, the budding Nazi and advocate of the regeneration of the peasantry. Virtually all textbooks on genetics discussed eugenics. Recognizing the lack of an adequate scientific basis for sterilization and eugenic legislation, Haecker and Richard von Hertwig venerated eugenics as a nationalist religion. Their position was that eugenic aims were desirable but more research was necessary. Geneticists clamoured for greater state subsidies for research.[77]

By far the most striking example of the concern with applied hereditary science was the textbook on human heredity by Baur, the anthropologist Fischer, and Lenz. Its joint authorship symbolized the spirit of co-operation among Weimar biologists. It was published in 1921 by Lehmann, who had long planned such a eugenic textbook as a result of discussions between Ploetz and Lenz during 1913.[78] An enlarged edition appeared in 1923. It provided an extensive survey of genetics, human racial variation, and inherited physical and mental diseases. Its second volume was a study of human selection by Lenz. The introduction emphasized how science could explain the rise and fall of civilizations, and provide cures for 'diseases in the body politic' and a solid scientific basis for population policy and racial hygiene. The book was also prescriptive. It recommended genetic counselling, a minimum of three children for those deemed fit, and the avoidance of alcohol and tobacco. Parents, doctors, teachers and priests should combine in instilling racial hygienic principles into children, who were to learn that they were a subordinate part of a great racial organism.[79]

[75] V. Haecker, 'Die Annahme einer erblichen Übertragung körperlicher Kriegschäden', *Archiv für Frauenkunde*, vol. 4 (1920), 1–15.

[76] E. Baur, 'Die biologische Bedeutung der Auswanderung für Deutschland', *Archiv für Frauenkunde und Eugenetik*, vol. 7 (1921), 206–8.

[77] V. Haecker, *Allgemeine Vererbungslehre* (Braunschweig, 1921).

[78] Ploetz papers, diary, 14 August 1913.

[79] E. Baur, E. Fischer and F. Lenz, *Grundriss der menschlichen Erblichkeitslehre und Rassenhygiene* (Munich, 1921).

The Mendelian basis for eugenics was rejected by Lamarckian biologists such as Paul Kammerer. He was an Austrian socialist, who sensationally committed suicide in 1926, after being accused of faking the evidence for species transformation in the midwife toad. He rejected Darwinism and selectionism as typifying the conservative and bourgeois nature of racial theories. It was mistaken to see the extermination of the weak and poor by sterilization, incarceration and immigration controls as the only way to rid society of degenerates. Instead a healthy and fit society could be achieved by improving social conditions, nutrition and education. The mutual aid of socialism could therefore benefit future generations. This amounted to a socialist programme for positive eugenics. Physical exercise could be productive eugenic work. It would be possible to eliminate all racial defects and criminality. Social challenges required new characteristics. He supported the League for the Protection of Mothers and Sexual Reform. With Eugen Steinach, the surgeon, Kammerer researched on transplanting animal glands for the purpose of rejuvenation, hoping to further peace and progress.[80] Kammerer shows how critics of racial hygiene were themselves working from biological premisses.[81] His reformist views were akin to those of a good many social hygienists like Grotjahn and Tandler. Few were the critics of racial hygiene who were not in some way eugenicists or committed to biologistic solutions for social problems. Despite great differences between eugenicists such as Grotjahn and Lenz, they unanimously urged the nation to adapt to the dictates of 'biological politics'.[82]

New disciplines

University reform was considered a key piece of social engineering. Radicals regarded university professors as a privileged elite, clinging to monarchism. Most professors looked back longingly to the Kaiserreich, when there had been lavish university funding. Professors considered that their role as culture bearers was crucial if Germany was to survive the crisis of defeat and plebeian disorder. Reformers wished to create a more democratic structure within the universities, and to modernize the curriculum by introducing socially relevant sciences. Conflicts arose between defenders of an elite but restricted intellectual order, and the avant-garde proponents of new specialisms.

The collapse of the monarchy was the signal for the introduction of a range of university reforms. There were academic experiments in most fields, as disciplines such as psychology and sociology emancipated themselves from the tutelage of traditional subjects such as philosophy and law. Medical faculties were arenas of social conflict. In Imperial Germany professors had resisted specialisms which lacked a basis in experimental science, and which did not deal with the body as a whole. This meant that the development of disciplines such as dermatology and

[80] P. Kammerer, 'Produktive Eugenik', *Die Neue Generation*, vol. 20 (1924), 161–6; H. Stöcker, 'Prof. Dr Paul Kammerer, Wien', *Die Neue Generation*, vol. 22 (1926), 263–5.
[81] P. Kammerer, *Das Rätsel der Vererbung* (Berlin, 1925), p. 144.
[82] R. Fetscher, 'Biologische Politik', *Dresdener Neueste Nachrichten*, (1 August 1924).

paediatrics was restricted. There was a rapid increase in appointments in socially relevant specialisms in the turbulent post-war years. Sixteen out of thirty universities first established chairs of dermatology between 1918 and 1922. Fifteen universities founded chairs of paediatrics and of dentistry between 1919 and 1921, and in 1919 there were three new chairs of ear, nose and throat medicine.[83] Appointments in social medicine, racial hygiene and in a range of related specialisms meant that eugenics marched into the university curriculum.

The intellectual and social turmoil in university life was exemplified by the universities of Berlin and Munich, for they were also centres of political upheaval. Appointments at Berlin aroused strong animosities as the university, having established itself as a privileged elite under the Hohenzollerns, resisted the democratic order. There were radical suggestions for chairs of sexual hygiene, social hygiene, medical insurance, nature therapy, medical psychology and psycho-analysis. The disputes had precedents in Imperial Germany when there was much difficulty over the intervention of the state as violating traditions of academic freedom, although the state had managed to force the medical faculty to accept certain specialisms. In Berlin this had occurred for hygiene, dermatology, paediatrics, and ear, nose and throat. But, if the proportion of full professors to other appointments is considered, the medical faculty became more elitist between 1900 and 1914.[84]

Berlin social hygiene

From November 1918 the SPD attempted to force the Berlin medical faculty to accept a range of new disciplines. Priorities were socially relevant medical specialisms, population policy and nature therapy. The Prussian Assembly in May 1919 supported a motion of the USPD socialist, *Lebensreformer* and doctor, Hermann Weyl, demanding chairs in homoeopathy, physical therapy and social hygiene in all universities. Haenisch, the Prussian Minister for Science, Art and Education, forced an outraged medical faculty to accept the appointment of the tuberculosis researcher Friedrich Franz Friedmann as assistant professor. He had developed an unconventional turtle serum for TB. The proposal of the chair for 'biological therapy' was popular but stubbornly opposed by the faculty. Haenisch was an ardent supporter of nature therapy, and in 1920 suggested three possible candidates. All were rejected as unqualified by the faculty. The faculty protested that although previous Prussian ministers had sympathies for lay 'quackery', they had still dutifully upheld objective scientific standards. In April 1920 the minister appointed Franz Schönenberger who was well connected in socialist circles. As Schönenberger was a qualified doctor, this marked a concession to the faculty,[85]

[83] Eulner, *Entwicklung medizinischer Spezialfächer*. A defect of Eulner's approach is to ignore 'fringe disciplines' as nature therapy or racial hygiene.
[84] Weindling, 'Theories of the Cell State', pp. 146–8.
[85] ZSTA M Rep 76 Va Sekt 2 Tit IV Nr 46 Bd 21.

and the fulfilment of the wishes of nature therapists for a chair for the scientific basis of therapy and for educating doctors in alternative therapies. Schönenberger was editor of the leading journal, *Der Naturarzt*, and his appointment aroused great expectations that at last the academic bastions of scientific medicine had been penetrated by a radical reformer.[86]

The concern with population policy stimulated demands for chairs of social and sexual hygiene. In December 1918, the state intended appointing a professor for sexual hygiene, and considered the socialist sympathizer (and eugenicist), Blaschko, in order to impress on the medical faculty the importance of population policy. The indignant faculty replied that apart from Blaschko's lack of scientific distinction, he lacked moral standards. They were outraged that he had suggested that there would be less prostitution, if, like the proletariat, the middle class engaged in pre-marital sexual intercourse. The faculty distorted Blaschko's opinion, that earlier middle-class marriage would reduce prostitution.[87] The broad support for population policies opened the doors to sexual reformers and eugenicists. For example, in 1922 ministerial pressure was exerted on the Berlin medical faculty to appoint the social gynaecologist, Liepmann, for teaching sexual psychology, and Hirsch for teaching social gynaecology. Hirsch took an intermediary position between social and racial hygiene, whereas ,Liepmann emphasized the psychological and psychosomatic aspects of disease. In 1921 Liepmann obtained a chair (Extraordinarius) in gynaecology, but it was only in 1929 that Liepmann was granted the teaching post in social gynaecology, and the opposition of the faculty was overcome.[88]

While racial hygiene found its patrons on the right, social hygiene threw in its lot with the rising tide of socialism. Grotjahn viewed Germany's defeat with equanimity. He rejected Pan-Germanist expansionism, and Nordic racism, but intensely believed that those peoples with German racial elements were born cultural leaders. His return to scientific pursuits thus had a nationalist rationale. Moreover, the declining birth rate induced a sense of mission into social hygienists.[89] Grotjahn opportunely joined the MSPD. At the same time the Berlin professor of hygiene, Flügge, pressed for a Seminar for Social Hygiene to be established. They had to overcome the conservatism of the medical faculty: the physiologist Rubner opposed the division of hygiene as an academic discipline. While Flügge dealt with the faculty, Grotjahn negotiated directly with the MSPD Minister of Education, Konrad Haenisch and with the under-secretary Carl Becker. On 10 April 1919 Grotjahn contacted Becker, expressing the hope that a

---

[86] K. Körberle, 'Zur Kontroverse zwischen Schulmedizin und Naturheillehre vor dem Hintergrund der Entwicklung der Hydrotherapeutischen Anstalt der Universität Berlin', *Wissenschaftliche Zeitschrift der Humboldt-Universität zu Berlin*, math.-nat. R, vol. 28 (1979), 309–15.

[87] ZSTA M Rep 76 Va Sekt 2 Tit IV Nr 46 Bd 21 Bl. 268; Bd 34 Bl. 33–5.

[88] P. Schneck, 'Wilhelm Liepmann (1878–1939) und die soziale Gynäkologie im Spiegel der Aktenbestände des Archivs der Humboldt-Universität zu Berlin', *NTM*, vol. 17 (1980),102–20; V.C. Grabke, 'Wilhelm Liepmann als sozialer Gynäkologe', med. Diss. FU Berlin 1969.

[89] Grotjahn, *Erlebtes*, p. 190.

Department of Social Hygiene could be established since it was necessary for rebuilding the physical strength and numbers of the population. It should link hygiene with statistics and social sciences.[90] It was to provide a scientific basis for public campaigns so that the state and municipalities could institute social hygienic welfare centres.[91]

To secure his appointment, Grotjahn pulled strings through the Prussian Finance Minister, Albert Südekum, who was a long-standing friend. To Ministerial Director Naumann, he emphasized that there was a strong demand for social hygiene among students, and that on 23 May 1919 the Committee for Population Policy had supported Abderhalden's demand for chairs of social hygiene. When Haenisch wrote to Südekum on 26 August 1919 requesting that funds be made available for the chair, he stressed how important it was that the coming generation of medical students be taught medical statistics and racial hygiene.[92] On 2 May and 9 July 1919 the minister requested the medical faculty to establish a chair of social hygiene. The faculty considered the possibilities: Gottstein was too old; Alfons Fischer had literary abilities but lacked scientific distinction; three young lecturers in hygiene (Hermann Dold in Halle, Ernst Gerhard Dresel in Heidelberg, and Joetten in Leipzig) had to first prove their abilities in experimental hygiene. In the event only Kaup and Grotjahn were suitable. But Kaup was regarded as a poor teacher and he held untenable political views. Grotjahn had published extensively, but his research had been limited to the problem of alcoholism.[93] For sixteen months the faculty resisted. Their stand was reinforced by an association[94] of professors of hygiene. The conservative Rubner, a long-standing opponent of social hygiene and eugenics, was dean of the faculty, and the pathologist Lubarsch, an ultra-conservative DNVP supporter, was also opposed. On 29 April the minister informed the faculty that a chair of social hygiene was to be established. The faculty continued to hope for a sweeping political change that could oust the socialist administration. On 19 May 1920 Grotjahn appealed to Haenisch, when the faculty refused to establish the chair. On 21 May Südekum, the Finance Minister, intervened, with Haenisch saying that Grotjahn was *sehr unglücklich* (very unhappy) that there had to be another election when they had initially accepted him. Despite continued protests, Grotjahn was appointed professor by the ministry on 14 June 1920.[95]

Grotjahn's appointment paved the way for further developments in social hygiene and eugenics. In 1922 Flügge was succeeded by Hahn, who combined bacteriology with an interest in social hygiene, including eugenics. Hahn and Grotjahn persuaded the ministry to appoint a medical statistician because of the priority of the declining birth rate.[96] Another branch of social hygiene which it

[90] ZSTA M Rep 76 Va Sekt 2 Tit IV Nr 16 Bd 22 Bl. 60–1.
[91] *sozialhygienische Zentralstellen.*
[92] ZSTA M Rep 76 Va Sekt 2 Tit IV Nr 16 Bd 22 Bl. 113.
[93] ZSTA M Rep 76 Va Sekt 2 Tit IV Nr 16 Bd 22 Bl. 102–5.
[94] *Fachgemeinschaft.*   [95] ZSTA M Rep 76 Va Sekt 2 Tit IV Nr 16 Bd 22 Bl. 399.
[96] ZSTA M Rep 76 VIII a Sekt 2 Tit X Nr 83 Bd 19 Bl. 268, 276, 308.

was hoped to establish in Berlin was occupational medicine. Flügge's assistant, Korff-Petersen, had lectured on occupational hygiene since 1919. In 1921 the Reich Minister of Labour pressed for a chair for the Bavarian, Franz Koelsch. Flügge suggested that it might be feasible to establish an independent institute for social and occupational hygiene under Koelsch and Grotjahn.[97] The resistance to social hygiene was typical of the opposition to other specialisms like dentistry or Pavlovian experimental psychology. By 1921 the old guard felt sufficiently confident to take a stand. The senate protested against any more 'technical professors in specialized disciplines because this contradicted the essence of the University'.[98]

The appointment of Grotjahn meant that eugenics succeeded in infiltrating the medical curriculum. Since 1914 Grotjahn had lectured on social hygiene and eugenics. His course on social hygiene from 1919 was divided into a first part where TB, alcoholism and nutrition were discussed, and a second part on the social hygiene of mother and child, the declining birth rate and eugenics. These lectures were complemented by courses on heredity by Poll, whom the medical faculty supported for a teaching post in heredity. This was not surprising given that conservatives were campaigning for chairs of genetics. In 1921 and 1922 he lectured on heredity and eugenics, and in 1923 on the biology of genius, talent and feeble-mindedness.[99] Berlin exemplified how MSPD politics and the conservatism of the university helped rather than hindered the teaching of eugenics.

Munich racial hygiene

In contrast to the moderate reformism of Berlin, the university of Munich remained a bastion of conservatism. It was as a result of the conservative nationalism of Gruber that new teaching posts established eugenics and racial hygiene as integral to medicine. In Munich the two hotbeds of racial hygiene were Gruber's Institute of Hygiene, and the German Psychiatric Institute. At the university Lenz came into conflict with Kaup, as a result of a difference of approach between the biological, or the economic as a basis of eugenics. On 11 June 1919 Lenz was appointed *Privatdozent* with the aim of teaching social and racial hygiene (which he deemed equivalent). He gave courses on medical statistics and reproductive hygiene, and on elementary health (based on gymnastics, games, sport and school health). After a traumatic time in the Austrian Office of Social Hygiene, Kaup took refuge at Gruber's institute. Kaup was concerned with toxicology and the socio-economic aspects of hygiene as a means of racial betterment, whereas Lenz's main interests were selection and the genetic basis of diseases and disabilities. In December 1921 Kaup argued with Lenz shortly before the former was to lecture to the Munich Society for Racial Hygiene. From January

[97] ZSTA M Rep 76 Va Sekt 2 Tit IV Nr 46 Bl. 139–45.
[98] ZSTA M Rep 76 Va Sekt 2 Tit IV Nr 46 Bl. 156.
[99] ZSTA M Rep 76 Va Sekt 2 Sekt 2 Tit IV Nr 46 Bl. 517.

1922 Kaup began to criticize racial hygiene from the perspectives of social hygiene, and argued against Lenz's combination of Mendelism and Nordic racism. He considered that Lenz was unrealistic in his plans for selective racial hygiene based on a belief in the potential for evolutionary improvement of the Nordic race. Kaup could not accept Lenz's demands for only selective social welfare benefits, and his belief in the futility of measures to improve the physical well-being of a population. Kaup had a Lamarckian approach to heredity, believing that welfare and exercise would benefit future generations. He attempted to combine Grotjahn's social hygiene and the eugenic views of Schallmayer by arguing for non-selective welfare benefits. He called this programme 'National Hygiene'.[100] Kaup's hostility to Lenz alienated Gruber. When Lenz was appointed Germany's first professor of racial hygiene on 1 April 1923 (although at the lower level of Extraordinarius), the tensions worsened. Kaup criticized as utopian Lenz's 'selectionist fantasies' and his belief in the possibility of breeding a noble super-race, and he considered Lenz's view that Germany was composed of three races to be mistaken.[101] Racial hygiene was thus divided over questions of methodology, analysis of current conditions, and expectations of future developments. Gruber retired from the chair of hygiene in 1923. Kaup had been led to expect that he would succeed Gruber in the chair of hygiene, but this did not occur. Whereas Kaup had long co-operated with social hygienists such as Grotjahn, Lenz turned against economic approaches to social hygiene on the grounds that they were 'Jewish'. From October 1924 there were public arguments between Kaup and Gruber. Kaup accused Gruber of blocking his career and of withholding his salary.[102] Gruber demanded that Kaup be disciplined by the Education Ministry.[103] On retiring, Gruber was hailed as 'the German doctors' true Führer', and in 1924 he was elected President of the Bavarian Academy of Sciences. In 1925 Karl Kisskalt was appointed professor of hygiene, and he combined racial and constitutional hygiene with bacteriology.[104]

The other major initiative in Munich was the founding of the German Psychiatric Research Institute in April 1918 by Kraepelin. Rüdin was appointed as head of a Genealogical Department. Before the war the Kaiser Wilhelm Gesellschaft (KWG) had rejected the idea of a research institute combined with a hospital. Kraepelin argued that a hospital was equivalent to a laboratory. American funding for eugenic research was also a model. The concern with war injuries, social disorders and nervous strain of troops and armies at the end of the war combined to favour the establishing of the Institute.[105] Institute reports denounced the 'murderous peace' as threatening the existence of a highly gifted elite, and

[100] I. Kaup, *Volkshygiene oder selektive Rassenhygiene?* (Leipzig, 1922).
[101] BHSTA Mk 35575 Fritz Lenz; Mk 35522 Ignaz Kaup; Munich University Archives, personal files on Gruber, Kaup and Lenz.
[102] I. Kaup, 'Nochmals Darwinismus und Rassenhygiene', *Münchener Neueste Nachrichten*, (4 November 1925).   [103] BHSTA Mk 17704 Gruber, Max.
[104] Munich University Archives, files on the Institute of Hygiene.
[105] E. Kraepelin, 'Ein Forschungsinstitut für Psychiatrie', *Zeitschrift für gesamte Neurologie und Psychologie*, vol. 32 (1915), 1–38.

stressed the practical relevance of research on the decline of alcohol consumption, syphilis, the family background of mental illness, and occupational psychology.[106] James Loeb (an American expatriate and patron of classical art and literature – immortalized by the Loeb editions of classical texts) gave generously. So too did Gustav Krupp von Bohlen und Halbach. It was only in 1924 that the KWG and the Bavarian state took over responsibility for the institute. Rüdin and, from 1924, Hans Luxenburger developed a eugenically based demography in order to establish the genetic patterns for inherited diseases. Rüdin conflicted with clinical approaches to psychiatry at Oswald Bumke's university clinic and with laboratory studies of nerve structure as a basis of mental illness.[107]

Eugenics profited from the atmosphere of political crisis. It had an appeal to both the left and right. Its scientificity offered an apparently objective basis for the solution of social problems. Eugenicists courted both the ultra-right – as in the case of Gruber in Munich – and the left, as Grotjahn's opportune entry into the MSPD shows. Eugenics was attractive to a broad range of medical specialisms such as hygiene and psychiatry, to biologists, to anthropologists and social scientists. It gave them a means of arguing for the social relevance of their disciplines, and fitted the mood of the times with the yearning for social order based on secure natural values.

Institutionalizing eugenics

Political parties supported demands for the teaching of eugenics. The DNVP petitioned on 18 February 1922 in the Prussian Assembly for the teaching of heredity as a specialized science in medical faculties.[108] The Prussian Committee on Racial Hygiene demanded more research on heredity and genetics. In 1922 the medical students' league[109] called for emphasis on racial hygiene as of vital importance for the future of the race and nation. University courses and a national institute had been long-standing demands of the Racial Hygiene Societies. The textbook of eugenics of Baur, Fischer and Lenz called for racial hygiene to be a compulsory subject in all German medical schools. This aim was restated by the German Racial Hygiene Society in October 1922.[110]

Racial hygiene and eugenics were introduced in a variety of guises. There were lectures on racial, social and sexual hygiene, human heredity and genetics, psychiatry, family research, European or German racial studies, and in demography. The lecture lists of German universities show that most eugenic lectures were provided for medical students, rather than for students of all faculties. Well over

---

[106] 'Zweiter Bericht über die Deutsche Forschungsanstalt für Psychiatrie in München zur Stiftungs- ratssitzung am 30. April 1921'.
[107] E. Rüdin, 'Familienforschung und Psychiatrie', *Die Naturwissenschaften*, vol. 9 (1921), 713–21.
[108] *Preussischer Landtag*, 1921/22, Drucksache Nr 2077, 18 February 1922 p. 2,433; *Preussischer Landtag* (21 February 1922), p. 7,333. [109] *Verband Deutscher Medizinerschaften*.
[110] F. Lenz, *Menschliche Auslese und Rassenhygiene* (Munich, 1921), pp. 216–22.

half of the lectures were given by specialists in hygiene. Increasing numbers of eugenics lectures were held by anatomists, anthropologists, and psychiatrists. Other lectures with a eugenic content were given by biologists and clinicians, as well as by historians and theologians, but these represented a far smaller percentage. Numbers of lectures each year rose rapidly between 1919 and 1924 when a high point was reached, to be exceeded only in 1932. These findings confirm the overwhelming medical dominance in the field of eugenics with a particular stress on public health and chronic diseases.[111]

Professors of hygiene were among the most active eugenicists. Courses began in the turbulent years between 1918 and 1920 and were generally repeated yearly (see table 6).

A national institute for research into human heredity was a long-standing aim of eugenicists. It had been suggested to the Kaiser Wilhelm Gesellschaft and by Gruber to the *Zentralstelle für Volkswohlfahrt* before the war, and scientists such as Abderhalden pressed for this at the Prussian Assembly and at the state Committee for Racial Hygiene. The Reich Ministry of the Interior discussed the planned institute in January 1923. The scheme was supported by the Prussian Ministries of Education and of Welfare. Family research conducted by doctors and anthropologists was to be a priority. The spokesmen for the Prussian Medical Committee on Racial Hygiene (Baur, Goldschmidt, von Luschan and the medical statistician, Roesle) pointed out that Great Britain, Sweden, Switzerland and the United States already had such institutes. A wide range of problems such as cancer, TB, mental diseases, and crime were to be investigated urgently, and a survey of the racial composition of Germany was to be launched. Another plan involved departments for cell biology, genealogy, racial anthropology, hereditary diseases and biological constitutions, and medical statistics. The Reich authorities decided that such an institute could not be established for the moment, but they promised to make funds available for posts in human heredity. They emphasized that it was necessary to co-ordinate hereditarian and demographic research.[112]

Underlying the fragmented initiatives of eugenicists was an ambitious plan for social reorganization. Co-ordinating research, establishing new appointments and institutes, and making eugenics part of the training for a rising generation of professionals were only preliminaries. The fruits of eugenic education and research were to feed and fortify all aspects of daily life, giving the nation renewed corporate identity and purpose. The aims and methods were scientific, but the crisis of defeat had transformed the nature of science.

Welfare eugenics

In response to the disintegration of the social order in 1918, medical officials pressed for draconian measures. They feared the effects of epidemic and chronic diseases,

[111] M. Günther, 'Die Institutionalisierung der Rassenhygiene an den deutschen Hochschulen vor 1933', med. Diss. Mainz, 1982.
[112] BAK R 86 Nr 2371 Bl. 196–9, 236–9; ZSTA P 15.01 Nr 9421.

Table 6. *University Lectures in racial hygiene, 1918–1920*[113]

Year	University	Professor	Title of lectures
1918	Göttingen	Rosenthal	National health care (social and racial hygiene)
	Berlin	Grotjahn	Racial hygiene and eugenics
1919	Freiburg	Fischer	Social anthropology
	Freiburg	Nissle	Social hygiene, including racial hygiene
	Halle	Drigalski	Social hygiene, politics, biology
	Heidelberg	Dresel	Social hygiene, including racial hygiene
	Leipzig	Döllken	Racial hygiene and criminal psychology
	Munich	Lenz	Social hygiene and racial hygiene
	Tübingen	P. Kuhn	Racial hygiene
1920	Dresden	P. Kuhn	Sexual, racial and social hygiene
	Giessen	Huntemüller	Heredity and racial hygiene
	Halle	Anton	Racial welfare and heredity
	Kiel	Kisskalt	Racial hygiene
	Cologne	Müller	Hygiene, including heredity
	Rostock	Reiter	Population policy, including race
	Tübingen	Basler	Racial physiology

sexual excesses,and a rise in mental disorders. The collapse of the political order was matched by a breakdown of the peoples' physical constitution. The nation seemed to be on the brink of racial extermination. The remedy advocated by medical officials was extensive medical controls. Their aim was to breed a healthy and fit future generation to compensate for the war losses.

State administrators were converted to eugenic values during the crisis of defeat and social disorder. Alarmed bureaucrats resorted to a biologically conceived nationalism. The Imperial Health Office condemned the Allies' *Hungerblockade* as 'a war of racial extermination against the German race'. Spectacular accusations were made against the Treaty of Versailles as a calculated Allied attempt at child murder. Health officials feared that the loss of dairy cattle would cause a massive surge of infant deaths. Officials asserted that 80,000 deaths were due to the *Hungerblockade* and that the German nation had 'lost' four million births due to the war.[114] The condition of German youth was so bad that the *Volkskörper* was *ruiniert*. Statisticians prophesied a disintegration of the race due to the declining birth rate. Family-oriented welfare measures and social hygiene were regarded as a means to rebuild the biological fabric of the race.[115] The Imperial Health Office

[113] See Günther, 'Institutionalisierung'.
[114] O. Krohne, 'Die gesundheitliche Not des deutschen Volkes', 4 January 1923, in ZSTA P Nr 9409 Bl. 101–5.
[115] ZSTA M Rep 76 VIII B Nr 2049 betr volksgesundheitliche Fragen während des Krieges 1918–19; BHSTA MF68014 Medicinalwesen.

diagnosed sickness as corrupting minds and nerves.[116] It pointed to the need to defend the family against 'epidemics' of abortions, VD and psychopathy. This official mentality idealized the family, nursing and racial purity. Experts in social hygiene aimed to root out and destroy degenerate characters. Their campaign in defence of the German family invoked terrifying threats of diseases, deaths and racial extermination.

Racial hygiene was nurtured within the protective womb of the state. In May 1920 a Committee for Racial Hygiene was established in Prussia. It was convened by the health official, Krohne, and enjoyed the support of Gottstein as Ministerial Director. The initiative in eugenics was seized by medical officers and university professors. Its membership was restricted to those eugenicists who were distinguished in the medical sciences.

The Prussian Committee for Racial Hygiene, May 1920
Geneticists: Baur, Bluhm, Correns, Goldschmidt and Poll
Medical statistician: Roesle
Gynaecologists: Bumm and Max Hirsch
Anatomist: Hans Virchow
Pathologist: Westenhöfer
Anthropologist: Luschan
Psychiatrist: Bonhoeffer
Physiologist: Abderhalden
Medical officers: Gottstein, Krohne and Beyer.

In 1921 the social hygienist Grotjahn replaced Abderhalden.[117] The committee shows how scientists were asserting that their work deserved state support as a national priority, and that they should dictate social policies. The Committee for Racial Hygiene was incorporated into the Prussian Health Council in 1921.[118] The USPD representative, Weyl, criticized the council's apparent impartiality as highly partial. Twelve members were civil servants. No members were communist or USPD parliamentary representatives. There was no nature therapist or homoeopath. As the only USPD party member was also director of the Berlin Youth Welfare Office, professional qualifications outweighed the political.[119] These criticisms also applied to the Prussian Committee for Racial Hygiene, which had Population added to its responsibilities.[120] The eugenicists continued to take an active, but controversial role, although some became disillusioned as when in 1926 the geneticist Baur protested to the Minister of Welfare that the Council was impotent.[121]

---

[116] 'Ein Krankheitsfieber hat eben die Menschen auch in ihrem geistigen, inneren Leben ergriffen und breitet sich immer weiter aus', ZSTA P Nr 15.01 Bl. 146 and 15.01 Nr 9408 Bl. 432.
[117] ZSTA M Rep 76 VIII B Nr 2072 Bl. 14 Abderhalden to Minister, 9 June 1920.
[118] *Landesgesundheitsrat.*
[119] *Preussischer Landtag* (77. Sitzung am 30 November 1921), p. 5,242.
[120] *Ausschuss j, Rassenhygiene und Bevölkerungswesen.*
[121] ZSTA M Rep 76 VIII B Nr 48 Die Ernennung und die Tätigkeit der Mitglieder des Landesgesundheitsrat für Preussen, Mai 1921 bis Juli 1927, Bl. 463, Baur on 30 January 1926.

Administrative, medical and eugenic interests coalesced. The Prussian Medical Department published a eugenic manifesto by Westenhöfer which had been presented first to the Berlin Racial Hygiene Society in 1919. This stressed positive eugenics and welfare.[122] These aims were pursued in the discussions of the Committee on Racial Hygiene, and in turn influenced legislation and policies. Meetings of the Racial Hygiene Committee were held quarterly. Goldschmidt recollected: 'We were to prepare legislation on such matters as abortion, help for large families, sterilization of defectives and so forth'.[123] In June 1920 the Committee discussed the racial hygienic legacy of the war. Baur and Westenhöfer presented papers on emigration and inner colonization in November 1920. Max Sering and Franz Oppenheimer, both theoreticians of rural colonies, were invited to comment. The Reich Ministry of the Interior approved the committee's recommendation that the state support such settlements. In January 1921 Hirsch and Bluhm led the discussion on abortion.[124] In 1921 Grotjahn and Poll initiated discussions on eugenics and income tax. They were joined by officials from the Ministry of Finance. That low income resulted in late marriage of such elite groups as the army and police was a cause for concern.[125] As part of the Prussian Health Council the committee debated marriage certificates, compulsory sterilization, rural settlement, genetic counselling and blood group research.

The obsession of medical officials with racial degeneration found an echo among the health experts of political parties in the state and Reich parliamentary assemblies. The USPD spokesman, Weyl, was an unrelenting critic of the lack of expenditure on welfare, because of the 'racial biological' crisis of the nation. The war casualties, psychiatric disorders, starvation and high disease rates were 'national' concerns, shared by all parties. To socialists, the degeneration in health was an index of social deprivation. To nationalists in the DNVP, the rise in nervousness and diseases represented a decline in national morale. Left and right agreed on the need for more education about health issues on a scientific basis. Population policy was a unifying bond between political parties.[126] Expert committees on racial hygiene meant that professional and eugenic groups took a substantial initiative in formulating health, welfare and population policies. The administrative and party political influence of professional and eugenic interests limited the extent to which party politics on a democratic basis could shape the Weimar welfare state.

---

[122] M. Westenhöfer, *Die Aufgaben der Rassenhygiene (des Nachkommenschutzes) im neuen Deutschland. Vortrag gehalten am 27. Februar 1919 in der Berliner Gesellschaft für Rassenhygiene* (Berlin, 1920), (= Veröffentlichungen aus dem Gebiete der Medizinalverwaltung vol. 10 no. 2).

[123] R.B. Goldschmidt, *In and Out of the Ivory Tower* (Seattle, 1960), pp. 230–2.

[124] ZSTA M Rep 76 VIII B Nr 2072 Beirat für Rassenhygiene; BAK R86 Nr. 2371 Bd 1 Bl. 153–66.

[125] 8. Sitzung des Beirates für Rassenhygiene, 15 October 1921, ZSTA M Rep 76 VIII B Nr 2001 Bl. 42–3.

[126] Weyl, in *Verfassungsgebende Preussische Landesversammlung Stenographische Berichte* (181. Sitzung 27 November 1920), p. 14151.

THE SOCIALIZATION OF HEALTH

Eugenic expertise

The priorities of social hygiene characterized state welfare policies during the 1920s. Social hygiene focused on the health of mothers and children, the combating of chronic diseases and psychiatric disorders, and the hope of improving the quality of future generations. Innovative experiments in social medicine and social work resulted in comprehensive schemes for family welfare, such as *Familienfürsorge*. The Weimar constitution gave the state and municipalities responsibility for welfare, so inaugurating a 'welfare state'. While it marked an end to the view that welfare was a private philanthropic concern best left to voluntary organizations, the welfare state was a complex construction of insurance, state, municipal and voluntary agencies.

The wartime aims of curbing abortions, combating chronic diseases and promoting large and healthy families remained a feature of welfare policies. Immense floods of behavioural disorders and diseases threatened to engulf the nation. Organic theories of the state flourished with renewed vigour in the post-war crisis of defeat. The new ideologies stressed the promotion of 'child rich' families, eugenics and a greater attention to maternal health. There was a shift away from utilitarian liberal economics to a welfare-oriented theory of the nation as an organic 'human economy'. Human welfare rather than profit was to motivate the economy. The finance-economy was an organism in which the state could regulate redistribution of wealth through welfare benefits. This organicist theory of state socialism was popularized by the evolutionary sociologist, Goldscheid. Its ecological emphasis on the limitations of natural resources, and on the value of life, made it readily adaptable as a means of justifying state regulatory measures in the fields of fiscal and welfare policies. In the crisis of capitulation and the collapse of the Imperial order, eugenic demands for the extension of public health measures and for positive schemes of racial improvement began to attain a new currency.[127]

Welfare experts projected an image of deteriorating social conditions. Their pessimistic analyses established the necessity of their services and an intellectual climate favourable to eugenics. The more disease and social deviancy that could be detected, the more experts and their remedial measures were needed. Norms of hygienic and orderly behaviour were to be inculcated into the population. Alarmed demographers predicted that the German *Volk* had lost its vitality and would die unless the will to have large numbers of children could be engendered into people. The Bavarian statistician, Friedrich Burgdörfer, feared an ageing population. He stressed the importance of promoting the 'racially healthy German family', and of measures to combat 'the rationalization of sexual life'. Eugenicists took up the

---

[127] P.J. Weindling, 'Eugenics and the Welfare State during the Weimar Republic', in W.R. Lee and E. Rosenhaft (eds.), *The State and Social Change* (Oxford) in press.

nationalist slogan of a *Volk ohne Raum* (a people without space) and pronounced that Germany was a *Volk ohne Jugend* (a people without youth). Eugenic welfare schemes were politicized as the means for the salvation of the social and moral order of the nation.[128] Education and persuasion to adopt a healthy lifestyle were backed up by an army of professional welfare experts, who could use techniques of public indoctrination and compulsory powers. Underlying the extension of state power was a growth of middle-class professionalism. The voluntary welfare services that had proliferated during the war were institutionalized as professional careers in social work.[129] Established professions such as medicine and midwifery also gained career opportunities. Infant and child health and welfare services were expanded.[130] In theory there was a socialization of welfare legitimated by a democratic constitution. In practice, the first beneficiaries of the welfare state were the middle-class welfare workers. At times, professionalized welfare acted primarily in the interests of clients; but all too often 'higher' social interests such as social control, surveillance and the health of the totality of the *Volkskörper* transcended the democratic rights of the citizen.

Professionalism, reinforced by official powers, meant that welfare defined new spheres for the exercising of coercion. Welfare raises the issue that Weimar democracy was not unstable just because of the anti-democratic extremism of the ultra-left and ultra-right. The new technocracy of professions and welfare administrators might be seen as erecting anti-democratic and coercive social structures by extending the welfare state. The growing influence of social hygiene, social biology and eugenics provided an ideology of professional expertise. State administrators were converted to eugenic values during the crisis of defeat and social disorder. Alarmed bureaucrats abandoned Naumannite ethical theories for a biologically conceived nationalism. The birth of the Weimar Republic provided favourable opportunities for public health experts and statisticians who had been pressing for social hygiene. Whereas most of the senior officials were removed, only eight per cent of technically qualified officials lost their posts.[131] There was enthusiasm for a technocratic approach to government, using the skills of those qualified in economics, sociology and medicine. Eugenics as an ideal amalgam of these disciplines became part of policies of socialization and democratization, offering scientific solutions to social welfare problems. Eugenicists gained leading positions in public health administration, and influenced the administrative and legislative priorities.

Eugenics appealed to a state concerned with social reconstruction and political stabilization. Eugenicists argued that the decline in the birth rate was especially

---

[128] F. Burgdörfer, 'Das Bevölkerungsproblem, seine Erfassung durch Familienstatistik und Familien-politik', diss, München, 1917; Burgdörfer, *Der Geburtenrückgang und seine Bekämpfung, die Lebensfrage des deutschen Volkes* (Berlin, 1928).
[129] R. Landwehr and R. Baron, *Geschichte der Sozialarbeit* (Weinheim and Basle, 1983), pp. 166–71.
[130] C. Sachsse, *Mütterlichkeit als Beruf* (Frankfurt-on-Main, 1986), 203–7.
[131] W. Runge, *Politik und Beamte im Parteienstaat* (Stuttgart, 1968).

pronounced among elite groups in the population. Given that the war had caused a disproportionate loss among the middle-class *Führerschichten*, it was feared that a lack of gifted leaders could jeopardize the nation's future. Liberal thinkers such as Max Weber and Naumann bequeathed an emphasis on the charismatic qualities of strong leadership. Eugenics can be seen as giving medicine charismatic authority. The elitist eugenic concern with the quality of the population was taken up by population and public health experts. Eugenically-minded doctors saw their profession as a leading social group, responsible for guarding the health and vigour of the nation. They claimed an essential role in schemes of national reconstruction. Eugenicists argued that one-third of the population was degenerate, and should be prevented from reproducing, whereas superior elements in the population should be encouraged to have large families. The declining birthrate continued to be a major factor in social welfare policies. A debate flared up between advocates of positive eugenic strategies concentrated on elite leading groups in the population, and those wanting benefits available to all as a type of 'national eugenics'.

A barrier to understanding the way that eugenics influenced social welfare during the Weimar Republic has been posed by an overly narrow understanding of eugenics as primarily the negative eugenics of compulsory sterilization and forced 'euthanasia' policies. This is not to deny that 'euthanasia' and sterilization were discussed. During the post-war political instability, demands were voiced for legislation for sterilization and 'euthanasia' in the interests of society and future generations. But these radical solutions posed a deep threat to democratic liberties, and were given a hostile reception by judicial officials supporting liberal concepts of the rights of the individual citizen. Negative eugenics was consequently rejected by state health administrations except when, as with contraception, it could be blended with voluntary consent. It was felt that positive eugenics was more in keeping with the reformed political structure and social needs of the nation. Positive eugenic welfare measures opened immense professional opportunities in state planning of a healthy and efficient society.

Centralization and professionalization

Underlying the campaign for positive eugenics was a militant professionalism, seeking to extend the scope of public health by adding a medical component to socialization programmes. In the political upheavals of 1919, medical campaigners for social hygiene had a clear aim: a national Ministry of Health headed by a doctor. The aim of such a Ministry had figured in earlier turning points in national history of 1848 and 1870. Yet in contrast to the earlier liberalism of medical reformers, the 1919 demands were for a strengthened state with interventive powers in the sphere of population policy and family health. Democratization did not necessarily mean that health care systems and the medical profession should be made democratically accountable. Instead it meant that doctors should be armed with extensive powers as medical officials.

The absence of democratic aims can be seen in left-wing doctors' demands during the revolutionary period of 1918–19. Although the soldiers' and workers' councils initially reflected a spontaneous mass desire for democracy, medical practitioners sought to extend rather than share their powers. For a fleeting moment, a central Ministry of Health under a doctor seemed to have emerged in November 1918. The doctor, Heinrich Stoffels, was appointed representative of the 'Council of Workers and Soldiers for all Sanitary Matters in the German Socialist Republic'. Yet Stoffels' power was in reality limited to Berlin, and Centre Party contacts suggest that he owed his position to his professional rather than political standing. He was undermined when the left-wing socialists of the USPD withdrew from the government.[132] The Majority Social Democrats (MSPD) preferred to work within the inherited administrative structure. In February 1919 the MSPD expert on social policy, Rudolf Wissell, wrote to Hugo Preuss, the Reich Minister of the Interior and author of the Weimar constitution, that Stoffels' appointment had no authority, and that the Reich did not wish to transfer health affairs to a single, autonomous authority.[133]

Concern among public health officials and Berlin doctors over the medical implications of demobilization in November 1918 was fixated on VD, and the threat this posed to the quality of the population. Socialist doctors serving the workers' and soldiers' councils demanded authoritarian extension of medical powers. Typical was the urologist Benno Chajes (a son-in-law of the revisionist socialist, Eduard Bernstein, and a socialist councillor in Berlin) who represented the Workers' and Soldiers' Council of Brandenburg. In December 1918 and January 1919 Chajes lobbied the MSPD Reich Chancellor, Philipp Scheidemann, over the inadequacy of state measures to prevent the spread of infectious diseases. Chajes demanded authoritarian powers as a medical officer. This was in line with the state decree of December 1918 for compulsory treatment for VD and a monopoly of the medical profession for all treatment of uro-genital diseases.[134]

From November 1918 there was a campaign by a broad coalition of medical reformers for a Reich Ministry of Health. This was demanded by the USPD doctor, Moses, who had taken a lead in the birth strike agitation, by Grotjahn, the eugenicist and director of the municipal office of social hygiene in Berlin, and by Hirschfeld, the doctor, sexologist and sexual reformer. Hirschfeld assigned a range of eugenic and social hygienic functions to the Ministry, which was to have control over welfare services that were to include preventive health measures. He emphasized that doctors should have the determining role in the state health service.[135] Doctors could overcome class divisions, and integrate the *Volksorganis-*

[132] I. Winter, 'Geschichte der Gesundheitspolitik der KPD in der Weimarer Republik', *Zeitschrift für ärztliche Fortbildung*, vol. 67 (1973), 455–72, 498–526; Labisch and Tennstedt, *GVG*, I, p. 58.

[133] D.S. Nadav, *Julius Moses und die Politik der Sozialhygiene in Deutschland* (Gerlingen, 1985), pp. 152–3.   [134] Nadav, *Julius Moses*, pp. 150–1.

[135] M. Hirschfeld, *Die Verstaatlichung des Gesundheitswesens* (Berlin, 1919); *Vorwärts*, (24 Jan. 1919); Wolff, *Magnus Hirschfeld*, pp. 170–1.

mus. Hirschfeld believed that biology had replaced theology and that hygiene was the basis of morality. At public meetings and in petitions, doctors demanded that the Medical Department of the Reich Ministry of the Interior, and the Reich Health Office be combined in a Reich Ministry of National Health, Social Insurance and Population Policy. It was to have strong powers because of the current crisis in the nation's health, and was to be headed by a minister supporting the socialist republic.[136] Their model was the Austrian *Staatsamt für Volksgesundheit*, which was strongly influenced by the racial hygienist Kaup. The implications of the proposals were to boost the power of the medical profession both in the sphere of the state and throughout society in that the healthy as well as the diseased should become the responsibility of the doctor as a state official.

This coalition of medical and sexual reformers was unsuccessful. The National Assembly debated the reform plans in March 1919, and on 2 April 1919 passed a law allocating responsibility for public health, mental hospitals and statistics to the Reich Ministry of the Interior; social hygiene, maternity benefits, war pensions and occupational medicine became the responsibility of the Ministry of Labour. The rationale for the administrative division of health was that of maintaining social order. The link with the Ministry of the Interior arose because medicine was seen in policing rather than therapeutic terms, with the control of disease and incarceration of the infectious as priorities. Insurance considerations accounted for the Ministry of Labour's responsibilities. On 16 April 1919 the Reich Ministry of the Interior torpedoed the Grotjahn-Hirschfeld-Moses proposals for a Ministry of Health. Carl Hamel, the official responsible for health matters at the Interior Ministry, was mildly sympathetic, but pointed to the obstacles posed by the *Länder*. The Reich Health Office – itself directed by a legally trained official – objected that a centralized ministry would not fit in with the constitution as this was a federation rather than a unitary state. The office cautioned that insurance questions were the province of the Ministry of Labour, and that any authority headed by a doctor would incur the wrath of the sickness insurance funds. This arrangement consigned the Reich to a weak role as merely registering national statistics and co-ordinating welfare legislation in the *Länder*.[137]

Grotjahn felt that it was a mistake to have divided insurance and pensions in the Ministry of Labour from health and welfare.[138] The demand was taken up by the USPD which petitioned the Reichstag for a central Ministry of Health headed by a doctor in October 1919 and November 1921. Grotjahn did not wish to see the USPD taking the lead in social hygiene. In a remarkable lurch to the left, the Naumannite Grotjahn rejoined the majority faction of the SPD in autumn 1919. He sought to use his position to become MSPD spokesman on health, and to inject eugenics and population policy into the party programme. In 1920 he presented a comprehensive health policy to a committee consisting primarily of members of

[136] ZSTA P 15.01 Nr 10948 Schaffung einer deutschen Reichsbehörde für das Gesundheitswesen; Nadav, *Julius Moses*, pp. 153–9.   [137] Nadav, *Julius Moses*, pp. 177–8.
[138] Grotjahn, *Erlebtes*, pp. 236–7.

the Socialist Doctors' Association. But the MSPD avoided discussion of health at its annual conference, because issues like alcoholism, nature therapy, vaccination and abortion were highly contentious. Grotjahn was advised to prepare the ground by private lobbying for support and by leaving out all controversial issues. He proposed nationalization of all hospitals, clinics and pharmacies, and for all medical personnel to be part of a comprehensive system of social insurance. He calculated that to mention eugenics explicitly would jeopardise an otherwise uncontroversial set of proposals. A Hamburg doctor, Andreas Knack, agitated for special clinics for monitoring hereditary fitness, and for educational measures to dissuade the degenerate from procreating. The policies proposed at the party conference of June 1922 had a number of eugenic features. These included 'parental advice clinics' to ensure that future generations would be healthy in body and mind, and reform of the care of 'degenerates'. The programme culminated in the demand for a Ministry of National Health, Social Insurance and Population Policy. That the main thrust of the programme was nationalization of all medical services showed how eugenics assisted the extension of professional powers. Control of social insurance was important for Grotjahn's plans for introducing a pro-natalist 'parenthood insurance'. The programme was accepted, but Grotjahn was isolated on the right-wing of the party, having opposed the fusion of the USPD and MSPD. It was indicative of the nationalism of Grotjahn that he preferred a coalition with the parties of the right to unification of the SPD.[139]

There were apocalyptic expectations that social hygiene would provide the basis of a rejuvenated social order arising from the ruins of defeated Germany. Social hygiene was publicized as a means of the nationalization of medicine, and for inculcating national values, self-respect and reason in the German people. It offered a common platform for conservative doctors and medical officers, and for radical reformers because social order and the increase of professional powers were unifying aims. Medical reformers had to overcome the suspicions of their conservative colleagues who showed their animosity to socialism by sporadic strikes in February and March 1919. Reformers claimed that they should be made responsible for overseeing what the Viennese eugenicist Tandler called 'organic capital of the state'. It was argued that in order not to alienate the conservative majority of the profession, socialization should be limited to a redrawing of the relations between the profession and the state, rather than being interpreted in a party political sense. New professional opportunities were a palliative to a belligerent and economically hard-pressed medical profession.[140]

The lack of a democratic concept of health care was a consequence of the nationalist and professional appeal of social hygiene. Alfons Fischer, the brains behind the Baden Society for Social Hygiene, petitioned for social hygienic reforms. For Baden he demanded a Department of Health headed by a doctor. On

[139] A. Labisch, 'Neue Quellen zum gesundheitspolitischen Programm der MSPD von 1920/22', *IWK*, vol. 16 (1980), 231–47; Grotjahn, *Erlebtes* pp. 242–3.   [140] Nadav, *Julius Moses*, p. 162–3.

a national level he persuaded the German Society of Public Health to campaign from July 1919 for a 'Health Parliament'. This was to be composed of public health experts in the field of social hygiene. It meant that health would not be so much the responsibility of a single minister as the collective responsibility of professional representatives. On 26 October 1919 a meeting of nearly one hundred experts in social hygiene was convened in Weimar. Here, Bumm, the President of the Reich Health Office, forcefully opposed the 'Health Parliament' as a vehicle for doctors committed to social hygiene attempting to gain dominance over other health and welfare associations.[141]

The *Länder*

The Weimar constitution, formally inaugurated in July 1919, was a symbol that Germany was a nation in which sovereignty was vested in the people. This impression was strengthened in that the constitution turned Germany into a welfare state. It defeated those officials and conservative groupings opposed to welfare as a state responsibility. Clause 119 of the constitution provided for the protection of the health of the family and of future generations. Yet while the constitution legitimized the claims of the social hygiene lobby, it did not provide for adequate protection of the individual when confronted by the guardians of state welfare. Confusion also reigned with regard to the responsibilities of the *Länder* and municipalities. Both pursued ambitious welfare programmes, spurred on by the sense of the need to alleviate the nation's socio-economic crisis. There was a political ambiguity to welfare. It was legitimated as much by biological idealization of the *Volkskörper* as by democratic ideals. The *Freikorps'* idealization of the family, nursing and racial purity were not so far removed from concerns of the welfare state.[142] Just as the MSPD resorted to the *Freikorps* to maintain political order, so doctors could exterminate supposedly hereditary characters resulting in behavioural disorders such as 'psychopathy'.

In contrast to the Reich Health Office's preference for continuity of its restricted monitoring functions, there was vigorous dynamism in the *Länder*.[143] The Prussian state offers an outstanding example. Its sheer size and extensive obligations posed immense challenges to politicians. The MSPD established a Welfare Ministry in 1919. But because political stabilization was a priority, the MSPD allowed the minority coalition partner, the Centre Party, to control the Ministry throughout its existence from 1919 until 1932. The Prussian Medical Department became part of the Ministry, along with a Department of Housing. The Medical Department's director was Gottstein, the expert in child health. That he replaced the bacteriologist Kirchner typified the transition in priorities from bacteriological

---

[141] Nadav, *Julius Moses*, pp. 166–7; Thomann, *Alfons Fischer*, pp. 130–7.
[142] Theweleit, *Männerphantasien*.
[143] G. Schreiber, *Deutsches Reich und Deutsche Medizin. Studien zur Medizinalpolitik des Reiches in der Nachkriegszeit (1918–1926)* (Leipzig, 1926).

control of infectious diseases to maternal and child welfare with an emphasis on preventive measures. The division of power between the MSPD and Centre opened the way for administration based on professional expertise and scientific objectivity. At the same time certain politicians in the Centre and socialist parties supported eugenics. Heinrich Hirtsiefer, the Centre Party's Minister of Welfare from 1921 until 1930, advocated a eugenic-based welfare programme.[144]

The process of the professionalization of the Prussian Medical Department had its roots in the pre-war German appointment of Kirchner as a medically qualified official. Gottstein's appointment as *Ministerialdirektor* in 1919 marked the entry of municipal expertise into central government. He had led the assault on bacteriology during the 1890s, and had pioneered welfare services in pre-war Charlottenburg. Gottstein ensured that the state fostered infant and child health, and school medical services in order to promote health and to weed out the degenerate. He supported state eugenic measures such as anthropometric surveys in schools, marriage certificates, and compulsory medical treatment for diseases such as VD.[145] At lower levels of the department there was continuity of personnel, ensuring a survival of values tinged by Imperial authoritarianism. Gottstein was succeeded in 1924 by Dietrich, who was also especially interested in child welfare having directed the imperial infant welfare campaigns since 1900. In 1926 Krohne became Ministerial Director, a position he held until his death in office in 1928. Krohne's responsibility for population questions, infant health and midwifery showed that in these spheres there was administrative continuity spanning the 1914–18 war and the formative years of the Weimar Republic. It meant that medical officials had a distinct set of loyalties that set them apart from other legally trained officials. This resulted in often striking conflicts in policy-making. The legally trained officials supported the rights of the individual in health matters. The medically trained officials supported the authority of their professional colleagues. That Krohne was head of the German and Berlin Societies for Racial Hygiene from 1922 showed how the combination of professionalism and welfare responsibilities contributed to the strengthening of eugenics at the heart of the state.[146]

The number of full-time state medical officers steadily increased. It meant that the Medical Department stood at the head of a semi-autonomous hierarchy of medical officials. By 1928 there were 133 full-time municipal and state medical officers, although there were still 294 part-timers. Similarly there were more part-time than full-time school medical officers. This meant that public health retained strong links to the rest of the profession. Gottstein established three Academies for Social Hygiene in Prussia, which provided training for medical officers. These included a strong element of eugenics in their curricula. The Academy at

---

[144] H. Hirtsiefer, *Die staatliche Wohlfahrtspflege in Preussen 1919–1923* (Berlin, 1924), pp. 70–3.
[145] A. Gottstein, *Das Heilwesen der Gegenwart, Gesundheitslehre und Gesundheitspolitik* (Berlin, 1924), pp. 224–34. [146] M. Stürzbecher, 'Otto Krohne', *Berliner Ärzteblatt*, vol. 92 (1979), 697–8.

Düsseldorf was dominated by Schlossmann's interests in infant welfare and population policy, although these were tempered by Teleky's concerns with occupational health.[147] Grotjahn took the lead at Charlottenburg in establishing a curriculum based on a biologistic concept of social hygiene. There were lectures in heredity (by Poll), population policy and eugenics, and anthropometrics. At Breslau, the anthropologist Mollison lectured on racial hygiene and biometrics.[148] These academics equipped doctors to take on posts in the expanding state health services. Grotjahn established good relations with Conti when he obtained qualifications so that he could work in infant and child health clinics. Professional aims cut across party political affiliations.[149]

The twin processes of professionalization and the advance of eugenics were paralleled in other *Länder*. The socialist administration of Saxony advocated such radical eugenic policies as sterilization. The basis of the Saxon measures was the Welfare Law of May 1918 which enabled state welfare measures and the co-ordination of state, municipal and voluntary agencies for infants, children, housing, TB and cripples.[150] In Baden, Alfons Fischer campaigned for an Office of Social Hygiene. His plan was rejected by the Baden Ministry of Labour, because it considered that no single authority had competence in health affairs. Fischer continued to campaign for piecemeal reforms such as child benefits and other measures which had eugenic motives.[151] However, the medical administrations of Baden, Bavaria, Hessen, Mecklenburg and Württemberg appointed officials who adopted eugenic measures in policies towards chronic diseases such as VD and TB, and in the targeting of social problem groups such as youth psychopaths. It is necessary to trace the process of policy formulation in each state to see how medical demands for intervention and eugenics were curbed by other authorities responsible for education, justice and welfare, as well as the extent to which party political and other concerned groups could block the pressure from the eugenicists.

Municipal health

Municipal health was a major area of welfare expansion in the 1920s. Cities saw welfare measures as a means of promoting corporate social harmony and stability. Konrad Adenauer, who had become mayor of Cologne in 1917 and a protégé of Naumann, saw welfare as a means of social corporatism and he drew on biology to

---

[147] E. Rodriguez Ocana, 'La Academia de Higiene Social de Düsseldorf (1920–1933) y el Proceso de Constitución de la Medicina Social como Especialidad en Alemania', *Dynamis*, vol. 3 (1983), 231–64.

[148] ZSTA M Rep 76 VIII Nr. 335 die Sozialhygienischen Akademien 1921–1928; M. Stürzbecher, 'Von der Sozialhygienischen Akademie zur Staatsakademie des öffentlichen Gesundheitsdienstes (1920–1944)', *Berliner Ärzteblatt*, vol. 82 no. 17 (1969), cited as offprint.

[149] Labisch and Tennstadt, *GVG*, II p. 393.

[150] Sächsisches Landesgesundheitsamt, *Einrichtungen auf dem Gebiete der Volksgesundheits- und Volkswohlfahrtspflege im Freistaat Sachsen* (Dresden, 1922).

[151] Thomann, *Alfons Fischer*, p. 130.

describe the city as an organism. Other Centre Party and SPD politicians were similarly motivated to promote welfare. Out of the wartime voluntary associations, there emerged authorities for comprehensive family welfare. Control of these was disputed due to rivalry between the caring professions. To the fury of social workers, Grotjahn successfully used his position as a member of the Reichstag to ensure that the Youth Welfare Law of 1924 gave health departments control over child health.[152] By way of contrast, there were exteme experiments in democratization. Health centres, organized by progressive sick funds in socialist municipalities such as Berlin or in the city-state of Bremen, were symbols of modern socialist medicine.[153] In addition to socialist attempts to 'embrace the whole family', women social workers were a progressive – and controversial – innovation; it was believed that family welfare ought to be a female enclave in city government.[154]

The post-war period saw the emergence of powerful municipalities. In 1920 Berlin was formed from seven surrounding cities. Other cities such as Hamburg and Frankfurt grew in area. City-administrators were imaginative in their social policies in areas to do with housing, sports and leisure facilities, and transport. Health was no exception. The municipalization of health care in Berlin provides an instructive example of conflicting motives. In pre-war Berlin the authorities had established offices for bacteriology and disinfection. The peripheral municipalities were pioneers in social hygiene with the work of such as Gottstein in Charlottenburg, Rabnow in Schöneberg, and Silberstein in Neukölln. But Berlin's administration resisted demands of a radical lobby of doctors such as Weyl campaigning for social hygiene. In 1915 a Municipal Medical Office, with one clinician and one expert in social hygiene (Grotjahn) was established. This office was virtually impotent. It had no powers over the policing aspects of public health, nor over school health and infant care with the many school doctors and nurses. Much of Grotjahn's time was spent on organizing food distribution.[155] In 1918 Grotjahn resolved to try and emulate the innovative municipalities for the planned authority of 'Greater Berlin'.[156] Municipal reform became entangled in the power struggle between the radical left and those forces supporting state authority. From 1918 until spring 1919 there was a strong Spartacist challenge in Berlin, and pressures for local autonomy and democracy within the city continued. In May and June 1919 it looked as if the centralized scheme would win the day. A grouping of state and municipal officials fought for a unitary medical authority to administer 'Greater Berlin'. It would have powers over what had once been independent

---

[152] For the background to the law see E. Harvey, *Youth Welfare and Social Democracy in Weimar Germany: the Work of Walter Friedländer* (New Alyth, 1987), pp. 22–8.

[153] E. Hansen, M. Heisig, S. Liebfried, F. Tennstedt, *Seit über einem Jahrhundert: Verschüttete Alternativen in der Sozialpolitik* (Cologne, 1981), pp. 97–101.

[154] D.F. Crew, 'German Socialism, the State and Family Policy, 1918–33', *Continuity and Change*, vol. 1 (1986), 235–63.

[155] Stadtarchiv Berlin Rep 00/ 1812 Medizinalamt der Stadt Berlin 1914–20.

[156] Grotjahn, *Erlebtes*, p. 193.

municipalities and would have control over what had hitherto come under the authority of the state police.[157]

Gottstein of the Prussian Welfare Ministry allied himself with the strongly anti-revolutionary Grotjahn, who served in the municipal Medical Office until April 1919, and then took over responsibility for sanatoria and the evacuation of sick children until October 1920. Grotjahn and Gottstein aimed to secure a centralized Office of Social Hygiene. This would take over the functions of the 'morals police', and sought a transfer of powers concerning, for example, welfare and schooling from other adminstrative departments. The plan was that the Health Office was to be headed by a doctor with responsibility for infant welfare, school medical services, Poor Law services and welfare. It was emphasized that hygiene as a science was a 'unitary whole', so a science-based adminstration had to be a centralized administration. In September 1919 the municipality still favoured Gottstein and Grotjahn's plans for centralization.[158]

Opposition to 'over rigid centralization' began to be voiced by medical officers from the peripheral municipalities which were to lose their autonomy. Silberstein argued that by its nature social hygiene had to be administered on a decentralized basis. The Ministerial Director Weber (the bacteriologist and organizer of Lingner's Hygiene Exhibition) argued against Gottstein that since districts had special needs over-centralization was impracticable. By March 1920 Weber's more decentralized schemes were winning, and were enacted in the socialist-sponsored legislation for Greater Berlin of 27 April. The central Office of Social Hygiene was left with responsibilities only for statistics, advice and monitoring the welfare measures carried out in the districts. This meant that the office was as bereft of real powers in Berlin as the Reich Health Office was in Germany as a whole. Even the districts were to carry out their own bacteriological investigations. The radical socialist doctors Rabnow and Weyl argued that such welfare measures as infant care had so many social and economic aspects that they should not be left to doctors. In November 1920 the administration of Berlin forced the health planners to implement measures on a decentralized basis in accordance with the democratic structure of Berlin. There was still some rearguard action by health officials arguing that it was not possible to provide hospital services, convalescent homes and bacteriology on a decentralized basis, and that the Youth Offices were usurping control of school and infant health services. But by 1922 the Health Office conceded that social hygiene was to be left to the districts. The dispute exposed the authoritarian views of Gottstein and Grotjahn, two of the most influential figures in social hygiene and state health measures. That the lines of battle were drawn between medical officials and politically elected representatives supported by a very few radical doctors, reflected the divisions over health policies in the state.[159]

[157] Stadtarchiv Berlin Rep 00 Nr 1812 Medizinalamt der Stadt Berlin 1914–20.
[158] Stadtarchiv Berlin Rep 01 HV GB Nr. 325 betr. die Deputation für das Gesundheitswesen, vol. 1, 1920–23.
[159] Stadtarchiv Berlin Rep 01 HV GB No 325 betr. die Deputation für das Gesundheitswesen. vol. 1 1920–23.

Berlin's six new administrative districts pioneered an exemplary range of welfare services. For example, Grotjahn's pupil, Bruno Harms, directed a proliferating range of clinics and social workers from the municipal hospital of Moabit.[160] Health centres and clinics abounded.[161] The 'decentralized' Weimar measures were to be reversed only in 1935 when public health officials forced through the unification of state and municipal medical services.

Grotjahn's successor in the municipal health department was the eugenicist and child health expert Gustav Tugendreich who had directed the infant welfare clinic in Schöneberg since 1901. In 1926 the eugenicist Drigalski moved from Halle to become director of the municipal health department. While eugenicists were inclined towards centralization, at a district level eugenics could also flourish. Grotjahn's students populated posts in the district health offices: the socialist Salo Drucker as medical officer in Wedding oversaw a range of services including school health, alcoholism, VD, psychopathy and innovations such as social cosmetics for alleviating scarred and disfigured faces.[162] Others of Grotjahn's students, such as the school doctor Georg Benjamin, did not agree with authoritarian biological values and plunged into radical politics for the KPD. Georg Löwenstein, medical officer in the Berlin district of Nowawes and Lichtenberg, is an example of a socialist doctor who, staunchly supporting the principle of local autonomy, nevertheless had allegiances to eugenics in the state-sponsored eugenic League for Regeneration. As secretary for the Anti-VD Society, and influential in the Red Cross, he had many ties to the Prussian state health administration. He led the campaign for special measures for the detention of youth delinquents and prostitutes.[163] In the working class suburb of Kreuzberg a special Health House was opened, enthusiastically supported by the socialist mayor, Martin Kahle. The House was welcomed for its contribution to eugenics.[164]

That eugenics could thrive in Berlin was all the more remarkable given that it was more radical than other municipalities. Most municipalities made substantial concessions to state control and professional interests. Welfare clinics were grouped into central welfare centres, in part staffed by doctors. But in order to avoid antagonizing the medical profession, clinics merely dispensed advice and welfare benefits. As there were overlapping municipal and state medical services, it was possible to agree on either municipal or state provision of services. In Prussia, the municipalities gained the upper hand. In Southern Germany, the initiative lay with state public health officials.[165] Towns and districts established departments of

[160] C. Pross and R. Winau (eds.), *Nicht Misshandeln. Das Krankenhaus Moabit* (Berlin, 1984).

[161] R. Schmincke, *Das Gesundheitswesen Neuköllns* (Berlin, 1929); M. Stürzbecher, 'Das Gesundheitsamt des Bezirks Tiergarten von 1920–1933', *Berliner Medizin*, vol. 16 (1965), 211–14.

[162] *Festschrift Haus der Gesundheit* (Wedding, 1982).

[163] S. Leibfried and F. Tennstedt (eds.), *Kommunale Gesundheitsfürsorge und sozialistische Ärztepolitik zwischen Kaiserreich und Nationalsozialismus – autobiographische, biographische und gesundheitspolitische Anmerkungen von Dr Georg Loewenstein* (Bremen, 1980).

[164] M. Kahle, 'Qualitative Bevölkerungspolitik', in *Das Gesundheitshaus. Einführung in das Aufgabegebiet der sozialen Hygiene unter besonderer Berücksichtigung der Gesundheitsfürsorge im Verwaltungsbezirk Kreuzberg der Stadt Berlin* (Berlin, 1925), pp. 7–19.

[165] Labisch und Tennstedt, *GVG*, I, pp. 67–80.

health, youth care and welfare. Most were opened between 1919 and 1921. By 1928 there were 828 such welfare offices. These directed often elaborate systems of closed institutions, and many types of social workers and health visitors. By 1928 there were 2,244 'family workers', and 675 of these were attached to health departments. Towns tended to keep these systems separate whereas in the countryside the responsibilities were amalgamated in a single district welfare office on the pre-war model. In towns co-ordination of civic and voluntary agencies might be undertaken by a co-operative *Arbeitsgemeinschaft*.

One function of the clinics was to identify patients for referral to closed institutions such as hospitals, sanatoria and asylums. Hospitals still carried the stigma of Poor Law institutions. Closed institutions also served custodial policing and eugenic functions. The unproductive and hereditarily unfit could be detained and 'humanely' prevented from having children. The cost of such institutions made them vulnerable to criticisms of excessive public expenditure on welfare, and yet such institutions could only cope with a small percentage of cases deemed to be 'in need'. Municipal welfare clinics and, where they were grouped together, welfare centres, could provide alternatives to incarceration. A visit to the clinic would invariably result in a social worker visiting the family. Clinics were cheap to run, and could be spread throughout the population. They dispensed beds, bedding, cutlery, and food supplements. They could also identify such degenerate species as alcoholics, psychopaths, the venereally diseased and the tubercular. The apparently fit who were actually carriers of hereditary diseases could be located as could those suffering from mild forms of mental disorders. Services were carried out by family social workers, and a medical officer had overall responsibility. The clinic was still the best means of tending to family welfare, and for carrying out surveillance on the population.

The ability of professional groups to manipulate municipalization was shown by the demands of the Socialist Doctors' Association. Their aims were two-edged in that they sought to reform the structure of the profession as well as to expand state health services. Eugenics was a central focus. After the war a new influx of doctors such as Grotjahn, who joined the association, saw eugenics as the basis of public health. Yet even the founder-member Zadek, who since the 1890s had been an SPD activist, integrated socialism and eugenics. He wrote in 1919 in a USPD paper that hygiene was socialism, concerned with the totality of society. A municipality was like a family, and its adminstrators had a parental responsibility to care for the citizens' welfare from cradle to grave. In order to attain the higher development of the people, socialist municipalities should implement preventive medicine to eradicate the weak and strengthen those with superior physical and mental capacities.[166] Left-wing socialist doctors were opposed to state centralization, and favoured a municipally based system. But they urged that doctors be given a privileged position in municipal health centres, and used eugenics as a rationale. In

[166] Nadav, *Julius Moses*, p. 179.

this way, eugenics was a barrier to democratization, because its scientific claims required professional expertise; and it justified greatly extending the scope of interventive authorities. A network of eugenically trained doctors and social workers began to spread in the social services.

The most radical initiatives drew on the tradition whereby doctors were the officials responsible to democratically controlled sickness funds. There was a wave of conservative doctors' strikes aimed especially against the sickness funds in 1920 and 1923. The plan for insurance-financed municipal health centres (*Ambulatorien*) was put into action in 1924. Support came from socialist insurance officials such as Kohn, who directed the Berlin Sick Fund. SPD experts in social hygiene such as Weyl and Moses gave important backing in the journal, *Der Kassenarzt*, and with Norbert Marx initiated the campaigns for these health centres by declaring them to be an alternative to a welfare policy based on population policy and the concept of the 'human economy'. Legislation of 1919 had curbed the veto rights of employers in sickness funds. The sickness insurance funds were keen to extend benefits to their members' families. In Berlin this occurred only in July 1924. The health centres marked a change from liberal traditions of 'free practice' to a socialist organization. They were staffed by socialist doctors, and had trade union support. The socialist doctor, Franz-Karl Meyer-Brodnitz, acted as intermediary between the unions and the *Ambulatorien*. In 1927 he took over the department of social hygiene of the German Trade Union Council. More radical were the communist plans for a 'proletarian health service' in health centres (*Gesundheitshäusern*). That all those socialist initiatives were staffed by conventionally trained professionals made them vulnerable to the view that eugenic theories were integral to modern preventive medicine.[167]

To some such as the Berlin medical officer Richard Roeder, the health centres offered the opportunity of making the medical profession more accountable. In 1925 he announced: 'Today everyone from a minister to a worker is subject to controls, and rightly so. Only the doctor is uncontrolled, and not even by colleagues, and the sick are expected to offer up their greatest possession, their health.'[168] The sickness insurance health centres claimed that they could offer a far more effective service than state clinics. Chajes – inspired by Grotjahn – cited VD as an outstanding example of the advantages of a family-oriented system of care which combined treatment and welfare. The other services of clinics, such as treatment for TB, alcoholics, infants, cancer and psychopaths, could also be more effectively provided. In 1928 the Berlin clinic for sexual advice and birth control was opened by Charlotte Wolff. Yet such clinics show the collectivist priorities of social hygiene as health care for the individual became a channel for imposing population policy and a range of social norms. Much depended on the quality of the advice. Some staffing the clinics were libertarian like the communist sexologist, Hodann. Others were highly authoritarian eugenicists like Chajes, who ran an

---

[167] Hansen, *Verschüttete Alternativen*, pp. 160–82.   [168] Hansen, *Verschüttete Alternativen*, p. 180.

occupational health clinic from 1925. At the same time professional contacts cut across political allegiances. Meyer-Brodnitz, the trade union doctor, and Löwenstein, the venereologist, worked in association with Grotjahn and other eugenicists. The insurance health centres were as vulnerable to eugenics as state systems of care. A system that was more comprehensive could be more comprehensively abused. The structure of the welfare state provided opportunities for eugenic measures at all levels, while not creating compensating mechanisms for representing the interests of patients and clients.

Population policies

Despite the disintegration of the social order during 1918, medical officials pressed for population policy with renewed vigour. In May and June 1918 the Reichstag had discussed measures to suppress abortion and contraception. The Chancellor emphasized public opposition to social and eugenic abortion. The tone remained characteristic of the restrictive moral codes of Imperial Germany. Yet there were intimations of greater emphasis on biology and reproduction. Pro-natalist opinions intensified during the final few months of Imperial Germany. By December 1918 a sharp reversal occurred: the Reichstag was debating the USPD's radical socialist proposals for liberalizing abortion and contraception. Other radical innovations occurred in the sphere of child health and preventive medicine. As women took a greater role in professional, administrative and political spheres, radical ideas on birth control, and the family were advanced by feminists and the left. But their radicalism clashed with militant pro-natalist schemes of positive encouragement to bear children and for eugenic controls in a state population policy. Eugenics was caught between the radical reformers and conservative nationalists. The medical profession, the churches and public health administrators pressed for comprehensive state controls and inducements to raise that birth rate.

   Population policy was a slogan that appealed to all political parties, as in keeping with the spirit of national reconstruction. Health and welfare reforms had a good chance of success if presented to parliamentary legislatures as means of achieving a population policy. Parties from the KPD to the DNVP were solidly in favour of raising the birth rate.[169] The Prussian parliamentary committee on population was reconvened under the chairmanship of the USPD socialist and doctor, Weyl, and then under the physiologist and DDP member Abderhalden. That he was succeeded by a number of doctors including Schlossmann and Struve (DDP) and Stemmler (Centre) opened the committee to accusations of professional bias. The committees received petitions from concerned groups including the Racial Hygiene Society, and individual doctors including Dreuw, the anti-salvarsan campaigner, and Boeters, a medical officer who was an advocate for sterilization.

---

[169] J. Lang (= DNVP Secretary), 'Wie treiben wir eine gesunde Bevölkerungspolitik?', *Deutsche Tageszeitung*, (11 December 1919).

Eugenicists were quick to seize the initiative. Abderhalden in the Prussian assembly during May 1919 proposed a comprehensive programme of eugenic welfare measures. These included measures to suppress prostitution, for health certificates prior to marriage, midwifery reform, municipal facilities to improve the physique of youth, playgrounds, combating alcoholism, care of 'illegitimate' children, and land reform. The ministerial officials Gottstein, Dietrich and Krohne met with the committee to discuss these measures.[170] They endeavoured to reconcile the pronatalist demands for quantity and the eugenic requirement of quality in state policies.

VD

The widespread incidence of chronic diseases threatened the health of families. Arising from demobilization was a spectre of soldiers spreading VD, so causing sterility in marriage, and blind and syphilitic infants. It was feared that the carefully planned wartime system of clinics, continual medical inspections and controls on soldiers had broken down. The response was a decree for VD treatment on 11 December 1918, and on 17 December there was a decree for diseased soldiers. The decree of 11 December gave public health officials powers to order compulsory treatment. Moreover, doctors were granted a monopoly of treatment for not only VD but for all diseases involving the genitalia. The decree thus fulfilled longstanding aspirations of the medical profession. Policing powers were transferred to public health officials. Instead of police controls over prostitutes, the decree allowed compulsory treatment for not only women but also men suspected of being infectious. It limited the right of patients to chose whether they wanted to be treated and how; and it struck a blow against the free competition of the so-called 'quacks'. While it signalled a victory for those campaigning for extension of public health, it was at the expense of individual liberties. As the socialist Gräf put it, the patient was viewed as a part of the body politic, and infection of another was a crime.[171]

Between 15 November and 14 December 1919 the Reich Health Office attempted a national survey on the extent of VD. The authorities estimated that they had information on only 50 per cent of VD patients, but calculated that there was a substantial increase in VD in cities. This seemed to justify continuing the strong measures against VD. The decree of 1918 was a symbol of medical coercion. In practice, it was less radical in its concept and effects than might have appeared. Compulsory treatment was already in force in Bavaria, Bremen (since 1901), Brunswick (since 1906), Dessau (since 1864), Lübeck (since 1879), and in Meiningen (since 1897). Some authorities regarded compulsory treatment as effective. But officials in other *Länder* such as Hessen in September 1920 described

---

[170] ZSTA M Rep 169 D II C Bevölkerung A Bd 1 Nr 1.
[171] *Verfassungsgebende Preussische Landesversammlung* (121. Sitzung am 25 Februar 1920), pp. 9,932–7.

the disorder among patients detained for treatment: incarcerated patients were trying to break out, and others – the reports alleged, especially the black French troops – were breaking into the hospitals. In 1921 Gottstein concluded that half the reports thought the measures a success, and the other half condemned them as ineffective.[172]

But it was the underlying principles rather than the actual effects which meant that VD remained a highly charged and emotive issue in the Weimar Republic. Blaschko, representing the Anti-VD Society, and allies in the public health administration pressed for a law regulating VD treatment and preventive measures. There was parliamentary pressure for the old morals police to be removed from the control of the criminal police and turned into an authority solely for the purposes of health care. In October 1920 legislation was drafted, and tabled at the Reichstag. The measures were drawn up in consultation with such academic experts as the professor of dermatology, Jadassohn, who strongly rejected the criticisms of salvarsan. Parents and teachers were to be obliged to ensure treatment by a doctor, and health authorities were granted compulsory powers. It was to be a crime punishable with a three year prison sentence for anyone knowingly having VD to have sexual intercourse. It would also be a crime to marry without giving notice that one had VD. Only doctors qualified in Germany were allowed to treat VD (on any part of the body) and all diseases of the sexual organs. Any other therapist offering treatment or distributing tracts about alternative therapies was liable to one year's prison or a fine of 100,000 marks. The sale of remedies for VD was restricted to the medical profession. If a patient discontinued treatment, the doctor would be obliged to notify the VD advisory clinic. Penalties were to be imposed for breast feeding by anyone with VD and all wet nurses had to produce a medical certificate to the effect that they did not have VD. Finally, there were to be public advisory centres for VD throughout the Reich, working in association with the health authorities.[173]

Many socialists such as the doctors Löwenstein and Moses regarded these measures as necessary. VD – like alcoholism and TB – was associated with poverty and overcrowding. These proposals provoked fierce opposition. Other socialists condemned the legislation as depriving individuals of rights over their bodies. Conservative moral reformers wanted a return to special measures for prostitutes and suppression of all contraceptives. The idea of compulsory treatment with salvarsan caused consternation among groups supporting nature therapy, and anti-semitism was a feature of opponents of salvarsan. Nature therapists, homoeopaths, 'biochemical practitioners' and other alternative types of medical practitioners bombarded state assemblies with petitions. They attacked the legislation as violating *Kurierfreiheit* – the patients' right to choose therapies – and derided medical science as itself quackery.[174] The stormy passage of the proposed legislation showed how unwieldy the legislative machinery of the Republic was.

[172] ZSTA P 15.01 Nr 11881 Verordnung vom 11 Dezember 1918.
[173] Reichstag, *Aktenstücke 1920/23*, Nr 5801, pp. 6,744–55.
[174] GSTA Dahlem, Rep 84a Nr 868.

The proposals were withdrawn in 1920 owing to the financial burden of advisory clinics on the *Länder*. The planned measure was introduced and debated during 1923, and after the elections of 1924 the legislation was reintroduced in 1925. But it was not until 18 February 1927 that the anti-VD legislation was ultimately passed with compulsory treatment intact. It marked a victory for the powers of health authorities. That for nearly ten years an important segment of health policy was shaped by an emergency decree shows the scant regard of public health authorities for legislative procedures.

Just as the legislation was in its final stages, a scandal erupted over the death of a seventeen-year-old, Elizabeth Kolomak, in Bremen. While in police custody she had been compulsorily treated with massive doses of salvarsan, and her family had been denied the chance of arranging private treatment. In December 1926 a book called 'Killed by Life' and purporting to be the girl's diary was published. In fact it had been greatly added to by the mother. But the point was made that 'loving care' which justified the system of medical controls could in fact be murderously brutal. Matters were made worse when it emerged that the girl might have been the victim of experimental treatment.[175] Democracy and medical progress were difficult to reconcile.

Tuberculosis

Underlying TB measures were concerns with the weakened constitution of the race. The rise in deaths from TB during the final years of the war, and post-war malnutrition and housing shortages caused widespread alarm. As with the attack on VD, the development of a network of state clinics was envisaged.[176] There was to be comprehensive registration of all TB cases. And as with the VD campaign, this entailed a loss of individual liberty for the sick, justified by the need to protect family health. The Centre Party representative Stemmler said that given that there was a hereditary disposition to TB in certain families, it was necessary to isolate the sick and prevent the infection of the healthy. The Prussian Assembly's Committee on Population Policy in 1923 pressed for co-ordinated national measures against TB with co-operation among medical officers, school doctors and TB clinics, and adequate numbers of clinics and sanatoria. Municipalities opposed the measures as an infringement of their rights. Adenauer, the mayor of Cologne, objected that the law gave the right to demand from municipalities payment for the costs of incarcerating patients. This infringed the financial independence of the municipality.[177] The TB Law of 1925 established autonomous authorities under professional control.

---

[175] E. Meyer-Renschhausen, 'The Bremen Morality Scandal', in R. Bridenthal, A. Grossmann and M. Kaplan (eds.), *When Biology became Destiny* (New York, 1984), pp. 87–108.
[176] ZSTA M Rep 76 VIII B Nr 4197 Bekämpfung der TB. Nr 4158 Berichte auf den Runderlass von 16 Februar 1920 betr Ausbau der Tuberculosefürsorge.
[177] *Preussischer Landtag 1921/23* (18 April 1923); *Preussischer Landtag 1921/23*, Drucksachen Nr 4990 and Nr 6141.

Prussian legislative measures for TB followed a similar course to those for VD, and there was a polarization of opinion over treatments, professional rivalries and patients' rights. Socialists favoured such alternatives as light, fresh air and nutritional therapies. There was a vociferous lobby of socialists supporting the turtle serum of Friedmann, who received the backing of Adam Stegerwald, the Minister of Welfare. Doctors were outraged. The liberal, Schlossmann, declared Friedmann's remedy to be an insult to German medicine, and demanded its boycott by the medical profession.[178]

Midwifery

Midwifery reform illustrates the ideological continuities but also the administrative pitfalls of population policies. Reform of midwifery dated back to ministerial discussions at the turn of the century. The midwife was to be given the status of an official, a minimum income was to be guaranteed, and her training improved; her responsibilities were to be extended to include advising mothers on feeding and infant care, and reporting on congenital malformations, syphilis and other infant diseases. In return for the rise in status, responsibilities and income, midwives would have to accept limitations on where they practised. This was to ensure an even distribution of midwives in town and country. The measures were intended in part to police midwives so that they would not undertake abortions and administer quack remedies, but also to satisfy the midwives' demands for professional status.[179]

During the war, the proposals for midwifery reform became bogged down because of the entrenched position of the Finance Ministry which blocked the necessary financial resources. In the republic midwifery reform accorded with the priorities of family health, and the need to improve the status of women. In October 1919 the Prussian Ministry of the Interior decided to give the midwife status as an official. By December 1919 plans for legislation were ready, establishing a system of district midwives; but discussions dragged on.[180] The measures were controversial as the state's priority of an even distribution of midwives clashed with the midwives' interest of practising in centres of population. The Prussian Assembly eventually passed the midwifery reforms in 1924. It resulted in an outcry as the numbers of midwives in Berlin were to be halved. The law was referred to the supreme constitutional court, which decreed that the Reich had to pass an enabling law. This invalidated the Prussian reform. As in Imperial Germany, midwifery reform failed because of liberal restrictions on state powers. The most that Prussia could do was within the framework of the traditional system.

---

[178] ZSTA M Rep 76 Va Tit X Nr 73 Bd 1 Friedmann; *Verfassungsgebende Preussische Landesversammlung* (20 February 1920, 27 November 1920); *Preussischer Landtag 1921/23* (18 April 1923).

[179] ZSTA M Rep 76 VIII B Nr 1443 betr die Regelung des Hebammengesetzes 1915–20.

[180] *Preussischer Landtag 1921/22*, Drucksache Nr 2731, Entwurf eines Gesetzes über das Hebammenwesen.

Midwives were given more training and responsibilities so that the length of time taken to qualify in Prussia was twice as long as in Bavaria.[181] Reform was limited to those spheres in which public health officials had discretionary powers. This typified the weakness of Weimar population policy. Given that midwives had a fundamental role in the reproduction of a fit and healthy population, and given the constitution's support for a rise in the status of women, midwives should have attained substantial gains. In fact the disruptive effects of the planned legislation, and financial shortages conspired to make any reform stillborn.

Marriage certificates

Health certificates prior to marriage became a priority as a way of breeding a healthy and 'high value' race. They were favoured as being without the problems of more radical negative eugenic measures such as sterilization. They were praised for their educative and health-promoting value, as well as for being a humane means of deterring the unfit from marrying. Those suffering from TB, VD, mental disorders and judged to be of an inferior constitution were to be dissuaded from marrying. As it was emphasized that the health examinations could only be carried out by a suitably qualified doctor, they also fulfilled professional aspirations. The Racial Hygiene Society continued to agitate for health examination prior to marriage. In April 1919 the wartime reports on certificates were referred by the Reich Ministry of the Interior for reconsideration by the Reich Health Council, as 'racial hygiene had increased in its significance for the nation's future'. The physiologist and DDP representative, Abderhalden, proposed such certificates to the Prussian Legislature on 23 September 1919, and in petitions to the mayor of Berlin; the lawyer and eugenicist Schubart presented proposals in January 1920 to the Reich and on 5 May 1920 to the Prussian administration; the doctor, G. Madaus, organized a petition in July 1920. The Reich Health Council met on 26 February 1920 when it heard reports from the professor of hygiene, Abel, and from Schubart. Abel cautiously recommended only a VD certificate. But Schubart wanted the state to provide a comprehensive examination free of charge.[182] The Reich Health Council called on a further nine outside experts. Five were eugenicists: the dermatologist Blaschko, Bluhm, Christian (all representing the Berlin Racial Hygiene Society), as well as the social gynaecologist, Hirsch, and Weber of the Society for Population Policy. Only Käthe Schirmacher saw the matter from a feminist perspective. The council marked a turning-point in official acceptance of the desirability of eugenic controls on marriage.

The result of the Reich Health Council discussions was that the Reichstag approved a law on 11 June 1920 for the distribution of a health education pamphlet

---

[181] ZSTA M Rep 76 viii B Nr 1416 Fortbildung der Hebammen 1918–22.
[182] ZSTA P 15.01 Nr 9379 Bl. 70–157; W. Abel, 'Zur Frage des Austausches von Gesundheitszeugnissen vor der Eheschliessung', *Öffentliche Gesundheitspflege*, vol. 5 no. 5 (1920), 145–62; P. Kuhn, 'Über amtliche Heiratsvermittlung', *Öffentliche Gesundheitspflege*, vol. 4 no. 7 (1919), 221–32.

to all intending to marry. It was drawn up in consultation with Blaschko, Schubart and the anatomist Schwalbe. It was suggested that their cumbrous scientific style be improved by a leading author such as Gerhart Hauptmann or Thomas Mann. Half a million copies of the pamphlet, called 'Points to Note for Those Marrying', were to be distributed by registry officials. This emphasized the personal value of health to the individual, and its importance for the breeding of future generations. In order to avoid eugenic perils, the 'holy duty' to marry a healthy partner was invoked. This was deemed the responsibility of the families of those marrying, but it was only the doctor who could give authoritative guidance. The betrothed should go to a doctor and heed medical opinion on the suitability of the marriage. The pamphlet warned that ill-health would bring an unhappy marriage, degenerate children, and impose burdens on the state. The pamphlet represented an important stage in the official recognition and support for eugenics, and boosted the authority of the doctor over marriage and procreation.

The pamphlet had its critics. Schubart complained of the delay until February 1921 before its distribution, and of the fact that it did not look official enough. But the pamphlet also won converts to eugenics. It cemented an alliance with registry officials who were enthusiastic about their new role as guardians of the nation's future health. The League of Registry Officials became an ardent supporter of eugenic measures, with its chairman, Edwin Krutina, active in discussions of marriage restrictions. Registry officials welcomed eugenics as extending the scope of their professional responsibilities. In 1921 officials reported that there was lively public interest in the advice given, although no engagements seem to have been dissolved.[183]

The Reich Health Council in February 1920 considered that educative measures were insufficient, and urged that there be compulsory medical examinations prior to marriage. It accepted that there was a need to replace war losses and to improve the quality of future generations. It saw that 'racial degeneration' could be reversed, if the mentally and physically unfit were prevented from marrying. It recommended that specialized medical 'Marriage Examiners' be appointed, and that there be compulsory exchange of certificates. It conceded that those marrying should be free to draw their own conclusions from the certificates. If the state was reluctant to make examinations compulsory, there should be at least a standard form introduced, and facilities provided to give the chance of screening. This was intended as a step towards compulsory procedures. Schubart proposed a law based on voluntary principles, with the exception that certificates were to be compulsory for minors. Most *Länder* were against compulsion, as they feared that there would be public opposition. Prussia and Mecklenburg were exceptions. In Prussia both the Committee on Racial Hygiene and state officials, taking the lead from *Ministerialdirektor* Gottstein, favoured compulsory and comprehensive examinations.[184] In 1921 the Prussian Ministry of Welfare suggested that the public were

[183] ZSTA P 15.01 Nr 9379 Bl. 210–51.   [184] ZSTA P 15.01 Nr 9379 Bl. 320–73.

becoming concerned about the fitness of future generations, and were prepared to accept legislation for health examinations. A number of possibilities were considered: that all males should be required to have a certificate that they were free from VD; that all marrying must undergo a health examination, and the refusal to do this would annul the engagement; that the certificates must be exchanged, but it was left to either partner to draw conclusions; and, finally, that a medical certificate had to be given to the registry official, who in the event of a serious illness would have to prohibit the marriage.

Prussian officials pointed out that marriage laws had precedents in several US states, but as the disqualification from marriage was for the certified mentally ill, the venereally diseased and those receiving Poor Law care, the vital ingredient of a eugenic medical examination was lacking. In Sweden the marriage law of 1915 had been extended in its scope by the VD law of 1919, so that medical officers and registry officials were informed of all cases of VD. The value of the certificates was that they could prevent infection of the spouse-to-be, and the birth of children of an inferior eugenic quality. There was also an important socialist experiment of the anatomist, Tandler, and Kautsky jun. in Vienna, where a marriage advice clinic was successfully established on a voluntary basis. These experiments were controversial as such clinics took on a wide range of functions including therapy, psychological counselling and advice on birth control. Innovative medical ideas were combined with interventive powers.

Negotiations with the Reich and Prussian Ministries of Justice resulted in a clash of opinions between the legal and the medical viewpoints. The judicial officials maintained that there must be no state interference with the individual's free choice in marriage. Moreover, the matter was one that required legislation on a Reich level. The Reich authorities declared that they were unwilling to act on the issue. On 12 October 1921 the SPD petitioned for health examinations before marriage.[185] Welfare-oriented eugenicists such as Muckermann and the Centre Party representative Fassbender campaigned in favour of compulsory health certificates.[186] Racial hygienists joined in. Lenz agitated for marriage certificates in Muckermann's journal, 'The Future Generation'.[187] With such pressure building up, the Prussian welfare officials added fuel to the fire when on 12 February 1922 Hirtsiefer, the Prussian Minister of Welfare, presented a memorandum on the need for health certificates. He favoured compulsory exchange of certificates, which he justified as an educational measure. There should be no legal prohibitions on marriage. The additional information that certificates would provide was in the interests of those marrying, and in accordance with the constitutional responsibility

---

[185] *Preussischer Landtag* (1921), Drucksache Nr 1203.
[186] M. Fassbender, *Des deutschen Volkes Wille zum Leben. Bevölkerungspolitische und volkspädagogische Abhandlungen über Erhaltung und Förderung deutscher Volkskraft* (Freiburg, 1917).
[187] F. Lenz, 'Einige wirtschaftliche Forderungen der Rassenhygiene zum Wohl der Familie', *Das kommende Geschlecht*, vol. 1 (1921), 155–62; Lenz, 'Das Gesundheitszeugnis vor der Verlobung als Familiensitte', *Das kommende Geschlecht*, vol. 2 no. 1 (1922).

of the state to care for future generations. According to Grotjahn's statistical estimates, there were 180,000 mentally ill, 90,000 epileptics, 120,000 alcoholics, 156,000 cripples, 30,000 blind, 18,000 deaf and dumb, and 300,000 with advanced pulmonary tuberculosis. These estimates raised the hope that certificates could prevent further cases. But the state reluctantly accepted the need to maintain individual rights.[188] The memorandum received the support of the Prussian Assembly's Committee on Population Policy. The Centre Party welfare expert, Fassbender, reported on the overwhelming medical evidence for such certificates. On 24 November 1922 the Committee voted that the *Landtag* should introduce legislation for certificates as a legal requirement, although prohibitions on marriage ought not to be mandatory. They recommended educational measures in schools on the value of marriage to health, and teaching and examination of medical students in hereditary science.[189] But in March 1923 the Reich Ministry of the Interior insisted on a wait and see policy. It meant that the initiative was taken by eugenicists and sexual reformers who established municipal clinics on the Austrian socialist pattern.[190]

Family allowances and taxation were debated as positive eugenic methods. In 1920 the French National Assembly set an example by passing laws to restrict abortion and contraception; it considered imposing financial penalties on the unmarried and on couples without children. The DNVP campaigned for benefits for 'child rich' families to guarantee the physical, mental and moral value of their offspring. Civil servants' organizations (with political links to the DVP and DNVP) clamoured for improved family benefits. In 1921 Krohne of the Prussian Medical Department initiated surveys of fertility among officials and the police. There was a stream of demands for improved family benefits from all political parties. The KPD championed the rights of the pregnant and the need for better care after birth. Maternity allowances were acted on only during emergencies such as the inflation. Long-term legislation proved to be impossible.

The plans for the socialization of health involved ambitious legislative programmes. The parliamentary impetus and Weimar constitution promised to provide a framework for an equitable and far-reaching system of welfare. But agreement proved difficult to achieve. There were conflicts among and within political parties, and between ministries (as for Finance and Welfare) and ministerial officials. Yet set against this was the consensus that health was a matter for promoting national unity. In 1924, *Ministerialdirektor* Dietrich concluded his speech on the budget with the exclamation that health care was a means of achieving 'a healthy and strong nation'.[191] Population and the declining birth rate were rallying cries for a medical and public health lobby which was keen to extend its power. Measures proposed amounted to a eugenic programme. But they

---

[188] *Preussischer Landtag* (1921/22), Drucksache Nr 2162, Denkschrift des Ministeriums für Volkswohl-fahrt über die Forderung von Gesundheitszeugnissen vor der Eheschliessung.
[189] *Preussischer Landtag* (1921/22), Drucksache Nr 3954.   [190] ZSTA P 15.01 Nr 9380 Bl. 5–23.
[191] 'ein gesundes, starkes Volk', *Preussischer Landtag* (18 October 1924).

incurred opposition that united radical and conservative opponents of state intervention, while a majority agreed on welfare systems that promoted the dominance of the medical profession. Each part of the welfare programme advanced scientific medicine as opposed to nature and other alternative therapies. The modernist atmosphere of the 1920s with its sexual explicitness and consumerism exacerbated the tensions. The churches, the medical profession and welfare bodies allied in moral purity campaigns against feminists and sexual reformers. It was the reactionary religious, professional and welfare lobbies that were drawn even closer to the bosom of the state.

The inflation

The inflation of 1922–3 countered the expansion of welfare. The wartime legacy of widows, orphans and war-wounded and the impoverishment of many meant that the cry was raised for extension of welfare facilities. At this time of great need, financial retrenchment necessitated cuts in welfare. Seen from a Social Darwinist perspective the reduction of welfare could be reinvigorating. In 1923 the Reich Health Office commented that high mortality rates meant that natural selection was taking place of weaklings and cripples, and that overall health statistics were not unfavourable.[192] Despite the closure of infant clinics and milk kitchens, infant mortality rates had worsened less than expected. Mothers were still able to breast feed, and the officials recognized that the declining birth rate reduced infant mortality. The Prussian *Ministerialdirektor* and eugenicist, Krohne, was concerned that the middle class and craftsmen were harder hit than workers.

However, inflation was not conducive to health. Medical officials recognized that the sickness statistics were incomplete as they did not register depression, physical weakness, weight loss or nervousness. The moral and economic basis for good health was lacking. Krohne feared that Germany would become a focus of infection in an epidemiological and moral sense.[193] This Prussian view was echoed in other states. While the Baden Ministry of the Interior was alarmed in January 1924 at the rapid deterioration in health, it was primarily concerned with the moral effect on the people's *Seelenleben* (spirit). The opinion of psychiatrists such as Hoche that patients were tending to become depressed and psychopathic was noted.[194]

Analyses by ministerial officials reflected more their conservative and professional prejudices than the underlying reality. The situation can be compared to the 1912 survey on the declining birth rate. Medical and local district officials forwarded reports which supplemented the bare bones of statistics with a great deal of qualitative observations. Generally comments focused on the condition of patients at clinics. If clinic facilities were cut, then so too was the source of observation. Observations also conflicted. The state administrator[195] of Aachen

---

[192] ZSTA P 15.01 Nr 9408 Bl. 430, Gesundheitliche Schäden.
[193] ZSTA P 15.01 Nr 9405 Bl. 93, June 1923–January 1924.
[194] ZSTA P 15.01 Nr 9405 Bl. 244–51.   [195] *Regierungspräsident.*

commented that for the second half year of 1924 there was increased chlorosis and TB among young working girls, and general malnutrition due to the high cost of food. The state administrator of Cologne suggested that youth wages were too high, and caused an increase in pleasure-seeking and drinking so bringing about the rise in attendance at VD and TB clinics. He did admit that 65 per cent of children went hungry without breakfast or a warm meal, and lacked underwear.[196] Moral convictions that blamed sickness on the afflicted or on incompetent mothers thus shaped medical judgements.

The widespread cuts in services were regarded with alarm. Cities such as Magdeburg reported on cuts in school meals and infant clinics. There were vivid details of the incidence of rickets, malnutrition, TB, dermatological conditions and of a rise in gonorrhoea and VD. By contrast, reports from predominantly rural areas such as Minden and Königsberg were positive. Whereas there was reduced milk supply in urban districts, rural provinces could maintain free milk for mothers. This reinforced the conviction that rural conditions were physically, morally and medically healthier.

Nature therapy and social medicine

Eugenic concerns with the quality and quantity of the population and future generations were a major incentive for the expansion of welfare services. The alliance of advocates of the welfare state and the medical profession constituted a powerful bloc at the centre of Weimar welfare. However, it is necessary to appreciate the continuing challenges offered to professional authority. Nature therapy had the backing of elements on both the political left and right. In response to the alliance of public health officials and the medical profession, nature therapists lobbied to maintain their rights. In January 1922 the *Verband für Volksheilkunde* organized a Congress for Population Policy and Welfare in Essen. They pointed out that the programme of state medical legislation threatened the rights of sickness funds and patients. The Association wished to uphold free scientific and therapeutic competition of the biological methods of healing.

Welfare measures retained elements of nature therapy. Positive health was the slogan of the 1920s welfare lobby. Air, light, a healthy diet and exercise were recognized as the basis of good health. School health services applied many of these natural forces to promote health. This was evident in gymnastics, sport, open air schools, and 'sun ray' ultra-violet therapies. It was possible to combine positive eugenic stress on natural fitness with nature therapy. Where nature therapy clashed with the medical establishment was over issues such as the professional privileges of doctors, and in the treatment of infectious diseases. The Parliamentary lobby supporting nature therapy was a constant obstacle to the extension of professional powers in the legislation for VD and TB.

There were very few advocates of social medicine who saw the potential hazards

---

[196] ZSTA P 15.01 Nr 9408 Bl. 10–34, November–December 1924.

of the abuse of medical powers. The socialist doctor Friedrich Wolf analyzed the risks of scientific medicine. He urged reform of all aspects of medicine by criticizing the authoritarian form of objective science and doctor-patient relations. As a young doctor he had participated in the free youth rally of 1912 on the Hohen Meissner mountain, and was impressed by Canadian health camps. In the 1918 revolution he joined the Workers' and Soldiers' Council in Dresden, and in 1920 became medical officer for the socialist council of Remscheid. He opened maternity clinics, factory crèches and a health park, and gave medical lectures to school children. When the *Freikorps* Lützow marched in on 13 March 1920 he became commander of the southern wing of the Ruhr Red Army. Disappointed at factionalism in the popular front, he joined the painter, Heinrich Vogeler, at the Worpswede artists' community. Influenced by syndicalism, they attempted to live a socialist style of life and work, an attempt that he later regretted as utopian and illusory. Wolf was outraged at the pro-natalist propaganda of the Kaiserin Auguste Viktoria-Haus, at the lack of help for mothers and at the mass starvation of children. Vogeler gave his home, the Barkenhoff, to the socialist welfare organization, *Rote Hilfe*, in 1923. It became the first communist children's home in Germany. It was a place where children, who were orphaned in the Ruhr fighting, could recuperate from the ravages of poverty. He decorated the house with socialist inspired murals, depicting poverty and the proletarian struggle. The authorities ordered that the murals be removed.[197]

Wolf expressed his criticism of degenerate consumerism in a utopian comedy, *The Black Sun*.[198] He then opened a rural medical practice as a nature therapist. He visited all patients by foot or on skis, kept a vegetarian diet, exercised vigorously, and wrote poetry and plays. He emphasized the need for doctor and patient relations to be a partnership, and for the patient to have knowledge of his or her body. In 1925 he began to write a book called 'Nature as Doctor and Helper', outlining his approach to nature therapy. He argued for medicine to be extended to include healthy housing, diet and working conditions. He envisaged a mass educational campaign for positive health by teams of doctors, gymnasts, cooks, social workers and gardeners. Rural camps were to be provided for the masses to recuperate and learn how to keep themselves healthy with gymnastics, baths and breathing exercises.[199] Wolf's weakness was that his devotion to rural communal cells as the basis of health, happiness and socialism was based on total rejection of science and urban life. His rural slogan of *Volk ohne Land* and plans for rural settlements of unemployed workers could be misinterpreted by nationalists. He joined the Association of Socialist Doctors in 1927 and the KPD in 1928. It was only after this that his work was to have a wider impact.[200] Wolf was one of the few radical critics of professional state medicine and eugenics. In their place, he

[197] D. Erlay, *Heinrich Vogeler* (Fischerhude, 1981).   [198] *Die Schwarze Sonne.*

[199] F. Wolf, 'Entwurf einer Volksgesundheitsschule', in Wolf, *Aufsätze 1919–1944* (Berlin, 1967), pp. 103–6.

[200] A. Oesterle, 'Naturheilkunde und Revolution' in *Volk & Gesundheit* (Tübingen, 1982), pp. 230–7; W. Jehser, *Friedrich Wolf* (Berlin, 1981), pp. 48–51.

advocated socialism and the people's right for choice in matters of health and family welfare. The democratization of health became ever more vulnerable to authoritarian political, professional and administrative forces.

'SEXUAL BOLSHEVISM'

The advance of doctors, psychologists and social workers into the sensitive realm of sexuality provoked far-reaching controversies. The professional reformers were divided in their attitudes to pro-natalism, abortion, contraception and homosexuality. Enthusiasts for the liberalization of sexuality from the stuffy conventions of Imperial Germany came into conflict with the authoritarian moral purity campaign, demanding stricter controls on sexual permissiveness and procreation. Nationalists feared an epidemic of dissolute sexual behaviour, occurring in the wake of demobilization and revolutionary upheavals. Progressives proclaimed sexual happiness as a basic human right to which all were entitled. They criticized the eugenic conviction that sexuality was merely a question of reproductive fitness and of the health of future generations. Biological values and professional interests penetrated both the left and right wing of the sexual reform movement.

Berlin was a centre of conflict between sexual reformers and moral purity campaigners. Pastor Ludwig Hoppe of Berlin wrote a savage attack on 'sexual bolshevism'. The pamphlet demonstrated that the revived moral purity campaign was linked to economic, political and medical issues. Sexual reform was stigmatized as promiscuity leading to VD and to physical and mental degeneracy. Economic considerations of the cost to the nation, especially to those who were fit and healthy, had a great impact during the economic crisis. The response to sexual bolshevism was to urge the state to promote healthy and prosperous families by welfare benefits and health education. Degenerate psychopaths should be located and detained, and 'valueless life' should be prevented by eugenic abortion and sterilization.[201]

The hysterical reactions to sexual reform were provoked by advances in female emancipation. The Weimar constitution granted women rights of equality in marriage, the vote and equal employment opportunities. Women entered political life and the civil service, and political parties took women's issues to heart. While these gains symbolized the democratic intentions of the founders of the republic, they were undermined by persistent, and in some ways worsening, social inequalities of women. About one-third of the labour force in the 1920s were women. They earned 30–40 per cent less than men. The excess of women to men (32.2 million women to 30.2 million men in 1925), and pro-natalism meant that there was much opposition to married women working.[202] To counter this,

---

[201] L. Hoppe, *Sexueller Bolschewismus und seine Abwehr* (Berlin, 1921) in ZSTA P 15.01 Nr 9352 Bl. 36–65; on police control of morality see 30.01 Nr. 5791 Sittlichkeitsregel.

[202] R. Bridenthal and C. Koonz, 'Beyond Kinder, Küche and Kirche: Weimar Women in Politics and Work', Bridental *et al., When Biology Became Destiny*, pp. 33–65.

socialists demanded further improvements in conditions at work for women. They campaigned for free medical services, maternity benefits and improved child welfare. Many of the demands of the League for the Protection of Mothers, such as for better ante- and post-natal care and for removing the stigma of 'illegitimacy' became standard. The USPD and KPD were starry-eyed over the Soviet Union's pioneering social legislation. Whereas in reality Soviet health policies were much influenced by German social hygiene, to German radical socialists communism symbolized true sexual equality in employment, free and safe abortion in hospitals, a health service for all, and the decriminalization of homosexuality.

Pro-natalism had widespread support among all political persuasions. Ideas of an organic community and concern with future generations exercised a strong emotional appeal. The Women's League (BDF) espoused *völkisch* ideas of selfless dedication to the family. In 1919 the BDF laid greater stress than ever on the vital duty of the woman to the family and nation. The programme proclaimed, 'The family is the highest and most intimate form of the lifelong human community'. The purity of family was held to be the basic condition of social health and national fitness. Women should be employed not on terms of equality, but 'according to their nature and their qualities'. Women should exert a 'motherly' influence over society. This view was inspired by the ideal of an organic *Volksgemeinschaft*, or community. The BDF supported the moral purity campaign against sexual libertarianism, pornography, abortion, VD and publicity for contraception.[203]

The BDF changed in its political complexion. Before the war liberal sentiments of the Progressive Party characterized bourgeois feminism. In Weimar the political make-up of the women's organizations was more complex. The DNVP was close to the Housewives' Unions and the League for Child Rich Families. Some feminists changed from radicalism to conservatism; an example was Schirmacher, who represented the DNVP. The right began to gain ascendancy in the BDF. Anna von Gierke combined DNVP politics with a leading position in training social workers. Liberal members of the BDF committee such as Marie Baum were replaced.[204] Democrats including the wife of Friedrich Naumann campaigned against depopulation and moral decay, and demanded improved health facilities and education for women. Suffrage and constitutional rights could have only a limited effect in improving conditions for women, given the entrenched pro-natalist lobby and socio-economic conditions which sustained gender inequalities.

The fears and fantasies of the right preyed on the extreme and the exceptional. Berlin became a symbol of decadence, as the metropolis achieved world renown for its uninhibited sexuality. On the one hand there was a welcome removal of taboos, as in the case of homosexuality, and acceptance of sexuality as individual satisfaction. On the other, there was commercialization of sex with cabarets and prostitution. Berlin became a law unto itself and could not be equated with the more rigid conventions in the rest of Germany. A combination of blatant

---

[203] Evans, *Feminist Movement*, pp. 236–8.   [204] Evans, *Feminist Movement*, pp. 247–8.

commercialism, promiscuity and avant-garde sexual reformers gave substance to the allegation of 'sexual bolshevism'. But the relations between poverty and prostitution, and the reality of women's conditions were harsher and more prosaic than that conjured up by lurid images of depraved sexuality associated with free love and communism. Accusations of epidemics of VD and abortions arose more from emotive nationalism and belligerent professionalism than from dispassionate and realistic observations.[205]

There was for a short time after the war a rise in the birth rate, but when the downward trend resumed the debate of moral versus economic explanations was resumed. Infant mortality declined, but rates of maternal mortality increased from 21.9 per thousand in 1913 to 47.0 per thousand in 1923.[206] The left argued that maternal mortality was due to poverty, inadequate and insanitary housing, whereas the right ascribed deaths in childbirth to a rising tide of abortions. This picture of depraved immorality is offset by the fact that a greater proportion of the population was marrying than ever before. It might be argued that popular reproductive behaviour was adjusting to modern norms with both partners working and practising birth control. Between the entrenched ideological extremes of the moral purists and sexual reformers, popular sexual behaviour went its way. The 1920s saw a growth of mass culture and mass consumerism. The cinema and cigarettes were frowned on by nationalists as symptomatic of the wave of degeneration. Gymnastics, sports, nature rambles, nudist 'free body culture', vivacious fashions in dancing, and jazz became popular. On the domestic front, fitted kitchens and bathrooms began to be part of the housing of the working class. There was a novel array of mass-produced household appliances such as fridges, pressure cookers and vacuum cleaners. Perhaps contraceptives were accepted as one more type of convenient domestic gadget, and so became part of this modern rational lifestyle.

Eugenics and birth control

Sexual reformers campaigned for a democratic, free and equal sexuality. Sexual tolerance, sex education, freely available birth control and abortion on demand were the objects of the sexual political struggle. The campaign had medical and welfare dimensions. There resulted a series of alliances between feminists and reformers with experts in medicine and social work. While there was some identity of interest between the welfare eugenicists and radical sexual reformers, the eugenicists tended to view matters in corporate biological terms, and to emphasize professional controls. Grotjahn was a typical blend of reformer and eugenicist. On the one hand he viewed the trend to smaller families as an unstoppable social

---

[205] G.L. Mosse, *Nationalism and Sexuality. Respectability and Abnormal Sexuality in Modern Europe* (New York, 1985).

[206] G. Schreiber, *Deutsches Reich und Deutsche Medizin* (Leipzig, 1926), p. 17.

process. On the other, he claimed that the doctor should be the Führer of the people in sexual counselling and family health.[207]

Abortion generated heated controversy. To the left, abortions were symptomatic of poverty, overcrowded housing and a lack of knowledge of birth control. To the right, abortions symbolized immorality and lack of self-control. Women were accused of succumbing to self-interest and consumerism, instead of heeding their duty to give birth to the next generation of Germans. Gynaecologists joined forces with the churches and conservative politicians to condemn the morality of women who had abortions and the 'quacks' who carried these out. Experts in 'social gynaecology' like Hirsch pronounced that most spontaneous abortions were caused by conditions at work or toxic substances such as lead. Radicals concluded that there should be improved working conditions and maternity benefits, whereas conservatives drew the conclusion that the New Woman ought to be returned to her natural place in the home.

There were renewed efforts to stamp out neo-Malthusian publicity and the selling of contraceptives. Manufacturers were infuriated at state interference in a free market. They complained that over zealous officials had prosecuted manufacturers of a wide range of irrigators and hygienic articles meant for purposes other than contraception. The Reich Health Office replied that whatever the intended purpose, they could be used either for contraception or abortion. It protested that while it accepted that contraceptives might be used within marriage, all commercial advertising and display still ought to be suppressed. Automatic vending machines and their location in public places such as railway stations prompted a series of clashes with the authorities.

The radical campaign for abortion gathered strength. The more that Stöcker's demands for female sexual emancipation were accepted, the more radical she became. She did not join any political party, but moved in the anarchist circle that had formed around Landauer who came to grief in the Munich Soviet. The League for Protection of Mothers continued to be one of the most active and radical of the sexual reform groups. It demanded sexual advice centres to provide free advice to juveniles, the single and the married, as well as the removal of penalties for abortion. Feminists protested that the clinics ought to have lay, women counsellors and ought not to be exclusively controlled by medical experts. In reaction to this there was a series of church-supported campaigns. It was in this context that 'sexual bolshevism' was attacked. Nationalists insisted on stricter censorship of literature and films, and there was a renewal of the anti-abortion campaign. In May 1922 the state of Bavaria demanded that the Reich outlaw birth control, sterilization and abortion.[208]

The Reich League for Child Rich Families emerged as a power on the right demanding the reconstruction and restoration to health of the *Volk*. Its origins

---

[207] A. Grotjahn, *Die hygienische Forderung* (Königstein and Leipzig, 1921).
[208] ZSTA P 15.01 Nr 9352.

were in the welfare organizations that proliferated prior to and during the war; Clause 155 of the Weimar Constitution promised healthy housing and economic benefits for the child rich. An *Ortsbund der Kinderreichen Frankfurts* (Local League for the Child Rich of Frankfurt) was established in 1919 and in the Rhineland an association of child rich families and widows spread. Between 1919 and 1924 these were fused together in a single body, which launched an emotive welfare campaign for taxation benefits, housing, welfare benefits, price reductions, gardens and allotments, rural settlements, help with schooling and training in sewing and household duties. The inflation intensified demands for food, housing and welfare benefits, and for a reform of the social insurance system through the introduction of a parental insurance.[209] Families with four children, and widows with three qualified as 'child rich'. The League had strong support in the DNVP and the churches. Many health experts sought to channel its demands towards eugenics. In 1924 a national meeting in Weimar heard lectures by Philaletes Kuhn, Muckermann and Andreas Thomsen on the 'dying of civilized races'.[210] Grotjahn publicized the need to provide economic subsidies for the child rich. He drew the attention of the state health authorities to the League's work, and paved the way for state subsidies.[211] Grotjahn's student, Hans Harmsen, was to organize a medical caucus within the League. Social hygienists focused on the issue of parental insurance. Other eugenicists who gave their support included Abderhalden, Rainer Fetscher, and Kuhn and the gynaecologist Kramer. Demographers such as Burgdörfer were also enthusiasts.[212] The League established a system of local medical experts who wrote tracts, lectured and gave advice on TB, infant health and generally on the health of the family and of future generations. These included the medical officers Engelsmann (Kiel), Stark (Karlsruhe), Schroeder (Obershausen), Vonessen (Köln), Herzfeld (Dresden) and Professor Hoffmann (Heidelberg). They ensured that the League's stress on pro-natalism blended with emphasis on health and eugenic qualities, and opposition to contraception. The League not only demanded benefits for the 'child rich' but also fought against the new sexual radicalism by arguing that the 'child poor' should be financially and morally penalized. There was much interest in the maintaining of large and healthy peasant families and rural settlement schemes.[213] That Krohne, the Prussian Ministerial Director, and Arthur Gütt, the ultra-nationalist public health planner, were active in the League, shows its force as a link between the pro-natalism of Imperial Germany and Nazi racial policies.

Eugenicists were quick to respond to the opportunities and problems of post-war society. They secured themselves a position as dispassionate experts, to whom the left and right, the state and voluntary organizations could turn for help. The

---

[209] *Elternschaftsversicherung.*   [210] *Aussterben der Kulturvölker.*
[211] Grotjahn, *Hygienische Forderung*, pp. 147–50.
[212] R. Fetscher, 'Die Bewegung der Kinderreichen', *ARGB*, vol. 14 (1922), 370–1.
[213] ZSTA P 15.01 Nr 26234 Bund der Kinderreichen Bl. 6–23; *Nachrichtenblatt des Reichsbundes der Kinderreichen.*

welfare eugenicists such as Grotjahn and Hirsch played an important role in placing eugenic issues on the agenda of a great variety of welfare groups. The quickness of the response to the political upheavals was shown by a petition on 'state children' by Hirsch of 13 December 1918. He detected a spirit of state socialism in all issues of social policy. He applied this to the declining birth rate, arguing that the pregnant and new-born had a right to state welfare facilities and that children's homes had to be established. The orphans and single-parent families resulting from the war made this especially important. The state's investment would find a return in terms of 'living capital' of healthier and happier lives.[214]

Eugenicists pressed for draconian controls to eradicate illegal abortions. In 1922 the Saxon Health Council and Reich Health Office demanded the registration of all pregnancies. They supported maternity benefits in the hope that these might contribute to turning the rising tide of abortions. In October 1924 Hirsch addressed the Prussian Committee on Racial Hygiene and Population. Krohne and Hirsch gave papers demanding legalization of eugenic abortion for hereditary diseases such as hysteria and feeble-mindedness. These abortions were to be carried out by trained specialists.[215] The liberalization of abortion was thus delivered to the control of professional experts.

Sexual reform

Berlin became an international centre for homosexual emancipation and for sexual reform. The sexual reform movement was a loose alliance of campaigners for the legal rights and improved conditions for women, homosexuals and other groups against whom discrimination was practised. The movement marked a transition from an ethically based morality to a scientifically condoned code of tolerance of sexual behaviour. Sexual scientism would be a more appropriate characterization of the movement than 'sexual bolshevism'. Many reformers were heirs to the monism of Haeckel and Forel, and they espoused a non-racialist type of eugenics. They felt that sexual happiness was essential for social well-being. The sexual constitution was seen in biological terms of heredity and environment. As sexuality was reduced to positive, analytical sciences such as anatomy and cell biology, it became the domaine of scientifically minded professionals. Advances in genetics, endocrinology and biochemistry were expected to yield understanding of reproduction and sexuality. Because biology was itself rich in psychic and social analogies, it did not mean that the new science was necessarily strictly determinist. Most sexual reformers emphasized that there was no absolute division between femaleness and maleness. Nor was there a strict demarcation between the hereditary constitution and environmental conditioning. Hirsch, Hirschfeld and Tandler considered that there was an immutable inherited genotype, but allowed

---

[214] M. Hirsch, 'Staatskinder. Ein Vorschlag zur Bevölkerungspolitik im neuen Deutschland', *Archiv für Frauenkunde*, vol. 4 (1919), 181–7.   [215] ZSTA P 15.01 Nr 9352.

great scope to the interaction of the individual with the natural and cultural environments with regard to the phenotype. Others like Kraus saw an interaction between the constitution and environment. As psychology became ever more scientific, it meant that emphasis on individual perceptions also had a role in any scientific analysis. There was agreement that at puberty and the early stages of maturity, environment was a paramount influence.[216]

Hirschfeld established an Institute for Sexual Science in July 1919 in Berlin. Monistic impulses were shown by there being a 'Haeckel Auditorium' with the inscription that 'Science is not there for its own sake but for all humanity'. The Institute offered marriage guidance and counselling for sexual problems, and undertook biological, sociological and ethnological research; but above all, it was renowned for the study and counselling of homosexuals. The Institute employed the radical social, medical and sexual reformers, Arthur Kornfeld and Hodann, and two venereologists, Bessunger and F. Wertheim. There were hopes that Steinach, the Viennese endocrinologist and pioneer of testicle transplants would join the Institute, but instead the physiologist H. Friedenthal was appointed. In 1919 Hirschfeld established a World League for Sexual Reform, which in 1921 organized an international congress in Berlin. Hirschfeld's campaign for sexual tolerance, pacifism, internationalism and popular enlightenment outraged the nationalist right. After turbulent beginnings, the Institute was registered with the state as the 'Magnus Hirschfeld Foundation'.[217]

Hirschfeld and the sexual reformers faced opposition from the medical profession and the public. A police report stigmatized the Institute as 'a homosexual citadel'.[218] On 26 January 1921 a state medical committee on homosexuality, composed of Krohne the medical official, and the Berlin medical professors Lubarsch, His and Bonhoeffer, condemned homosexuality as 'psychopathic'.[219] Hirschfeld was the victim of physical violence. The *Schutz- und Trutz-Bund* sabotaged his lectures. After a lecture in Munich in October 1922 on Steinach's operation for rejuvenation by testicle implants, he was so badly beaten up by anti-semites that his death was reported in the press. While death threats were made by the right, there was substantial socialist support for Hirschfeld's work, and for his public lectures on 'the right to love'.[220]

Hirschfeld conceived the Institute as a place primarily for scientific research, with counselling as a subsidiary function. Research concentrated on the hereditary and 'psychobiological' aspects of sexuality. Attempts were made to establish the organic basis for sexual behaviour, and to consider the eugenic and demographic implications. The Institute contained a medical department, library and archive. There was a sexual advice clinic, and treatment was administered with X-rays and

[216] M. Hirsch, 'Sexualwissenschaft und Konstitutionswissenschaft', *Archiv für Frauenkunde*, vol. 9 (1923), 75–80.
[217] C. Wolff, *Hirschfeld*, pp. 178–82; ZSTA P 70 In 1 Institut für Sexualwissenschaft Bd 1–7.
[218] ZSTA P 15.01 Nr 9352.   [219] ZSTA M Rep 76 viii B Nr 2076 Homosexualität.
[220] Wolff, *Hirschfeld*, pp. 197–200; M. Hirschfeld, *Race* (London, 1935).

artificial sunlight. Artificial human insemination was carried out on occasions. During the Institute's first year it claimed to have been visited by 4,000 people, and to have given 1,250 lectures. It was also a mecca for foreign doctors and for those attracted by the free atmosphere of Berlin, such as Christopher Isherwood. A crowning glory was when in 1923 the Soviet Commissar for Health, Nikolai Semaschko, visited the Institute.[221]

The Weimar emphasis on reproductive sexuality continued to stigmatize homosexuality as 'unnatural' and 'degenerate'. The Scientific-Humane Committee, chaired by Hirschfeld, attempted to counter this. Its strategy was to recruit professional advocates for the cause from the ranks of doctors, biologists and lawyers. They were meant to give the campaign respectability, by linking the reform to the force of biological arguments about heredity and sexual variation. Vulgarity, sentimentality and mass agitation were strenuously avoided, although there were other more democratic initiatives. The aim of the campaign was to convince the makers of public opinion, such as the clergy, doctors and lawyers, that homosexuality was natural.[222]

Sexual reformers were quick to use the cinema to put their message across. In 1919 Hirschfeld joined the cast of a film, produced by Richard Oswald, called 'Other than the Others'.[223] The scenario was about a young violinist, who was blackmailed because of homosexuality and committed suicide. His friend was saved by the advice of a physician, played by Hirschfeld, and lived to make a new identity for himself and to campaign for the welfare of others. Its showing in May 1919 provoked howls of protest from the right and from the conservative psychiatrists Kraepelin and Moll.[224] Hirschfeld also produced a film in 1919 called 'The Laws of Love'.[225] This provided a scientific account of the evolution of sexuality from the simplest organisms to mankind, and proved that the 'third sex' deserved better treatment. This was rather like the work of the naturalist author, Boelsche, transposed to the screen. Biology and medicine were regarded as the basis of the emancipatory campaign. This was both a strength and a weakness, in that Hirschfeld's use of eugenics made homosexuals vulnerable to discrimination based on racial biology.

Biology was a two-edged weapon in the fight for sexual liberation. Hirschfeld's colleagues were enlightened progressives by the standards of the age. But they were captives within a eugenic and biologistic framework. This can be illustrated by the views of sexual reformers like Kronfeld, Hirsch and Hodann. Having studied biology with Haeckel (to whom he dedicated his first publication), Kronfeld trained as a psychiatrist. After distinguished war service, when he was awarded the Iron Cross first and second class, he joined a revolutionary soldiers' council in

---

[221] C. Wolff, *Hirschfeld*, pp. 172–89.

[222] H.-G. Stümke and R. Finkler, *Rosa Winkel, Rosa Listen* (Reinbek bei Hamburg, 1981).

[223] *Anders als die Anderen*.

[224] Wolff, *Hirschfeld*, pp. 190–5; J.S. Hohmann, *Sexualforschung und -aufklärung in der Weimarer Republik* (Berlin and Frankfurt-on-Main, 1985), pp. 107–27, 258–76.   [225] *Gesetze der Liebe*.

Freiburg. He then worked at Hirschfeld's Institute, where he opened a department for sexual psychology. His work took him in the direction of psychotherapy, but he continued to draw on eugenic theories as well as Kretschmer's theories of psychosexual constitutional types. In 1926 he set up his own practice, joined the Association of Socialist Doctors, and became the first lecturer in psychotherapy at the University of Berlin. He supported a movement for 'individual therapy', which was in sharp contrast to the mental hygiene movement. The contrast can also be seen in attitudes to schizophrenia: whereas Rüdin's approach was hereditarian, Kronfeld's was based on associationist psychology.[226]

The main forum for the science of sexology was the 'Medical Society for Sexual Science and Eugenics in Berlin', founded in 1913 by Eulenburg. Monthly discussions of the biological basis of sexuality were published in Hirsch's 'Archive of Woman Studies and Eugenetics'. This represented the liberal wing of the eugenics movement, 'eugenetics' being a distinctive term introduced by Hirsch as more scientific. The membership of the group was even more overwhelmingly medical and male than in other varieties of eugenics, although there were diverse approaches within the Society. Hirsch, a member of the Prussian Committee on Racial Hygiene, was concerned with population policy, and published transcripts of the Committee's discussions. Others were more interested in the physiology and psychology of sex. Some, like Hermann Rohleder, saw the solution to the nation's problems in artificial human insemination, a technique which Rohleder had been pioneering since 1907. The theories of sexual periodicity of Wilhelm Fliess were a perennial topic of discussion. Others such as the Gestalt philosopher, von Ehrenfels, demanded eugenic morality.

There was a lively interest in biological research on simple marine organisms and associated philosophies of such as Driesch and Hartmann. There emerged a distinctive emphasis on the inherited constitution. Mendelian concepts of an inherited genotype were seen as important but not as the whole story. There were doubts about the application of genetics to humans. Lingering Lamarckism made many feel that the inherited constitution interacted with environmentally conditioned parts of the body. The Berlin professor of medicine, Kraus, typified the interest in applying the theory of an inherited constitution to diagnosis and therapy. He linked research on glands and hormones to Gestalt theory uniting psychology and physiology. He wished to shift the emphasis in viewing disease from the local malfunction of individual organs to the whole person. He urged that there were subjective and individual elements in the reaction to all stimuli and processes. Qualitative individual factors of feeling and instinct were part of the individual Gestalt. By invoking the Gestalt theories of Ehrenfels, Kraus was drawing on an alternative current in eugenics, as well as on the Berlin philosophical school of Gestalt psychologists such as Kurt Koffka, Wolfgang Köhler and Max

---

[226] I.-W. Kittel, 'Arthur Kronfeld (1886–1941)', *Psychologische Rundschau*, vol. 37 (1986), 41. M. Hodann, *History of Modern Morals* (London, 1937), pp. 1–21.

Wertheimer.[227] Kraus' philosophy shows how Weimar modernism was rooted in monism and idealist traditions. The society proclaimed sexology as a modern *Naturphilosophie*.

Scientific control and therapy for the pathological was a major concern of the sexual reformers. The euthanasia proposals of Binding and Hoche were discussed, but there was greater interest in more moderate procedures such as eugenic abortion, sterilization, and transplants or implants of animal testicles for rejuvenation or therapy. Advances in surgery, endocrinology and the theory of constitutional medicine linking anthropology with clinical research stimulated the discussions. Scientists were ever more convinced that psychosexual behaviour was determined by the sexual glands. A basis was found in C.E. Brown-Séquard's discoveries of the role of the glands in sexual maturation, a process called 'inner secretion', and of the possibilities of injecting substances from animal testicles for rejuvenation. From 1919 Sergei Voronoff's experiments on implanting monkey testicles for rejuvenation aroused much interest in France and the USA. The Austrian surgeon Steinach developed techniques for testicle transplants, which were pioneering in their surgical techniques, and valuable for the treatment of the war wounded and those who had had their testicles amputated because of TB or cancer. The social benefits of his work were publicized in an Austrian government film in November 1920. It was hoped that Steinach's experiments on castrating animals would provide a basis for sexual therapy.[228] Rejuvenation transplants raised serious problems of tissue composition and grafting techniques of animal on human skin. Some anatomists such as Hermann Stieve rejected the sexual specific functions of the interstitial cells. Others claimed that testicle transplants could 'cure' homosexuality. Hirschfeld spoke in November 1920 on how Steinach's experiments confirmed his 'third sex' theory of variation.[229] Steinach had suggested that histological findings on the testicles of homosexuals showed that there were features comparable to those in female glands at puberty like an excessive number of Leydig cells. Hirschfeld confirmed this, but interpreted it as a variation on the normal.[230]

Medical enthusiasm for having discovered the biological basis of sexuality and ageing meant that an atmosphere of confidence in solving sexual problems through medical counselling and surgery was generated. Eugenicists' attempt to establish a scientific basis for sexual reform was two-edged. On the one hand the intentions of many eugenicists were genuinely reformist. They wished to relieve the burden of moral guilt and social pressures on groups such as homosexuals. The choice of a

---

[227] F. Kraus, 'Geschichte und Wesen des Konstitutionsproblems', *Archiv für Frauenkunde*, vol. 9 (1923), 81–95.   [228] D.N. Hamilton, *The Monkey Gland Affair* (London, 1986).

[229] M. Hirschfeld, *Künstliche Verjüngung, Künstliche Geschlechtsumwandlung. Die Entdeckungen Professor Steinachs und ihre Bedeutung volkstümlich dargestellt* (Berlin, 1920).

[230] M. Hirschfeld, 'Hodenbefunde bei intersexuellen Varianten', *Sexualwissenschaftliches Beiheft, Archiv für Frauenkunde*, vol. 7 (1921), 173–4.

scientific strategy had points of weakness, since once racial categories permeated science, then science could change from a means of emancipation to a justification for persecution.

Health education

The aims of reviving the *Volkskraft*, and enforcing moral and healthy behaviour inspired the work of health educators. The economic crisis and national priorities prompted co-ordination of health education under a national committee. The Dresden Hygiene Museum offered expertise in mounting health exhibitions, and enjoyed the financial resources of the bequest of the Odol manufacturer, Lingner. The achievement of Lingner had been to replace printed literature by visual representation. While he intended that individuals should learn about their own bodies for themselves, by the 1920s the aim was to be collective instruction of the masses. Health education thus followed the shift from individualism to corporate organicism. The museum aimed to promote 'the national hygiene of the social organism', and to avoid working in the interest of industrialists.[231]

A transition occurred from voluntary to state-sponsored organizations. The Society for National Hygiene[232] which had organized local health education groups was superseded by a state body. In 1919 a Prussian Committee for Hygiene Education was convened. It included the nucleus of welfare-oriented eugenicists: Gottstein, Grotjahn, Krohne and Abderhalden. Other members were representatives of welfare organizations, such as the conservative Berlin internist, His, for TB, and Blaschko for VD. In June 1919 they met to consider whether there should be a national health education organization as a means of tapping the resources of the Dresden Museum. The Reich government was favourable and Abderhalden contacted Alfons Fischer of the Baden Social Hygiene Society. Fischer had been empowered by the German Society for Public Health to co-ordinate a national social hygiene organization.[233] In October 1919 a Reich Committee for Health Education was established, and state and provincial bodies followed.

The Saxon authorities and the Dresden Museum were enthusiastic. During the war, the museum had mounted travelling exhibitions on topics such as war relief and infant care. Between 1919 and 1921 one million people visited the travelling VD exhibition. The museum had a sense of its national role in disseminating the laws of orderly, hygienic behaviour. By November 1919 the Reich Committee for Health Education had been convened under the chairmanship of Carl Neustätter, the director of the Hygiene Museum, and Reich funds were allocated. The sickness insurance funds, welfare bodies, trade unions and womens' organizations were represented. The aims, methods and personnel of the health educators were restricted to the medical profession; the Hygiene Museum was in an influential

---

[231] STA Dresden MdI Nr 1539 Lingner Stiftung.
[232] Deutsche Gesellschaft für Volkshygiene.
[233] ZSTA P 15.01 Nr 9370 Bl. 1–7 Der Reichsausschuss für hygienische Volksbelehrung.

position, but demands by the medical historian, Karl Sudhoff, that the museum was to have absolute control over all initiatives in health education were rejected.[234] The Dresden Hygiene Museum was suffering an internal crisis. It had talented advisers like Sudhoff, staff, exhibits and boundless confidence in its role, but lacked a building. In 1917 a fatal decision was made to invest Lingner's shares, left in trust, in government war loan stock. Now the museum had to appeal for funds from the Reich, states, and industrialists. It sought the support of eugenicists. In 1920 Philaletes Kuhn, the professor of hygiene who had lost his job in Strasburg, came to Dresden, and tried to convert the museum to racial hygiene. He made fervently nationalist appeals to the Reich in tones emphasizing racial regeneration. But the museum opportunely decided to switch its allegiance from the right-wing racial hygienists to other SPD-oriented eugenicists. It was more in keeping with the socialism of 'Red Saxony' and the prevailing national politics. Grotjahn was cultivated as a warm friend of the museum. He ensured that the Parliamentary Committees on Population Policy passed resolutions calling for support of the museum. He contacted the USPD spokesman on hygiene, Moses, in order to mobilize left and trade union support. In June 1922 the museum proudly announced that it had won the backing of Pater Muckermann, the Jesuit biologist and eugenicist, who had previously been a critic of the museum. It meant that the museum had accommodated itself with the Centre-Left alliance that was to dominate Weimar eugenics. The museum in 1922 declared as its aims 'ensuring national fitness, and the physical and mental health of future generations'. These were the slogans voiced throughout the welfare-oriented system of public health.[235]

The Reich Committee for Health Education also had to compromise with the left. Initially, the committee's views were those of the ultra-right with stirring appeals in 1919 for 'strong men and vigorous women' to regenerate the family. The committee was hampered by the political and professional problems of admitting nature therapists and alternative therapists, who were clamouring for parity and representation in the movement to socialize medicine. The Reich Committee continued to be cautious in its dealings with the left. Whereas Grotjahn was acceptable, Weyl was rejected as a 'red rag', and a representative of the medically conservative Anti-Quackery League, Carl Alexander, was co-opted.[236]

The Hygiene Committee continued the policy of the Dresden museum by sponsoring visual rather than literary propaganda. Travelling exhibitions for VD and TB were launched. Constructivist art gave a powerful means of visual display of scientific and demographic information. Symbolic representations (known as isotypes) corresponding to statistical values and quantities vividly illustrated health and social conditions. The social hygienist, Teleky, appreciated their potential when first used in Austria. Exhibitions were populated by vivid representations of

[234] ZSTA P 15.01 Nr 9370 Bl. 28–73.
[235] STA Dresden, Sächsische Gesandtschaft Nr 1042 Hygiene Museum; MdI Nr 1539 Lingner Stiftung.   [236] ZSTA P 15.01 Nr. 9371 Bl. 5–8.

the declining birth rate in terms of rows of babies or pictures of idyllic families shrinking in size, and of hereditary alcoholism with lines of bottle-swinging men.

The greatest innovation was the sponsorship of films. There was a parliamentary furore over Hirschfeld's educational film, 'Other than the Others', when the Centre Party representative, Fassbender, attempted to have strict censorship imposed. There was a spate of 'moral films'[237] from 1919 which dealt with such topics as homosexuality, abortion, drug addiction and prostitution. These commercial productions combined social criticism with commercialism, and in varying degrees with voyeuristic scenes. There was obvious public relish for how respectable professors could fall victims to opium or prostitution, and for the portrayal of doctors as abortionists.[238] Socialists argued that pornographic films on sexual perversions could not masquerade as 'educational' if there was state production of films.[239] A compromise was reached when in 1921 contracts were made by health educators with Ufa, Deulig and other film companies. The first film commissioned was on 'Dangers of the Summer Heat for Infants'. There followed in 1921 a humorous comedy, 'Malchen – the Innocent from the Countryside',[240] which illustrated urban health risks. The Reich Ministry of the Interior made 20,000 marks available for commissioning films in 1922.[241] The Anti-TB League sponsored 'The White Plague' in 1922. The film company, Ufa (*Universum Film Aktiengesellschaft*), established a medical film department which made public health propaganda films such as 'Infant and Cripple Welfare' and 'Small-pox Prevention'. Ufa had been founded in 1917 when General Ludendorff ordered the War Ministry to co-ordinate film production in order to raise national morale. The Ufa cartel was financed by industrialists such as Krupp who had an interest in war production. That its films served conservative moral and eugenic ends was intentional as the company was meant to curb the harmful American influence, to educate, and to improve the quality of German films. The Anti-VD League with characteristic initiative sponsored an Ufa-produced film which enjoyed much popularity.[242]

Films soon came to serve eugenic purposes. The doctor, and Ufa producer, Kurt Thomalla became especially interested in eugenic films. With Kronfeld he presented medical films to the Berlin Society for Sexual Science and Eugenics in 1922. Such films had a dual role to communicate science to university students and to the medical profession, and to reach the general public. Films such as Steinach's on biological researches on the sexual glands were justified as presentations of scientific knowledge, but they met with a stormy response from the censorship authorities and from the moral purity lobby. Fassbender and Muckermann considered that films and visual materials had to balance a variety of aims. The public was attracted by the human and entertainment aspects, but the underlying

[237] *Sittenfilm.*   [238] Hohmann, *Sexualforschung*, pp. 256–83.
[239] *Verfassungsgebende Preussische Landesversammlung* (24 October 1919).
[240] *Malchen, die Unschuld vom Lande.*   [241] ZSTA P 15.01 Nr. 937 Bl. 36, 50, 87–96.
[242] *Die Geschlechtskrankheiten und ihre Folgen*, ZSTA P 15.01 Nr. 9372 Bl. 72–6.

aims of racial and social hygiene should not be lost from sight.[243] During the 1920s there were to be a series of confrontations with the censorship authorities when sexual reformers adopted the film as a medium for converting the public to greater tolerance of homosexuality and for promoting greater awareness of the eugenic risks of sexually transmitted diseases. Films became a major flashpoint in the controversy over sexual reform and family welfare.

'Psychopaths'

The collapse of the authority of the state, church and family was seen as unleashing a wave of mental disorder. Educationalists and psychiatrists detected widespread incidence of 'feeble-mindedness', 'neuropathy', and, the most disturbing of all, 'psychopathy'. They warned that psychopathic children would grow into a future generation of criminals, prostitutes and vagabonds. Psychopathy was a term used to denote mental abnormalities that stopped short of insanity, and that could be attributed to heredity manifested in 'degenerative anti-social behaviour'. The interpretation of psychopathy as an inherited disorder was built into the pre-war mental health law. Psychiatrists had resisted the attribution of breakdown and shock to the experience of war, and preferred such diagnoses as schizophrenia because this stressed the hereditary weak constitution of the patient. The morals and health of youth were at the centre of the concern to control psychopathy. Pastor Hoppe, the scourge of 'sexual bolshevism' established a 'centre for youth sexual protection'.[244] After the war, Bavaria and Prussia organized measures in response to demands by the German Association for the Welfare of Youth Psychopaths.[245] A survey of treatment facilities for psychopaths was held by Prussia in September 1920, and special clinics were encouraged by a decree of November 1921. A symptom of psychopathy was rootlessness, necessitating special measures for young vagrants. The provincial reports emphasized the links between social and mental disorders. Some administrators saw clinics as a means of dealing with political extremists, putschists and revolutionaries. Clinics were to be centres of control. Other experts were sceptical, arguing that 'psychopaths, who are cleverer and more cunning than the average person, will avoid the special clinics'.[246]

Clinics worked in association with the new youth welfare officers,[247] school nurses and doctors, and the families of the mentally disordered. Here was an ideal area for co-operation between doctors and educators. The aim was 'comprehensive care'. The pattern was repeated in many towns with school children and youth as the main targets. Special departments for youth psychopaths were established such

---

[243] M. Fassbender, 'Jugendschutz und Jugendwohlfahrt in der deutschen Gesetzgebung', *Das Kommende Geschlecht*, vol. 3 no. 3 (1924), and 'Das Wissen und Wollen der beiden Geschlechter', vol. 3 no. 4 (1924); ZSTA 15.01 Nr 9370–1.   [244] *Zentrale für Sexuellen Jugendschutz.*
[245] Deutscher Verein zur Fürsorge für Jugendliche Psychopathen; ZSTA M Rep 76 VIII B Nr 1850 Bl. 169; ZSTA P 15.01 Nr 9384 Psychopathen-Fürsorge 1920–25.
[246] D.F. Happich, 'Die Not unserer Psychopathen', *Die Innere Mission*, vol. 15 (1920), 81.
[247] *Jugendämter.*

as that — ominously (because of its role as a Nazi extermination centre) — at the *Landes Heil- und Erziehungsanstalt Hadamar*.[248] Between 1920 and 1927 fifty-eight homes and advisory clinics were established for psychopathic youths.[249] In 1923 the chairman of the Society for Special Education,[250] Egenberger, estimated that 25 per cent of all youths were psychopaths. He believed that 'the question of degeneration and decadence is a question of national survival'. Psychopathy raised the problem of the mental health of broad segments of the population. Egenberger was part of a group of educators in Munich who were especially concerned with organic degeneration. They had links with psychiatrists such as Max Isserlin, who established a Neurological Therapy and Research Institute for Children and Youths, and with the eugenicist Rüdin and the German Psychiatric Institute. Rüdin considered psychopathy to be an intermediate condition between the diseased and the normal. Consequently, most psychopaths were outside custodial institutions. The society, the Reichstag and states urged the need for central collation of statistics.[251]

The organic approach of Munich psychiatrists was distinct from a more educationally oriented Berlin group of such as Ruth von der Leyen (of the Association for the Care of Youth Psychopaths),[252] the socialist Walter Friedländer, and Friedrich Wilhelm Siegmund-Schultze (who developed the concept of a 'psychopathic constitution' and became the first director of the Berlin Youth Office). The Berliners constituted a liberal and progressive wing of youth welfare. They had a biologistic and state-oriented approach, but their efforts were directed towards rehabilitation.[253] Friedländer, a founder of the Workers' Welfare organization,[254] pioneered 'social pedagogy' and 'family care' in the Prenzlauer Berg Youth Office. He abandoned the concept of 'psychopath care' in favour of 'therapeutic education', preferring education to incarceration.[255] He ensured that the Prenzlauer Berg district of Berlin was a model of integrated youth welfare and health services by co-operating with the health department of the communist medical officer, Alfred Korach, in the provision of such facilities as Kindergarten, free milk, orthopedic centres and recuperation for tubercular children. The aim was to extend medical surveillance of physiological development to systematic monitoring of psychological development by systems of mass observation.[256] This pioneering experiment in dealing with mental instability in the community rather

[248] later to be the 'euthanasia' centre.
[249] ZSTA M Rep 76 VIII B Nr 1850 Einrichtung von Fürsorge- und Beratungsstellen für psychopathische Kranke 1920–1923.   [250] *Gesellschaft für Heilpädagogik.*
[251] ZSTA P 15.01 Nr 9384 Bl 341.
[252] *Verein zur Fürsorge für Jugendliche Psychopathen.*
[253] W. Jantzen, *Sozialgeschichte des Behindertenbetreuungswesens* (München, 1982).
[254] *Arbeiterwohlfahrt.*
[255] E. Harvey, 'Sozialdemokratische Jugendhilfereform in der Praxis: Walter Friedländer und das Bezirksjugendamt Berlin Prenzlauer Berg in der Weimarer Republik', *Theorie und Praxis der sozialen Arbeit*, (1985), 218–229.
[256] Harvey, *Youth Welfare and Social Democracy in the Weimar Republic: The Work of Walter Friedländer* (New Alyth, 1987), pp. 59–61.

in closed institutions laid the foundations of the child guidance clinic, and established an influential model of community care.

In contrast to 'progressives' such as Friedländer and von der Leyen, the hereditarian and authoritarian approach gained in influence during the 1920s. It was represented by such as Werner Villinger, the doctor in charge of the Hamburg Youth Office from 1926–34 (and later 'euthanasia' adjudicator). Concepts of social order and biologistic and mystic concerns (for example, with the 'divinity of childhood') formed a bond between psychiatrists and youth social workers. Pastor Happich of the Hephata asylum illustrates how concerns with heredity and social order reached the welfare institutions of the *Innere Mission*. In 1920 he revealed motives for the fear of degeneration when he quoted what he regarded as evidence of the link between psychopathy and bolshevism:

A twelve year old psychopath provided conclusive evidence when he said 'I know what I want to be when I am 17, I will be a Spartacist leader. That's what I'm suited for.' He knew exactly what those of his type have become.

The pastor was to lead the campaign for sterilization of mental defectives.[257]

Attitudes towards cripples were similarly motivated by fears of anti-social and delinquent behaviour. Cripples were a major post-war concern. There were large numbers of disabled ex-servicemen, and the war had also scarred the civilian population, in that the rise in TB had left many deformed children. As with TB victims, the priorities for cripples were to be preventive medical measures aimed at the younger generation. These problems were not without undertones of social control and eugenics. Physical disabilities were correlated with mental retardation and delinquency. There was especial concern with hereditary mental illness. In October 1919 the Prussian Parliamentary Committee on Population met to discuss provisions for cripples. They planned early location of cripples, treatment of curable conditions, occupational training, and institutionalization for cripples according to their needs. Homes for cripples had a dual welfare and eugenic function, in that they were regarded as a 'humane' means of preventing the inferior members of the race from procreating. The Prussian Cripples Welfare Law of 1920 required that negative psychological traits be noted. Physical abnormalities were signs of potential social deviance.[258]

Hereditary data banks

Demands by eugenically minded doctors for demographic data on hereditary diseases in families extended medical powers in the sphere of social welfare. The

---

[257] 'Die Not unserer Psychopathen', *Die Innere Mission*, vol. 15 (1920), 81; P. Göbel and H.E. Thormann, *Verlegt – Vernichtet – Vergessen . . .? Leidenswege von Menschen aus Hephata im Dritten Reich* (Schwalmstadt-Treysa, 1985).

[258] C. Poore, 'Der Krüppel in der Orthopädie der Weimarer Zeit. Medizinische Konzepte als Wegbereiter der Euthanasie', *Argument*, Sonderband 113 (1984), 67–78.

aim was to correlate records of medical, school and criminal authorities. Hereditary data-banks[259] would be used as the basis for research on the inheritance of diseases, mental disorders and crime, and of positive qualities such as leadership, fitness and genius. Doctors argued that it was not enough to locate only the sick and their parents, because the healthy could be carriers of latent pathogenic genes. Medical experts demanded the screening of total populations. For this the support of local, provincial, state and Reich authorities would be necessary.

Demands for health passports and hereditary data banks date from before 1914, and were linked to a long-term process of expansive medical professionalization. Psychiatrists and eugenicists took a lead in instigating data banks as a means of controlling crime and delinquency. When in May 1918 the German Psychiatric Institute was founded by the psychiatrist Kraepelin, armed with substantial municipal and state funds, its research was linked with administrative needs, as in its study of the mental health of war invalids, and with the problem of the 'anti-social'. Kraepelin's pioneering research on *dementia praecox* as an adolescent psychosis was combined with a Pan-German sense of war as healthy.[260] The Institute claimed official status, and stressed its aim of protecting the public from the dangerous and burdensome mentally ill. Its Genealogical Department under Rüdin established a massive data bank with records of asylums, hospitals, parishes, prisons, and information collected through interviews with families. Rüdin's aim was hereditary prognosis, so as to enable preventive medical schemes to be implemented. By calculating the Mendelian ratios and patterns of inheritance, it was hoped that effective genetic counselling could be provided. The racial hygienists Gruber and Rüdin praised the pioneering work on population and health statistics by the human geneticist Weinberg in Württemberg, where eugenicists drew on a long-standing system of family records to analyze the inheritance of diseases. Human genetics was the scientific underpinning of the demand for compulsory marriage certificates and marriage advice clinics. Control of the degenerate would allow positive cultural and moral values to flourish.[261]

Criminal biology was one of the first areas in which it was expected that social hygiene and hereditary biology would shed light on social conditions. In 1919 Rüdin joined forces with Theodor Viernstein, a Bavarian medical officer, for research on the families of prisoners at Straubing. School records were used to provide details of the intelligence of convicted criminals. On 15 January 1920 the Ministry of the Interior gave its approval.[262] The Director of the Bavarian Ministry of Justice, Richard Degenow, supported the introduction of a system of graded punishment, based on biological analysis of a criminal's instincts and character. The Bavarian Health Council, on which sat racial hygienists such as

259 'Erbkarteien'.
260 R.W. Whalen, *Bitter Wounds. German Victims of the Great War, 1914–1939* (Ithaca and London, 1984), pp. 61–5.
261 E. Rüdin, 'Familienforschung und Psychiatrie', *Die Naturwissenschaften*, vol. 9 (1921), 713–21.
262 BHSTA Mk 11158 Psychiatrische Angelegenheiten.

Gruber, approved a biological questionnaire to establish ancestry, diseases and behaviour. In 1924 the Bavarian Ministry of Justice decided to have a central Criminal Biological Record Office[263] based at the Straubing prison. The *Kultusministerium* ordered schools and parish registries to co-operate. In 1921 Rüdin began compiling a 'total register of the biological population'.[264] In 1926 the Reich Ministry of the Interior gave the Genealogical Department official status and rights to consult state and criminal records. It was to supply information to prisons, police, and law courts. The material was overseen by doctors, anthropologists and psychiatrists, and used for biological research, in areas such as twin studies. In 1928 it was decided to transfer these records to the German Psychiatric Institute.[265]

Criminal biological surveys were organized in other states on the Bavarian pattern. In 1923 the Dresden eugenicist, Fetscher, began to use Saxon criminal records for research on sexual deviants. In 1925 he gained the support of the Saxon Ministry of Justice for a comprehensive *Karthothek* on the anti-social. Regular grants of between 5,000 and 8,000 RM per year were made until 1933. He worked in conjunction with the police and other state and municipal authorities, commenting 'that the records of welfare offices often include biologically significant data'. Such information was to be of value for marriage counselling, career advice and for the juvenile court, and in distinguishing those prisoners who could be re-educated from those who were hereditarily incurable. In 1925 he emphasized the value of the data for sterilization. The Labour and Welfare Ministry requested that they be allowed to consult the survey in order to pass on information to welfare and youth offices. Psychiatrists such as Rüdin consulted the data. By 1930 Fetscher had data on 800,000 individuals from 70,000 families. He recorded mental and physiological disorders, alcoholism, character, indebtedness, and for women, details of pregnancies, menstruation and menopause. The aim was to produce a *Psycho-biogramm* relating physical to mental qualities using the typology of Kretschmer who related physical type to character. Research on the organic basis of personality was combined with racial hygiene.[266] Criminal biological surveys indicate how eugenics diminished individual moral responsibility, replacing this by hereditary determinism.

'The Rhineland bastards'

Moral purity campaigners, health educators, and advocates of negative eugenics joined forces to defend racial purity when French troops marched into the

---

263 'kriminal-biologische Sammelstelle'.
264 T. Viernstein, 'The Crimino-Biological Service in Bavaria. Outline of its Organization and Aims', RAC, BSH/24/Series 4/Box 9/folder 619.
265 BHSTA Mk 11779 Erbbiologische und kriminalbiologische Untersuchungen der Strafgefangenen; BAK R 86 2374 Bd 1 Bl. 328–9.
266 R. Fetscher, 'Zweck und Aufbau Erbbiologischer Karteien', *Die Medizinische Welt* (November 1933), 1,610–4; STA Dresden Justizministerium Nr 1587 Erbbiologische Karteien.

Rhineland. The Treaty of Versailles was resented by nationalists as bleeding Germany of scarce demographic and economic resources which were vital to sustain the race. The Treaty caused the 'loss' of 10 per cent of the population. The burden of economic reparations was loathed as damaging to the nation's health and prosperity. Medical officials were alarmed at possible effects on infant health owing to the loss of dairy cattle. The professor of paediatrics, Adalbert Czerny, was criticized by the Prussian medical department for not having put the medical case against reparations more forcefully at the Paris negotiations.[267] The Treaty spurred health officials into monitoring its damaging effects on the nation's health. The medical profession mobilized against the Treaty by holding public meetings, such as that at the University of Berlin in December 1922.[268]

The reaction to the occupation was coloured by racism. In April 1919 the German delegation asked for black troops to be excluded from the occupying forces; this was unacceptable to the Allies. A force of 85,000 allied soldiers was stationed in the Rhineland. Because of German violations of the demilitarized status of the Rhineland, and because of delays in reparations, the French enlarged their zone of occupation on 6 April 1920.[269] Only a small proportion of the troops were Asian, African or Caribbean in origin. But German propaganda grossly exaggerated the numbers, and created a mythology of animal hordes brutalizing civilized Germans. Chancellor Müller was indignant at the impropriety of 'Senegal negroes occupying Frankfurt University and the Goethe House'. Lurid accusations of rape and robbery were made. Politicians defended the 'dignity of the white race' and of German culture against 'the black curse'. All parties, except the USPD, protested in the Reichstag against the deployment of non-white troops. The socialist President Friedrich Ebert denounced the injustice of an occupation by a 'lower culture'. Some (but not all) feminist socialists denounced the occupation as an 'unnatural' threat to the female sex. Others pointed to the health risks posed by the blacks. Stöcker demanded passive resistance against the continuing economic and military war being waged by the Allies against the German people.[270]

Pamphlets and newspaper stories were run on the 'Horror on the Rhine'.[271] The occupation brought home to Germans that imperialism was a thing of the past: no longer could the German overseas possessions be justified on the basis of the superiority and civilizing benefits of German culture and science. The troops had the effect of transforming this cultural imperialism into biologistic nationalism.

[267] ZSTA P 15.01 Nr 9403 Gesundheitliche Schäden der Kriegs- und Nachkriegszeit, 1920–22 Bl. 17; A.M. Lockau, *The German Delegation at the Paris Peace Conference* (New York, 1941), p. 39.

[268] 'Kundgebung der Deutschen Ärzteschaft zur gesundheitlichen Notlage', *Klinische Wochenschrift*, vol. 2 no. 2 (8 January 1923), 53–9. Orations included: W. His, 'Der Niedergang der Lebenshaltung des Deutschen Volkes', pp. 53–6; H. Dippe, 'Die Deutsche Ärzte am Krankenbett des Deutschen Volkes Schicksalsfrage', pp. 56–8; P. Krautwig, 'Deutsche Kinder in Not, des Deutschen Volkes Schicksalsfrage', 58–9.

[269] S. Marks, 'Black Watch on the Rhine: A Study in Propaganda, Prejudice and Prurience', *European Studies Review*, vol. 13 (1983), 297–334.

[270] H. Stöcker, 'Ruhrbesetzung, und waffenloser Widerstand', *Die neue Generation*, vol. 19 (1923), 1–4.   [271] R. Pommerin, *Sterilisierung der Rheinlandbastarde* (Köln, 1979), pp. 7–18.

The popular racist reaction went beyond what could be tolerated by the state and respectable politicians. A 'German Emergency League against the Black Curse' was founded to combat 'the decline of the white race'. The German Foreign Office considered it so extreme as to discredit the German case, and so no official support was given. The League's founder, Heinrich Distler, was accused of embezzling funds collected for propaganda. The authorities regarded Distler as thoroughly disreputable, for such reasons as having infected his wife with syphilis.[272] Doctors, however, rallied to Distler's cause and spoke on the medical implications of the 'black curse'. The Prussian section of Distler's League was headed by Frau von Konopacki-Konopath; her husband, an official in the Ministry for Reconstruction, was also active in the League. (That they were to organize the Nordic Ring in the mid-20s indicates how the 'black curse' mobilized defenders of racial purity.) The Foreign Office preferred scientific experts in racial hygiene. It selected the anthropologists Martin (professor at Munich) and Fischer to put the German case in Sweden. Günther, the Nordic propagandist, expressed his concern that 'negro blood was running in the veins of Germans, especially due to the "Black Curse" on the Rhine'. Anthropological science was thus invoked to defend Germany's national integrity.[273]

The authorities were concerned that the occupation was a threat to public health and morality. It was at this level that health officials betrayed racist anxieties, and showed the biologistic nationalism underlying public health measures. Krohne typified the reaction of public health officials. He accused the French of a sadistic lack of regard for human life. Inflation, milk shortages and economic dislocation were causing a rise in TB. Above all, it was the damage to the health of the future generation that alarmed him.[274] Health officials accused the occupiers of having a degenerative effect on morals. They condemned the troops as rapists and spreaders of VD, thereby causing sterility among native Germans. The French and Belgian military authorities opened special licensed brothels in order to show that they had the problem under control.

Health propaganda was a nationalist weapon to be invoked against the French in addition to racial prejudice. The French troops were accused of spreading influenza, skin diseases, TB and worms. Professors of hygiene pointed to the potential hazards of such tropical diseases as malaria.[275] Welfare became a means of continuing subversion against the occupiers. The Prussian Finance Ministry conceded that it gave grants for infant welfare clinics in the Saar only because of their propaganda value against the French. The occupying forces began to compete in the distribution of welfare supplements so as to pacify the population, especially youthful dissidents.[276] The supposed ravages of TB and VD, and the shortages of

---

[272] BHSTA MInn 72853 Notbund gegen die schwarze Schmach.
[273] Pommerin, *Rheinlandbastarde*, pp. 18–20, 27.
[274] O. Krohne, 'Versailles, Ruhreinbruch und Volksgesundheit', *Deutsche Allgemeine Zeitung* (23 February 1923).   [275] Marks, 'Black Watch', p. 301.
[276] ZSTA M Rep 151 IC Nr 9074 Bl. 152.

milk, food and fuel meant that clinics were regarded as vital. The Prussian authorities were outraged that municipal medical and welfare facilities could not be sustained.[277] Poverty and disease were exacerbated by the economic burdens of the occupation. But the problems of chronic diseases were shared with other areas of Germany and officials admitted that morbidity and mortality rates in the Rhineland were no worse than elsewhere.[278] Nationalist hostility against the foreign oppressors was a convenient surrogate for the explanation of economic inequalities in German society.

The eugenic awareness of the Germans was heightened by the birth of between 500 and 800 babies of mixed-racial origins. Medical officers counted up and reported on the numbers of 'illegitimate' children and the proportion of white to non-white.[279] With the black troops stigmatized as syphilitic and idiot criminals, state officials were confronted by demands for the sterilization of the mulatto children. Some officials were concerned 'with the racial purity of future generations'. Sterilization was considered by Bavarian officials in the Ministry of the Interior during 1927.[280] The demands were rejected by the Reich Minister for the Occupied Territories who considered that German mothers would oppose sterilization of their children. The Reich Health Office denied that mulatto children were a racial hygienic peril, and pointed out that the sterilization would be illegal.[281] The medical reaction to the Ruhr occupation shows how the human costs of the post-war calamities was a major issue in determining social policies. It reflected a generalized view of medicine's involvement with public morality and order. The ferocious public reaction revealed how widespread *völkisch* racism was becoming. However, the medical administration remained capable of separating the eugenic concern with the health of 'future generations' from *völkisch* racist propaganda.

Sterilization

There was agitation for – and implementation of – sterilization as a remedy to the threats posed by the physically and mentally degenerate. There had long been a minority of eugenicists favouring sterilization for criminals and the insane. They were spurred on by the US sterilization laws, and by the support of psychiatrists.[282] Sterilization was regarded as humane, modern and scientific. But there were

---

277 ZSTA M Rep 76 VIII B Nr 2833 Hygiene in Schulen 1922–4, Bl. 230.
278 ZSTA P 15.01 Nr 9422 Gesundheitsverhältnisse im Einbruchsgebiet 1923–27.
279 ZSTA M Rep 76 VIII B Nr 2056 Folgen des feindlichen Ruhreinfalls; Rep 151 I C Nr 9074 Bevölkerungspolitik; ZSTA P 15.01 Anstalten Nr 9404.
280 Sterilization was supported by Geheimrat Dr Dieudomé.
281 BHSTA MA 107830 Farbige Truppen; G. Lilienthal, '"Rhinelandbastarde", Rassenhygiene und das Problem der rassenideologischen Kontinuität', *Medizinhistorisches Journal*, vol. 15 (1980), 426–37.
282 The *Archiv für Kriminalanthropologie* carried articles on sterilization in 1913; Holmes, *Bibliography of Eugenics*, pp. 496–514.

differences of opinion among eugenicists as to whether there should be compulsory or voluntary sterilization, and whether social indications were admissable. In 1922 the Racial Hygiene Society supported voluntary sterilization of the hereditarily sick, but recognized that compulsory measures were scientifically and socially premature.[283] The more academically-inclined racial hygienists felt that sterilization might jeopardise the implementation of positive eugenic measures by the state, but in the turbulence of post-war Germany a vociferous lobby campaigned for compulsory sterilization. The campaign was treated seriously by state officials, and by doctors. Surgically, vasectomy was reckoned to be a simple operation. There were considerable medical and social issues relating to the extent and nature of hereditary diseases and medical authority at stake.[284]

Some doctors simply used their professional prerogative and went ahead with sterilizations. Lenz reinforced the academic campaign for sterilization by arguing in a handbook of gynaecology that eugenic sterilization did not constitute criminal assault.[285] Gütt, who became the architect of Nazi public health, was an active campaigner for sterilization in 1919. There was an unknown quantity of sterilizations carried out in these years. Most doctors were discreet about a measure which might bring prosecution. But there was one exception, who gave maximum publicity to the eugenic sterilizations that he had initiated, in order to campaign for compulsory sterilization. This 'sterilization apostle' was Heinrich Boeters, who was medical officer in Zwickau in Saxony. Despite Boeters' eccentricities, that he was a medical officer indicated the permeation of public health by eugenics. Since 1921 he had referred patients, mostly children, to a distinguished surgeon and director of the state hospital in Zwickau, Heinrich Braun, for sterilization. Braun covered himself by obtaining a certificate from a psychiatrist that in each case the malady was hereditary, and that he had obtained written consent of both parents or of the guardian.[286] That in 1924 Braun was elected president of the German Surgical Association shows that he was not regarded as having breached professional standards.[287] Boeters added that operations were also carried out at private gynaecological clinics in Aue and in Zwickau. A minimum of nineteen and a maximum of sixty-three patients were sterilized by Boeters.

Boeters' sterilization campaign provoked conflicts with the Saxon authorities. In April 1922 the local administrator commented that Boeters was on the verge of nervous collapse, and that an additional medical officer should be appointed.[288] Boeters magnified his actions, pretending that he had authorized as many as 300 sterilizations. If others did not follow his example, he predicted that the nation

283 Leitsätze der Deutschen Gesellschaft für Rassenhygiene, 14 and 15 October 1922, points 27 and 28.
284 Noakes, 'Nazism and Eugenics', p. 81; Bock, Zwangssterilisation, pp. 45–51.
285 F. Lenz, 'Erblichkeitslehre und Rassenhygiene (Eugenik)', in J. Halban and L. Seitz (eds.), Biologie und Pathologie des Weibes, (Berlin and Vienna, 1924), pp. 803–68.
286 H. Braun, 'Die künstliche Sterilisierung Schwachsinniger', Zentralblatt für Chirurgie vol. 51 (1924), 104–6.   287 'Heinrich Braun', in Grote (ed.), Selbstdarstellungen, vol. 5 (1925), pp. 1–34.
288 STA Dresden Kreishauptmannschaft Zwickau Nr 2752, 1922–23 betr. Bezirksarztstelle in Werdau; MdI Nr 15182 Bezirksärzte 1908–11 for Boeters' career.

would be populated by degenerates, and Germany would cease to be a civilized nation. His aims were characterized by an authoritarian concern with social order, and demands for a racial dictator. In October 1923 he claimed that if he had been listened to twenty years before there would be 'quiet and order in the nation'. Boeters urged his medical colleagues to sterilize idiots, the feeble-minded, epileptics, the blind, deaf and dumb. He recommended sterilization especially for children with learning disabilities, and for those in institutions such as the mentally ill so as to permit their release. Women and girls who gave birth to illegitimate children should be examined as to their mental state, and if degenerate should be sterilized. Hereditary criminals could be released after sterilization. The operation should be performed only by doctors with adequate training in surgery and gynaecology. Sterilization of those of high eugenic value should be an offence under the law of assault.

Boeters was a tireless propagandist. He sought to convert state officials and the public to sterilization. After exhausting the patience of the Saxon authorities, he turned his attention to the Reich. On 8 October 1923 Boeters offered the Reich Health Office large quantities of his newspaper articles. The Saxon authorities warned that Boeters had been suspended, and that official contact with him was inadvisable.[289] They regarded Boeters as mentally deranged, and suspected that he was suffering from paranoia. He was showing the same lack of inhibitions in his dealings with superiors as in his sterilization campaign.[290] They considered him to be incapable of a balanced view of the legal and scientific aspects of sterilization. But they emphasized that Boeters had not been suspended for instigating the Zwickau sterilizations – indeed they welcomed these as having triggered off socially and eugenically important discussions. Boeters pursued a vendetta against the authorities, claiming that since 1924 the Saxon Foreign Office had sabotaged his attempts to publish in scientific journals and newspapers and to deal with other authorities. He alleged that the right to consult his personal files was denied. Late in 1925 Boeters was retired 'owing to a weakening mental capacity' and officials warned of his 'querulous delusions'.[291]

Although Boeters was dismissed as a crank, eugenic sterilization was given serious consideration by the authorities. Sterilization was first discussed by the Prussian Health Council in 1921. At this time it was referred for further expert advice; the authorities regarded the politically unstable situation as grounds for postponing any decision. On 16 July 1923 the Thuringian Ministry of Trade requested the Reich for a legal opinion on whether voluntary sterilization could be introduced into Germany. It was in Saxony that the most radical sterilization proposals were formulated. Although Saxony had a strongly socialist government, as in Prussia health was in the hands of nationally-minded experts. The Saxon

[289] ZSTA P 15.01 Nr 9347 Bl. 246, Massnahmen gegen den Geburtenrückgang 1919–1924.
[290] ZSTA P 15.01 Nr 9347 Bl. 314.
[291] ZSTA P 15.01 Nr 9347 Bl. 192; Reichsjustizministerium 30.01 Nr. 6094 Unfruchtbarmachung von Verbrechern, Bl. 79

Health Council discussed sterilization in October 1923, and January, March and May 1924. The committee included a number of racial hygienists drawn from the ranks of psychiatry, such as Ferdinand Stemmler (the director of the state mental hospital of Arnsdorf), Bumke and Nitsche, and the professor of hygiene, Kuhn. (Nitsche was to be 'T4' Ober-Gutachter in the Nazi medical killing of mental patients.) They considered sterilization as a 'humane' and cost-effective measure for schizophrenics, manic-depressives, alcoholics, psychopaths, the hereditary feeble-minded and those with a criminal disposition. The surgeon Braun was invited to the session in March 1924, much to Boeters' resentment. Stemmler drafted a law justifying sterilization on the basis of racial hygiene. His premise was that culture inhibited selective processes in society. He proposed a commission of a lawyer, a psychiatrist and a doctor trained in racial hygiene. Citing the evidence of Rüdin and Schallmayer, he claimed that sterilization was appropriate for psychiatric diseases such as schizophrenia, epilepsy, Huntington's chorea, and hereditary crime, but in other diseases such as manic-depression it was deemed harmful. The Saxon Committee supported sterilization as a voluntary measure, but with the decision taken on the advice from a doctor and a psychiatrist. The methods should be either by operation, or by X-rays, a technique first used by Ochsner in Chicago in 1899.[292] The Saxon Ministry of Justice gave the verdict that sterilization contravened the law of assault. But they urged that the concept of health should not be seen in individualistic terms, but as associated with the collectivities of the family and nation. Sterilization would then have preventive justification. The law of assault should not apply so far as a mentally ill or criminal person was concerned. In June 1924 the proposals for voluntary sterilization were referred to the Reich Health Office.[293]

On 1 December 1923 the Prussian Ministry of Welfare convened a meeting of its Racial Hygiene Committee. The Berlin professor of psychiatry, Bonhoeffer, and the legal official Moser provided expert opinions. Others present were all eugenicists: the geneticists Goldschmidt and Poll, the social hygienists Grotjahn and Hirsch, the pathologist Westenhöfer, and the official Krohne. Bonhoeffer condemned Boeters' proposals as an unsuitable basis for legislation and administration.[294] Bonhoeffer recommended further hereditary biological and clinical research. There should be study of the results of Swiss and US legislation, which was of interest for criminology and therapeutics. He considered that eugenics should be strictly limited to hereditary diseases and medical conditions. If there was ever to be sterilization, it should not be compulsory, and only state administrative bodies should be responsible for evaluating and instigating the operation. They discussed the possibility of extending sterilization to criminals and the anti-social.

[292] F. Stemmler, 'Die Unfruchtbarmachung Geisteskranker, Schwachsinniger und Verbrecher', *Allgemeine Zeitschrift für Psychiatrie*, vol. 80 (1924), 437–68; ZSTA P 15.01 Nr 9349 Bl. 14–26.
[293] ZSTA P 15.01 Nr 9349 Bl. 315.
[294] K. Bonhoeffer, 'Die Unfruchtbarmachung der geistig Minderwertigen', *Klinische Wochenschrift*, vol. 3 (1924), 798–801.

Grotjahn spoke out against compulsion, and concluded that more clinical and medical experience was necessary.[295] At the very least, these verdicts amounted to calls for additional research. Socialists in the Prussian *Landtag* responded by calling for welfare measures to improve women's experiences of pregnancy and birth, so as to avoid degenerate offspring. The socialist representative, Frau Kunert, praised the work of the Racial Hygiene Society in attacking the root causes of degeneracy.[296]

The implications of these early discussions were that medical and public health authorities could administer eugenic sterilization. But there was a crucial source of opposition, stemming from the legal officials of the ministries of justice. The Reich Health Office was directed by a legally trained official, Franz Bumm, who moderated the office's position to condoning only welfare-oriented eugenics.[297] In October 1923 the Health Office pointed out the US legislation had met with massive opposition. While the science of heredity suggested that sterilization could be effective in reducing the numbers of mental and physical degenerates, racial hygiene had not provided conclusive proof for every aspect of the problem. Moreover, there were legal, religious and political barriers. Finally, such remedies could not be condoned either by the afflicted individual or their families. Given that social disorders and nervous stress were rife in the nation, the time did not seem appropriate. The office decided to initiate inquiries in the USA on the basis of Géza von Hoffmann's 1913 book on US eugenics.[298] In response to continual pressure by Boeters and the Saxon proposals, the Reich Health Office concluded in January and March 1924 that the sterilization issue was not yet ripe for discussion.[299] The Prussian Ministry of Justice could see the justification for sterilization on a medical and social basis, but not for eugenic sterilization. Its attitude and the law itself, were determined by the concern for protecting the interests and rights of the individual patient. The Ministry ventured to criticize the laws of heredity as controversial, and cited the anti-eugenic tract of the biologist Oscar Hertwig.[300]

Despite the efforts of the Saxon authorities to lobby newspaper editors in order to convince them that Boeters was mentally unstable, he published a dramatic series of newspaper articles. He wrote incessantly in national and local papers, in specialist journals and wherever he could find either a sympathetic or a gullible editor. Significantly, in 1925 he published in the monthly bulletin of the Protestant *Innere Mission*.[301] He held a series of public meetings. He drafted a series of laws, called the *Lex Zwickau*, to urge sterilization instead of institutionalization of the

---

[295] Leitsätze, Ausschuss für Bevölkerungspolitik und Rassenhygiene von 1 Dezember 1923 in BAK R86 Nr 2374 Bd 1 Bl. 353–5; ZSTA P 15.01 Nr 9357 Bl. 195.
[296] *Preussischer Landtag* (1921/24), Drucksache Nr 7483.
[297] K.-D. Thomann, 'Das Reichsgesundheitsamt und die Rassenhygiene', *Bundesgesundheitsblatt*, vol. 26 (1983), 206–13.
[298] G. von Hoffmann, *Die Rassenhygiene in den Vereinigten Staaten von Nordamerika* (Munich, 1913).
[299] ZSTA P 15.01 Nr 9347 Bl. 322–3.   [300] ZSTA P 15.01 Nr 9349 Bl. 84.
[301] ZSTA P 15.01 Nr 9348 Bl. 9–34; ZSTA M Rep 76 VIII B Nr 2001 Bl. 211, Boeters in *Bausteine. Monatsblatt für die Innere Mission*, vol. 57 no. 1 (1925).

eugenically degenerate. He argued that his demands were becoming milder. He had initially proposed to sterilize all mothers of 'illegitimate' children, and now he targeted only those with hereditary diseases.[302]

In 1925 a magazine, *Das Tagebuch*, pointed out that the 'sterilization apostle Boeters' had lost touch with reality. Whereas he claimed that he had sterilized 300 patients, they could only document nineteen cases. His scientific delusions proved that he was sick, as he claimed to have discovered a new theory of heredity, and he had proposed to sterilize aggressive women because the German woman was by nature passive. Details of the cases suggested that the adolescents and children treated would have benefited from special education. In the case of a nine year old, a school doctor had diagnosed hereditary feeble-mindedness, but the costs of special education were too high, and so she was referred to Boeters. A fourteen year old had been withdrawn from an asylum where she was being educated. It was disturbing that Boeters' actions had not been condemned by the authorities.[303]

Boeters exerted continual pressure on the Reich. In January 1925 he addressed a large meeting in Berlin, when he clashed with Moll, the expert on medical ethics, and the eugenicist Hirsch. Their criticisms provided the Reich Health Office with ammunition. They dismissed the Saxon voluntary proposals and Boeters' compulsory proposals again in February 1925. The Reich officials said that the public meetings had shown how Boeters' views were too controversial among the medical profession. As Hodann informed several reformers, a basis for racial hygienic sterilization in medical science was still lacking. It was still unclear which conditions were inherited and what benefits could result from education and social conditioning.[304] No other European state had compulsory sterilization. But officials conceded that voluntary sterilization was a possibility. This marked the end of the first wave of sterilization proposals, but an undercurrent of hereditary research continued throughout the 1920s, so that by 1930 there was consensus that a scientific basis for sterilization had been achieved.

Euthanasia

The widespread anguish at the defeat, political turmoil, mass starvation and sickness during the crisis of 1919–24 broke down precepts of humanity and benevolence. The national collapse and foreboding of the extermination of the German *Volk* provoked the conception of hitherto unthinkable extremes of radical eugenic measures, justified by national survival. Compulsory sterilization and medical killing or 'euthanasia' were the ultimate forms of negative eugenics. Medical killing of 'valueless life' as a solution to national social ills was prescribed

---

[302] Copies of various formulations (at least three) of the *Lex Zwickau* abound in official files as ZSTA P 15.01 Nr 9347 or BAK R 86 Nr 2374.
[303] ZSTA P Nr 9348 Bl. 57; O. Kraus, 'Der Fall Boeters', *Das Tagebuch* (7 March 1925).
[304] M. Hodann, 'Rassenhygiene', *Die Neue Generation*, vol. 21 (1925) 123–4.

by doctors and lawyers, and provoked widespread discussion.[305] In 1920 the lawyer Karl Binding and the psychiatrist Alfred Hoche published a book on 'the destruction of life that is no longer worth living'.[306] A second edition was published in 1922. The tract was hailed as expressing the feelings of many as a result of war and its aftermath.

The transition from euthanasia (a term which derived from the Greek for 'fine death') at the request of a suffering individual, to compulsory, bureaucratized and professionalized forms of medical killing was symptomatic of the demise of liberal individualism. During the 1890s euthanasia had been discussed in terms of whether a doctor might abet and allow a terminally ill patient to die at the request of the patient. Such 'mercy killing' represented an individualistic concept of euthanasia as the right of the individual to choose when to end their life. In 1895 Adolf Jost published a 'social study' of euthanasia, suggesting that the incurably ill had the right to choose death, and that this was of benefit both to the dying and to society. This introduced the concept of death in the interests of the 'health' of the 'social organism'. He coined the concept of *negativen Lebenswert* to express the subjective and objective factors that justified the termination of life.[307]

While Jost's approach was conceived in terms of a balance between individual rights and society, eugenics shifted the emphasis away from the individual and on to the extermination of 'useless life'. Incurable illness became equated with degeneracy. The concept of incurability was extended to include those with a life expectancy of many years.[308] In 1911 Hegar, the Freiburg gynaecologist, who previously advocated sterilization and castration, argued for the social and racial benefits of euthanasia as a means of fortifying the fit and strong by ridding them of the burden of the weak and dying. The Monist League debated euthanasia proposals, suggested by a terminally ill TB victim, in terms of the individual and social value of suffering.[309]

The war destroyed the value attached to individual life, shifting the emphasis to collective national survival. There were new supporters of a eugenic view of euthanasia. In 1915 Alexander Elster argued for euthanasia since it was in the interests of society to maintain the health of only the fit. Hoche also took steps towards the justification of compulsory euthanasia. In 1915 he wrote of the end of atomistic individualism, and of the transformation of the nation into an organism of a higher order. He argued that the *Volk* was an organism of a higher order with rights above those of the individual.[310] He began to change his attitude to euthanasia during the war, when he suffered the loss of a son. In a university oration

[305] R.J. Lifton, *The Nazi Doctors. Medical Killing and the Psychology of Genocide* (New York, 1986).
[306] K. Binding and A.E. Hoche, *Die Freigabe der Vernichtung Lebensunwerten Lebens. Ihr Mass und Ihre Form* (Leipzig, 1920).   [307] A. Jost, *Das Recht auf den Tod. Sociale Studie* (Göttingen, 1895).
[308] K. Nowak, *'Euthanasie' und Sterilisierung im 'Dritten Reich'* (Göttingen, 1984), pp. 43–4.
[309] Roland Gerkan, (letter to Wilhelm Ostwald on euthanasia), *Das monistische Jahrhundert*, vol. 2 (17 May 1913), 169–73.
[310] A.E. Hoche, *Krieg und Seelenleben*, (Freiburg-in-Breisgau and Leipzig, 1915).

of 6 November 1918, he still opposed terminating the lives of the incurably ill. But by 1920 he was arguing that doctors were responsible for the welfare of the totality of the social organism, and that exterminating the lives of harmful or useless members was necessary.[311] Many agreed that war casualties and the nation's lack of resources, food and Lebensraum justified euthanasia. It was claimed that it was wrong to sustain worthless lives of the sick and deranged, while worthwhile lives of starving children were being lost.[312] During the war mental hospitals had suffered severe cuts in rations, and there was death from malnutrition on a substantial but incalculable scale. Such informal but lethal neglect of the mentally ill was to be formally justified in terms of 'therapeutic' benefits for the health of the fit and of future generations.

It was in response to the post-war crisis that the Freiburg phalanx of anti-socialist eugenicists radicalized their anti-socialist Darwinism and supported medical killing with a medical and social rationale. Binding had been professor of law in Leipzig, but had retired to Freiburg. His positivistic theory of legal norms based on historical precedents and social requirements challenged concepts of individual rights. The state was the guardian of the law, and whatever the state decreed was right, even if it contravened morality. He distinguished between those patients able to give consent, when the patient's will was to remain paramount, and those 'incurable idiots' unable to give consent and for whom he advocated a commission – a physician, psychiatrist and lawyer. This form of tribunal was to remain a key feature in attempts to bureaucratize eugenic controls. The notion of expert panels with power over life had been developed during the war for medical abortions.

Hoche had been professor of psychiatry in Freiburg since 1902. He specialized in neuropathology. He had a deep personal conviction of the insignificance of the individual as a product of ancestral generations. His materialist emphasis on heredity led him to oppose Freud. He had experimented on executed criminals in order to show that the spinal cord could conduct electricity. The defeat of Germany alarmed him. Left-wing students tore down his portrait because of his nationalism, and they threatened to storm his home. He felt vulnerable as a psychiatrist. Because he feared that irate patients attacked doctors who did not support claims for war pensions, he invariably kept a pistol at hand during consultations.[313] Hoche combined professorial elitism with economic concerns by linking the convictions that doctors always had the right to sacrifice life in the interests of the majority, and that the completely idiotic were an immense burden on the economy. Euthanasia was a 'national duty' to prevent the 'nation's degeneration'. He estimated that there were 500,000 'idiots' with 'valueless' lives, and a further 10,000 congenitally crippled. Euthanasia represented the reverse side of the ideology of the 'human economy'. If society was to ensure that life was to be

---

[311] Nowak, 'Euthanasie', p. 47.
[312] C. Burchardt, 'Euthanasie – "Vernichtung Lebensunwerten Lebens" im Spiegel der Diskussionen zwischen Juristen und Medizinern von 1900 bis 1940', med. Diss. Mainz 1981, pp. 50–3.
[313] A.E. Hoche, Jahresringe (Munich, 1935), pp. 216–7, 223.

of productive value, unproductive lives of 'human ballast' should be eliminated as an oppressive burden on the fit and healthy. Binding and Hoche re-defined euthanasia from being a curative ending of a tormented life to being a curative value for the social organism, and refuted the charge that this was murder. Euthanasia was envisaged for the incurably mentally ill who no longer had the will to live. Hoche divided the mentally ill into those with 'acquired mental death' such as schizophrenia and a syphilitic 'softening of the brain', and those born with abnormalities. It was necessary to distinguish between patients having a rapport with their environment, and those incapable of any feelings such as piety or gratitude. The decision was to be taken by two doctors.[314]

Binding and Hoche triggered off a wide-ranging medical, legal and theological discussion. Euthanasia attracted the attention of many newspapers. Students completed dissertations on the merits of euthanasia. On 19 November 1920, the judge Karl Klee argued in a lecture to the Society for Forensic Medicine that the killing of the anti-social and the worthless was a legitimate measure of social hygiene. In the same year a work was published under the pseudonym of Ernst Mann, called 'The Moral of Power'. In a fictitious state doctors subjected people to an annual medical inspection, and referred the infirm and the suffering to the medical police. This utopian vision extended compulsory euthanasia to organic diseases like cancer and TB. In 1922 the same author, whose real name was G. Hofmann, published on the 'Release of Humanity from Suffering'.[315] He demanded the elimination of the mentally ill and infirm, and of crippled children at birth. Too many cripples and sick were bad for national morale, and were an immense economic burden. The Karlsruhe *Ärztetag* of 1921 discussed, but rejected, legalization of euthanasia. This surfaced in a 1922 petition to the Reichstag for the killing of the mentally ill and of crippled children. In 1922 Councillor Borchardt from Liegnitz published a draft law for the killing of the mentally ill.[316] Following this format of an ideal law, the medical officer Boeters, in 1923, and Ludwig Lemme in Heidelberg considered that the unfit were a morally unjust burden on the fit, and that the state might kill 'valueless life' that had degenerated to the level of a plant or animal.[317]

Staunch opposition arose. Euthanasia was denounced as murder, as contravening the essence of law, which was to sustain life, and as open to abuse. Dr Wauschkuhn of the Berlin-Buch asylum pointed out that definitions of incurability were elastic; the fear might arise that what was expected to be a short stay in an asylum might have fatal consequences. In 1920 Ewald Meltzer, the Director of the Saxon asylum of Grosshennersdorf, sent 200 questionnaires to parents of so-called idiot children. Of 162 replies, only nineteen favoured

[314] Binding and Hoche, *Lebensunwerten Lebens*; E. Klee, *'Euthanasie' im N.S. Staat. Die Vernichtung des 'Lebensunwerten Lebens'* (Frankfurt a. M., 1983), pp. 20–2.

[315] E. Mann, *Die Erlösung der Menschheit vom Elend* (Weimar, 1922).

[316] Borchardt, 'Die Freigabe der Vernichtung Lebensunwerten Lebens', *Deutsche Strafrechtszeitung*, vol. 9 (1922), 206–10.   [317] Klee, *'Euthanasie'*, p. 26.

euthanasia for their children. Many neurologists attacked Binding and Hoche for undermining the humanitarian medical ethos of care and cure. It was wrong to assume that the mentally ill had a low level of vitality. There was a grave risk of misdiagnosis, of poisoning doctor-patient relations, and of arousing popular hostility against all medical institutions.[318] Grotjahn argued that medical techniques of controlling pain were so effective as to render euthanasia unnecessary. In 1925 the asylum director, Dr (theol.) Martin Ulbrich, wrote on the problems of the incurably mentally disabled, and of their 'vegetable-like' existence. His verdict was that they were the results of sin, and they were warnings to the rest of society to remain virtuous. There was thus a duty to care for the incurable.[319]

Medical killing and Nazi racism

The early plans for euthanasia were a response to the terrifying conditions of post-war Germany. But the rift between euthanasia as a eugenic extreme and Nazism had still to be bridged. The elimination of the sick and infirm was a cure for society as a whole. The discussions occurred in a medical and legal context rather than in a racist context, and show the force of an independent strain of biologistic opinions. The political extremism of post-war Germany precipitated hitherto undreamt of measures as biology supplanted humanitarian ethics. Compulsory sterilization and 'euthanasia' were the medical counterparts of the *Freikorps* and the first full flush of Nazism. There was a surge of racist nationalism. The publisher Lehmann provided a link between Hitler, *völkisch* racism and racial hygiene. Hitler's *Mein Kampf*, written in 1924, shows a grasp of Darwinian natural selection as a basis of evolution; biological examples of the sterility of hybrids were cited to justify struggle between races. Yet although presented by Lehmann with a copy of the Baur, Fischer and Lenz textbook of human heredity, Hitler showed ignorance of modern Mendelian views on heredity in his support of the dated idea of blending inheritance of parental characteristics in the offspring. He might have come across the idea of sterilization in a memorandum by Gütt, which was in the possession of Ludendorff. Hitler condemned 'humane' intervention in the process of sexual selection – suggested by Ploetz's racial hygiene – as Jewish and pacifist. Hitler did suggest sterilization of the mentally ill, and medical tribunals to select those fit for settlement. *Mein Kampf* stressed the need for Germans to restrict mating to only those of Aryan stock. It prophesied that inter-marriage would bring about racial degeneration with physical and intellectual regression, compared to 'a slow but surely progressing sickness'. While revealing the fear that unless Germany hit back against Jews and the Allies the nation would perish, Hitler does not seem to have grasped the anthropologists' point that there was no such entity as a pure German race. Nor had he as yet understood the medical debates on 'euthanasia'. Eugenicists

---

[318] E. Meltzer, 'Das Binding'sche Problem', *Klinische Wochenschrift*, vol. 2 (1923), 1911.
[319] Nowak, *'Euthanasie'*, pp. 55–7, 58–60.

such as Lenz paid greater attention to sterilization and marriage certificates than to euthanasia, as the priority of eugenicists was control of fertility. Euthanasia was dismissed by Lenz and other racial hygienists as irrelevant to eugenic fertility controls in 1923, although Lenz recognized its value for malformed babies.[320] The intellectual rift between Nazism and racial hygiene was matched by eugenic experts' disdain for the dictator as a psychopath.[321]

The aftermath of the war saw innovations that set an agenda for the future development of the welfare state on eugenic lines. At the same time there was a hardening of the biologistic and racist hostility to humanitarian welfare. With hindsight, national socialism was the most ominous product of the post-war crisis, but at the time the priority of eugenicists was to ensure that the extension of welfare institutions and the socialization of health care was used to advance the cause of improved health of future generations. Ambitious schemes for comprehensive family welfare were to dominate the Weimar period. The expansion of the welfare state had conflicting rationales, ranging from radical socialism and feminism to patriarchal conservatism. Eugenicists competed for power to manage and control this expansion. It was remarkable how the welfare state was able to grow, despite severe economic difficulties and inflation. This was because of the dynamic forces of professionalization and patriotic social reconstruction. The tentacles of social hygiene probed every sinew of everyday life from sexuality to the rationalization of industrial work. As long as the expansive welfare system was democratically accountable, or at least run by professionals having a humane and benevolent sense of duty to the sick, then social hygiene was at least benign if not of positive benefit. Once the professional and social ideologies became more authoritarian, then safeguards would no longer operate to protect the existence of the sick, the disabled and those with unconventional lifestyles. The expansion of custodial institutions, health centres, and networks of social work, initiated by the movement for post-war reconstruction, could be turned to coercive and authoritarian ends once the political and ideological barriers to imposing compulsory sterilization and euthanasia were removed.

[320] G. Koch, *Euthanasie, Sterbehilfe. Eine dokumentierte Bibliographie* (Erlangen, 1984), pp. 26, 40.
[321] G. Bock, *Zwangssterilisation im Nationalsozialismus* (Opladen, 1986), p. 26; review of Binding and Hoche in *ARGB*, vol. 14 (1922), 211.

6

Weimar eugenics

There was a brief interval of stability and recovery during the mid-1920s when daringly innovative art and culture gathered momentum. There was confidence in the economic and technical capacities of science as a basis for planning and production in modern society. Many industries were modernized in line with theories of efficient and rationalized production. Domestic consumer demand rose for novel products such as electrical appliances, gramophones and radios, as well as for cosmetics and mass-produced clothing. The public enjoyed mass entertainments like the cinema and sporting events. A self-conscious modernism became fashionable. Exposure to American culture and industrial products was accompanied by the rationalization movement in industry, by the culture of 'new sobriety' (*Neue Sachlichkeit*) and by adoption of a consciously modern lifestyle suited to the accelerating pace of urban life.[1] Critics of modernism linked consumerism to the decline in the birth rate, and to physical degeneration resulting from nervous stress and consumer excess, as in the case of indulgence in alcohol and tobacco and overspending on consumer luxuries. Much of the eugenicists' efforts went into ensuring that industrial and urban society would retain organic values associated with the family.

Intellectually, these were years of experimentation. Weimar culture attained a legendary brilliance. Among the artistic movements were expressionism, ecstatic utopianism, bitingly critical social realism, Dadaist irrationalism, and the surrealist discovery of the unconscious. Intellectuals revelled in a sense of elitist superiority, and condescendingly agitated for improved education and living conditions for the proletariat.[2] Intellectual euphoria for scientific solutions to social problems infected science, medicine and welfare measures: social work, public health and sexual counselling were developed in a spirit of avant-garde modernism. Whereas

---

[1] J. Hermand, 'Unity within Diversity? The History of the Concept of "Neue Sachlichkeit"', in K. Bullivant (ed.), *Culture and Society in the Weimar Republic* (Manchester, 1977), pp. 166–183.

[2] S. Lamb, 'Ernst Toller and the Weimar Republic', in Bullivant (ed.), *Culture and Society*, pp. 71–93.

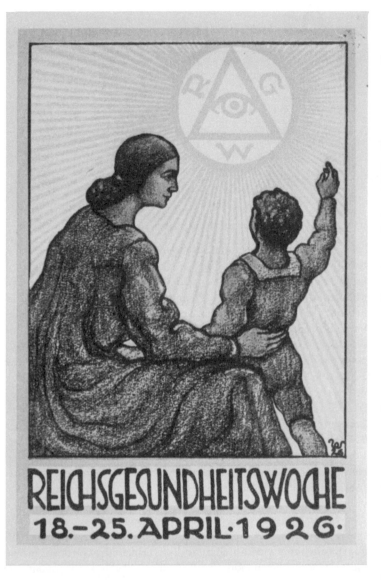

6 The Reich Health Week, postcard designed by O. Weigelt and printed by G. Martini, Stuttgart. The Health week was designed to promote public awareness of health as based on medical science. It was the idea of the socialist doctor, Julius Moses, but was boycotted by left-wing controlled sickness funds. Innovative methods of health education utilized during the Reich Health Week included the use of films, radio talks, sporting events, and shop window displays.

conservatives idealized the remnants of the traditional social order, the artists and social critics attacked bourgeois conventions as pathological and diseased. Experts in social hygiene and eugenics attempted to reconcile these antitheses on the basis of positive health. As rationalization required experts to dictate what was rational, social hygiene and welfare services took on this role in domestic life.[3] But the position of the modernist elite was precarious. This was partly because there were inherent contradictions within the brave new Weimar world. Consumerism and the vision of rational economic planning could only be reconciled during a period of economic buoyancy. Once the boom ceased there resulted a clash between the heightened consumerist appetite for mass-produced goods and entertainments, and the growth of an all-embracing system of state welfare.

At first sight there seemed to be a radical break between the archaic culture of Wilhelmine Germany and Weimar modernism. The break was less clear if organicism is recognized as a link between the old and new Germanies; this was indicated by the survival of eugenics. Ideas of positive health drew on organicist biology and nationalist ideology. Eugenicists blended organicist traditions with social planning and consumerism. They advocated greater personal hygiene, sport and outdoor leisure pursuits. Eugenicists linked their plans to the new psychiatry and sexual reformism, while defending hereditarian concepts which reflected a commitment to conservative values and to social stratification on the basis of hereditary worth.

That organicist values remained deeply rooted in German social and economic thought can be seen in the rationalization movement in German industry. Rationality was cast in an organicist mould. Corporatist concepts of state co-ordination of industry and unions continued in the spirit of post-war social reconstruction. These were legitimated by an organicist ideology of the *Berufsstaat*. National cohesion was to be sustained by an ideal of a 'social partnership'.[4] The factory was compared to a productive organism. Machines were depicted as organic extensions of the human body. This theory of *Organprojektion* suggested that technology had a harmonizing and cultural potential. It required a suitably adapted workforce skilled in specific functional tasks and yet imbued with organicist and nationalist values.[5] There was a marked preference for the welfare-oriented ideas of 'Fordism' – that there should be rationalization without social conflict – over the Taylorist drive for specialization and industrial efficiency.[6] There was a consensus among doctors, managers and officials that the term 'Taylor system' should be avoided, because of its connotation with de-skilling, monotony and intensification of the labour process. A German science of work was to have

[3] A. Grossman, 'The New Woman, the New Family and the Rationalization of Sexuality. The Sex Reform Movement in Germany 1928–1933', PhD dissertation, Rutgers University, 1984.
[4] *soziale Arbeitsgemeinschaft.*
[5] J. Herf, *Reactionary Modernism, Technology, Culture, and Politics in Weimar and the Third Reich* (Cambridge, 1984), pp. 157–9.
[6] H. Ford, *Das Grosse Heute und das Grössere Morgen* (Leipzig, 1926).

distinctive basis in organicist concepts of the 'human economy'.[7] Fordist ideals of a clean and sober workforce, and of social integration rather than confrontation suited German conditions where the state had a key interventionist role. Fordism was able to overcome some of the antipathy of the *völkisch* right because between 1920 and 1927 Ford was an outspoken critic of Jewish internationalism.[8] Industry supported the idea that German capitalism was inherently different to Western capitalism; class tensions could be reduced through corporatism. Many industrialists also had doubts about Western democracy and international co-operation. They looked to the state for arbitration in industrial relations, and formed massive conglomerate trusts to regulate national markets.

Given the limitations of natural resources and of Germany's defeat as a great power, science was to provide substitutes for the loss of raw materials and colonial sources of supply. The state remained keen to sponsor efforts to advance the scientific basis of production, industrial organization and management.[9] The 1920s saw key sectors of German industry modernize and rationalize production to an advanced level. The importance of social medicine was recognized: for as the pace of industrial production quickened, the greater were the risks of industrial accidents and diseases. Experts in social medicine such as Teleky in the Ruhr and Koelsch in Bavaria found opportunities in industrial health. Such new technologies as electrical rock drills in mining increased the risks of dust diseases; in 1926 came compensation legislation for silicosis. Experts were required as industrial medical officers, medical inspectors of factories, and hygienists and toxicologists to establish and monitor 'safe' levels. Firms based on more advanced technologies, as in the chemical industry, employed medical officers to screen workers' health. The Taylorist drive for efficiency and intensification of work was a stimulus to studies of fatigue and of the physiology of muscular contraction. But scientists regarded mechanistic physiology as outmoded. The eugenic concern with adaptation, constitution and mental capacity was well suited to the comprehensive welfare-oriented approach characterizing Weimar social policy.

Biology was an integral part of the movement to rationalize industry. Scientific management was interested in a biologically based psychology for the selection of fit and productive workers. This movement for vocational selection, known as 'psycho-technics', urged total screening of the workforce.[10] As the status of applied science rose, openings were created for applying social biology. Rationalization found an ally in hereditarian biology. Professors of hygiene and physiology co-operated with industrialists in the establishing of the Kaiser Wilhelm Institute for Occupational Physiology. Psychiatrists at Kraepelin's Munich Institute and

[7] C.S. Maier, 'Between Taylorism and Technocracy', *Journal of Contemporary History*, vol. 5 (1970), 27–61.
[8] Poliakov, *Anti-Semitism*, pp. 245–50; F. Lenz, review of 'Henry Ford: Der internationale Jude', *ARGB*, vol. 15 (1923), 434–46.
[9] R. Brady, *The Rationalisation Movement in German Industry* (Berkeley, 1933), pp. 3–11.
[10] P. Hinrichs, *Um die Seele des Arbeiters* (Cologne, 1981); R. Schmid, *Intelligenz- und Leistungsmessung. Geschichte und Funktion psychologischer Tests* (Frankfurt-on-Main, 1977), pp. 145–50.

eugenicists like Fetscher advocated a biologically grounded industrial psychology. They were keen to gain acceptance for the screening of workers[11] in order to select and advise on the suitability of particular biological types for particular jobs. They argued that medical supervision could weed out those workers who were unsuited to tasks because of predisposition to such diseases as TB or to neuroses. The techniques acquired by the medical profession in promoting military efficiency were transferred to industry. Studies were made of the physiology of work, and anthropometric techniques were to classify the 'racial' characteristics of occupational groups.[12] Hirsch took an interest in the special hazards for working women. Tandler's *Zeitschrift für Konstitutionslehre* contained studies of the physique and 'constitution' of a variety of population groups such as gymnasts, students, and apprentices in a variety of trades. Kaup's index of height and weight, Kretschmer's correlations between physique and character, and Reichel's addition of chest size, were used to compile 'constitutional indices' for different occupations. The professor of hygiene, Karl Bernhard Lehmann (the brother of the Pan-Germanist publisher and also a committed Pan-Germanist), stressed how racial factors could not be influenced by social conditions and nutrition. Verschuer sought to analyze the genetics of different constitutional types. His researches on the genetics of tuberculosis posed a barrier to the recognition of – and compensation for – industrial diseases such as silicosis and asbestosis. Rather than accepting these as distinctive fibroses of the lung caused by toxic substances at work, these were subsumed in the concept of a constitutional predisposition to lung diseases. The eugenicists saw how total screening of the population could be linked to economic efficiency, and could further the eugenic aim of locating the hereditarily unfit.

The Weimar occupational health system enlarged the scope of screening, medical certification and evaluation of health risks with the appointment of medical inspectors of industry. The social hygienist Teleky was appointed as the first Prussian provincial medical inspector of factories in the Rhineland in 1921, and director of the Academy of Social Hygiene at Düsseldorf. In 1925 compensation legislation was extended to cover eleven new occupational diseases. The German Trade Union Congress (ADGB) was forced to defend its members' interests by appointing medical experts. In 1926 the Grotjahn student Meyer-Brodnitz was appointed as its medical adviser. He recommended unification of the sprawling insurance system and a socialization of health services. Trade unions and sickness funds should do more to educate workers on health risks and to promote welfare services. Socialization required that levels of medical expertise in public health services be raised, whereas employers wished to rely on the more conservative independent general practitioners as 'certifying surgeons'.[13] At the

---

[11] 'Berufsberatung'.

[12] For example, E. Brezina and V. Lebzelter, 'Über Habitus und Rassenzugehörigkeit von Wiener Schmieden und Schriftsetzern', *Zeitschrift für Konstitutionsforschung*, vol. 13 (1927), 1–41.

[13] D. Milles, 'Chancen und Blockaden. Der Aufschwung gewerbehygienischer Anstrengungen und die Herausprägung des Berufskrankheitenkonzepts in der Weimarer Republik', in Milles and R. Müller, *Berufsarbeit und Krankheit* (Frankfurt-on-Main, 1985), pp. 84–110.

same time experts in occupational hygiene sought to keep science 'free' from the influence of trade unions and political parties. They indicated a way in which an economy could be modernized without becoming embroiled in political entanglements.[14] The arguments for producing more children of better quality were – in part – responses to the need for an adequate industrial labour supply, and schemes for rural settlement were justified by nationalist concepts of economic self-sufficiency. Eugenics reinforced the movement for a planned deployment of the nation's scarce resources.

Social conflict was to be reduced by planning based on applied social science. Ideas arose for social surveys conducted by research teams which included biologically minded psychologists, anthropologists and health experts. Planning for health went with the idea of a planned economy by an interventionist state. A spirit of utopian planning seized architects and designers, state and municipal officials, and doctors and social workers. They looked forward to an urban environment where efficient expenditure of effort could allow the population to manage the tasks of work and domestic life, as well as providing recreation and welfare facilities. More effort went into reform of domestic life than in intervention in the process of production in the workplace. Although many eugenicists such as Grotjahn, Hirsch, Kaup, and Krohne had experience of the medical hazards of mines and workshops, they focused their attention on the family or at least on such questions as the special problems of working mothers. Medical services needed to be expanded irrespective of the chequered fortunes of German industry.

Housing reform was indicative of the attempts to construct an ideal environment. From 1925 modern architecture mushroomed in most cities but especially in Berlin and Frankfurt. While the functionalism of the Bauhaus symbolized the concern with rational efficiency, there were also expressionist architects who continued the garden city and utopian 'back to the soil' movements. There were settlement schemes dominated by primitive and monumental symbols, such as the utopian folk communities. Visionary planning of housing estates drew on ideals of an organic community.[15] Within the home rational design was to ensure economy of effort. Fitted kitchens and bathrooms were designed to promote cleanliness and efficiency. The idea of positive health inspired planners to prevent TB and infant mortality by personal hygiene, improved nutrition and environmental improvement. Nature was invoked as an invigorating and healing force. Inside and outside, light and air were priorities with gardens, balconies and open spaces. Community centres were a focus, and there were amenities like crèches and clinics, hospitals and sports facilities. The pioneer of prefabrication, Max Taut, saw the architect's main task as that of an organizer, solving biological, social, technical and psychological problems.[16]

Medical reformers saw the housing problem as the key to improved health and a

[14] MPG Arbeitsphysiologie Gen II 8 Bd 3 1918–22 Meeting of 29. 8. 1919.
[15] W. Pehnt, *Expressionist Architecture* (London, 1973).
[16] S. Willett, *The New Society* (London, 1982), pp. 124–8.

buoyant birth rate. Housing attracted the attention of eugenicists who, in contrast to modernist architects, favoured more traditionally designed single family houses with gardens, as conducive to the rearing of large and healthy families. Maximizing fresh air with playgrounds and sports facilities would prevent rickets and TB. Urban conditions were as far as possible to be 'ruralized'.[17] Grotjahn and Harmsen considered that overcrowding contributed to the declining birth rate, and was a cause of not only illness but also of youth delinquency and crime.[18] Modern culture attempted to blend the urban, professional and scientific with organic social values and the priorities of the family. While the inevitability of rationalization as part of the nation's development was accepted, efforts continued to channel people's energies into working to sustain healthy families, rather than just for personal consumer gratification. Although marriage rates were increasing (1928 was a boom year), the birth rate continued to decline. The declining birth rate which had been a phenomenon of the upper classes now spread to the industrial proletariat. Ever higher estimates of abortion rates were produced, and experts in social hygiene worried about the 'rationalization of sexual life'. At the same time the modernists had their critics. Nationalist forces were regrouping, and oriented themselves to the values of motherhood, the peasantry and national traditions. Traditionalists and moderns were poised to clash over population and welfare policies.

MOBILIZING THE PUBLIC

The public's appetite for advice literature and products for better health was recognized as immense and largely unsatisfied. Commercial and professional interests competed to fulfill the demands of the rapidly expanding market for health. Eugenic education was meant to modify the market forces of consumerism and rationalization in order to sustain healthy families. Eugenicists urged the expansion of welfare measures and the promotion of a positively healthy lifestyle. Positive eugenics characterized the relatively more prosperous mid-20s with intensified health education and propaganda. The reasons were partly financial, in that education and associated activities like gymnastics were cheaper than providing welfare supplements and improving living conditions, and partly ideological in that the eugenic mentality was meant to inspire more orderly behaviour and a sense of national duty. A voluntaristic and democratic code of eugenics had to rely on education in order to infuse a new 'will' to regenerate the German family into the population.[19]

A eugenic education organization was established to counter the degenerative

[17] Grotjahn, *Hygienische Forderung*, pp. 152–7.
[18] H. Hirtsiefer, *Die Wohnungswirtschaft in Preussen* (Berlin, 1929); V. Noack, *Kulturschande – Die Wohnungsnot als Sexualproblem* (Berlin, 1925); de Laporte, *Wohnungsnot und Sittlichkeit*, = Schriften zur Volksgesundung.
[19] A. Grotjahn, *Die Hygiene der menschlichen Fortpflanzung* (Berlin and Vienna, 1926), p. 338.

effects of consumerism on physique and on the birth rate. The German League for National Regeneration and Heredity[20] was founded in Berlin on 16 March 1925, its statutes were publicized in May and its first major meeting was on 3 September 1925. The eight founders were state officials (Arthur Ostermann, Otto Stölzel and the registry officials Edwin Krutina and Hans Wander), welfare and public health experts (Christian of the Reich Health Office, and Behr-Pinnow), the publisher Alfred Metzner and the editor Konrad Dürre. The League offered a means of linking the interest groups from which the founders were drawn, and for reaching a wide public audience. The term *Aufartung* had a basis in the post-inflationary economic concept of *Aufwertung* or revaluation. The idea of regeneration conveyed the optimistic spirit of social reconstruction that prevailed during the mid-20s. *Aufartung* was free from *völkisch* racial connotations, and it sounded more German than *Eugenik*. Its aim was the health of future generations, which it termed *Zukunftshygiene*. While publicity stressed science and the future, it also appealed to nationalist sentiments with its slogan: 'Protect German Heredity and thus the German Type!'.

The League for Regeneration was even more closely involved with the state welfare apparatus than the Racial Hygiene Society. The initial impetus came from registry officials who had since 1920 distributed health education literature. In October 1924 the League of Registry Officials[21] approached the Racial Hygiene Society with the suggestion that they co-operate. Nothing came of this and instead the registry officials sought support from a more evangelical organization. The secretary of the League was an ardent eugenicist. Like many converts he practised what he preached and regarded the mental and physical health of his own family in racial terms. In order to bring the blessings of eugenic education to the public, he established contact with Metzner for distributing publications for registry officials. Metzner became treasurer and published the league's journal, *Eugenik*, and family ancestry books.[22] The *Familienstammbuch* contained eugenic advice and inspiring words on the need to breed a strong race. Ostermann supported extension of the responsibilities of registry officials. Krutina was a tireless lecturer and educator for eugenics, which he saw as a means of providing more specialized training for registry officials. He also lobbied for extending state registration requirements.[23]

The League represented an effort to create a broad-based public opposition to the sexual reformers, and especially the League for the Protection of Mothers. The veteran infant health campaigner, Behr-Pinnow, became chairman of the League for Regeneration. He was converted to eugenics from the moral viewpoint that motivated his crusade against the League for the Protection of Mothers in Imperial Germany, but Behr-Pinnow still had the League for the Protection of Mothers

[20] *Deutscher Bund für Volksaufartung und Erbkunde.*
[21] *Reichsbund für Standesbeamte*, founded in 1920.
[22] *Zeitschrift für Volksaufartung und Erbkunde*, vol. 1 no. 1 (15 January 1926).
[23] E. Krutina, *Chronik eines guten Bundes*, (Berlin, 1942); 'Edwin Krutina †', *Das Standesamt*, vol. 6 (1953), 241–2.

and Sexual Reform (a 1920s addition) as his *bête noire*, with eugenicists and sexual reformers fighting for control of marriage advice clinics. Behr-Pinnow's influential position in welfare organizations meant that he renewed the attempt to convert welfare experts to eugenics. He aimed to influence not only doctors, but also teachers, priests, organizers of sporting events and all those active in social welfare.[24] Eugenics was to permeate the expanding spheres of leisure and consumerism.

Education and positive eugenics were major concerns of the League for Regeneration. However, it also recommended negative eugenic methods such as sterilization and preventive detention. In 1925 Behr-Pinnow commended Boeters for having initiated the discussion on sterilization. He hoped that more doctors would join the campaign. But it was necessary to provide a sure scientific basis for sterilization. In 1929 he argued that although sterilization was technically illegal, no one had been prosecuted when it was justified on the basis of genetics. He advocated the sterilization of mentally subnormal children before they entered special schools. The League's aims from 1925 included the demands that the physically and mentally degenerate should not be allowed to procreate. Through selection of parents with a good quality pedigree, the whole nation's quality could be improved. Behr-Pinnow considered that there was only a German *Volk*, not a German race, while regretting that the allied 'vultures' had caused the territory of the German state to be far smaller than the *Volk*. A sign of the lack of anti-semitism was the league's choice of the Goldschmidt-Rothschild Bank for its finances.

Behr-Pinnow accepted the racial classifications of Günther, Fischer and Lenz that Germany was a composite of the Nordic, Mediterranean, Alpine and Dinaric races, as well as Kretschmer's correlation of physique and character. Behr-Pinnow regarded the Nordic race as endowed with superior spiritual and physical qualities, facts which accounted for German achievements in science, technology and in social organizations. He cited the insituting of TB and infant welfare clinics as an example of a French innovation, but one only correctly applied in Germany. Behr-Pinnow regarded the declining birth rate as a sign of the degeneracy of the French nation. As in 1912, he continued to accuse socialism of being a cause of the declining birth rate. He attacked the Russian Revolution as having 'sterilized the nation' by removing the cultured elite and the nation's *Führerschaft*. He supported Lenz's scheme for resettling selected child rich families on special eugenic small-holdings. He advocated the instilling of eugenic consciousness through the family. But he was keen to introduce a system of marriage certificates for men and to increase the responsibilities of registry officials in ensuring that only the healthy should marry. He cited the work of the municipal medical officer, Drigalski, in Halle as a model of racial screening prior to marriage, while Behr-Pinnow placed great hope in the effects of education. Registry officials should give families advice, and work in conjunction with health offices and eugenically minded doctors. Behr-

---

[24] Rott papers, Behr-Pinnow to Rott, 24 February 1926.

Pinnow's writings show that behind the League lay deeply held racial biological and nationalist convictions.[25]

The vice-chairman and, from 1930, chairman of the League for Regeneration was the Prussian public health official, Ostermann. He had moderate SPD sympathies. His support ensured an abundance of official subsidies especially from Prussia and the Reich, and the use of state machinery for distributing the League's propaganda. The *Ministerialdirektor* and chairman of the Racial Hygiene Society, Krohne, kept his distance from the League, although he and Ostermann were in a commanding position in the eugenics movement. The annual subsidies of 6,000 marks in 1926 rising to 10,000 marks in 1928 from the Prussian Welfare Ministry and 5,000 marks from the Reich Ministry of the Interior represented half of the League's total annual income.[26] It received substantially more from the state than did the Racial Hygiene Society.[27] The Prussian Ministries of Welfare, Education and of the Interior supported the eugenic aims of the League and urged officials to raise eugenic consciousness in their localities.[28] That meetings were often held in the Prussian Welfare Ministry indicates how the League was an extension of the state welfare apparatus. The Reich Health Office joined at the instigation of the medical statistician, Roesle.[29] The League attempted to gain support on a local level. Bremen's medical officer Tjaden and the Hamburg professor of anatomy, Poll, urged that there be state recognition of the League. Tjaden supported the educational work of the *Bund*, but had doubts about the aim of excluding the mentally deficient from procreation.[30] Drigalski, the Berlin medical officer, was unable to obtain municipal support for the League.[31] The situation suggests that local health officials were out of step with local authorities in their allegiance to eugenics.

Those at the head of the League declared that the Racial Hygiene Society had failed to reach broad sectors of the public. This was because it lacked a popular journal. The membership of the Racial Hygiene Society had mixed feelings. Some thought that the League was superfluous. Others were ready to co-operate with it, as in a better position to popularize eugenics. Lenz welcomed its foundation but mischievously pointed out in the *Archiv* that the term *Erbkunde* – genetics – could be confused with *Erdkunde* – geography.[32] This was a clever response to the accusation that 'racial hygiene' could be confused with *völkisch* racism. Most

---

[25] C. v. Behr-Pinnow, *Die Zukunft der menschlichen Rasse. Grundlagen und Forderungen der Vererbungslehre* (Berlin, 1925); Behr-Pinnow, *Menschheitsdämmerung?* (Berlin, 1929).

[26] ZSTA M Rep 76 VIII B Nr 2073 Bl. 121; Nr 2074 Bl. 301, 373, 429; ZSTA P 15.01 Nr 9421 Bl. 229 for details of state subsidies.

[27] Berlin Racial Hygiene Society was granted 1,000 marks in 1929. ZSTA Rep 76 VIII B Nr 2074 Bl. 300.

[28] BAK R 86 Nr 2371 Bd 2 Bl. 367; Förderung rassenhygienischer Bestrebungen: 23 Februar 1926.

[29] BAK R 86 Nr 2371 Bd 2 Bl. 334.

[30] STA Bremen V2 Nr 1536 Deutscher Bund für Volksaufartung.

[31] Landesarchiv Berlin Rep 42/Acc 1743 Nr 9018; Stadtarchiv Berlin GB 877.

[32] F. Lenz, 'Ein "Deutscher Bund für Volksaufartung und Erbkunde"', *ARGB*, vol. 17 (1925), 349–50.

eugenicists liked the idea of a more popular journal. But it was hated by the Munich publisher Lehmann as not *völkisch* and it rivalled his own efforts in the popularization of racial hygiene. He denounced the League as a subversive clique of Berlin Jews.[33] The monthly journal was widely distributed, even to members of the Berlin Society for Racial Hygiene. 5,000 copies of its journal were printed as copies were distributed by state and voluntary agencies.[34] It claimed support as far afield as among the Germans of Siebenbürgen in Rumania. The journal projected an image of eugenics as one concerned primarily with health and heredity. By the time it fused with the German Racial Hygiene Society in the autumn of 1932, the League had 600 members, whereas the Racial Hygiene Society had only 500.

The League for Regeneration held many conferences on eugenic themes such as marriage, taxation and schooling. The speakers were drawn from the established nucleus of eugenicists. A typical example was the conference of October 1928, attracting an audience of over 700. The speakers were Baur, Fischer, and Grotjahn on 'eugenics and the people'; Lenz, Löwenstein (of the Anti-VD Society), and three school teachers on 'eugenics and schooling'; Muckermann, Ostermann, the Hamburg anthropologist Walther Scheidt, and Krutina on 'eugenics and the family'. These speakers, all experts in either eugenics or public health, typified the Weimar consensus on eugenics and welfare. The League provides insight into the importance of the popularizing of ideas of health and biology for the welfare state.

HEALTH PROPAGANDA

The 1920s were a golden age of health education and propaganda as a result of the shift from state policing to professional educational agencies. Much hope was placed in health education for school children, as well as in health promoting activities such as gymnastics and sports. The health educators were aware that unless they invented new methods of communication the public's interest would dwindle. The gospel of better health was propagated with a missionary zeal. Health was projected as something of national and economic value. By following the prescribed laws of hygiene, benefits would accrue to both the individual and society.

The pre-war efforts at health education were based on expressing scientific ideas in simple lectures and in cheap pamphlets; but during the Weimar period an effort was made to appeal to the public's taste for entertainment, fashion and consumer goods. A national hygiene museum, with origins in Lingner's International Hygiene Exhibition of 1911, co-ordinated efforts. Exhibitions large and small on health and homecraft were continually being mounted and circulated around the country. Medical scientists relentlessly advocated better health for the labouring masses. In October 1925 the Emergency Fund for German Science sponsored a

---

[33] M. Lehmann, *Verleger J.F. Lehmann* (Munich, 1935), pp. 403–4.
[34] *ARGB*, vol. 26 (1932), 99.

week of lectures on medicine for the working people, which was staged in the Ruhr.[35] A climax came with two national events held during 1926: these were the Gesolei, health, welfare and exercise exhibition, and the Reich Health Week in April 1926. These were major tests for innovative methods of health propaganda offered by the radio and cinema. Health publicity material became visually attractive through the use of such modern media as cartoons and entertaining, being presented as popular literature in the style of romances and adventure stories. Statistics of the declining birth rate and degeneration were presented by the ingenious use of scale models and pictures. Graphic isotypes of prams and coffins representing birth and death rates showed that unless current trends were halted the nation would become senile and die.

Educating youth

The modernization of the school curriculum allowed for increased teaching of biology. Biology was a means not only of conveying the facts of life, but also of objectifying stereotypes of the normal family and reproductive behaviour. School biology as a means of teaching the facts of life was supported in the Prussian Assembly of 1919.[36] In 1924 there was a petition in the Prussian Assembly for eugenic education in schools. Krohne and other ministerial officials supported this.[37] In 1925 Prussia introduced 'social hygiene' into the curriculum. Teachers were asked to show with tact the importance of sexual hygiene for the welfare of the individual and society. Parents, youth workers and the churches were to be alerted as to their responsibilities for health education. Other states such as Hamburg in 1928 and Saxony in 1932 followed the Prussian example. Pupils were to be taught the laws of reproduction, heredity and hygiene. They were to be made aware of their responsibility for the next generation. Girls were to learn their special duties for health care and motherhood.[38]

The school biology curriculum was to include study of the laws of cellular life and of the 'cell state', the ecology and formation of social groups, heredity and sexual hygiene. The subject was to awaken in pupils the love of nature and of the *Heimat*, and a reverence for all living creatures and for the natural order. The environmental and economic relevance of biology was to be stressed. Biology was seen as character-building, and as relevant to awakening a sense of civic responsibility. Teachers were to use film-strips, photos and films, and to lead expeditions, in order to arouse enthusiasm for nature. Pressure for educational reform came from the German Society for Scientific and Mathematical Education. It argued that biology was an essential subject linking the sciences and the

---

[35] *Medizinische Wissenschaft und werktätiges Volk* (Berlin, nd).

[36] *Verfassunggebende Preussische Landesversammlung* (71 Sitzung 24 October 1919), pp. 5,665–8; also *Preussischer Lantag* (228 Sitzung 24 March 1923), p. 16, 354.

[37] ZSTA M Rep 76 VIII B Nr 2074 Bl. 70, 31 January 1924.

[38] I. Scheele, *Von Lüben bis Schmeil. Die Entwicklung von der Schulnaturgeschichte zum Biologieunterricht zwischen 1830 und 1933* (Berlin, 1981), pp. 256–7.

humanities. Its members were convinced that the laws of heredity and eugenics ought to be common knowledge. They wrote textbooks which covered Mendelism, cell theory and evolution. The society considered that eugenics should be taught in the context of the laws of heredity, so as to instil in pupils a sense of responsibility to the nation and race. The curriculum should include: 1. Positive and negative human selection. 2. The birth rate and maintaining the population size. 3. Marital fitness and health, and the value of marriage certificates. 4. The perils of alcoholism and VD for the germplasm. The aim was to inculcate political values: 'The soul of the pupil is to be filled with the spirit of order in all life, and of humanity's dependence on nature'.[39]

School doctors and sport teachers were encouraged to undertake health education, sports and gymnastics being fashionable ways of promoting positive health. Doctors were urged to set an example by joining sports clubs, and the specialized medical discipline of *Sportarzt* developed. Among this new breed of medical specialists were racial hygienists such as Astel. School sports were to be combined with education and the inculcation of the ideal of the dynamic *Vitalrasse*.

Mass education

Administrators, doctors and teachers joined forces on the Reich Council for Health Education. The culmination of their efforts was the Reich Health Week which began on 18 April 1926. This can be traced to English and America precedents but the idea of a German Health Week was the brain-child of Moses, the SPD health spokesman. Moses suggested it in 1924 to the Sickness Insurance Association which had eleven million members.[40] They envisaged it as a co-ordinated project of sickness funds, welfare organizations, trade unions, doctors and public health experts. It reflected the Weimar spirit of social co-ordination and the shifting emphasis to preventive medicine.

Moses' suggestion aroused more enthusiasm on the right than on the left. The communists boycotted the plans, whereas Georg Schreiber of the Centre Party and Haedenkamp of the DNVP gave their support. Many sickness insurance funds opposed the idea, but the public health authorities were enthusiastic. The Reich Ministry of the Interior and the Reich Health Educational Council assumed a co-ordinating role, ensuring that the Health Week would reinforce nationalist ideals. The main organizers were to be the 1,000 state medical officers and 300 municipal medical officers. Bumm, the president of the Reich Health Office, emphasized the need to involve the clergy, teachers and the Red Cross. The social hygienist Harmsen of the evangelical *Innere Mission* pressed for the clergy to take a leading role in health education. Haedenkamp, representing the medical profession, welcomed the week as an opportunity to involve independently practising doctors as well as public health officials. These developments show how conservative forces manipulated health propaganda.[41]

---

[39] Scheele, *Lüben*, pp. 264–72.   [40] *Hauptverband der Deutschen Krankenkassen*.
[41] ZSTA P 15.01 Nr 9411 Reichsgesundheitswoche.

A striking feature of the Health Week was the multiplicity of propaganda methods. These included medical lectures, evening entertainments, films, exhibitions, posters, educational pamphlets, shop window displays, opening ceremonies of new medical institutions, school classes, sermons, theatre and cinema events, concerts, radio lectures, sports events, allotment propaganda and newspaper reports. A newsletter was issued from December 1925 to co-ordinate local committees, and there was central distribution of educational materials. The week opened with a ceremony in the *Aula* of Berlin University on 18 April 1926. It was acclaimed as a grand success.[42]

The Health Week prompted the introduction of regular radio talks on hygiene on the national station, *Deutsche Welle*. The first was given by Dietrich, the Prussian health official. Other talks were given by social hygiene experts such as Grotjahn. The talks were on the first and third Friday of each month from 8 until 9 in the evening. They continued as a regular feature of health education, and were also used for continuing education of doctors.[43] The Health Week encouraged the making of films and filmstrips. A precursor was the 1925 film, 'Ways to Strength and Beauty',[44] which was based on the principle of a healthy mind in a healthy body. It proclaimed the health and beauty of the naked body, and involved such state institutions as the Prussian School of Physical Education, and many other schools of dance, gymnastics and physical education. The Health Education Council commissioned the short films, 'Prevent Wet Feet', 'Air Properly' and 'Hatschi'. As visits to the cinema had rocketed to two million per day, the council claimed a major success when cinemas agreed to show short films of fifteen minutes. The film company, Ufa, was keen to collaborate on health films, and it produced a short film, 'Hygiene in Domestic Life'. For the Health Week it produced a one hundred-minute feature film, 'Fritzchens Werdegang'. The Reich Health Office also sponsored a film on 'Work and Health', with the Bavarian occupational health expert, Koelsch, as the main adviser.[45]

In March 1926 Krohne chaired a discussion on establishing a Reich Office for welfare films. Although this was not formed, it provided the opportunity for admitting to the Health Education Council the German League for Racial Regeneration and the German Racial Hygiene Society as well as the Reich Committee for Gymnastics and the Society for Occupational Hygiene. In 1927 Ufa produced a spectacular film on the history of evolution, 'Natur und Liebe'. At this time the Berlin and German Racial Hygiene Societies were planning a film to popularize racial hygiene. In spring 1927 the first specifically eugenic film had its premiere. Thomalla was commissioned as director: he was a doctor and the Reich Health Education Council's film specialist. In the early 1920s he made biological films for Ufa and had been involved in Hirschfeld's projects. He was responsible for

---

[42] D.S. Nadav, 'Zur Einberufung der Ersten Reichsgesundheitswoche im Jahre 1926', *Die medizinische Welt*, ns. vol. 27 (1976), 1,069–72.   [43] ZSTA P 15.01 Nr 9412.

[44] *Wege zu Kraft und Schönheit*.

[45] ZSTA P 15.01 Nr 9412; 15.01 Nr 10658 betr medizinische Filme 1921–27.

advising the Anti-VD Society on its film 'False Shame'[46] in 1928, which was criticized as being propaganda for the medical profession. He wrote the script for 'The Curse of Heredity'. It had two sub-titles: 'Those Who should not be Mothers' and 'A Film of Love and Duty'.[47]

The eugenicists were much pleased with the film. They praised it as a work of brilliant popularization and as an undoubted 'hit'.[48] But the critics were not. The *Film-Echo* commented 'that a work of art was intended, with the spirit of love and duty and the demonic power of fate; but a mediocre film resulted'. Thomalla continued to be the Health Education Council's main director of films. In 1927 he was commissioned by the council to produce another Ufa feature film on health, a cartoon and three 'shorts'. His work on the racial hygiene film was thus part of a broader role as the link between health education, the medical profession and a booming film industry. The takeover of Ufa in 1927 by the DNVP politician, Alfred Hugenberg, confirmed the nationalist orientation that was reflected in the health films.

The health educators co-operated with the Racial Hygiene Society and League for Regeneration. Gottstein and Krohne combined their official positions on health education councils with the advocacy of eugenics. Much effort was spent on popularizing the laws of heredity both directly and indirectly through organizations such as the Anti-VD Society; its socialist secretary, Löwenstein, supported eugenic concepts of health education. It was argued that the laws of heredity should be popularized in such a way as to arouse a sense of personal responsibility to the family and nation. Health officials encouraged the Societies for Racial Hygiene and for Regeneration to participate in the Health Week. The physiologist, Abderhalden, and Kahl, president of the Union for Health, demanded that the public be informed about population policy, sexual ethics, VD and the need for moral restraint. Medical officers were to undertake this as well as advising mothers on child care.[49]

The GE-SO-LEI exhibition

Exhibitions were a great public attraction. They were partly an entertaining spectacle but also fulfilled a thirst for knowledge and a personal curiosity about the body. The Dresden Hygiene Museum gained a public reputation with exhibits centred round the Visible Man and the Visible Woman. The museum began to include a eugenic component in its many touring and large-scale exhibitions and literature. Of those on its staff, Neustätter was especially favourable to eugenics. Fetscher contributed popular pamphlets on hereditary science and racial hygiene. A major offshoot of the Museum was the national hygiene exhibition, the Gesolei. Plans for the exhibition were started in 1924 by the paediatrician, Schlossmann,

[46] *Falsche Scham.*   [47] ZSTA P 15.01 Nr 9374 Bl. 213.
[48] Kroll, 'Eugenik/Rassenhygiene', p. 176; BAK R 86 Nr 2371 Bd. 2 Bl. 394–400.
[49] ZSTA P. 15.01 Nr 9449 Bl. 211.

who had not forgotten the educational creed of Lingner while he had been in Dresden. The Gesolei exhibition held in Düsseldorf during the summer of 1926 was a major shop window for social hygiene and, potentially, for eugenics. The name GE-SO-LEI stood for *Gesundheit, soziale Fürsorge und Leibesübungen* (health, welfare and exercise) which were popular catch-words. The exhibition was held in Düsseldorf partly because of the city's enterprise in social hygiene, and partly as a municipal attraction. The Dresden Hygiene Museum supported the exhibition as a 'national duty' because Düsseldorf had been occupied by the French, and because of the need to counter separatist and communist tendencies.[50] That the Gesolei attracted seven and a half million visitors shows the popularity of health issues in the 1920s.

Many Gesolei exhibits had a eugenic component. The Saxon display included a section on prisons with photographs and tables from Fetscher's eugenic criminal biological survey.[51] The League for Child Rich Families combined publicity for eugenics with evangelism for larger families. An exhibit on eugenics and heredity was supervized by the familiar Weimar eugenic nucleus of Grotjahn, Krohne, Lenz, Muckermann, the Munich anthropologist Martin, the Leipzig hygienist Kruse, and such local public health officials as Carl Coerper.[52] The Gesolei prompted much controversy. The socialist doctor, Hodann, claimed that the section on 'Population Policy and Racial Hygiene' had been badly placed, where it was easily overlooked. He accused the exhibition of yielding to the powerful interests of *Alkoholkapital*. Others complained about the poor publicity poster, and the badly researched and out-of-date statistics.[53] The eugenic exhibition was used in the next year by the Racial Hygiene Society at the Berlin Central Institute for Education in April and May 1927. This venture was supported by the Hygiene Museum and League for Child Rich Families. Many school children and welfare organizations visited the exhibition resulting in a total of 5,000 visitors, and 750 copies of the guide were sold.[54] The year 1926 also saw a travelling exhibition on 'Man in Health and Sickness'. The overall aim was to show how to remain healthy and prevent disease. Visitors were advised about the need to avoid hereditary poisoning, due to such causes as lead, mercury, alcohol, tobacco, syphilis and TB. The need for marriage advice clinics and for healthy couples to have four children was emphasized. Heredity and racial hygiene became a standard part of travelling exhibitions.[55]

In 1927 the finances of the Dresden museum building were settled, and a foundation stone was laid. The permanent exhibition was planned in three sections. The centre of the museum was to be about the human body. The left wing of the

---

[50] ZSTA P. 15.01 Nr 9376 Bl. 125.   [51] STA Dresden MdI 17222 Gesolei.
[52] Others were Bachmann and Robert Lehmann.
[53] 'Nochmals "Kritische Bemerkungen zur Gesolei"', *Der Sozialistische Arzt*, no. 3 (1927/8), 52–3.
[54] Kroll, 'Eugenik/Rassenhygiene', pp. 174–5.
[55] Ausstellung für Erbkunde und Eugenik, 24 April–15 May 1927, Berlin, Potsdamerstrasse 120, BAK R86 Nr 2371 Bd 2 Bl. 394–400.

building was to be on nutrition and the right on the health care of future generations. This included exhibits on pregnancy, the cell and heredity, marriage advice, racial hygiene, qualitative and quantitative population policy, birth, and infant and school health. It meant that a substantial proportion of the new museum had a eugenic rationale. In 1930 an international hygiene exhibition marked the opening of the national museum. There were a number of eugenic displays, including one on mental hygiene. The Reich League for the Child Rich had a major section, and its display and catalogue were organized by the Reich statistician, Burgdörfer.[56] The catalogue argued that the German nation was becoming excessively old due to the declining birth rate. Its displays graphically showed how the young were shouldering excessive insurance burdens of old age and sickness insurance instead of bringing up children. No longer did the museum focus on promoting individual self-awareness. Now, it intended to make the individual aware of obligations to family, ancestral *Sippe* and *Volk*, with the individual depicted as the product of heredity and of 'spiritual and mental forces of the greater whole'. Laws of integration and heredity were shown to permeate the construction and functioning of the body. The public was exposed to the rhetoric of the cell state in a deterministic and authoritarian form. The body was proclaimed as 'a symbol' of national unity and productivity. But there was no universalist law for all humanity. It was explained that psychology and physiology gave rise to specific combinations. Racial anthropology, psychology and eugenics showed that there were distinct racial psychological and physical types.[57] Fetscher showed how diseases and sexual deviancy could be correlated with physique. He catalogued the hereditary conditions of physique, skin, nerves, internal diseases and mental diseases.[58] The march of medical science was used to refute the liberal utilitarianism of 'the greatest happiness of the greatest number' and to justify an elitist creed of struggle, duty and self-denial.[59]

Health education passed into the hands of specialized educators, backed by state resources. Lingner's hope for a museum as an 'academy of the people', in which the individual was free to choose and select from spectacular exhibits, was not realized. But entrepreneurs did cash in on the health craze. The public appetite for exhibitions and consumer goods was indicated by the appearance of privately owned exhibitions. A *Volksmuseum* set up by Eduard Hamrer travelled the country under the name of 'Man'. There were exhibits on embryology, social hygiene, racial types and homosexuality. The exhibition was advertized as 'for adults only'. It was closely watched by the authorities. In Stuttgart in 1925, the exhibition had 15,000 visitors. The medical officer said that material on alcoholism, VD, and TB

---

[56] F. Burgdörfer, *Familie und Volk, Sonderschau des Reichsbundes der Kinderreichen Deutschlands und zum Schutze der Familie, e.V. auf der Internationalen Hygiene Ausstellung Dresden 1930* (Berlin, 1930).

[57] R. v. Engelhardt, 'Der Körper als Ganzes', in M. Vogel (ed.), *Der Mensch* (Leipzig, 1930), pp. 253–65.

[58] R. Fetscher, 'Körper und Lebengestaltende Faktoren', in Vogel (ed.), *Mensch*, pp. 340–56.

[59] Engelhardt, 'Der Mensch als Gestalter der Welt', in Vogel (ed.), *Mensch*, pp. 403–13.

was instructive but all other exhibits ought to be removed as unscientific and morally offensive. Other commercial rivals were a Munich anatomical and hygienic exhibition called *Anhyga* and a Society for Welfare and Health, which brought exhibits from the Dresden museum and used the exhibition for the commercial purposes of selling medicines and sticking plasters.[60] Products fortified with vitamins were another typical result of the growing pharmaceutical industry. Just as health educators exploited the consumer boom, so entrepreneurs exploited the growing market for health care knowledge and products.

There were many warnings as to how the public might tire of the gospel of health, and how it might misunderstand the intended message. Educators were urged not to breed a nation of hypochondriacs. Lenz was concerned that too much sensitivity to health could induce personal weakness. Yet the educators were not deterred. Their campaign was placed on a chain of command: from scientific specialists educating doctors, from the doctors to nurses, social workers and voluntary first aid workers, and from these to the population at large. Lingner's view of consumerism as the basis for openness and self-help in health care was replaced by an authoritarian structure of educators, backed up with scientific insight in how to manipulate mass psychology through propaganda. Films, exhibitions, and other techniques of health propaganda served to intensify the idea that biological health was the basis of family life and society. Social efficiency and public participation were key elements. They caught the mood of the times with their attempts to combine popular fashions and consumerism with medical and eugenic ideals.[61]

THE STRUGGLE FOR POPULATION

The movement for planning reinforced demands for population policy. A barrage of medical, demographic and economic evidence on the effects of the declining birth rate maintained that Germany was 'a nation without youth'. Industry required a fit and healthy work-force. Mothers were subjected to officially supported propaganda in favour of large, 'child rich' families. By way of contrast sexual reformers emphasized that women were being exploited as 'reproductive machines' to satisfy the inexorable demands of the capitalist economy. Most eugenicists stood between the pro-natalist and sexual reforming factions with their conviction that more children of higher quality was the solution to national problems.

A major flashpoint of controversy was the issue of abortion. Progressives argued that abortion was a matter of class discrimination since the wealthy could buy the services of a doctor. Conservatives saw abortion as murder resulting from immorality and as contributing to the declining birth rate and hence to the death of

---

[60] ZSTA P 15.01 Nr 9377 Deutsches Hygiene Museum.
[61] H. Berger and F. Ebner, *Der gegenwärtige Stand und die Organisation der hygienischen Volksbelehrung* (Berlin, 1929), (transactions of ministerial conference of 10 December 1927).

the nation. Commentators formed the impression that numbers of abortions were rising. The more progressive eugenicists argued that responsibly used contraception was a rational means of preventing the suffering and death resulting from illegal abortions. Radicals demanded that abortion on social indications should be legalized. This outraged the conservative establishment who intensified pronatalist propaganda. The conservative elite of the profession combined nationalism with professional hostility to abortion as practised by 'quacks' and midwives. Illegal abortions thus represented the worst abuses of uncontrolled medical monopoly. Given that feminist views of reproductive self-determination were widespread and accorded with the higher degree of economic autonomy gained by women, a clash between the sexual reformers and conservatives occurred. The state-supported population policy thus came into headlong conflict with the movements for sexual reform.

The state's position was indicated in 1925 by the Reich Health Office's memorandum on Germany's need to increase births, in order to replenish the weakened population resources. This was drafted by Carl Hesse, the office's medical expert on social hygiene, who was a cautious moderate in matters of eugenics. The need for a vigorous nation meant that free abortion would be too great a risk. A repeal of the abortion penalties was regarded as inopportune. It was the policy of the Reich to increase and fortify the nation's weakened population reserves. The office stressed that only the medically qualified had any right to carry out abortions, and then only if the life of the mother were threatened. It would be racial suicide if women no longer wished to be mothers. To offset these trends state support for the 'child rich' was recommended.[62]

The position of the eugenicists was that abortion had to be prevented by positive welfare measures to improve the economic position of families and especially that of unmarried mothers. In October 1924 the Prussian Committee for Population met to discuss the admissibility of abortion on eugenic grounds. Its concern with positive welfare was shown by a memorandum of the geneticist Baur on foreign racial hygienic legislation and the impact on population policy of rural settlement schemes. In November 1925 the Prussian Committee for Population and Racial Hygiene reappraised the question of eugenic abortion. The meeting was on 'The Increase of Abortions from the Standpoints of the Nation's Health and Racial Hygiene'. The speakers were Grotjahn and the medical officer Lönne. Grotjahn used the spectre of a rising tide of abortions to justify the registration of pregnancies of single mothers-to-be. He argued that there should be more welfare facilities for the 'illegitimate'. Whether hereditary diseases required eugenic abortion was discussed. It was suggested that abortion could be undertaken in cases of retinitis pigmentosa, amaurotic familial idiocy, schizophrenia, epilepsy, feeble-mindedness, Huntington's chorea, manic-depression, the Pelizaeus-Merzbacher

[62] BAK R 86 Nr 2369 Bd 1 Bevölkerungspolitik 1919–1929, Hesse to Reich Ministerium des Inneren, 23 March 1928.

disease, and degenerative hysteria. The legal situation prompted much discussion, as it was suggested that eugenic abortion could be interpreted as legal. The committee agreed that there should be milder laws, better statistics, more intensive health education, and improvements in infant and child care.[63]

The consequences of this policy were that the state monitored areas of health and hygiene associated with sexuality and reproduction. Hygienic products, especially cures for menstrual pains, were carefully vetted so that they should not be abortifacients. It was agreed that there should be extensive anti-abortion propaganda, using the channels of welfare clinics, women's organizations and crèches.[64] While in theory the Weimar constitution guaranteed personal liberties, in practice the central state authorities were biased against sexual reforms and the free choice of the individual in reproductive matters. This contrasted with the trend among sickness insurance funds and socialist municipalities to support the movement to make contraceptive advice freely available. Thus a division arose between the central state on the side of pro-natalism, and the municipal and sickness insurance agencies siding with the sexual reformers. The state's attitude was shaped by reliance on professional experts, whereas the lower tiers of government had greater contact with popular opinion and living conditions.

The sexual political campaign for individual rights to control fertility gathered force. The League for the Protection of Mothers continued to take a radical line on these issues. The league had the support from outstanding leaders in the movement for sexual enlightenment such as Hodann, and a growing and active membership. Its journal, *Die Neue Generation*, was written in a direct and frank style, which ensured a wide readership. The population policy serving state, church, and industrial interests continued to be the major enemy. Evidence was cited of the poverty, disease and neglect of children in 'child rich' families. The wretchedly sick and impoverished state of mothers with many children was vividly depicted.[65] As a leading feminist and lay organization, the league set the tone for a coalescing of popular birth control organizations, scientifically minded sexual reformers and left-wing political parties.[66]

The position of 'social hygiene' became controversial. Those eugenicists with strong allegiance to hereditary biology and professional controls found themselves in difficulties in socialist organizations. The lay sexual reformers became more powerful. A major break occurred when Grotjahn was pressured out of SPD groupings. This marked a turning point in the relations between the social hygienists and the SPD. Grotjahn had entered into the SPD in order to gain a platform for his biologically based programme of social hygienic reform, and he campaigned for a minimum of three children per family. This pro-natalism was

[63] ZSTA P 15.01 Nr 9348 Bl. 126–63; Nr 9349 Bl. 331–3.
[64] F. Baum, 'Ueber den praktischen Malthusianismus, neo-Malthusianismus und Sozialdarwinismus', Diss., University of Leipzig, 1928.
[65] Auguste Kirchhoff, 'Etwas vom "Kindersegen"', *Die neue Generation*, vol. 24 (1928), 267–74.
[66] Grossmann, 'New Woman', pp. 150–5.

rejected by political activists, so pushing the eugenicists towards the right while allowing an alliance of socialists and sexual reformers to coalesce. In September 1926 the Committee on Workers Welfare of the SPD organized a meeting on population policy.[67] The Frankfurt politician, Max Quarck, spoke on socialism and population policy. Other speakers included the socialist doctors Moses, Raphael Silberstein (a Berlin medical officer), Knack, Karl Kautsky jun., as well as women trade unionists and feminists. That Grotjahn was a conspicuous absentee meant that this socialist initiative marked a decisive break between SPD and academic social hygiene. A radical alliance was established, called ARSO (*Arbeitsgemeinschaft sozialpolitischer Organisationen*). Trade unionists, feminists and socialists such as Martha Ruben-Wolf mounted the platform on its behalf.[68] The alliance developed links with the KPD since it had begun to take an interest in women's issues, contraception and the 'sexual political struggle'. Grotjahn and other social hygienists like Fetscher reacted by turning towards the pro-natalist agitation of the Reich League for the Child Rich, which took up Grotjahn's scheme for a parenthood insurance.

In the mid-20s political agitation for abortion law reform reached a high pitch. Maternal mortality rates were rising and were attributed to a rise in illicit abortions.[69] Estimates of an increasing number of abortions were taken as explanations of the declining birth rate. The estimates were impressionistic and indicated a political stance rather than any reality. Those figures based on individual practices or on sickness insurance statistics have a greater authenticity and suggest that most abortions were carried out in the major cities such as Berlin and Hamburg. The position of the doctor was also unclear, although the 1927 Reich Supreme Court ruling did allow termination when a mother's health was seriously at risk. Leaders of the medical profession in the *Ärztevereinsbund* opposed liberalization of the law. They were concerned that doctors were ready to comply with demands from their patients and sought to enforce stricter moral standards. They launched a public campaign in defence of the German family. The authorities acknowledged that maternal health was adversely affected by professional incompetence, and steps were taken to improve the training in obstetrics for medical students. The tightening up of medical standards was seen as central to the birth rate question.

Alarmed state officials reported on the mass meetings organized for free abortion and for publicizing contraception. Medical officers viewed such meetings as signs of degeneration, for their ideas threatened the health of the *Volkskörper*. The Society for the Suppression of Quackery assumed a vigilante role, supplying the state with accounts of meetings. Organizations sprang up with names like 'Peoples'

---

[67] *Hauptausschuss für Arbeiterwohlfahrt.*

[68] BAK R86 Nr 2369 Bd 1 contains official reactions to radical initiatives for sexual reform.

[69] ZSTA P 30.01 Nr 6232 Die Abtreibung 1925–1931; C. Usborne, 'Abortion in Weimar Germany – the Discourse among the Medical Profession', unpublished manuscript.

League for the Protection of Mothers and Sexual Hygiene', or 'League for Sexual Hygiene and *Lebensreform*', 'League for German Birth Control', 'Association for Birth Control', and the 'Society for Proletarian Free Thought'. These were channels for selling contraceptives, as the laws on public indecency could be avoided by selling through brochures and lectures. Here neo-Malthusian ideology coincided with commercialism. By 1924 these associations had established themselves as counselling and lay-dominated associations for sexual advice and reform. Their activities included bulk-buying of contraceptives and distribution to members. They adopted an anti-capitalist and anti-professional rhetoric. Homoeopaths and lay practitioners played a key role. In 1924 Saxony, with its high level of population density and industrialization, saw the emergence of a League for Sexual Reform in Chemnitz and an Association for Sexual Hygiene in Dresden. They claimed a combined membership of 13,000. They were attacked as communist and quack organizations.[70] Some made a point of excluding the educated middle class, and were lectured to by autodidact workers. Others were steered by middle-class sexual reformers. Hodann, a medical officer and sexual counsellor of Hirschfeld's Institute for Sexual Science, was a frequent speaker. They published pamphlets and news-sheets with titles like 'Love and Life', and organized lectures on topics like 'Happiness in Marriage', or 'Forced Birth and Poverty', or 'Love without Consequences'. Lectures vividly presented – often with film-strips and slides – the facts of embryology, pregnancy and birth. Methods of birth control and the need for contraception were highlighted. They argued for sexual advice centres rather than marriage advice clinics.

The police kept track of the movements of peripatetic lectureres, and reported to public health officials that birth control campaigners were often swindlers and nature therapists. The police warned campaigners of the need for restraint and to avoid contravening the laws of assault, indecency or of using the title of *Arzt*. They made sure that minors did not attend the meetings, and stopped the showings of films and the distribution of pamphlets. In 1928 the Stuttgart police seized the books by Hodann, and they were later to prosecute the radical doctors Else Kienle and Friedrich Wolf.[71] Films attracted the hostility of police censors. In 1926 the Bavarian authorities unsuccessfully tried to ban the film 'Crusade of Women',[72] which included a scene of a woman teacher being raped by an idiot. The film aimed to show the dangers of back-street abortion.[73] The Dekawe film, 'Must a Woman become a Mother?'[74] incurred the wrath of the Reich Health Office in 1926. The medical official Hesse condemned the film as 'amoral and depraving'. Although it showed the harmful consequences of abortion, the film argued that social need was a greater force than law. The film was banned by the censors.[75] The Soviet pro-

---

[70] Grossmann, 'New Woman', pp. 112–7; H. Lehfeldt, 'Die Laienorganisationen für Geburtenregelung', *Archiv für Bevölkerungspolitik*, vol. 2 (1932), 63–87.
[71] ZSTA M Rep 76 VIII B Nr 2004 Bl. 7–14.   [72] *Kreuzzug des Weibes*.
[73] ZSTA P 15.01 Nr 9349 Bl. 418.   [74] 'Muss die Frau Mutter Werden?'
[75] ZSTA P 15.01 Nr 9348 Bl. 62–65.

abortion film, 'Sonja Petrova', in which Semaschko, the health commissioner, played a medical prosecutor, provoked deep disgust on the part of a medical officer sent by the authorities to report on sexual reform meetings.[76]

In 1928 the sexual reform agitation reached a climax with the founding of the first national organization for sexual reform. This was the Reich League for Sexual Hygiene[77] which claimed to have 400,000 members. That year Hirschfeld promoted the World League for Sexual Reform, and sickness insurance funds opened a series of birth control clinics. These pioneered birth control for social rather than medical or eugenic reasons. They showed a heightened degree of politicization, and were consciously populist mass movements. They declared war on the state and professional welfare organizations.[78] The Association of Socialist Doctors became active in campaigns for birth control. Reorganized in 1924, their membership climbed from 626 in 1928 to 1,500 in 1932. That they gained the membership of Friedrich Wolf and Hodann, and of such long-standing sexual reformers as Theilhaber, meant that this association achieved a position of genuine influence over the initiatives on the left. A consequence was the galvanizing of conservative forces in the profession for a renewed onslaught on the radicals.[79]

In many ways the officials and more conservative elements among the profession felt that they were a beleaguered minority. Statistical indicators suggested that the sexual reformers were winning. The birth rate continued to fall, and the authorities felt that the numbers of abortions were rising throughout the twenties. Some estimates put the number as high as one million abortions in 1930. Most medical associations and particularly specialists such as gynaecologists rejected the reformers' demands. In this context the intermediate position held by doctors such as Grotjahn and Hirsch could be seen in a more positive light. The medical profession grasped the opportunity to increase their status by acting as guardians of public morality. It was only women or socialist doctors and a few enlightened health officials such as Roesle who argued that illegal abortions posed a far greater threat to health and life, than would be the case if abortion were legalized.

The state, medical profession and churches allied against the onslaught of the sexual reformers.[80] Their efforts were co-ordinated by a number of health and welfare organizations: the Reich Council for Health Education, the welfare-oriented League for Regeneration, the evangelical Union for Health,[81] and the League for Child Rich Families. The travelling exhibitions of the German Hygiene Museum presented the official view.[82] They opposed the materialism of socialism,

---

[76] ZSTA M Rep 76 VIII B Nr 2004 Bl. 226; M. Ruben Wolff, 'Introduction to the Russian Film about Abortion', in N. Haire (ed.), *The Sexual Reform Congress* (London, 1930), pp. 238–9.

[77] *Reichsbund für Sexualhygiene.*

[78] Grossmann, 'New Woman', pp. 150–60 for 1928 as turning-point.

[79] Thomann, 'Weg', pp. 158–63.

[80] C. Usborne, 'The Christian Churches and the Regulation of Sexuality in Weimar Germany', in J. Obelkevitch, L. Roper and R. Samuel (eds.), *Disciplines of Faith* (London, 1987), pp. 99–112.

[81] *Arbeitsgemeinschaft für Volksgesundung.*

[82] ZSTA P 30.01 Nr 6216 Bewahrung der Jugend von Schund und Schmutz Literatur.

birth control and nature therapy by renewing emphasis on national ideals of duty and moral restraint.[83] Attempts were made to recapture the public's attention by offering entertainments, festivals and strong doses of moral propaganda. Some of the educative propaganda was relatively uncontroversial. The Anti-VD Society subsidized the dramas *Die Schiffsbrüchigen* in 1925, and *Olaf* in 1926. Two films were distributed: 'Ought we to be Silent?' and 'False Shame'. These served purposes of health education, while warning the public of the dangers of quackery and sexual promiscuity. Other initiatives reinforced ethical and moral values. In 1925 the physiologist and family welfare campaigner Abderhalden launched an initiative to popularize ethical ideals in a newly formed Medical and Popular League for Sexual Ethics. He claimed a membership of 600 doctors and 1,000 lay people. He produced a journal, *Sexualethik*,[84] aimed at medical officers, school doctors, teachers, the clergy and lawyers. There was much co-operation with Harmsen and the Union for Health. The venture received official subsidies, and the journal had about 4,000 subscribers.[85] The League for the Child Rich and Protection of the Family[86] continued to campaign for welfare measures to avert 'the catastrophe of the German family'. Its demands for welfare benefits for large families were supported by a broad coalition ranging from the radical eugenicists Fetscher and Grotjahn to DNVP doctors, such as Haedenkamp and the Nazi sympathizer Gütt, and demographers such as Burgdörfer and Zahn. Other enthusiasts included school teachers, medical officers, and university academics. Affiliated organizations included the nationalist social purity organization, the *Schutz- und Trutz-Bund*. Welfare and the protection of moral standards were regarded as medicines for a sickening body politic. The League for the Child Rich adopted the slogan, *zu unserer Kinder Heil!*

Medical aims were highlighted by Harmsen who as a pupil of Grotjahn had completed a dissertation on the declining birth rate in France. He combined commitment to moral purity campaigns from 1919 with medical and demographic expertise. He became the secretary of the Union for Health. Its president was Kahl and chairmen were the physiologist, Abderhalden and the Centre Party representative, doctor and Caritas organizer, Fassbender. The union was founded in November 1924 and reinforced in March 1926, by incorporating the Society for Population Policy. It stepped up public agitation and had an immediate impact at the Gesolei exhibition campaigning under the slogan 'pure and German!' The union had the support of groups concerned with hygienic issues such as TB, VD, and alcoholism; eugenicists from the German Racial Hygiene Society; moral purity organizations concerned with youth and with the moral standards of public entertainment; political parties and nationalist groupings; and state officials such as Saenger, the President of the Prussian Statistical Office, and Burgdörfer of the

[83] ZSTA P 15.01 Nr 26234 Bund der Kinderreichen 1928.   [84] later called *Ethik*.
[85] ZSTA P 15.01 Nr 9449.
[86] *Reichsbund der Kinderreichen Deutschlands zum Schutze der Familie*.

Reich Statistical Office. It was a coalition of 120 groups.[87] Its major funding came from the *Innere Mission* and the Reich Ministry of the Interior. Thousands of copies of its newsletter and propaganda leaflets were distributed. The Union engaged in a moral propaganda that lent itself readily to eugenic ideas. The declining birth rate and national decay were key slogans.

Harmsen exemplifies the role assumed by doctors in directing campaigns for moral purity. He initiated the series of pamphlets on population and welfare with one on France. Subsequently the Centrist Fassbender wrote on 'the German Nation's Will to Live', Wichern wrote on sexual ethics, and Fetscher on heredity.[88] Harmsen organized a series of conferences fusing church welfare with eugenics. The Child Rich had an exhibit for the Gesolei organized by Fetscher, and a series of popular pamphlets edited by Burgdörfer and von Loesch. These denounced the 'two child system' as certain to result in the death of the *Volk* in 300 years, pointing out that under the system such national leaders as Bismarck and Hindenburg would never have been born.[89] Harmsen achieved great popular success with his campaign for a German Mothers' Day as a celebration of the family. Children were asked to honour and support not only their own mother but all German mothers. He submitted a memorandum to the state on behalf of the Union for Health. A Mothers' Day had been proclaimed in the United States on 9 May 1914. Certain German towns had had a Mothers' Day since 1923, and it was popular among the 'Southern Germans' of the Italian South Tirol. It would be of especial value in the fringe areas of Germany as a means of national integration.[90] Harmsen found support from commercial interests in the Association of German Flower Sellers. The year 1927 marked a high point in the campaign for a national Mother's Day, which flourished due to the combination of commercial, medical and religious interests.[91]

The Mother's Day was the antidote to the problems of abortion, contraception and decadence. The state, churches and social purity organizations favoured a moral solution to what they regarded as primarily moral problems. The collectivist rhetoric of national health and the body politic was meant to inculcate selfless devotion to the family and nation.[92] Such ideological campaigns avoided costly positive solutions in terms of welfare measures such as orphanages, parenthood insurance and land reform. Consumerism and technological advance meant widespread distribution of contraceptives. Antiseptics meant that even the illegal abortions might be less hazardous. Mass democracy required mass education to reinstate the moral standards and a sense of duty to the nation. By the late 1920s sexual reform had forced its way on to the centre of the political stage.

[87] ZSTA P 15.01 Nr 9348 Bl. 112–8; 30.01 Nr 5793 Sittlichkeitsvergehen Bl. 37–41 Satzungen 11 Mai 1925.   [88] *Schriften für Volksgesundung.*   [89] Burgdörfer, *Familie und Volk*, pp. 35–7.
[90] ZSTA P 15.01 Nr 9449 Bl. 69–84.
[91] K. Hausen, 'Mütter zwischen Geschäftsinteressen und kultischer Verehrung. Der "Deutsche Muttertag" in der Weimarer Republik', in G. Huck, (ed.), *Sozialgeschichte der Freizeit* (Wuppertal, 1980), pp. 249–80.   [92] Harmsen, 'Mütter', pp. 271–5.

MARRIAGE CLINICS

Marriage advice clinics were an attempt at reconciling eugenics with democratic values and the psychological, medical and social needs of the population. The clinics institutionalized and professionalized the ideas of reproductive hygiene, with professionally trained staff screening the health of young couples and issuing marriage certificates on the basis of hereditary fitness. It was a strategy based on education rather than compulsion. Those deemed unfit for parenthood were to be dissuaded from having children. Those of high eugenic value were to be educated on the need to have at least three children. But this delicate compromise between professional authority and popular need failed. The clinics developed into a battlefield between eugenicists and feminists. Eugenicists insisted that the clinics be strictly for advising those about to marry as to whether they were suited for having children, and should propagate the gospels of negative and positive eugenics. They were condemned as repressive by feminists and radical sexual reformers, who wanted the clinics to dispense contraceptives and offer sexual advice, especially to adolescents.

As with virtually all the innovations in Weimar eugenics, the hereditary clinics owed their origins to forerunners during the crisis of 1919–24. During 1921 Austrian socialists discussed such clinics as a means of preventing VD, and in March 1922 a clinic was opened by the anatomist Tandler and Karl Kautsky jun. in Vienna. It was the first such clinic to be municipally funded.[93] By 1923 'family advice' or marriage clinics were established by eugenicists in Munich, Halle and Dresden. By 1925 there were hereditary counselling clinics run by Weitz at the university policlinic of Tübingen and by the anthropologist Fischer at the Freiburg Anatomical Institute. There were also radical alternatives arising from the sexual reform movement. Hirschfeld opened a clinic at the Berlin Institute for Sexual Science in 1919; others were sponsored by the League for the Protection of Mothers and for Sexual Reform. The League established 'Marriage AND Sexual Advice Clinics', first in Hamburg in 1924 and then in Bremen, Frankfurt-on-Main, Mannheim and Breslau. The socialist doctors and eugenicists, Knack and Georg Manes, were behind this initiative in Hamburg. Knack hoped that a sexual advice clinic could screen for VD and prevent abortions.[94] Unlike the more conservative eugenicists, they regarded advice on contraception as a major responsibility of the clinic.

The Hamburg Sexual Advice Clinic was viewed with much anxiety by medical officers and racial hygienists, who requested information about the clinic. In reply to the Danzig medical officer, Dr Pfeiffer of the Hamburg Health Office denied any connection with the clinic. Although it was supported by the Hamburg Municipal Sickness Insurance, Pfeiffer attributed this to confusion between preventive

[93] Sablik, *Tandler*, p. 280. K.v. Soden, *Die Sexualberatungsstellen der Weimarer Republik, 1919–1933* (Berlin, 1988).   [94] A.V. Knack in *Die Ortskrankenkasse*, no. 6 (1923).

medicine and birth control. His hope was that such clinics might serve a useful ethical function. This typified the concern of the medical profession to appropriate the clinics as an additional means for medical prescriptions of lifestyle.[95] Racial hygienists became interested in the ventures. During October 1924 Drigalski requested information on the Hamburg clinic; he himself had established a marriage advice clinic in Halle where he was medical officer. Drigalski was due to address the German Society for Racial Hygiene on 18 October and, with Eugen Fischer, was to speak on racial hygiene family advice clinics. He wished to know what type of questionnaire was in use in Hamburg, and what type of advice was given. Pfeiffer inspected the clinic and reported to Drigalski that despite certain good features the clinic was too much influenced by the Viennese clinics which advocated birth control.[96] Drigalski agreed, regretting the participation of the sickness insurances and the excessively liberal concept of 'sexual advice'. Drigalski's clinic in Halle was limited to screening those intending to marry for TB, VD, anaemia, epilepsy and psychopathy.[97] He wished to circulate Pfeiffer's report to 'reliable' members of the Racial Hygiene Society, as it would help in their assessment of the League for Protection of Mothers. He despised the Hamburg clinic for claiming to be eugenic, and hoped that the anthropologist Scheidt would start a truly eugenic clinic.

Pfeiffer's inspection of the clinic and its records showed that 85–90 per cent of clients came to avoid unwanted pregnancies. Most wanted advice on whether to continue or interrupt their pregnancies because of their already large families, personal sickness or a sick or alcoholic husband, lack of housing or unemployment. In consultations women were advised to see their doctor for the fitting of an occlusive pessary. The sickness insurance would pay for this when medically prescribed. The doctor in attendance argued that eugenics meant that children should be conceived only at the most convenient times for the parents, so that only 'children of joy' should be born.[98] The dispute between Drigalski and the Hamburg sexual reformers continued to fester. The radicals (represented by Wilhelm Kaufmann, secretary of the World League for Sexual Reform) demanded non-medical advice centres, whereas Drigalski insisted on the primacy of the medical practitioner.

With medical officers coming to favour marriage certificates and eugenics, municipal and state support marked the next stage of development. Dresden provided an example of an experimental clinic that was sponsored by the sickness insurance funds but was run on eugenic lines. In 1923 Kuhn established a clinic to provide student medicals at the Technical University. Fetscher developed this into a clinic for hereditary health examinations. He linked this clinic to health education

---

95 STAH Medizinal Kollegium II U15 Sexualberatungsstellen 1924–29 Stade to Pfeiffer 6 October 1924; Pfeiffer to Stade 26 October 1924.
96 STAH Med Koll II U15, Drigalski to Pfeiffer 6 October 1924; Pfeiffer to Drigalski, 1 November 1924.   97 STAH Med Koll II U15, Drigalski, 30 October 1924.
98 STAH Med Koll II U15, Pfeiffer report, 20 October 1924.

on the dangers of VD, alcohol and TB for future generations. Another eugenic initiative was at Kiel under Josefine Hober. The Racial Hygiene Society renewed pressure for legislation for marriage certificates and added a demand for clinics. As the Reich authorities considered that a law for compulsory certificates would be unconstitutional, the matter was discussed at the Prussian Health Committee on Racial Hygiene on 18 July 1925. Krohne, now director of the Health Department, used the authority of the state to ensure that eugenics should be the priority in marriage advice. In February 1926 Prussia issued a decree enabling municipal authorities to establish clinics. These were to be administered by doctors, and their function was to educate and screen those intending to marry.[99] The Racial Hygiene Society wanted registry officials to bring the clinics to the attention of those proposing to marry, and recommended eugenic advice on contraception. In March 1926 Hirsch suggested guidelines including compulsory certificates.[100] Standard procedures and forms were agreed.

In June 1926 Berlin's first municipal marriage advice clinic was opened with much ceremony at Prenzlauer Berg. This was run by the socialist doctor and school medical officer Karl Scheumann, and by the communist doctor Korach. They offered advice on health and hereditary aspects of marriage. A medical certificate of fitness for marriage was issued; this bore the insignia of the municipality.[101] This district had a number of model welfare facilities, as for youth care. Marriage advice was part of progressive municipal welfare. By 1928 there were 224 such clinics in Prussia. Other states such as Bremen and Saxony followed the Prussian example, and insisted that such clinics be staffed only by doctors.[102] The main aim of the clinics was to reduce numbers of abortions by educating on birth control. The gynaecologist Hugo Sellheim advised that eugenic aims ought also to be included. The Protestant *Innere Mission* objected to contraception, but accepted the need for eugenic advice.[103] Many thousands of pamphlets on eugenics were distributed by the clinics.

The Prussian decree of 19 February 1926 allowing state marriage advice clinics was welcomed by eugenicists. It should be seen as part of a package of progressive legislation, such as the Law for the Protection of Mothers of 1927, extending maternity benefits and antenatal care. 'Preventive care' was to be provided by analyzing the capacity for a couple to have children on the basis of their health, and on the laws on heredity. The eugenicist Hirsch lectured on the marriage clinics to a favourably inclined Berlin Medical Society in March 1926. The society urged that a medical examination be made obligatory for both partners; but there should not be

[99] For the text of the Prussian decree see *ARGB*, vol. 19 (1927), 205–14.
[100] ZSTA M Rep 76 VIII B Nr 2001 Bl. 153–65, 187–95.
[101] F.K. Scheumann (with foreword by Krohne), *Eheberatung. Einrichtung, Betrieb und Bedeutung für die biologische Erwachsenenberatung* (Berlin, 1928); Scheumann, *Eheberatung als Aufgabe der Kommunen* (Leipzig, 1932).
[102] Denkschrift des Sächsischen Arbeits-und Wohlfahrtsministeriums über Ehe- und Sexualberatung, 21 December 1927.
[103] R. Fetscher, 'Eheberatung in Sachsen', *Eugenische Rundschau*, (1928), 60–8.

any ban on marriage or need to reveal the results of the examination. They stressed that the examination ought to be carried out by a qualified professional. They recommended that medical students be given lectures on the laws of heredity and the pathology of marriage. They wished for a national law to ensure these points. Other medical chambers such as that at Stettin echoed these opinions.[104]

The eugenicists joined forces with the medical profession and registry officials to agitate for provision of professionally run clinics.[105] In January 1927 Schubart, a lawyer and racial hygienist, petitioned the Reichstag for a clinic in each university town, and in every town with over 100,000 inhabitants. In June 1927 public health experts banded together in a Union of Public Marriage Guidance Clinics. This was in reaction to attacks from Kaufmann representing lay sexual advice clinics. These were condemned as 'political', unlike the municipal clinics which were to be administered on a scientific basis. The Union was organized by Drigalski who in 1926 moved from Halle to Berlin (with Grotjahn's backing) as municipal medical officer. The vice-chairman was the Hamburg geneticist, Poll. Other founders were Korach (as secretary), Scheumann of the clinic at Prenzlauer Berg, Fetscher, Kautsky jun. and Grotjahn. It was supported by a number of municipal medical officers. By this time there were about one hundred clinics. The association wished to extend these clinics on the basis of sexual science, which they regarded as an offshoot of social hygiene and eugenics. This was aimed as much at radical sexual reformers as at the conservative forces opposed to such clinics. Drigalski wished to exclude all lay advisers from the running of these clinics. Their aim was to keep 'the development of marriage guidance on healthy lines, and to avoid previous mistakes'.[106] They launched a publicity campaign against clinics which were set up by 'unqualified dilettantes', by which they meant feminists, sexual reformers and birth control campaigners. There were criticisms of the scope of the clinics, as officially they were limited to those who were engaged to be married. The examination at the clinic included a blood test (for syphilis) which meant that five marks would be paid by the sickness fund.

The state decree was criticized by the sexual reformer Hodann who condemned the decree's emphasis on science and marriage as an attack on the movement for birth control. He pointed out that most clients would come after they had started to have sexual relations. He therefore doubted whether the facts of heredity could really force an engaged couple, who were in love, to part. Hodann argued that the primary function of such clinics ought to be birth control – something excluded by the Welfare Ministry decree – and sexual psychological counselling, a topic ignored by the decree.[107] After the Prussian decree of 1926 the League for Protection of Mothers established sexual advice centres at Friedrichshain in Berlin, and then at

---

[104] ZSTA Rep 76 VIII B Nr 2001 Geburtenrückgang.
[105] Grotjahn, *Fortpflanzung*, pp. 253–671, 'Die eugenische Beratung durch den Arzt'.
[106] ZSTA M Rep 76 VIII B Nr 2001 Geburtenrückgang 1921–28 Bl. 290–312.
[107] M. Hodann, 'Über Notwendigkeit und Aussichten der Eheberatung', *Die Neue Generation*, vol. 22 (1926), 337–9.

Wilmersdorf, Kreuzberg and, with the participation of Hodann, at Reinickendorf. The Friedrichshain municipality and the Berlin *Ortskrankenkasse* supported the initiative of the league. The municipality hoped that the clinic might help to solve the problems of the 8,000 psychopathic families for which they were responsible.[108] Of 368 consultations, 163 were for birth control. Proof that there was a popular demand for birth control refuted the Union of Public Marriage Advice Clinics, which asserted that only one woman client in ten did not want children. At the league's clinic, contraceptive caps were fitted and then refitted every four weeks. Coitus interruptus was regarded as a cause of feelings of great anxiety in .women. The clinic criticized doctors who refused to advise on contraception for seriously ill, poor and exhausted women. It was pointed out that in 'child rich' families children were often malnourished, sick or deformed. Certain women whose husbands were alcoholics or tubercular were able to obtain eugenic abortions. The other clients often came as couples. They required sexual counselling and therapy in the case of problems such as frigidity and abnormal sexual practices. Clients were screened for VD and alcoholism. Legal advice was provided in cases of violence and other matters necessitating divorce. Literature recommended included van de Velde's controversial book, *Ideal Marriage*. The right to know about important processes in one's own body was claimed as a political principle.[109] The same pattern emerged for other sexual advice clinics. Hodann stated that at the Clinic for Sexual Advice and Birth Control in Berlin-Reinickendorf only 4 out of 712 visitors wanted eugenic 'marriage advice'.[110] The League for the Protection of Mothers had a number of parliamentary allies, which included the socialist representatives Eduard David and Siegfried Weinberg. This ensured that such issues as marriage certificates and sexual advice remained politically contentious.

Most controversial was the question of whether contraceptives should be provided. Grotjahn argued that contraception was a matter for individual doctors in their practices and opposed the opening of birth control clinics. Above all, the issue was whether these clinics ought to be exclusively for those marrying or whether they should be general sexual advice centres. More radical was the demand that contraception be paid for by sickness insurance funds. Other sexual reformers criticized as naive the eugenicists' view that merely dissuading someone from marriage would solve the problem of hereditary diseases. Such people would probably indulge in extra-marital sex, and so undergo additional health risks. They accused the state of greatly overrating the importance of heredity, and of underrating the extent to which improved social conditions could improve the

---

[108] 'Eröffnung der Ehe- und Sexualberatungstelle in Berlin', *Die Neue Generation*, vol. 22 (1926), 211–14.

[109] Hedwig Schwarz, 'Erfahrungen der Ehe- und Sexualberatungsstelle Friedrichshain', *Die Neue Generation*, vol. 24 (1928), 310–2, 348–50.

[110] M. Hodann, 'Fürsorgestelle für Sexualberatung und Geburtenregelung in Berlin-Reinickendorf', *Die Neue Generation*, vol. 27 (1931), 117–18.

health of children of unhealthy parents. Herta Riese of Frankfurt recommended sterilization as the best course of action for two abnormal partners intending to marry. She argued that contraceptive techniques could not be withheld from the people: these were a technology, and as with any technology, people were entitled to be advised as to its best use. But one thing was certain. Just as states abused technologies to wage war, so state authorities could not be trusted to advise on sexual matters.[111] This linking of sterilization to the role of hereditary clinics marked a new stage in the polarization between sexual reformers and racial hygienists.

The League for the Protection of Mothers and the sickness funds were successful in establishing a radical alternative form of organization to the more authoritarian professionally staffed, state-approved and municipally controlled clinics. The league could draw on traditions of feminism and lay agitation. The more radical funds combined party political links with a sense of accountability to their members. Politically radical organizations such as ARSO were intermediaries in the campaign for proletarian birth control. In 1928 a clinic financed by the sickness insurance funds opened in Neukölln with an aim primarily to provide birth control advice to workers for social rather than medical reasons. Five other birth control clinics were established in 1928. The progressive Berlin sickness funds argued that marriage clinics had only very limited appeal, whereas contraceptive provision and advice fulfilled a real popular need. The sickness funds were particularly concerned to attract greater numbers of the unmarried to their clinics.[112]

Hodann attempted to establish participatory forms of collaboration between lay counsellors and socialist doctors. This was shown by an innovative programme for the training of physicians as counsellors. Lectures were held by such experts as Stoeckel on the history of birth control, Ernst Gräfenberg on the IUD, Kurt Bendix of the Berlin sickness fund on the diaphragm, and other doctors on such topics as X-ray sterilization, surgical sterilization and artificial insemination.[113] These topics show the dilemma of the sexual reformers. They depended on contraceptive techniques that were being pioneered by doctors supporting eugenics. These techniques were often accompanied by an over-enthusiastic faith in technological solutions to social problems, and remained open to abuse. The trend even among radical groups was towards a scientific approach to birth control.

The marriage advice clinics occupy a crucial place in a transition which saw eugenics shift from being the concern of an educated elite to providing the rationale of expert planners supporting a state-imposed population policy. The clinics initiated a type of specifically eugenic institution designed to cope with large

---

[111] H. Riese, 'Die wahren Aufgaben der Eheberatungsstellen', *Die Aufklärung*, vol. 1 (1929), reprinted in Hohmann, *Sexualforschung*, pp. 151–6.
[112] K. Bendix, 'Birth Control in Berlin', in Haire, *Sexual Reform*, pp. 659–61.
[113] Grossmann, 'New Woman', pp. 153–62.

sectors of the population. That they were introduced on a municipal basis was typical of the relatively decentralized structure of Weimar welfare provision. What emerged were conflicting types of eugenics. One grouping was an alliance between medically qualified eugenicists and state officials. They attacked the popular alliance of lay sexual reformers which included SPD and KPD organizations, sickness funds and socialist doctors. Yet both groupings accepted forms of medical expertise, and biologistic and hereditarian concepts. The officially approved clinics also extended their role. Scheumann suggested that they provide 'biological family advice',[114] and Fetscher advocated their role as 'hygienic advice centres', advising on all aspects of health in adult life.[115] The clinics occupied a central position among the welfare services: after 1933 the evaluation of the population according to hereditary and racial categories became the central aim of public health and welfare. The *Eheberatungsstellen* were precursors of the Nazi clinics for *Erb- und Rassenpflege* (hereditary and racial welfare).

THE NATIONAL INSTITUTE

The authority of eugenicists over welfare institutions and issues was reinforced by the rapid growth of research on heredity, which drew on the prosperity of the mid-1920s. A crucial instance of the assertive claims by geneticists can be seen in the foundation of the Kaiser Wilhelm Institute for Anthropology, Human Heredity and Eugenics. It was established in 1927, and was a response to the demand for a national eugenics institute; this dated back to government discussions during 1921 which had their roots in pre-war schemes of Gruber, Kaup and Ploetz. The institute was later portrayed as a precursor of Nazi eugenic policies during the Third Reich. This was how in 1936 its director, Fischer, depicted its genesis.[116] But the origins and obligations of the institute derived from distinctive features of Weimar eugenics, and of the newly defined social role of science after 1918. The institute must be understood with regard to the hopes for a spirit of national co-ordination whereby scientific experts should dictate the development of social policy, and establish norms for a healthy family life.

The welfare orientation of Weimar eugenics was reflected in the contacts of researchers on heredity with Soviet eugenics.[117] Under Semaschko as Commissar

[114] *biologische Familienberatung.*
[115] *hygienische Beratungsstellen.* R. Fetscher, 'Eheberatungsstellen als Teil der Gesundheitsfürsorge', *Fortschritte der Gesundheitsfürsorge*, vol. 4 no. 3 (1930), 76–7.
[116] E. Fischer in *25 Jahre Kaiser Wilhelm Gesellschaft zur Förderung der Wissenschaften*, 3 vols. (Berlin, 1936), vol. 2, pp. 349, 355–6; E. Fischer, 'Das Kaiser-Wilhelm-Institut für Anthropologie, menschliche Erblehre und Eugenik', *Zeitschrift für Morphologie und Anthropologie*, vol. 27 (1927), 147–52; P.J. Weindling, 'Weimar Eugenics: The Kaiser Wilhelm Institute for Anthropology, Human Heredity and Eugenics in Social Context', *Annals of Science*, vol. 42 (1985), 303–18.
[117] L.R. Graham, 'Science and Values: the Eugenics Movement in Germany and Russia in the 1920s', *American Historical Review*, vol. 82 (1977), pp. 1,133–64, 1,136, 1,137; Graham, *Between Science and Values*, (New York, 1981), pp. 221–3; M.B. Adams, 'Science, Ideology and Structure: The Kol'tsov Institute 1900–1970', in L. Lubriano and S.G. Solomon (eds.), *The Social Context of Soviet*

for Health, Soviet eugenics and population genetics flourished. Not only did Soviet scientists visit Germany, but German medical scientists such as the pathologist Aschoff and the neurologist Vogt planned co-operative research. Comparisons deserve to be drawn between Weimar eugenics and British, Scandinavian, and United States eugenic movements, as these all contained social reformers who were keen to eliminate such social problems as poverty and illness while disengaging eugenics from ideologies of racial purity. Italian eugenics was characterized more by pro-natalist sentiments than by racial ideology.[118] The institutionalization of eugenics as a science resulted from changes in the professional expectations of geneticists, and in the scope of scientific activity. Biological laws of development, natural selection and inheritance were to provide proven standards on which to base legislation, socio-economic planning and counselling services. Eugenics changed from being the creed of an introverted nationalist grouping to becoming an integral part of social medicine and welfare. The shift occurred in conjunction with an enlarging of the scope of genetics to embrace social and demographic values and a creed of utility. The Weimar state relied on professional and scientific expertise, and geneticists rose to the challenge of restoring the biological fabric of the defeated and starving nation.

An indication of the extent to which eugenics affected biomedical research is provided by the Kaiser Wilhelm institutes. Eugenic dimensions to research were emphasized by Vogt's Institute of Brain Research. At the Institute for Experimental Therapy, Hans Reiter (who was later to take a leading position in public health during the Third Reich) researched on heredity and environment in child development. Baur's Institute for Plant Breeding at Müncheberg opened in 1927. He pioneered applied genetics for agriculture, and he regarded this as having implications for human heredity, rural resettlement and the nation's economy. Typical of the Kaiser Wilhelm Institutes was that funding came from both state and private sources. Baur's seed fund was subsidized by the publisher Lehmann and the banker Jakob Goldschmidt. That a scientific enterprise should attract *völkisch* and Jewish support shows the complexity of the interests involved in Weimar genetics

---

Science (Boulder and Folkestone, 1980), pp. 173–204; P.J. Weindling, 'German-Soviet Co-operation in Science. The Case of the Laboratory for Racial Research 1931–1938', *Nuncius*, vol. 1 (1987), 103–9.

[118] On British eugenics see: G. Searle, *Eugenics and Politics in Britain* (Leyden, 1976); C. Webster (ed.), *Biology, Medicine and Society 1840–1940* (Cambridge, 1981); M. Freeden, 'Eugenics and Progressive Thought: a Study in Ideological Affinity', *The Historical Journal*, vol. 22 (1979), 645–71; G. Jones, 'Eugenics and Social Policy Between the Wars', *The Historical Journal*, vol. 25 (1982), 717–28; M. Freeden, 'Eugenics and Ideology', *The Historical Journal*, vol. 26 (1983), 959–62. On Scandinavia see: N. Roll-Hansen, 'Eugenics before World War II. The Case of Norway', *History and Philosophy of the Life Sciences*, vol. 2 (1981), 269–98. On US eugenics see D. Pickens, *Eugenics and the Progressives* (Nashville, 1968); G.E. Allen, 'The Misuse of Biological Hierarchies: The American Eugenics Movement, 1900–1940', *History and Philosophy of the Life Sciences*, vol. 5 (1983), 105–28; D.J. Kevles, *In the Name of Eugenics. Genetics and the Uses of Human Heredity* (New York, 1985). On Italy and Spain see C. Pogliano, 'Scienza e Stirpe: Eugenica in Italia (1912–1939)', *Passato e Presente*, vol. 5 (1984), 61–97; R. Alvarez-Pelaez, 'Introduccion al estudio de la Eugenesia espanola (1900–1936)', *Quipu*, vol. 2 (1985), 95–122.

and eugenics. Two major pillars of eugenic research were the Kaiser Wilhelm Institutes for Biology and for Psychiatry. The foundation of an Institute for Anthropology, Human Heredity and Eugenics was neither an isolated occurrence nor an aberration in policies to support pure research, but the keystone in a grand eugenic edifice. Under Correns the Institute for Biology exerted a benign influence on eugenics, and Goldschmidt and Bluhm served on government racial hygiene committees.[119]

The Rockefeller Foundation facilitated the expansion of German hereditarian science into areas of social relevance. From 1925 some of its officials supported a 'Human Biology Program'. This integrated a number of spheres in biology and medicine, and was related to what the officials perceived as a social crisis of poverty, crime and inherited disease. It amounted to a modernized type of reform eugenics in line with the advances in biology and medicine. The Rockefeller's Trustees had their doubts about the support of eugenics and mental hygiene. But the official, Embree, who was at that time in charge of the medical sciences, went on a European tour in December 1926. This was ostensibly to prepare a nurse training programme, but instead he developed his contacts with German biologists in an attempt to pursue human biology.[120] A number of German eugenicists benefited from Rockefeller funds. These included Poll, who was active in the League for Regeneration, Bluhm, for research on heredity and alcoholism, Nachtsheim, for Mendelian research, the statistician Siegfried Koller, and Fetscher and Grotjahn among the social hygienists. While the Rockefeller Foundation was dismissive of Davenport's Eugenic Record Office, believing that it lacked scientific rigour, it was attracted to research on the genetic and neurological basis of mental traits such as crime and mental disease. Substantial investments were made in German psychiatry and neurology, and new buildings were provided for the Institute of Zoology in Munich.

The *Kaiser Wilhelm Gesellschaft* (KWG) had a major eugenic commitment in Rüdin's genealogical-demographic Department of the German Psychiatric Institute. In 1924 the KWG took over joint responsibility with the Bavarian state for maintaining the psychiatric institute. The most substantial Rockefeller funding was to go to the German Psychiatric Institute. The contacts between the Rockefeller Foundation and Kraepelin had been forged by a scion of the Kuhn-Loeb bankers, James Loeb, who encouraged research on criminal biology.[121] Loeb interested Abraham Flexner, who approached the Rockefeller Foundation. In November 1925 the Trustees agreed to contribute $2,500,000, with a further

[119] O. Vogt, 'Neurology and Eugenics. The Role of Experimental Eugenics in their Development', *Eugenics Review*, vol. 24 (1932), 15–18; H. Stubbe, *Geschichte des Instituts für Kulturpflanzenforschung Gatersleben* (Berlin, 1982), pp. 12–14; G. Zirnstein, 'Zur gesellschaftlichen Stellung der wissenschaftlichen Pflanzenzüchtung in Deutschland während der zwanziger und dreissiger Jahre des 20. Jahrhunderts', *NTM*, vol. 9 (1972), 60–9.

[120] Weindling, 'The Rockefeller Foundation', pp. 119–40; R.E. Kohler, 'A Policy for the Advancement of Science: The Rockefeller Foundation, 1924–29', *Minerva*, vol. 16 (1978), 480–515.   [121] E. Kraepelin, *Lebenserinnerungen* (Berlin, 1983), pp. 209, 219.

$75,000 in 1926. They were convinced that 'Munich is probably the best place in Europe to foster an outstanding institute devoted to investigation in psychiatry'. They were impressed by the support from the city of Munich and state authorities for a criminal biology data bank and district surveys of inherited diseases.[122] US and Soviet recognition of the innovative capacity of German research show how the international scientific community accepted hereditarian science and medicine as benefiting mankind by tackling the roots of social problems.

During the 1920s concern with social deviancy and hopes of its scientific control and cure made a hospital as legitimate a scientific facility as a research station. Scientists required the co-operation of state, municipal and school authorities. Eugenicists like Verschuer needed schools and hospitals to provide the records of many hundreds of twins for research into hereditary diseases. Rüdin's research on hereditary biology had the backing of the Bavarian Ministries of Justice and the Interior, as well as the co-operation of medical authorities and institutions. He established impressive standards for the genealogical reconstruction of families for the purpose of genetic research. In 1925 Fetscher began a similar *Erbbiologische Kartei* supported by the authorities in Saxony. Prussia authorized the compilation of such records from 1927, which significantly was the year in which the Kaiser Wilhelm Institute for Anthropology was established.[123] These research models, which applied the science of heredity to social problems, determined the organization and scope of the institute. Long-standing demands for a national research institute for eugenics and the new directions in the organization of Weimar science, account for the responsiveness of the KWG and of state authorities to the proposal for an institute for human heredity. The institute was rapidly established after it was first suggested in 1925 by Muckermann, the Jesuit biologist and expert on welfare issues.

The founding of the institute

It might seem paradoxical that the national eugenics institute should have been the brain child of a Roman Catholic. Muckermann had training in cell biology at the University of Louvain and was inspired by the Catholic opponents of Haeckel, such as the entomologist, Erich Wasmann. He joined the Jesuits in 1896 and combined studies of theology and biology in Jesuit colleges in the USA and in the Netherlands. From 1916 he became a tireless crusader for family welfare. In 1919 Muckermann had been antagonistic to eugenics as he disapproved of the concept of degeneracy, preferring the term *Anderwertig* to *Minderwertig* (i.e. of otherness to degeneracy). But by 1922 he joined the committees of the Berlin and German Racial Hygiene Societies while involved in family welfare work. His change of heart on eugenics was symptomatic of the recognition of the importance of

[122] RAC 1.1./71/9/56.
[123] For surveys of the 'anti-social', BAK R 86 Nr 2374 Bd 1 Bl. 328–9; ZSTA M Rep 76 VIII B Nr 2074 Bl. 346.

eugenics for social welfare. Muckermann's influence cannot be ascribed solely to his energy as an organizer, but must be explained in terms of the structural conditions of social welfare administration and the balance of political power in Prussia and the Reich.[124] The Centre Party had shed conservative Catholics to the DNVP, and it took a role as intermediary between more liberal-minded bourgeois Catholics and workers. Welfare was important to its strategy of social integration. It also strengthened its hold on appointments in welfare and public health. Not only was the Ministry of Welfare under a Centre Party minister (Hirtsiefer), but also in 1928 Heinrich Schopohl, a Catholic and Centre Party man, became *Ministerialdirektor* of the Health Department. Schopohl was to preside over the sterilization discussions in the early 1930s. Muckermann's influence must therefore be seen in the context of the Centre Party's control of welfare. He was on excellent terms with politicians such as the Bavarian *Staatspräsident* and Hirtsiefer, doctors such as Schopohl, scientists such as Fischer and pro-eugenic Catholic theologians such as Joseph Mayer. The authorities in Baden, with its substantial Catholic population, were regarded as crucial. Muckermann assumed the important role of a middleman between the eugenicists, state officials and religious and secular welfare organizations.

In 1925 Muckermann suggested to the geneticist Nachtsheim (who worked in Baur's Institute at the Agricultural University in Berlin) that there was a need for a national eugenics institute. Baur mobilized the support of geneticists, while Muckermann took charge of recruiting support among state authorities and general public.[125] The close relations between the state and welfare organizations explain why Muckermann was in a position of influence which far exceeded his capacities as a biologist. He aimed to collect one million marks for the eugenic institute. During 1926–7 he gave hundreds of lectures and undertook extensive fund raising. The KWG had traditionally relied on donations from wealthy industrialists to support research in pure and applied science. It was indicative of the shift in the organization of science and medicine in the Weimar Republic that industrialists gave far less to the institute than the Reich and Prussian administrations. Muckermann had initially hoped to use his links with Ruhr industrialists to good ends, but contacts through the Centre Party with state, municipal and insurance fund officials proved far more lucrative. Between 24 April 1926 and 2 August 1927 considerable amounts of money were raised (see table 7).[126]

[124] Technical University Berlin archives, Muckermann MS 'Aus meinem Leben'; F. Glum, *Zwischen Wissenschaft und Wirtschaft und Politik* (Bonn, 1964), p. 284; H. Muckermann, 'Erblichkeitsforschung und Eheschliessung in der Zukunft', *Bericht der Verhandlungen des bevölkerungspolitischen Kongresses der Stadt Köln, Pfingstwoche von 17.–21 Mai 1921* (np, nd), pp. 73–97; K. Nowak, *'Euthanasie' und Sterilisierung im 'Dritten Reich'* (Weimar and Göttingen, 1984), pp. 107–11; K.-E. Lönne, *Politischer Katholizismus im 19. und 20. Jahrhundert* (Frankfurt a. M., 1986).

[125] H. Nachtsheim, 'Die Notwendigkeit einer aktiven Erbgesundheitspflege', *Gesundheitspolitik*, vol. 21 (1964), 323.

[126] MPG Generalverwaltung 2411, Finanzierung 18.6.1926–2.9.1927. Nr 2412, Finanzierung 17.9.1927–30.12.1931.

Table 7. *The financing of the Kaiser Wilhelm Institute for Anthropology, Human Heredity and Eugenics*

Type of donor (and number, if known)	Reichmarks
Private and industrial (16)	23,200
Municipal (7)	8,725
Provincial insurance funds	
(*Landesversicherungsanstalten*) (21)	15,868
Provincial and rural district funds	
(*Landkreis und Provinz*) (9)	56,700
Prussian Minister for Science	200,000 + site worth
	200,000
Reich Minister of the Interior	500,000

In addition to state donations, other donations of 5,000 marks or more came from:

Province of Upper Silesia	20,000
Province of the Rhine	10,000
Province of Westphalia	7,500
Rural district of Beuthen	5,000
Municipality of Essen	5,000
Province of Silesia	5,000
Schaffgott'sche Works Chemnitz	5,000
Julius and Hans Thyssen	5,000

The Kaiser Wilhelm Gesellschaft remained an independent corporation administered under the auspices of the Reich authorities. This greatly annoyed federal state administrations who had responsibility for scientific education and medicine. Thus the Anthropological Institute had national status as a Reich institution, but its location was problematic. Negotiations with the Baden Ministry of the Interior collapsed, preventing its establishment under Fischer in Freiburg. Other eugenicists wished for the funding to be spread on a regional basis so as to facilitate local population studies.[127] Berlin was chosen as the location due to the presence of the immense statistical resources of the Reich administration. Close scientific co-operation was envisaged with the Biological Institute of the KWG, and support from municipal medical institutions was ensured. The experts in social hygiene, Drigalski (the municipal medical officer of Berlin) and Grotjahn, were on the governing board of the anthropological institute. It meant that the social problems of Berlin with its mass unemployment and political violence impinged on the activities of the institute.

The anthropological institute was seen as having a dual scientific and social role.

[127] F. Lenz, 'Das deutsche Forschungsinstitut für Anthropologie, menschliche Erblehre und Eugenik in Berlin-Dahlem', *MMW*, vol. 74 (1927) 1764; H.W. Siemens, 'Vererbungspathologie und Klinik', *MMW*, vol. 74 (1927), 1,407.

The Senate of the KWG hoped that the institute would counter dilettante racism.[128] The emphasis on the scientific image of eugenics was conveyed by the use of the term *Eugenik* in the title of the institute in preference to *Rassenhygiene*. This was a direction favoured by the Berlin group of the Racial Hygiene Society, which adopted the term *Eugenik* in 1931. Scientificity was reinforced by the fact that the opening of the institute coincided with the Fifth International Congress of Heredity; this was organized by Nachtsheim and massively subsidized by the Reich. Baur organized a section on racial hygiene and eugenics, and invited Ploetz to hold a lecture indicating the lack of substantial state support for eugenics. The 1927 genetics congress marked the end of over a decade of isolation of German biology – and of German eugenics. During the mid-1920s Germany was admitted to the International Federation of Eugenic organizations, to the League of Nations and to the Health Office of the League, which included a section on eugenics.[129]

The organization of the institute

The institute had three departments. Fischer, as director, headed the department for anthropology, chose the other staff and determined research priorities. Muckermann headed the eugenics department, and Verschuer led the department for human heredity. Muckermann underwent secularization, enabling him to relinquish his Jesuit vows while remaining a priest. The Prussian state awarded him the title of professor and recognized his academic credentials. Muckermann and Fischer came from the Catholic peripheries of Germany, Muckermann hailing from Westphalia and Fischer from Baden. It was only later that Fischer left the Catholic Church. Verschuer's religious beliefs were evangelical. Nationalist impulses pervaded research on inherited diseases. In keeping with the spirit of the co-ordination in science, the institute had close links to the university. Fischer's appointment was combined with a university chair in anthropology, and the institute took over the university's anthropological collection. Fischer stressed the relevance of his work to public health and to judicial proceedings, one activity of the institute being to establish paternity in legal cases.

The scheme depended on Fischer's accepting the post of director. In July 1926 he confided to Schemann, that his appointment was a condition for the foundation of the institute: 'This pistol is at my chest'.[130] Fischer's approach to anthropology was based on biological heredity. He relied less on craniometry and other anthropometric methods, and more on genetics, and the mapping of racial variation in terms of biological characteristics such as blood groups, inherited diseases and other traits

[128] Schemann papers, Fischer to Schemann 17 September 1927; MPG Generalverwaltung 2043; K. Nemitz, 'Antisemitismus in der Wissenschaftspolitik der Weimarer Republik. Der "Fall Ludwig Schemann"', *Jahrbuch des Instituts für deutsche Geschichte*, vol. 12 (1983), 377–406.

[129] H. Nachtsheim, 'Der V. Internationale Kongress für Vererbungswissenschaft', *Die Naturwissenschaften*, vol. 15 (1927), 989–95; ZSTA M Rep 76 VIII B Nr 2073 Bl. 308; Goldschmidt, *Ivory Tower*, pp. 232–3; Ploetz papers, Baur to Ploetz, 28 March 1927.

[130] Schemann papers, Fischer to Schemann, 11 July 1926.

which could be explained in hereditarian terms. Family reconstruction was thus a major feature of the biological methodology. Initially Fischer had praised the benefits of racial inter-breeding, as in his classic study of the Rehoboth intermarrying of settlers and natives in South West Africa. Later Fischer accepted Gobineau's emphasis on racial purity and, as both Schemann and Fischer worked in Freiburg, the foundations were laid for a symbiosis between academic anthropology and Gobineau's racist theories.[131]

Muckermann was as much a propagandist as a researcher. He promoted a 'broad church' approach in his efforts to overcome sectarian differences between eugenicists. He attempted to reconcile negative eugenic advocates of sterilization with the positive eugenic advocates of social welfare. His solutions tended to be couched in nebulous terms such as the need to instil 'a new racial consciousness'. Eugenics was a gospel of health and morality which would reinvigorate the family. His emotive phrases blurred over what were often substantial differences on eugenic issues. His research focused on 'the normal family', and on groups selected for positive eugenic qualities. He studied rural populations with large families and low infant mortality. He analyzed the fertility of 5,000 university professors. There followed studies of 4,800 army officers and of 39,000 Prussian police and officials.[132]

The department of human heredity, headed by Verschuer, concentrated on twin studies. He examined 700 pairs of twins with regard to the issue of the inheritance of mental qualities. He found 150 pairs of criminal twins, and researched on the inheritance of tuberculosis and cancer. This work was supported by the Reich Ministry of the Interior, the Prussian Ministry of Welfare and the Rockefeller Foundation. In 1927 Verschuer recommended sterilization for the mentally and 'morally' subnormal, and he emphasized the biological basis of class structure. He condemned democracy as a quantitative rather than a qualitative social system, which posed undue financial burdens on the natural elite.[133] Wolfgang Abel, an anthropologist, researched into the inheritance of physiognomy. Blood group research was a priority. I.G. Farben financed an experimental project on the determinants of cranial form using vitamins and toxic substances.

Fischer, Muckermann, Verschuer and their co-workers linked their scientific research with eugenic schemes that were selective and authoritarian in their political implications. They placed as much emphasis on eugenic education as on research, emphasizing the links between theory and practice. From 1927

---

[131] On Fischer's backing of Schemann see Nemitz 'Antisemitismus', pp. 399, 401–2.
[132] H. Ebert, 'Hermann Muckermann', *Humanismus und Technik*, vol. 20 (1976), 29–40; D. Grosch-Obenauer, 'Hermann Muckermann und die Eugenik seiner Zeit', med. Diss, Mainz 1986. For examples of Muckermann's many eugenic publications see: H. Muckermann, 'Wesen der Eugenik und Aufgaben der Gegenwart', *Das kommende Geschlecht*, vol. 5 (1929), 1–48; BAK R 86 Nr 2370 Vererbungsforschung, for research on differential fertility in 1931; MPG 2404 Tätigkeitsbericht; Nowak, '*Euthanasie*', pp. 33, 40, 107–11.
[33] K.-D. Thomann, 'Otmar Freiherr von Verschuer – ein Hauptvertreter der faschistischen Rassenhygiene', in Thom and Spaar (eds.), *Medizin*, pp. 38–41.

Muckermann invited Fischer and Verschuer to co-edit the journal *Das kommende Geschlecht* (the future generation) which was distributed by the Prussian state to officials and medical officers. By 1932 Fischer had given three courses to Prussian medical officers on eugenics. Muckermann undertook a marathon lecture programme on eugenics for the Berlin Racial Hygiene Society, and encouraged the foundation of eugenic groups. The institute provided the leadership of the German and Berlin Racial Hygiene Societies. This marked a shift away from the directing role of state officials. In 1928 Fischer succeeded Gruber on the editorial board of the *Archiv*, and was president of the German and Berlin Racial Hygiene Societies from 1928 until 1933. Muckermann and Verschuer were secretaries of the societies, which met at the institute. Fischer and Muckermann were deeply involved in the League for Regeneration presided over by Behr-Pinnow and the state official Ostermann. State officials placed great reliance on the directive role of the scientific elite to provide guidance on social issues. Ostermann and another medical official, Tschammer von Quaritz, went so far as to call for biologically based laws.[134]

At a time of financial crisis, eugenicists offered the state positive reasons for the dismantling of welfare institutions, and for the drafting of sterilization legislation. Verschuer argued that social policy and economics should be based on racial hygiene. From 1928 he publicly attacked the welfare state: social insurance was a burden on the economy and reduced the capacity for work. Welfare supported the degenerate and work shy at the expense of the industrious. Lenz agreed that there was an imminent new dawn in social thought with society being reconstructed on the basis of biological differentials.[135] The institute boosted confidence in the science of eugenics. Whereas previously, legislation had been hampered by doubts as to whether there was a firm enough scientific basis for eugenics, the confidence and dynamism of the institute did much to dispel such questioning. Fischer wrote to Schemann that 1930 was to be an important year not only for science but for 'our' *Volk*. The work of the institute was to be on 'patriotic matters'.[136] Politics and economics were to be subordinated to biological laws.

The Kaiser Wilhelm Institute for Anthropology, Human Heredity and Eugenics was shaped by the distinctive development of the organization of Weimar science. The integration of social utility with scientific research was encouraged. Contemporary standards in German science suggest that there was no necessary demarcation between hereditarian biology and eugenics, even if the researchers differed in the extent of their eugenic commitments and in their social philosophies. State funding and support played a major role. But the anti-democratic sentiments

[134] ZSTA M Rep 76 VIII B Nr 2073 Bl. 373; Nr 2074 Bl. 467, 480; Ploetz papers, Fischer to Ploetz, 29 October 1928; Behr-Pinnow, 'Vererbungswissenschaft und Eugenik', *Arbeitsgemeinschaft für Volksgesundung. Mitteilungen*, no. 17 (14 June 1929).

[135] O. v. Verschuer, *Sozialpolitik und Rassenhygiene*, (Langensalza, 1928); published also in *Nationalwirtschaft* and in Friedrich Mann's *Pädagogische Magazin*; reviewed by Lenz in *MMW*, vol. 75 (1928), 1854.

[136] Schemann Papers, Fischer to Schemann, 24 December 1929.

of Fischer and Verschuer show that the state was funding a group of scientists who wished fundamentally to reconstruct the political and economic basis of the Weimar society. The innovations in Weimar biology were both a product and a challenge to the political and economic conditions under which the republic laboured. Institutes were bastions of scientific expertise, erected to defend the *Volk* against chronic poverty, dissolute morality and sexual reform, and they fomented opposition to the welfare state.

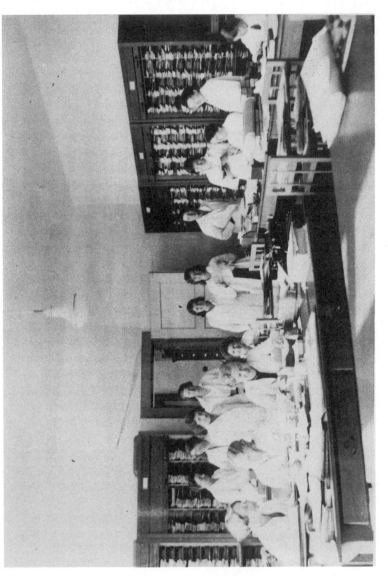

7 Secretarial assistants of Ernst Rüdin at the German Psychiatric Institute, Munich, circa 1930. The eugenicists developed ambitious plans for area surveys of medical, social and demographic records during the economically depressed years from 1929. The psychiatrist, Rüdin, had used genealogical records in order to demonstrate the inheritance of schizophrenia in Mendelian terms. The scientific surveys were to form the basis of systematic collection of data of human heredity in Nazi Germany. The photo is reproduced by permission of Professor Edith Zerbin-Rüdin.

7

The sick bed of democracy, 1929–1932

The slump and medicine

The Great Depression shattered the economic basis of the welfare state. The financial foundations of social security and sickness insurance were swept away, when in the wake of the Wall Street Crash of autumn 1929 the Central European banking system collapsed in the spring and summer of 1931. Local authority initiatives in housing and welfare were especially vulnerable as some had been supported by municipal savings banks and American loans.[1] State welfare authorities were subjected to a ruthless axeing of funds by retrenchment-minded ministers. The edifice of the Weimar welfare state – a soaring but unfinished modernist construction by planners and social hygienists – came crashing down into the abyss of National Socialism.

Weimar Germany had always lacked secure economic foundations. Agriculture – still employing one-third of the workforce – was in a state of chronic depression. Modernization and efficiency of such industries as chemicals meant overproduction. Business cycles meant that there were years when unemployment was high, as in 1926 when two million were jobless. A few medical studies of the effects on health of unemployment were made by doctors at the labour exchanges. They assumed that increased welfare benefits could prevent lasting harm to the health of workers and their families.[2] In 1929 it seemed as though here was yet another economic down-turn which would have a purgative effect on excesses in wages and production and would be followed by recovery. But by 1931 Germans were in a state of panic at the economic calamity. It meant that after an initial period of non-reaction, there was a massive over-reaction in the sphere of welfare with savage cuts to all services. Municipal welfare experts pointing out that needs were greater than

---

[1] H. James, *The German Slump* (Oxford, 1986), pp. 85–109.
[2] P. Trüb, 'Die vertrauensärztliche Tätigkeit beim Arbeitsamt in Duisburg, ihre Organisation und Ergebnisse', *Reichsarbeitsblatt*, no. 28 (15 May 1930), II, 435–45; K. Dohrn, 'Die gesundheitliche Folgen der Erwerbslosigkeit', *Der Öffentliche Arbeitsnachweis*, no. 4 (1927), 337–40.

ever clashed with economists who stressed the need for stringent retrenchment and selectivity in health and welfare administration.[3] Numbers of health and social workers were reduced, clinics were closed and benefits were cut. Doctors observed an increase in neurosis and suffering. The psychiatrist Viktor von Weizsäcker observed that instead of war there was depression, and instead of escape to the Heimat there were neurotic expectations of dependence on state welfare and insurance systems.[4] The mayor of Leipzig diagnosed the situation as 'the sick-bed of capitalism'. Liberal and democratic values seemed to be in their death-throes.

The crisis was manipulated by diverse social groups. 1927 had seen the introduction of unemployment insurance and of an eight-hour day. The electoral victories of the SPD in May 1928 had given it the chance to expand social insurance. Employers, especially in heavy industry, exploited the economic crisis to reverse these trends by engineering wage and social insurance cuts. They pressed for dismantling the mechanisms of social arbitration established by the welfare state. The political climate saw a rise in authoritarianism. Parliamentary procedures were undermined by a dictatorial system of emergency decrees. The Chancellor between 30 March 1930 and May 1932, Heinrich Brüning, hoped for an authoritarian coalition as a 'national government'. Brüning was the Centre Party leader and governed with the support of an increasingly disaffected SPD. His main political ally was the ultra-conservative President, Paul von Hindenburg, and his government was one of experts rather than politicians. He relied on presidential emergency decrees. Brüning's policy of deflationary cuts exacerbated the unemployment and mass poverty. He was succeeded by Franz von Papen, a Catholic aristocrat, who resigned from the Centre Party and entered into a coalition with the right. His policy of a 'new state' aimed to cripple socialism. At the same time the NSDAP was increasing its share of the vote from 18.3 per cent of votes cast in September 1930 to 37.3 per cent in July 1932, gaining strong support among the Protestant middle class. The mood generated demands for corporate and authoritarian management of social problems. Politics became more polarized and violent, and the SPD launched a last ditch campaign to mobilize a popular defence of the republic under the banner of the 'Reich Flag Black, Red and Gold' movement.

Whereas the post-war crisis of 1918–1923 was characterized by the slogan of 'reconstruction' or Aufbau, the economic crisis of 1929 instigated a reverse trend of Abbau with the dismantling of social institutions. The state was in a dilemma: as needs grew resources diminished. Between 1929 and 1932 unemployment rocketed from 1.8 to 5.6 million. The tax revenue per person fell from 65.4 marks to 27.2 marks in 1930. The upshot was that clinics closed and social security benefits were cut. Stuttgart was exceptional in that it continued to build during the depression; a hospital for skin diseases and a midwifery school were built.[5] Welfare

---

[3] T. Paulstich, Sparsamkeit und Zweckmässigkeit in der Wohlfahrts- und Gesundheitsverwaltung (Leipzig, 1932).
[4] V. v. Weizsäcker, Soziale Krankheit und soziale Gesundung (Berlin, 1930), p. 12.
[5] James, Slump, p. 100.

had been based on principles of state subsidies for municipalities, which became burdened by having to support the long-term unemployed. Whereas the Reich authorities had hitherto been weak in the spheres of health and social policy, there were now attempts at centralized control. In July 1932 Papen deposed the Prussian government by decree, and became *Reichskommissar* with full powers of control. This ended the Centre-SPD coalition in Prussia under which welfare had prospered. Hirtsiefer was replaced as Welfare Minister. The Prussian Ministry of Welfare was dismantled on 1 December 1932, when the health department reverted to the Ministry of the Interior.

Political events were succumbing to the right-wing forces of Hindenburg, the army, heavy industry and Junkers demanding protective tariffs. Coinciding with authoritarian politics and industrial relations was an attempt by professionals to exert dictatorial powers. Doctors were aware that in a situation of high unemployment and widespread suffering, they combined powers of officials and judges in that they certified benefits, so affecting the economic position of millions.[6] Doctors used the situation to campaign against the controls of sickness funds. Professional leaders attacked the expansive 'imperialism' of the sickness funds. Since regulations of 1923 restricted the numbers of sickness insurance doctors to a ratio of one physician for 1,000 patients, access to insurance practice was difficult. Young doctors demanded *Lebensraum* in which to practise. There was outrage when in July 1930 the government imposed a fee of 50 Pfennig to be paid by the patient in order to reduce the financial obligations of the insurance funds. It had the effect of reducing patient visits and thus the income of insurance doctors.[7] In this atmosphere there was a renewed campaign against lay practitioners, against the rising numbers of women doctors, and against the high percentage of Jewish doctors in cities and particularly in Berlin.[8] Numbers of women doctors rose from 1,225 in 1925 to 5,123 in 1933. Anti-feminism, anti-semitism and anti-socialism were welded together by economic pressures.[9] This resulted in sympathy for authoritarian politics. Professional insecurities thus contributed to the middle-class backlash against Weimar democracy.

The combination of nationalism and professional politics was to result in the ending of the liberal tradition of the self-administration of the municipalities and sickness insurance.[10] Leaders of the profession joined such organizations as the

---

[6] Weizsäcker, *Soziale Krankheit*, p. 2; E. Straus, *Geschehnis und Erlebnis. Zugleich eine historiologische Deutung des psychischen Traumas und der Renten-Neurose* (Berlin, 1930).

[7] M.H. Kater, 'Physicians in Crisis at the End of the Weimar Republic', in P.D. Stachura (ed.), *Unemployment and the Great Depression in Weimar Germany* (Basingstoke, 1986), pp. 49–74.

[8] Statistics on 'Jewish doctors' derive from Nazi censuses and so were used to justify boycotts and dismissals; see W.F. Kümmel, 'Die Ausschaltung rassisch und politisch missliebiger Ärzte', in Kudlien, *Ärzte*, pp. 56–81.

[9] E.M. Klasen, 'Die Diskussion über eine "Krise" der Medizin in Deutschland zwischen 1925 und 1935, med. Diss., University of Mainz, 1984, pp. 46–60; K. Frankenthal, *Der dreifache Fluch; Jüdin, Intellektuelle, Sozialistin* (Frankfurt-on-Main, 1981).

[10] S. Leibfried and F. Tennstedt, *Berufsverbote und Sozialpolitik 1933. Die Auswirkungen der nationalsozialistischen Machtergreifung auf die Krankenkassenverwaltung und die Kassenärzte* (Bremen, 1979), p. xv.

Stahlhelm and were active in the DNVP. A leading protagonist of these attitudes was the chairman of the German and Prussian medical officers association, Gustav Bundt, who from 1928 represented the DNVP in the Prussian *Landtag*. During the crisis demands began to be voiced for a 'Reich Medical Officers' Law' which was to reinforce the powers of the medical officer as a state official.[11] There was a sense of a simultaneous economic, ethical and scientific crisis in the profession. The social hygienist Schlossmann diagnosed a professional malaise due to a 'technicization' of medicine resulting from panel practice. He urged that the scope of medicine be extended from therapy to general care and preventive medicine to guard the nation's health. Others, such as the medical historian Paul Diepgen and the Berlin internist His, spoke of a 'proletarianization' of the profession. Demands intensified for the dismantling of social insurance. The solutions were seen in terms of reinforcing the autonomous status and authority of the doctor. Underlying this specifically medical response was a widespread fear among the middle classes of pauperization. Authoritarian values amounted to a defence of class identity. The profession's attack on sickness insurance and municipal welfare, and the associated attempts to institute a *Reichsreform* to displace federal states such as Prussia, amounted to a rejection of liberal institutions. The middle class opposed the liberal legacy of the federated Reich, which it perceived as corrupted by socialism. The Nazi onslaught against the corruption of liberal individualism gathered support.

The economic crisis brought about a change of heart on welfare. The mid-twenties dream of equal rights and improved living standards ended. Positive measures with equal entitlement for all in need were too costly. Eugenicists abandoned strategies of custodial institutions for detention of the unfit and positive eugenic welfare measures. The economic crisis coincided with what was perceived as a demographic crisis. Differential fertility raised the spectre that those in the population of high eugenic worth were dying out. The nation would be populated by a mass of degenerates.[12] Eugenicists responded to the authoritarian atmosphere of retrenchment by advocating selection and survival of the fittest as the means of national salvation. Such welfare-oriented eugenicists as Grotjahn, Harmsen and Muckermann shifted the balance from positive to negative eugenics. They became crusaders for sterilization, cost-cutting and stringent selectivity in benefits. Medical advocates of sterilization such as Rüdin gained prominence. From a position of objective, science-based values, these professional experts offered the nation clearly formulated guiding principles. A brief age of scientific dictatorship had dawned.

Public health and welfare experts advocated ruthless policies of selective benefits. On the positive side, there was an urgent need to sustain 'child rich' families of high eugenic quality. Eugenicists were outraged by the series of cuts in the income of officials, believing them to be damaging to a group which was carrying out great biological and social work. Following the example of fascist

---

[11] Labisch and Tennstedt, *GVG*, I, pp. 102–16.
[12] F. Burgdörfer, *Der Geburtenrückgang und seine Bekämpfung* (Berlin, 1928); also in *VGM*, vol. 218 no. 2 (1929).

Italy, demands increased for a bachelor tax and measures to ensure that rural populations remained economically viable. Above all, the ideological reserves of national patriotic duty were to be invoked to strengthen the family. Eugenicists incited the Reich League for Child Rich Families to intensify its campaign for a parenthood insurance, and so build up public pressure for a population policy. Sterilization and reduction of benefits to a minimum were the reverse side of the policy. Discussions of sterilization from 1929 emphasized the need to base welfare on a graduated scale of economic and eugenic values. The unproductive should be prevented from incurring further costs to the nation, whereas the fit and healthy were to receive extra benefits. The positive values that accompanied sterilization demonstrate the attraction of this measure as a means of freeing resources to benefit the racially valuable elements in the population.

Biologically conceived remedies replaced political solutions to social problems. Popularizations of eugenics pleaded for a return to 'natural' solutions to social problems. In 1927 the geneticist Goldschmidt published a popularization of biology, called *Ascaris*, which sold 15,000 copies by 1933. He considered that the scientist was in a position to draw conclusions for humanity as would a breeder for the improvement of his stock. The 'feeble-minded' and the deaf and dumb would not survive in nature. It was mistaken of society to allow the procreation of poor hereditary stock. He recommended measures to protect the nation's 'genetic treasury' such as institutionalization or sterilization of all with bad hereditary traits. Children should learn that only those of eugenic value had any attraction or merit. Eugenicists argued that natural selection should be allowed to operate throughout society, to counter the degenerating effects of urban life and of humanitarian welfare. It is in this context that biological studies which showed domestication as the cause of physical degeneration and pathological behaviour should be understood.[13] Biologists expressed in scientific terms broader concerns of the economically vulnerable bourgeoisie.

Women were regarded by such eugenicists as Hirsch as 'the biological capital of the *Volk*'. The family was the 'germ cell' of the nation. The secretary of the Reich Health Council, Christian, contributed to the rising tide of 'biological thought'. In the official organ, the *Reichsgesundheitsblatt*, he warned in Spenglerian terms of a decline of the West because of the neglect of the biological basis of society. The decline could only be prevented if biology was given primacy over economics with the restoration of the natural laws of survival of the fittest. The rise of degenerates threatened the future existence of the 'culturally creative natural Führer'.[14] It seemed that a fitter, healthier society would result from allowing free reign to natural selection. Biologists were in a position to justify the cutting of welfare expenditure. For their part economists and such conservative politicians as Brüning spoke of the 'healing' and 'purging' effects of crises in strengthening the economy.

[13] R. Goldschmidt, *Die Lehre von der Vererbung*, 2 vols. (Berlin, 1927), II, pp. 203–17. Goldschmidt, *Einführung in die Wissenschaft von Leben oder Ascaris* (Berlin, 1927).
[14] Thomann, *Fischer*, pp. 211–12.

Eugenicists pointed out that they were in a position to accelerate selective processes, for the birth rate – that barometer of national 'will' – had sunk to a dangerously low point. With the impending ruin of Germany's hereditary stock, the country stood on the verge of eugenic as well as economic bankruptcy.

The crisis of population policy

The retreat from expansive welfare programmes was in sharp contrast with the post-war determination to maintain welfare institutions at all cost. For the first few years of the economic crisis the lobby for expansion of family welfare measures maintained its position. During 1929 the state-subsidized Reich League for the Child Rich intensified the pressure on Severing (the Reich Minister of the Interior from 1928 until 1930) for increased welfare benefits by deploying Burgdörfer's arguments that only the child rich saved Germany from a rapid decline in the birth rate.[15] The league continued to lobby leading officials and politicians with the support of the *Bayerischen Volkspartei*.[16] As a result of a second meeting with Severing in April 1929, the formation of a committee for family welfare benefits was provided.[17] Pressure was maintained in the Reichstag from the *Bayerischen Volkspartei* and Centre Party for family welfare benefits. The Prussian minister, Hirtsiefer, accepted the priority of instituting Grotjahn's model of a family insurance scheme. In December 1929 the Reich authorities responded to the Prussian sponsored analysis by Burgdörfer of the demographic and social crisis, by establishing a Reich Committee for Population Questions.[18] This type of professional think-tank was to suffer the fate of its predecessors organized by the Prussian state. The last of a series of Prussian memoranda on the birth rate was issued in October 1928.[19] Initially the advice of outside experts was an attractive expedient in that the state could be seen to be considering extensive welfare measures. Then the professionals became an embarrassment as they disagreed among themselves, and their demands could not be reconciled with the immediate needs of officials and politicians. The committee was the responsibility of the Reich Ministry of the Interior and of the Reich Health Office, neither of which had much power over family welfare policy. That the Reich and not Prussia had taken the initiative was a sign of the attempt to impose central direction over the expansive local authorities.

Behind the establishment of the committee were political contacts between the eugenicists and the SPD. Dehmel, a doctor who specialized in marital problems, contacted Grotjahn in November 1929 on the need to convince 'comrade

---

[15] ZSTA P 15.01 Nr 26235 Bl 2, 91, 2 January and 1 March 1929; Hans Konrad of Reichsbund to Reich Minister of the Interior.

[16] F. Burgdörfer, 'Stehen wir vor einer Wendung des Geburtrückgangs', *Bundesblatt für den Reichsbund der Kinderreichen Deutschlands*, vol. 9 no. 6 (1929).

[17] ZSTA P 15.01 Nr 26235 Bl. 93.   [18] *Reichsausschuss für Bevölkerungsfragen.*

[19] *Der Geburtenrückgang in Deutschland. Seine Folgen und seine Bekämpfung. Denkschrift des Preussischen Ministers für Volkswohlfahrt*, in ZSTA P 15.01 Nr 26233 Bd 1.

Severing' that such a committee was necessary. For Dehmel, its objectives were establishing eugenic enabling powers for the Reich, introducing parental insurance and initiating a housing programme.[20] Severing was reluctant to include eugenicists on the committee. Communists and Nazis were also excluded, although there was much interest in the population policy of the Italian fascists. Severing considered that national survival was at stake, and that protection of motherhood took priority over party politics. It meant that professionals dominated the new body. The Reich Health Office recommended the economists Wolf, Schuhmacher, Herkner, Mombert, Oldenburg, and Spielhagen (a social insurance expert), and the demographers von Bortkiewicz, Burgdörfer, Roesle and Prinzing. But the office did wish to include the eugenically oriented social hygienists[21] as well as the gynaecologists Stoeckel, Sellheim and K. Winter, the paediatrician Czerny, and the moral purity campaigners Seeberg, Fassbender, Spranger and Thomsen. This grouping represented the well-entrenched coalition of eugenicists and nationalist-minded welfare experts, who like Grotjahn and Engelsmann had strong links with the Reich League for German Families and other welfare organizations.[22] Only Marie Lüders, one of the few women officials, could be taken as representing a progressive position on welfare.[23] The chairman of the committee was the social hygienist Gottstein. Grotjahn chaired a group on health questions, Sellheim chaired a second group on educational and ethical problems, and a third, chaired by the paediatrician Rott, was to consider economic policies.[24] Eugenicists were in a dominant position.

On 20 January 1930 the Committee for Population met to consider policies to increase the desire to bear children, and to improve care before and after birth. Severing introduced the discussion by emphasizing the need to achieve unanimity on these controversial issues. Improved measures to allow working women to have children were necessary. Grotjahn pointed to the growing burden of the elderly and to the economic risks of a decline in the numbers of youths entering the labour market. He concluded that the German population was in crisis. Sellheim demanded extended maternity services and benefits. Rott encouraged measures to decrease infant mortality. It added up to a call for a positive population policy, despite the national emergency.[25] The sub-committees pursued the need for positive measures. On 13 March 1930 Rott proposed improved reproduction on the basis of better clinical services and midwifery, especially for premature babies. On 8 May 1930 Burgdörfer, the demographer, demanded taxation reforms to benefit the child rich: bachelors should be made to contribute to the needs of

[20] Grotjahn papers, Dehmel to Grotjahn, 27 November 1929.
[21] Gottstein, Grotjahn, Harmsen, Kaup, Polligkeit, Engelsmann, Konrad, Eugen Fischer, Baur, Muckermann, Christian, Lenz.
[22] There was an alternative list of Würzburger, Adam, Behr-Pinnow, Poll, Ostermann, Marie Lüders, and the gynaecologists Engelsmann and Niedermayer.
[23] Mombert, Prinzing and Pfaundler declined to serve.
[24] BAK R86 Nr 2369 Bd 2 Bl. 223, 258; ZSTA P 15.01 Nr 26233 Geburtenrückgang Bd 2.
[25] BAK R86 Nr 2369 Bd 2.

families. There were papers by Kaup and Popitz, presenting a further shopping list of costly measures. On 9 May Hirsch demanded improved conditions for pregnant working women. In June moderate support for birth control was expressed providing it was administered by doctors.[26] On 13 December 1930, a meeting on family and housing was held. This opened with a hefty attack on the Reich's act of introducing a bachelor tax on 16 July 1930 without having consulted the committee. Tjaden, the Bremen medical officer, spoke on housing and health: child rich families needed hygienic housing and an extensive range of subsidies. Financial considerations were subordinated to the priority of inducing 'the will to bear children'.[27] The committee, with its growing demands for welfare benefits, was becoming an embarrassment to the cost-conscious state. For their part, committee members became disgruntled that they were not being taken into account in the state's management of the economic crisis. Nearly a year elapsed until a further meeting was planned on taxation. On 13 June 1931 Kaup, the veteran eugenicist, addressed the committee, demanding that the money raised by the bachelor tax should be used to benefit large families. But there should be no benefits to alcoholic parents and others with hereditary disabilities. Such people should be permanently incarcerated. On 5 July 1931 a further meeting condemned the effects of the cutting of child benefits. A resolution was passed condemning the financial cuts imposed in 1930 and 1931 as injurious to the family and destructive of the national will to bear children.[28]

Grotjahn, long an advocate of family allowances, was deeply hurt by the cuts. He complained to Gottstein about the reduction of child benefits for officials, and that once again the committee was not consulted. Grotjahn and Gottstein had resigned on 8 June 1931. Burgdörfer remonstrated that Grotjahn was being short-sighted as such an expert committee at least had the chance of edging things in a more promising direction.[29] Rott attempted to win Grotjahn back for a meeting on 10 July to discuss the reduction of child benefits. The meeting demanded that families with two or more children should have their allowances restored, since most German families could hardly survive.[30]

The Committee for Population maintained the will to have a positive policy despite the economic crisis. Official support for pro-natalism was shown by the offer by the Prussian state of a porcelain cup on the birth of a twelfth child. When money was lacking, a certificate for the 'child rich mother' was presented. The state was unable to support such luxuries as family allowances, improved maternity services and welfare benefits. The policies of pro-natalism, differentials in welfare

---

[26] Grossmann, 'New Woman', p. 234.

[27] See also Grossmann, 'New Woman', pp. 355.

[28] M. Stürzbecher, 'Zur Geschichte von Mutterschutz und Frühsterblichkeit', *Gesundheitspolitik*, vol. 8 (1966), 227–40.

[29] BAK R86 Nr 2369 Bd 2 Bl. 223, 258; Grotjahn papers, Burgdörfer to Grotjahn, 11 June 1931, Cornelia Hoetzsch, 1 July 1931.

[30] Grotjahn papers, Rott to Grotjahn, 29 June and 10 July 1931.

benefits and sterilization were not part of Brüning's deflationary crisis management; but demands for implementation of these policies increased. Welfare subsidies were giving way to authoritarian and illiberal measures. Papen's condoning of compulsory labour schemes and sterilization shows that the welfare state was becoming part of an authoritarian political structure. As a growing rift between the eugenicists and the state opened, they turned to authoritarian political parties, denouncing democracy and individualism as threats to the viability of the race. The rising tide in favour of sterilization was set in motion by campaigners for benefits for the child rich. The positive and negative eugenic policies were part of the same strategy to ensure that welfare benefits were restricted to groups of high eugenic quality. There were common underlying shifts in values. Positive measures for the child rich attacked individualism as a denial of responsibility towards the genetic future of the nation.

Doctors from all parties felt a common sense of outrage in that the state's deflationary policy of high rates of taxation and wage cuts were inflicted on the body politic without regard to implications for health and population policies. In November 1930 Moses, the socialist Reichstag representative, asked leading medical experts about the effects of unemployment on health. Given that social hygiene was determined by income, housing, food and clothing, it could not be divorced from general politics. Moses cited Naumann's view that nutrition was the basis of health. He argued that social policy should not be determined by the finance economy but by regard for the human economy. This could be achieved if doctors were involved in the legislative process. Doctors reported that malnutrition and depression were having a damaging effect on family life. Moral effects such as lethargy and irritability were condemned along with expenditure on labour and alcohol. Unemployment was taken as a factor in degeneration, not only for the afflicted worker and the family, but also for the *Volk*. Infants were regarded as suffering most in unemployed workers' families. Very few observers attributed specific diseases to the economic crisis: a rise in diphtheria was pointed out but TB cases and general mortality rates seemed unaffected. Better housing and nutrition were regarded as the best immunisation against sickness and disease.[31]

Doctors pointed to parallels between the Depression and wartime disease and malnutrition. Just as in these earlier crises, broad sectors of the population were now suffering from physical deterioration. Moreover, the economic crisis was comparable to the war as a collective experience for the medical profession in that it again felt 'called' to provide solutions to social ills. Where the situation now differed was that the politically conservative majority of the profession was to augment its position at the expense of liberal institutions, patient rights, individual rights for the integrity of a person's body and reproductive autonomy, and by turning against socialist and Jewish colleagues.

[31] J. Moses, *Arbeitslosigkeit. Ein Problem der Gesundheit* (Berlin, 1931).

Sterilization

Eugenicists such as Fetscher and Grotjahn argued that sterilization should no longer be regarded as a contravention of the law of assault, provided that it was carried out by an expert in medical eugenics.[32] This showed a profound reversal in liberal values, with professional authorities overriding the rights that had hitherto guaranteed individual integrity. In 1927 Grotjahn had demanded that the Prussian Health Council introduce sterilization on eugenic grounds. It was part of a campaign to remove the liability of doctors for operations and treatment carried out in good faith.[33] It meant that while nature therapists would be subject to civil laws, doctors would be free from legal redress by patients. Eugenicists were convinced of the necessity and of the technical feasibility of mass sterilization. The two stumbling blocks – the state and the public – became positive supports after 1929. The problem of how one could impose sterilization on the 'unfit' in a democratic society required legislation which could reconcile sterilization with democratic principles. In order to attain sterilization legislation, eugenicists had to compromise and accept voluntary principles requiring the patient's consent. Eugenicists such as Fetscher favoured compulsory sterilization of hereditary criminals in practice, but their public pronouncements were voluntaristic. In any case eugenicists knew that professionals could exercise indirect measures of coercion with persuasion, withdrawal of welfare benefits, and incarceration.[34]

During the mid-1920s, the constant barrage of sterilization proposals by Boeters meant that compulsion was viewed with caution by the authorities. That sterilization was very much a politically extremist demand with racialist overtones was clearly shown by the demands for sterilization of the mulatto children in the Rhineland. In March 1927 the DNVP asked for information about the numbers of children whose fathers were from the occupying troops. Replies showed that about one-third were of mixed race. The Bavarian official Sperr, who was responsible for the Pfalz, argued in July 1931 that only sterilization could maintain the purity of the race.[35] A number of key professional groups lobbied for sterilization. The Criminal Biological Society, representing a biologistic attitude to crime prevention, enthusiastically demanded sterilization. The ever-sympathetic Saxon Health Council recommended a change in the law of assault in 1928 removing medical operations from civil jurisdiction. In October 1928 the Reichstag committee on legal reform considered compulsory sterilization of criminals, as a result of a petition by Dr Zapf of the conservative *Deutsche Partei*.

[32] R. Fetscher, 'Zum Entwurf eines Sterilisierungsgesetzes', *Deutsches Ärzteblatt*, no. 33, (1932) cited as offprint.
[33] J. Noakes, 'Nazism and Eugenics: the Background to the Nazi Sterilization Law of 14 July 1933', in R.J. Bullen (ed.), *Ideas into Politics* (London, 1984), pp. 75–94.
[34] Bock, *Zwangssterilisation*, p. 50.
[35] ZSTA M Rep 76 VIII B Nr 2056 Folgen des feindlichen Ruhreinfalls, Bl. 125–36.
[36] GSTA Dahlem Rep 82a Nr 869 Bd 5 Bl. 35.

The Reich Health Office advised against compulsion because of instances of cruelty in the US sterilization laws and because of residual gaps in the science of heredity.[36] The biological rather than moral view of mental disorders was shown by the founding of a German Society for Mental Hygiene in 1928. The society was chaired by the psychiatrist Sommer of Giessen who was the veteran sponsor of research on the family and heredity. The aim of the organization was to encourage preventive measures, arising from an understanding of the biological causes of mental illness. This approach was dominated by Rüdin who began a professional and public campaign for sterilization.[37] Mental hygiene stood for the introduction of racial hygiene into psychiatry. Medical officers became increasingly in favour of sterilization. In 1929 Bundt petitioned the Reichstag concerning legalizing sterilization on behalf of the German Association of Medical Officers. This received much publicity in newspapers, although the Reichstag did not respond.[38]

Behind the demands of the criminal biologists, mental hygienists and medical officers lay a nucleus of eugenicists. Fetscher, Lenz, Harmsen and Rüdin were fervent advocates of sterilization. In 1929 Rüdin published a monograph on 'psychiatric indications for sterilization'. He argued that on the basis of heredity, mental illness could be predicted, and averted, by sterilization. On 28 February Muckermann addressed a meeting of the committee of the Berlin Racial Hygiene Society. Muckermann and Fischer (both Catholics) placed the interests of the family and *Volk* above that of 'inferior' individuals.[39] There was renewed discussion of sterilization among state authorities, as on 4 July 1929 by the Prussian Health Council's Committee on Population Policy. Those present were Bluhm, Christian, Fischer, Grotjahn, Harmsen, Muckermann and Rüdin. They rejected compulsion, as Rüdin said, 'for tactical reasons'.[40] On 14 November there was another meeting between the Racial Hygiene Society and ministerial officials. But opinions were still divided among eugenicists. When Rüdin lectured to the Berlin Racial Hygiene Society on 24 June 1929 on the psychiatric value of sterilization, there were still some critics of sterilization in the society. Sterilization did not appear again on the lecture programme of the Berlin society until January 1932 when the moderate Luxenburger spoke on the prevention and care of psychiatric disorders. By way of contrast the Munich Racial Hygiene Society petitioned the Reichstag to modify the criminal code so that voluntary sterilization would be legal if carried out by a doctor to counteract a severe threat to the health of the patient or offspring. This clause, formulated by Rüdin, was criticized by Lenz because he thought that for the time being the Reichstag might reject the whole principle of eugenic sterilization, whereas a change in the political firmament was

[37] E. Rüdin, 'Psychiatrische Indikation zur Sterilisiering', *Das kommende Geschlecht*, vol. 5 no. 3 (1929) 1–19; also published as pamphlet (Bonn, 1929); reprinted by the Committee for Legalising Eugenic Sterilization as *Psychiatric Indications for Sterilization*, (London, nd).

[38] GSTA Dahlem Rep 84a Bd. 5 Bl. 86–90.   [39] BAK R86 Nr 2371 Bd 2.

[40] BAK R86 Nr 2371 Bd 2 Bl. 154–61.

imminent.[41] The impact of the economic crisis caused the German Racial Hygiene Society to adopt voluntary sterilization of the degenerate as part of a programme of differential welfare benefits on 18 September 1931. Sterilization for the fit and healthy was to be illegal. Eugenic sterilization was linked with education and welfare benefits, its aim to raise the birth rate.[42]

In Dresden, Fetscher campaigned for sterilization in the local branch of the Racial Hygiene Society. He benefited from sympathetic public health authorities who favoured modification of the law of assault – the legal barrier against sterilization. But there was no need to wait for the cumbersome democratic process of law reform. Fetscher carried out fifteen eugenic sterilizations paid for by the Dresden sickness insurance fund in the course of hereditary counselling. He argued that the cost of sterilization was only a fraction of the cost of institutional care for a disabled child.[43] In 1930 he made a survey of attitudes to sterilization in welfare offices of ninety-five towns with over 10,000 inhabitants. Nineteen towns did not reply, fifty-three opposed sterilization, seventeen were in favour and six more positively advocated it. 112 persons were already sterilized: eighty-three for illness, and the rest for social and eugenic reasons.[44] Fetscher claimed that in 10 per cent out of 3000 cases in the Dresden Marriage Advice Clinic, contraceptive methods were recommended to prevent reproduction for medical, eugenic or social hygienic reasons.[45] In June 1931 the authorities in Offenburg prosecuted three doctors for 'social sterilizations' as constituting criminal assault. Socialists in the Reichstag petitioned for sterilization of hereditary criminals. In February 1932 the psychiatrist Nitsche of the Forensic-Psychiatry Association of Dresden submitted a resolution for the sterilization of criminals. Eugenicists felt that the day was dawning for decisive action on the admissibility of eugenic sterilization.[46]

In other countries demands for eugenic sterilization legislation were reaching a high point. The welfare-oriented eugenicist, Felix Tietze, convinced the Austrian League for Regeneration and Heredity of the value of sterilization for mental defectives, providing individual rights were maintained. In July 1928 the Eugenics Society in London initiated a campaign for sterilization.[47] In Denmark sterilization proposals were tabled in October 1928. Underlying these initiatives was a growing international mental hygiene movement, which emphasized eugenic preventive methods as medically administered solutions to psychiatric and social problems. The first world mental hygiene conference, held in Washington in 1930, and the

[41] F. Lenz, 'Ist Sterilisierung strafbar?', *ARGB*, vol. 25 (1931), 232–4.
[42] 'Leitsätze der Deutschen Gesellschaft für Rassenhygiene (Eugenik), 18 September 1931', *Deutsches Ärzteblatt*, vol. 61 (1932), 214.
[43] R. Fetscher, 'Zur Ehe- und Sexualberatung', *ARGB*, vol. 25 (1931), 308–17.
[44] Nowak, *'Euthanasie'*, p. 42.
[45] 'Die Eugenik im Dienste der Volkswohlfahrt', *VGM*, vol. 3 (1932), 701.
[46] Lenz, 'Ist Sterilisierung strafbar?'; ZSTA P Reichsjustizministerium 6094 Unfruchtbarmachung von Verbrechern Bl. 54.
[47] F. Tietze, 'Sterilisierung zu eugenischen Zwecken', *Volksaufartung, Erbkunde, Eheberatung*, vol. 4 (1929), 169–212.

Third International Eugenics Congress of 1932 were high points of solidarity among those advocating sterilization as a solution to costly welfare expenditure.[48] Sterilization for social and eugenic purposes was gaining in scientific respectability.

Church welfare experts were confronted by pressure for sterilization. Muckermann and Luxenburger gave countless lectures to Catholic welfare organizations, social workers and educationalists. Josef Mayer, the theologian at the *Institut für Caritaswissenschaft* and editor of the journal *Caritas*, published a work in 1927 on the 'flooding of the earth with criminals and degenerates'. He organized a Caritas conference in 1929 on eugenics and welfare at which he justified sterilization. However, while there was a Catholic eugenic lobby, most Catholic eugenicists were reticent about the thorny question of sterilization. Muckermann concealed his opinions under vapid rhetoric about the quality of the future generations.[49] Protestants were more outspoken. Harmsen brought the gospel of sterilization to Protestant welfare organizations.[50] He adopted the position of a conservative sexual reformer. The Union for Health that he administered was largely supported by conservatives, but he also had contacts with the campaign for sterilization and birth control. Harmsen and Muckermann's advocacy of eugenics to church welfare experts was highly controversial. Harmsen calculated that 300,000 needed to be sterilized. Given that a substantial proportion of homes and hospitals were run by Christian welfare organizations, the links between the churches and sterilization were of ominous significance. A culmination of the fusion of eugenics and welfare was the congress organized by the *Innere Mission* in 1931. Harmsen spoke on the feeble-minded; the deeply Christian eugenicist, Verschuer, spoke on the laws of heredity; and Pastor Happich spoke on the anti-social. They refuted accusations that Christian charity had resulted in a proliferation of the unfit, by sanctifying sterilization as a welfare measure.[51]

Sterilization was regarded as a medical innovation that united a broad front of medical practitioners of widely divergent social convictions. In May 1932, the Second German Conference on Mental Hygiene heard calls for sterilization from Rüdin and his Munich co-workers, and from other educational and psychiatric interests involved in the sterilization campaign represented by Fetscher, Harmsen, and Mayer. This was indicative of the new respectability of sterilization. Many health officials and welfare experts attended the conference.[52] In Berlin the welfare and youth authorities had passed a resolution calling for the sterilization of the anti-

---

48 G. Mann, 'The Third International Eugenics Congress 1932 (Unser Bild)', *Medizinhistorisches Journal*, vol. 15 (1980), 337–9.

49 Rüdin papers, Luxenburger correspondence, Muckermann to Luxenburger 18 May 1932, on Muckermann's ethical problems.

50 V. Ortmann, 'Probleme der Geburtenregelung in Deutschland in den Jahren 1914–1932 besonders im Lichte der Protestantischen Anschauungen', med. Diss, University of Hamburg, 1963.

51 H. Harmsen, *Praktische Bevölkerungspolitik* (Berlin, 1931); Harmsen, 'Gegenwartsfragen der Eugenik', *Die Innere Mission*, no. 2 (1931); ZSTA P 15.01 Nr 26243.

52 H. Roemer (ed.), *Bericht über die Zweite Deutsche Tagung für psychische Hygiene in Bonn am 21 Mai 1932* (Berlin and Leipzig, 1932).

social. Politically, there was a wide spectrum in favour of sterilization as a eugenic measure. Sterilization purely for contraceptive purposes was the object of much hostility among those concerned with the overall social context of reproduction and sexuality. Among socialists in favour of eugenic sterilization were Henrietta Fürth, who was a veteran feminist and commentator on marriage questions, and Hertha Riese, who was a Frankfurt sex counsellor. Riese claimed that sterilization had a rejuvenating effect on many of the hundred cases that she dealt with during 1931. Socialists regarded sterilization as a technique for solving the problem of mass poverty and a way to avoid burdening society with unwanted and congenitally sick children. The number of sterilizations was substantial during the 1920s: over the twelve years until 1931, 1,200 women were sterilized at the Freiburg gynaecological clinic. The sickness fund paid for sterilizations at Dresden, but not for other forms of contraception.[53] Welfare experts such as Fetscher, while themselves not socialists, attempted to influence SPD politicians and administrators.[54] The KPD regarded sterilization as acceptable on both medical and social grounds, provided that individual consent was guaranteed. Socialists were divided over the issue of eugenic sterilization. Certain doctors and welfare experts who supported state socialism on a technocratic basis, advocated eugenic sterilization, but such demands were never to be party policy. Eugenic sterilization was enthusiastically advocated by the NSDAP and DNVP. SPD supporters like Moses conceded by 1932 that given that the Nazis were supporting sterilization, this could no longer be regarded as 'progressive'. The change of heart was too late to discredit sterilization, because of the popularity of parties of the right.[55]

The DNVP included sterilization in its programme. But it was the Nazis who most effectively made an impact with the issue. Hitler renewed calls for sterilization for hereditary diseases in 1931. He proclaimed it as 'the most humane act for mankind'. The Nazis insisted on the need to do away with false sentimentality. Sterilization was necessary on a large scale, and not just for a few very extreme cases. This earned praise from the eugenicists Lenz and Rüdin. Hitler's calls were echoed by other party faithfuls such as Alfred Rosenberg, Walter Gross, the agriculturalist Darré, and the children's clinic doctor and Nazi medical organizer, Conti. The doctors, Hans Burkhardt and Martin Staemmler, wrote Nazi tracts in favour of sterilization and contributed to the journal of the Nazi Doctors' League, *Ziel und Weg*.[56]

The demands culminated in the Prussian Health Council session on 2 July 1932 on 'Sterilization in the Service of Welfare'. The political context was the overt authoritarianism of the Papen regime, which had virtually no Parliamentary support. The meeting illustrates the balance of forces on the sterilization issue. The meeting was attended by twenty-three selected members of the Health Council,

[53] Grossmann, 'New Woman', pp. 445–54.
[54] H. Fürth, *Die Regelung der Nachkommenschaft als eugenisches Problem* (Stuttgart, 1929).
[55] Bock, *Zwangssterilisation*, p. 55.
[56] H. Burkhardt, *Der rassenhygienische Gedanke und seine Grundlagen* (Munich, 1930).

thirty-six further experts, eight representatives of welfare organizations, and eleven representatives of Reich and Prussian Ministries. Thirty-seven out of seventy-eight participants were medically qualified. Eugenically minded doctors and biologists were in the majority. Four socialist doctors supported sterilization. They were Chajes, who was Grotjahn's successor, the health official Ostermann, the socialist gynaecologist Hirsch, and Scheumann, the marriage counsellor. They argued that eugenic sterilization ought to be combined with sterilization on social grounds. Those with Centre Party affiliations were the chairman Schopohl, one of the speakers Muckermann, and Wester, who alone rejected sterilization as 'brutal force' in which the doctor was equivalent to an executioner. The DNVP Prussian *Landtag* representatives, von Watter and Haedenkamp, were doctors, as were the newly elected Nazis Conti and Diehl (who collaborated with Verschuer on TB research). One woman doctor, Clara Bender, argued against the premiss of a need for population policy, and condoned sterilization solely for the purposes of preventing human misery.[57] Other leading eugenicists were the geneticists Baur, Bluhm, Fischer, Goldschmidt and Verschuer and the welfare experts Harmsen and Drigalski. The eugenicists from the Kaiser Wilhelm Institute in Berlin were thus represented in force, and were the single largest interest group.

Schopohl's introduction set the discussion in the context of health, population and welfare politics. The terrifying severity of the economic crisis had to be met with radical eugenic measures in order to reduce the costly burden of welfare. Muckermann began with the observation that Germany was not just an ageing society with a disproportionate lack of youth, it lacked healthy youth. He recounted the vast numbers and costs of the mentally subnormal. Moreover, his own and other surveys of differential fertility showed that the only families with an increasing birth rate were those who sent their children to special schools. He rejected the view that 'valueless life' should be exterminated, but nor should it be allowed to procreate freely. Although much had been done to reduce the costs of institutional care – from 3.42 marks to 2.42 marks per day in the Rhineland – this was not enough. Only sterilization could save the tax burden on the hereditarily healthy, and transform Germany into a nation of healthy youth.

The lawyer Eduard Kohlrausch reviewed the heritage of liberal laws, according to which eugenics was not a state responsibility, and citizens had sovereign rights over their bodies. It was necessary to secure a compromise between eugenic needs and individual consent. He saw that the application of scientific eugenics depended on a political situation, which would inevitably 'change over time'. The meeting was asked to support a range of positive educational, tax and welfare measures to benefit those of high eugenic value. The first to open discussions was the Nazi doctor, Conti, who claimed that if the liberal principle of consent was preserved, sterilization would be pointless, since for eugenics to be successful it had to tackle

---

[57] Bock, *Zwangssterilisation*, p. 51; H. Schopohl, 'Die Eugenik im Dienste der Volkswohlfahrt', *Volkswohlfahrt*, vol. 13 (1932), 469–97.

systematically the question of the racial composition and heritage of Germany. In reply Schopohl said that doctors in the Prussian Health Council had been discussing eugenics since the early 1920s. Moreover, the meeting should consider only eugenics and welfare, and exclude racial questions. None of the introductory speakers had used the term 'racial hygiene' or mentioned Ploetz or the Racial Hygiene Society. Fischer clearly grasped the significance of the meeting when he stressed that hereditary biology and eugenics were known only to a very few experts. It was up to these experts to advise economists, lawyers and politicians. Indeed, this is what Krohne had attempted to do in his time. Eugenics, Fischer insisted, had been in existence much longer than the NSDAP.

Later in July 1932 the Nazis captured a massive 37.4 per cent of the vote in a general election. While the Nazis remained out of office, their success reinforced authoritarian trends in social policies. Papen took direct control of the Prussian administration. As a result of the meeting on sterilization a committee was convened to revise the conclusions. This included Fischer, Muckermann and the psychiatrist Johannes Lange. It recommended that:

1. eugenic education and research be increased;
2. sterilization replace institutionalization, but only on a voluntary basis;
3. negative and positive fiscal eugenic measures be introduced and that there be a graduated system of welfare.

Those unable to carry out economically productive work should have a lower standard of care than those whom care could restore to fitness for work. On the positive side there should be measures to sustain peasant life, as 'each farmstead is a fruitful source of national vitality'. Factory workers and craftsmen should have houses with enough ground for growing vegetables. A draft sterilization law was prepared for those suffering from hereditary mental illness or feeble-mindedness, epilepsy or any other hereditary disease, or who were carriers of a latent disease. An application could be filed by the heads of welfare institutions, the relevant welfare association or doctors. Sterilization required the consent of the person, parents or guardian, and would be judged by a tribunal of two doctors and a lawyer expert in wardship law related to mental disorder.[58]

With the Prussian Health Council agreeing that a Reich law was necessary, the Prussian authorities needed further public and medical support. The meeting attracted the attention of Sir Horace Rumbold at the British Ministry of Health, who requested details of the draft law.[59] On 3 November 1932 the Reich Minister of the Interior, Wilhelm Freiherr von Gayl, received four representatives of the medical profession who demanded a sterilization law by emergency decree.[60] On 8 September Schopohl gave a radio talk on the need for a sterilization law, because 'the time was ripe for action'. Sterilization fitted the authoritarian political climate, and was justified as part of a system of differentiated welfare. On 25 September the

[58] 'Die Sterilisierung im Dienste der Volkswohlfahrt', *VGM*, vol. 38 (1932), 628–740.
[59] BAK R 86 Nr 2374 Bd 2 Bl. 44–5.   [60] ZSTA P 15.01 Nr 26248 Bl. 22.

Prussian authorities met members of the German Medical Association,[61] who accepted the necessity of the proposals. On 7 November the Medical Association and the *Hartmannbund* demanded a law which drew practical consequences from the present hereditary biological situation for the German people. This petition echoed the discussions of the Prussian Health Council. In November 1932 the Württemberg medical chamber urged that voluntary proposals be supplemented by compulsion. On 10 December there was a renewed discussion in the Reich Ministry of the Interior during which the economic urgency for sterilization was stressed. Here, also, compulsion was envisaged.[62] The medical chamber of Prussia demanded action. But administrators were soon to be overtaken by events.

ABORTION LAW REFORM

The economic crisis intensified not only demands for eugenic sterilization but also the movement for sexual reform in the context of a debate on the costs of poverty and unemployment to the nation. The sexual reformers disseminated populist forms of eugenics to a broad public and challenged the medical establishment. Sexual reformers popularized the eugenic rationale for abortion and contraception in the interests of the quality of motherhood, economic survival and personal fulfilment. There was a mass campaign for the abolition of the criminal statute against abortion, the infamous clause 218. In February 1929 the worsening social conditions were blamed for rising abortion rates. The cutbacks on housing and employment made women's position worse with regard to work and welfare. State propaganda for 'the blessings of children' was starkly contrasted to images of starving, pregnant, proletarian women in the work of artists such as Kollwitz and authors such as Friedrich Wolf.[63]

Women were especially vulnerable to the economic crisis. The cuts in welfare and the campaign against married women working increased the burden of domestic duties. Conservatives waged a war against 'double earning households'. Married women were dismissed from employment in order to take them off the labour market. Pro-natalist ideology was a conservative response to the problem of unemployment. The Reich Health Education Council intensified its campaign for health care in a domestic context. It publicized Hindenburg's remark that the aim of the state was to promote health. Exhibitions were organized on such topics as housework. Classes on childcare, health and nursing were provided for unemployed women, and welfare work was offered in the voluntary labour service.[64] In June 1930 the sexual reformers of ARSO held a conference to counter

---

[61] *Deutsche Ärztevereinsbund.*
[62] ZSTA P 15.01 Nr 226248 Bl. 119–21; Bock, *Zwangssterilisation*, p. 81.
[63] A. Grossmann, 'Abortion and Economic Crisis: The 1931 Campaign Against Paragraph 218', in Bridenthal (ed.), *Biology*, pp. 66–86.
[64] K. Hausen, 'Unemployment also Hits Women: New and the Old Women on the Dark Side of the Golden Twenties in Germany', P.D. Stachura (ed.), *Unemployment and the Great Depression in Weimar Germany* (Basingstoke, 1986), pp. 78–120.

the authoritarian implications of the Dresden Hygiene Exhibition. Grotjahn and the pro-natalist League for the Child Rich were relentlessly attacked by Julian Marcuse, Käte Frankenthal and Friedrich Wolf as betraying socialism by supporting welfare benefits for the 'child rich' and opposing birth control and abortion.[65] Social hygienists such as Grotjahn were frequent speakers on the population problem on the radio. The KPD responded with a campaign that shifted medical politics away from the workplace to the home.[66] Abortion and birth control can be regarded as popular responses to the economic crisis, representing a type of 'self-help' strategy for economic survival and improving personal health. Commentators had the impression that by 1931 rates of abortion exceded live births. The result was that popular needs were manipulated for professional and party-political purposes.

The reality of the situation regarding abortions is virtually impossible to judge. Some estimated that there were one million abortions each year in Germany.[67] It may have been the case that women were less inclined to accept a pregnancy passively. The effect of the belief in the rising numbers of abortions was that it strengthened the conservative conviction of imminent racial suicide. Lay abortionists, who were gaining competence and could be technically innovative, were condemned as a social menace by the medical profession on account of cases of death, sterility or septic infections. Yet underlying this accusation was professional animosity because abortionists were drawn from groups that posed unwelcome competition to doctors. Doctors frequently carried out abortions, from a mixture of motives. The law which allowed abortions if there was a severe threat to the health of the mother meant that it was at the discretion of the profession to decide what constituted a severe threat. Medical confidentiality enabled abortions to be carried out with relative frequency. Berlin practitioners were renowned for greater indulgence to patient demands for abortions than their rural colleagues. The concentration of women doctors in Berlin (virtually a fifth of all German women doctors) may have helped to create a more sympathetic climate. In 1931 Grotjahn published details of a medical practice which showed that a doctor in a small town performed 426 abortions in one year. Grotjahn wished that the medical profession resist patient pressure for abortions, and that the profession should exert greater authority over birth control and abortion.[68]

The rhetoric of the public campaign on the abortion issue should be seen more in a political light than as reflecting the real incidence of abortions. The lay birth control movement organized mass meetings, popular journals and mobile clinics for family planning. What occurred amounted to a clash of cultures, politics and professional interests on the birth control and abortion issues. The slogan of *Sexualnot*, literally sexual deprivation, was used as an emotive indictment of

[65] Grossmann, 'New Woman', pp. 225–9, 327; ZSTA P 15.01 Nr 26235 Bl. 225–34.
[66] Grossmann, 'New Woman', p. 268.
[67] S. Peller, 'Abortus und Geburtenrückgang', *Medizinische Klinik* (1931) offprint.
[68] A. Grotjahn, *Eine Karthothek zu §218* (Leipzig, 1932).

economic deprivation, militarism and state coercion. Attacks on coercive motherhood[69] show how political rhetoric was used for popular protest. Neo-Malthusianism was linked with socialism in an attack on state and bourgeois professional authority. The gynaecologist Else Kienle considered that a state which did not provide basic resources had no right to demand children be brought into the world. Arguments for repeal of clause 218 were extended into an indictment of the failure both of the Weimar social system and of scientific medicine to respond to social problems of poverty and to women's needs. The campaign began in February 1929 with a meeting organized by ARSO, the umbrella organization of the sexual reformers. But it was only in 1931 that the climax of the mass campaign was reached.[70]

The Centre Party Chancellor, Brüning set an authoritarian tone on social questions. This was reinforced by the Pope's encyclical on Christian marriage, *Casti conubii* of 31 December 1930; it was aimed more at the abortion campaign than at eugenic demands for sterilization. Indeed, there was some confusion as to whether the encyclical actually condemned sterilization, as it spoke approvingly of legitimate eugenic concerns with general welfare. Lenz argued that the encyclical condemned only castration and abortion, but left open the possibility of eugenic sterilization 'in the general interest'.[71] The encyclical imposed an absolute prohibition on non-marital sex and abortion, and criticized female emancipation. The SPD was tied to what in terms of welfare and social reform was a highly reactionary regime. The KPD appreciated that here was an opportunity for politicization and mass mobilization. On 21 January 1931 the Papal initiative was countered by a broad pro-abortion coalition. Communists, pacificists, Stöcker's League for Protection of Mothers and Sexual Reform, and intellectuals such as Einstein gave enthusiastic support. The arrest of the radical doctors, Else Kienle and Friedrich Wolf, in Stuttgart on 19 February 1931 created a sensation. Kienle's outrage at the authoritarian treatment of prostitutes by male doctors developed her feminist consciousness. She and Wolf were charged with having performed over one hundred abortions. The campaign in their defence gathered further support from liberal and socialist groups. Meetings, demonstrations, petitions and rallies followed in a militant campaign sponsored by the KPD, radical socialists and feminist activists during the height of the unemployment crisis.[72]

The arrest of Kienle and Wolf in 1931 was denounced as the result of persecution by their medical colleagues. Wolf said that Kienle and himself were the only doctors in Stuttgart campaigning for birth control and sex education. Wolf had referred those patients who in his opinion were entitled to an abortion under the existing law to Kienle. He argued that hunger and poverty were medical factors

---

[69] *Zwangsmutterschaft und Gebärzwang.*
[70] Grossmann, 'New Woman', pp. 225–9; BAK R86 Nr 2369 Bd 1; ZSTA P 30.01 Nr 6231 Die Abtreibung 1925–31 and ZSTA P 15.01 Nr 26233 for pamphlets and reports on sexual reformers.
[71] F. Lenz, 'Die päpstliche Enzyklika über die Ehe', *ARGB*, vol. 25 (1931), 225–32.
[72] Grossmann, 'New Woman', pp. 252–3; ZSTA P 15.01 Nr 6232 Die Abtreibung 1931–34, Bl. 27–9.

that could worsen a disease such as TB, an argument rejected as inadmissible by the medical chamber of Württemberg. With relish, Wolf pointed out that the Catholic eugenicist Muckermann was under Papal pressure to recant his views on eugenic abortion. He attacked the medical profession as in alliance with a reactionary political establishment, proclaiming that the masses must overthrow medical power.[73]

The KPD found sexual policies valuable in increasing its influence over sexual reform organizations, and in winning women's votes at what it perceived as the crisis of capitalism. It welcomed the abortion campaign as a mass movement which broadened its campaign strategy from the workplace to welfare and the home and provided links with intellectuals. Abortion highlighted the effects of poverty and lack of social services for working women. Yet concerted action by the KPD and SPD was immensely difficult, as Carl Credé complained to Wolf in April.[74] By June 1931 the KPD's unity policy had failed. A unity conference, in fact, had the reverse effect with the KPD accusing other organizations of being fronts for 'SPD treachery' or for contraceptive manufacturers. Other groups accused the KPD of exploiting the sexual reform movement.

The abortion campaign was remarkable in giving birth to the popular forms of radical culture of 'agitprop' theatre and 'sexpol' manifestos. Poems by Berthold Brecht, Weinert and Kurt Tucholsky, serialized novels and films took up the theme of abortion as a metaphor for class and sex oppression.[75] In 1929 Brecht and Erwin Piscator developed the idea of didactic plays designed for staging outside the conventional theatre. Piscator's touring collective mounted a *Zeitstück* on the abortion law, called 'Women in Need';[76] based on the novel by Credé, an SPD doctor who had also been prosecuted for performing abortions. Another theatre collective toured with Wolf's abortion play, 'Cyanide'.[77] This was hailed as a new 'Before Dawn', a reference to Hauptmann's seminal play. Wolf's drama was a piece of social realism, prefaced by medical estimates of the numbers of abortions, and concluding with the statement that, 'A law that turns 800,000 mothers into criminals every year is no longer a law'.

Wolf was among the few voices for alternative social values. He had become an advocate of nature therapy and of dietary reform, and his rejection of bourgeois values led him to join the KPD in 1928. Breakfast with him could be a torture for a Soviet comrade, who was denied salt, coffee and tea, and subjected to black bread and raw vegetables.[78] In 1928 Wolf published a book called 'Nature as Doctor and Helper'[79] in which healthy housing, diet and working conditions were demanded. Many points were transposed to 'Cyanide'. His play was an attack as much on the

[73] 'Die ärztliche Macht hört auf, die Massen haben das Wort'. ZSTA P 15.01 Nr 26235 Bl. 225.
[74] *Cyankali von Friedrich Wolf Dokumentation* (Berlin and Weimar, 1978), p. 315.
[75] *Cyankali von Friedrich Wolf*, pp. 459–82.   [76] *Frauen in Not.*
[77] *Cyankali von Friedrich Wolf*, pp. 459–82.
[78] A. Oesterle, 'Naturheilkunde und Revolution. Das Beispiel Friedrich Wolfs', *Volk & Gesundheit*, pp. 230–237.   [79] *Die Natur als Arzt und Helfer.*

medical profession as on the law. A scene shows a doctor giving a certificate for an abortion to an upper-class lady, but denying a worker certificates for sick pay. When Hete, a working girl pleads for an abortion certificate, she is dismissed with the warning not to go to back-street abortionists who use cyanide or instruments causing fatal pueperal fever. The play ends with Hete dying on stage from having taken cyanide.

The campaign clashed with medical authoritarianism, undermining the traditions of *Lebensreform* and self-help to which Wolf still gave voice. Doctors took a leading role. Hodann (the medical officer, communist sympathizer and sexual reformer) travelled the country denouncing sexual oppression. In 1930 the Bavarian authorities expressed alarm that someone with the authority of a doctor could so mislead the people.[80] Other active left-wing doctors included Frankenthal (who was outraged at the SPD's conservatism on the abortion issue), Martha Ruben-Wolf, Hirschfeld, the gynaecologist Liepmann, Peller and Kurt Bendix (the chief doctor of the Berlin Sickness Fund). Socialist and Jewish doctors were prominent campaigners, so heightening conservative animosity. The medical response included a eugenic element as a rationale for allowing medically carried out abortion for the sake of healthy motherhood.[81] Conservative sexual reformers were also involved, such as Harmsen of the Union for Health. Although he opposed abortion, he campaigned for medical control of sterilization and contraception. Sterilization can be seen to have been an acceptable medical solution to the problems of abortion and birth control, where self-help and lay control were pre-eminent. The KPD formulated a position that preferred medical controls to those of lay birth control organizations. However compassionate and sympathetic, the role of communist doctors such as Emil Hoellein and Hodann was to suggest that medical counselling on contraceptive techniques and medical abortions were eugenic solutions to such social problems as the declining birth rate.[82] The KPD was more concerned with improving the welfare of working-class mothers and reviving the flagging birth rate rather than with personal sexual satisfaction.[83] Ultimately, Frankenthal observed that the campaign failed to see the political crisis into which Germany was plunging.[84]

Public attention was distracted away from the risks of placing eugenics and racial hygiene in the hands of an authoritarian state. Indeed, the campaign might be regarded as useful in weakening the grip of pro-natalism, so that it could be replaced by racial hygiene, selective welfare, eugenic abortion and sterilization. While the difference between eugenic abortion and abortion as an individual right was great, the two positions could be confused and conflated. Abortion on demand

---

[80] Stadtarchiv München, Hodann file.
[81] ZSTA P 15.01 Nr 26233 Report on Komite für Geburtenregelung February 1924; Grossmann, 'New Woman', pp. 406–57 'The Eugenics Discourse in Sex Reform'.
[82] Grossmann, 'New Woman', pp. 224, 275.
[83] S. Hahn, 'Positionen der Kommunistischen Partei Deutschlands zur lebensbewahrenden Aufgabe der Medizin in der Zeit der Weimarer Republik', *Zeitschrift für die Gesamte Hygiene*, vol. 28 (1982), 468–71.   [84] K. Frankenthal, *Der Dreifache Fluch* (Frankfurt-on-Main, 1981), p. 164.

meant further medicalization in that criminal 'back-street' abortionists would be replaced by medical specialists. Eugenic abortion, as suggested by Hirsch, the social gynaecologist, would give the doctor power to terminate pregnancy for the diseases of poverty such as TB. Social justifications for abortion could include the eugenic argument that society was being saved from the burden of unwanted and hereditarily degenerate children. The KPD and abortion campaigners lacked a theory of reproduction other than in terms of orthodox medicine. There were restrictions on abortion, as well as professional controls, in the Soviet Union. Marxism failed to produce a theoretical alternative to eugenic sexual reform. Eugenics thrived in this crisis atmosphere as a medically regulated solution to problems of personal and mass poverty.

RACIALIZING THE SCIENCES

Until the late 1920s officials and welfare experts continued their strenuous efforts to separate medical and welfare-oriented eugenics from nationalist ideologies of racial purity. Racial hygiene as a concept was in disrepute among state officials. Ploetz was a marginal figure in the eyes of the authorities. When Muckermann spoke of eugenics, he traced its origins to Galton rather than to Ploetz.[85] In the sterilization discussions, even the term 'racial hygiene' was taboo. During the economic depression resistance to fusing eugenics and hereditary sciences with racial thought began to crumble. This was evident in a growth of enthusiasm for Gobineau's Aryan ideology and the techniques of blood group research, culminating in 'total' biological surveys of Germany in the early 1930s.

The economic crisis of 1929 marked the beginning of a boom in racial anthropology. University lectures began to increase on a variety of topics including human anthropology, racial studies, family biology, heredity and racial hygiene, all of which amounted to eugenics. National research projects were launched.[86] But this up-swing of eugenics caused a polarization of opinions over whether racial studies were scientific or a cover for right-wing racialism. When the Nordic racist Günther gained a chair in Jena in 1930 there were heated controversies. For the first time, opposition forces to racial biology and hygiene bonded together in reaction to the links being forged between racial sciences and Nazism.

The growing sensitivity to state-funded racial sciences was shown by the angry response to a grant from the Emergency Fund for German Sciences to the Gobineau propagandist, Schemann. In 1926 Schemann had applied for research funds for a study of 'Race in the Humanities. Studies on the History of Racial

---

[85] It was only in 1929 that Muckermann read Ploetz's book on racial hygiene; see Ploetz papers, Muckermann to Ploetz, 21 December 1928.

[86] E. Lehmann and R. Beatus, 'Der Unterricht in der Vererbungswissenschaft an den deutschen Hochschulen', *Der Biologe*, vol. 1 (1931/32), 89–96; E. Lehmann, 'Vererbungslehre, Rassenkunde und Rassenhygiene', *Der Biologe*, no. 9 (1938), 306–10.

Thought'.[87] He was warmly supported by Fischer, then still at Freiburg, who expected a 'strictly scientific book' which would give anthropology public recognition. In 1929 Schemann's study of racial epochs in history appropriately bore the imprint of Lehmann, the medical and *völkisch* publisher. There were many pointed *völkisch* references to the corrupting influence of Jews and Marxists on the current government. Schemann's foreword, which gave fulsome thanks to the Emergency Fund, triggered a hefty socialist attack. The left was already vigilant as to the Emergency Fund's grants to Nazi sympathizers. Funds had been awarded to the Greifswald mathematician, Theodor Vahlen, who had been dismissed for hauling down the black-red-and-gold republican flag. The SPD doctor and Reichstag representative, Moses, was scathing in his criticism of Schemann's grant: 'Any Mr Hitler can come along and demand funds for a pamphlet against Jewry and Rome'. As a result, the SPD minister Severing forced the fund to accept five Parliamentary nominees on its central committeee responsible for grants. It was a last-ditch effort to make the sciences democratically accountable. On 11 December 1929, the Emergency Fund withdrew Schemann's research grant 'because of political opinions expressed in addition to valuable scientific research'. It still accepted that the main body of Schemann's work was scientific.[88]

Moses condemned the Research Fund as biased in its overall policies. He considered that the Fund had neglected sciences such as social hygiene, sociology and social policy, which could contribute to the nation's 'social, cultural and physical development'. His justification was based on Ostwald's monistic view of science and society as a single natural entity. Moses argued that in the current financial crisis money should be given only to the socially most valuable sciences, rather than to pure science. It was an opinion that was itself based on biologistic premises, and which allowed the Emergency Fund to increase funding for national anthropological surveys. The Fund's organization was strengthened by an improved committee structure, and it was renamed the German Research Society.[89] Opposition to racist anthropology ironically reinforced scientific and medical eugenics and supporting institutions at a time of authoritarian trends in government.

Fischer was aware that, for as long as the Centre – SPD coalition survived, his position as head of the national eugenics institute in Berlin required compliance with government social policies, and caution in the adoption of racist ideas. He reprimanded his spiritual Führer, Schemann, for having denounced the government as degenerate. Fischer supported the view that Schemann could no longer receive government grants through the Emergency Fund. Indeed, Schemann's

---

[87] The end product was L. Schemann, *Die Rasse in den Geisteswissenschaften. Studien zur Geschichte des Rassengedankens*, 3 vols. (Munich, 1928–32).

[88] K. Nemitz, 'Antisemitismus in der Wissenschaftspolitik der Weimarer Republik: Der "Fall Ludwig Schemann"', *Jahrbuch des Instituts für Deutsche Geschichte*, vol. 12 (1983), 377–407.

[89] *Deutsche Forschungsgemeinschaft*; J. Moses, 'Die Notgemeinschaft der wahren Wissenschaft', MS in Nemitz, pp. 403–7; MPG Generalverwaltung Nr 2043.

völkisch beliefs jeopardized the whole of the Reichstag grant to the Emergency Fund.[90] Fischer at this point was pursuing ambitious plans of large-scale practical eugenics. His plan was for an anthropological survey of the German people to be supported by the Emergency Fund. It was to include blood groups, racial characteristics such as the form of the nose, hereditary diseases and fertility. Fischer could claim that his work placed human variation on truly scientific foundations of biology. But his scheme involved many controversial academic issues and personal rivalries as he was also chairman of the Berlin Racial Hygiene Society. He considered himself a *Realpolitiker*, duty bound by his institutional position to use official resources for the implementation of eugenics.[91]

The biology of blood

Plans for racial biological surveys were rooted in the formative period 1919–24, and drew on advances in research on hereditary diseases and serology. During the First World War, the Polish serologist Ludwik Hirszfeld had carried out an anthropological study of blood group types. This work, based on earlier studies with Emil von Dungern at Heidelberg, was on the specificity of blood proteins of 8,000 Allied troops of many nationalities, who were bottled up at Salonika. Hirszfeld discovered that in European peoples blood group A predominated, and in non-European type B was dominant. He generalized about two distinct European and non-European races, and claimed to have established a biochemical index of race.[92] In Vienna (and from 1922 at the Rockefeller University) Karl Landsteiner researched on the biochemistry of blood. This work, together with Hirszfeld's research, identified distinct blood group types. It was shown that blood types were inherited according to Mendelian rules. These innovations laid the basis for establishing a 'biochemical index of race'. There arose the possibility of large-scale surveys of blood types, with their distribution being mapped. International research projects were initiated, particularly in Germany and the Soviet Union. It was expected that blood types could give a more reliable indicator of race than skull or other external physical characteristics. The biological anthropology of the 1920s looked to human genetics and serology. Biological properties were to explain not only ethnic types but also predisposition to diseases. Serological analysis thus offered the possibility of a preventive medicine based on racial biology.

During the 1920s techniques for testing blood groups were improved so that it was possible to organize large-scale surveys of their racial distribution. German researchers were concerned with the increase in blood group B in the Eastern areas. Research was carried out on the blood of 'racially pure' rural groups. This was

[90] Schemann papers, Fischer to Schemann, 17 September 1927, 15 June and 12 December 1929.
[91] Schemann papers, Fischer to Schemann, 15 June 1929.
[92] W.H. Schneider, 'Chance and Social Setting in the Application of the discovery of Blood Groups', *Bulletin of the History of Medicine*, vol. 57 (1983), 545–62; M. Jaworski. *Ludwik Hirszfeld. Sein Beitrag zu Serologie und Immunologie* (Leipzig, 1980).

suggested in 1923 by the Society of Naval Doctors at Kiel. As with so many branches of eugenics, serology could trace its roots to the turbulent crisis of post-war collapse and inflation. Research groups for mapping the distribution of blood groups in rural areas were launched by the naval doctor, Paul Steffan in conjunction with the anthropologist, Reche. Felix Bernstein (a mathematician) suggested that group O was the original blood of all human beings, and A and B were later mutations. He worked in association with the eugenicist and statistician, Weinberg, and the serologist, Fritz Schiff.[93] Serology was pioneered by a group of innovative scientists with Jewish backgrounds – Bernstein, Hirszfeld (a Catholic convert), Landsteiner, Schiff, Weinberg and possibly Steffan – but it was appropriated by racist nationalists.[94]

The anthropologist, Reche, set out to justify his racial convictions on the basis of blood groups. While at the Colonial Institute in Hamburg and in Vienna from 1924–26 he sympathized with the *völkisch* strain in anthropology. He was the chairman of the Leipzig Eugenics Society from 1927, the same year he gained a chair at the Grassi Anthropological Museum in Leipzig, and was associated with the Lehmann circle of racists. He took the lead in establishing a Society for Blood Group Research, the aim of which was to carry out a national survey by dividing Germany and Austria into 800 districts with blood taken from 500 children in each district. The society hoped to recruit doctors as well as priests, archivists and teachers for its project, which was publicized in Ploetz's *Archiv*.[95] Members included the eugenicists Baur and Fischer, the Nordic racists Lehmann, Philaletes Kuhn, Hanno Konopacki-Konopath, and the architect Paul Schultze-Naumburg, as well as ultra-conservative Austrian politicians such as the sometime *Bundeskanzler* and police-chief Johannes Schober; but serologists of Jewish descent were conspicuously absent.[96] In 1928 a journal for racial physiology[97] was launched by Lehmann to publicize blood group surveys.[98] At the same time applications for research funds were increasing. Reche attempted to float the scheme for a national blood group survey that was to combine techniques drawn from a variety of sciences such as biochemistry, history and policing.[99] In 1928 an international section for sero-anthropology was established at the Amsterdam anthropological congress, and interest grew in the relevance of serology for immunology and blood transfusions. There was especial concern over blood group sampling in the Soviet Union with massive surveys carried out in the Ukraine and Caucasus. The purpose of these surveys was to locate racially distinctive groups. The German

---

[93] F. Bernstein, 'Zusammenfassende Betrachtungen über die erblichen Blutstrukturen des Menschen', *Zeitschrift für Induktive Abstammungslehre*, vol. 37 (1925), 237–70. I am grateful to Bill Schneider for help with sources.
[94] Ploetz papers, diary, 3 January 1907 for a comment that Steffan was Jewish or half-Jewish.
[95] 'Die Deutsche Gesellschaft für Blutgruppenforschung', *ARGB*, vol. 19 (1927), 446–7.
[96] 'Mitgliederverzeichnis', *Zeitschrift für Rassenphysiologie*, vol. 2 (1930), 193–6.
[97] *Zeitschrift für Rassenphysiologie*.
[98] O. Reche, 'Zum Geleit', *Zeitschrift für Rassenphysiologie*, vol. 1 (1928/9), 1–5.
[99] STA Dresden Nr 10209/49.

hygienist in the Soviet Union, Heinz Zeiss, encouraged surveys on populations of German extraction as in Southern Russia and the Ukraine; others took charge of the German settlements in Rumania and Hungary.[100]

In February 1927 the Prussian Health Council attempted to settle the question of the practical application of blood group research. Poll evaluated the proposed national survey, and advised on caution in funding what was still a controversial area of research because of its novelty.[101] A grant was refused by the Prussian state.[102] In December 1927 the Emergency Fund was critical of blood group research for anthropological, racial and constitutional studies. They had received independent proposals for surveys by Bernstein and Reche. Fischer argued that Bernstein's plans for research on occupational groups were mistaken. Instead there should be area studies and more research on the composition of blood. The Reich Health Office supported Fischer's view that there was no need for large scale surveys. Instead, the geneticists Baur and Lenz recommended that a commission for anthropological surveys be set up, and Goldschmidt demanded laboratory research on the genetic mechanisms of the inheritance of blood groups. The upshot was that Bernstein's application was rejected, and that Reche was invited to join a research team headed by Fischer.[103]

The initially negative evaluation of Reche's plans by the Reich health experts had repercussions at a local level. On 29 October 1926 Reche requested support from the Württemberg authorities for a survey of 22 districts and 500 children from each. The Württemberg medical authorities recommended that those districts with full-time medical officers (Stuttgart, Ulm, Heilbronn and eight rural districts) should co-operate and that the results be processed at Tübingen where there were laboratory facilities. The Ministries of Justice and the Interior supported the plan because of its value in paternity and criminal cases, although the *Kultusministerium* had doubts. Support also came from the Mecklenburg authorities. But the negative evaluation by the Reich in March 1927 meant that Reche's plans were abandoned by the Württemberg authorities. The school authorities of Saxony, Bavaria and Baden also reacted negatively. The way was clear for other schemes which had the support of leading scientists.[104]

The defeat of Reche's plan for a national survey created an opportunity for Fischer. In February 1928, at the meeting of the Emergency Fund for German Science, Fischer presented plans for a national anthropological survey. He argued that little was known of the hereditary and racial composition of the German *Volk*. Instead of age-group or occupational surveys, Fischer recommended studies of stable rural populations. Genealogical and historical reconstructions of the rural

[100] P. Steffan, 'Die Arbeitsweise der Deutschen Gesellschaft für Blutgruppenforschung', *Zeitschrift für Rassenphysiologie*, vol. 1 (1928/9), 8–10.
[101] ZSTA M Rep 76 VIII B Nr 2074 Bl. 185–7.
[102] ZSTA M Rep 76 VIII B Nr 2074 Bl. 373, 22 January 1927, application by Reche.
[103] ZSTA P 15.01 Nr 26242, meeting of 17 December 1927.
[104] HSTA Stuttgart, E 151 K VII Nr 15600 Blutgruppenforschung, and E 151 K VI Nr 374 Kaiser Wilhelm Gesellschaft.

populations would add substantially to the bare bones of anthropological statistics on skull shape, and hair and eye colour. The aim was to provide a multi-faceted anthropological picture. Everything from blood groups to photographs had to be included. The new direction in research had already been begun by Scheidt and Wriede in studies of peasants from lower Saxony. The survey would show the distribution of degenerative and pathological characteristics such as the incidence of consanguinity in marriage and the declining birth rate. Doctors were to be recruited to supply pathological data from hospitals. The survey would have an immense eugenic value.[105]

Fischer recommended that there be seven directors of local research teams. The initial seven anthropologists were: Otto Aichel of Kiel (chairman of the local Racial Hygiene Society), Theodor Mollison (professor at Munich), Reche, Karl Saller (at Göttingen), Scheidt (at Hamburg), and Georg Thilenius (the Hamburg professor of ethnology). They agreed to be selective in the choice of population groups. Fischer picked Westphalia, as having a peasantry of high eugenic value.[106] Other research was on degenerative physical traits and diseases. The results were published in a series, *Deutsche Rassenkunde*, which was written in a clear and direct style so as to have broad public appeal. It was planned that 'total' surveys of sixty-three districts would be published.[107] The proposal earned praise from the authorities as 'an ideal work of German research'. It complemented state-supported criminal-biological and psychiatric surveys such as those carried out in East Prussia.[108] Fischer's plans were acceptable to municipal authorities. In Berlin the medical officer Drigalski assisted the survey by permitting tests on school children and allowing the use of laboratories.[109]

Fischer was judicious in selecting co-workers. He excluded all Jewish eugenicists, geneticists and serologists, but he included the liberal-minded Vogt. While the tone of his plans verged on ideas of a racial mystique, he managed to preserve the scientificity of the enterprise. In August 1928 the authorities asked for reassurance that the anthropological research would not be used in public discussions of the Jewish question. His grant applications had made disparaging references to the Aryan and Nordic racial anthropologists, Günther and Schemann. Their work was condemned as impressionistic and subjective. Fischer's plan was to be strictly scientific and comprehensive. Between 1927 and 1932 he attempted to develop a distinctive eugenic strategy that was biologistic and oriented to national demographic problems, but which drew the line at Aryan racism.[110]

Fischer attempted to out-manoeuvre Rüdin, who posed a threat in the eugenics movement, as a more vehement advocate of sterilization and state controls. Rüdin did not figure in Fischer's original plan of 1928 but he had subsequently to be

[105] ZSTA P 15.01 Nr 26242 Vererbungslehre Bl. 48.
[106] BAK R 73 Nr 169 Rassenforschung.   [107] BAK R73 Nr 169 Fischer, 18 August 1929.
[108] ZSTA M Rep 76 VIII B Nr 2074 Bl. 430, 436.
[109] ZSTA P 15.01 Nr 26242 Vererbungslehre Bl. 119.
[110] BAK R73 Nr 169 18 August 1928 NDW to Fischer.

included in the project, because his ambitious plans for hereditary biological surveys were very similar to Fischer's. Rüdin enjoyed improved research facilities when the German Psychiatric Research Institute had a new building financed by the Rockefeller Foundation in 1928. He strengthened his position in 1929, when he extended his research projects despite the economic crisis. He received grants of 10,000 marks from the Bavarian Minister President, 12,000 marks from the Reich Labour Ministry, 3,000 marks and a loan of 100,000 marks from the Berlin Provincial Insurance Office, and 30,000 marks from the city of Munich. Eugenicists claimed that they were tackling the root causes of poverty, crime and disease, and pointed out that welfare relief was a short-sighted palliative. Rüdin's grants were for compiling hereditary genealogies of population groups. Data were drawn from psychiatric and medical institutions, homes for the blind or for 'cretins', and hospitals and special schools for the mentally ill. Rüdin was rapidly expanding his research staff, who scoured the country areas for relatives of those under investigation, enlisted the support of the local clergy and conducted interviews and physical examinations. His quantitative and qualitative topography was expected to be of practical value in that it would reveal the actual incidence of mental illness in a district, rather than just those patients who happened to be under treatment in a mental hospital.

By contemporary standards of research on human biology Fischer's master plan was innovative and impressive. The Rockefeller Foundation proved to be an enthusiastic source of funds. It considered that Fischer's scheme was unrivalled in its comprehensiveness and in its inter-disciplinary approach. The Foundation agreed to pay 10,000 marks for five years from 1930. The sum was matched by the Emergency Fund. The Rockefeller Foundation sponsored serological and neuro-histological research on the organic basis of mental disease. Fischer's plans appealed to Rockefeller officers who were interested in co-operative and applied research on the natural basis of society. Their commitment to Fischer was to prove an embarrassment for them after 1933.[111] There was increasing emphasis on 'hereditary pathology' in Fischer's research plan. He decided to examine not just racial characteristics, but also the biological effects of migration, industries and endemic diseases over several generations. Erich Kallius of the Heidelberg Anatomical Institute pointed to the importance of studying latent pathological characteristics. He singled out TB as a case where the hereditary disposition needed to be clarified, as he was convinced that welfare methods were mistaken. This opinion was supported by the eugenicist Siemens, who had clinical experience as a venereologist, and by Vogt, who wished to use municipal facilities for hereditary surveys in Berlin.[112]

The authoritarian aims of Fischer's project are suggested by its co-ordination with the funding of criminal biology. As Rüdin and his Munich colleague

---

[111] Rockefeller Archive Center 6.1/1.1/4/46; Weindling, 'The Rockefeller Foundation and German Biomedical Science 1920–1940', pp. 119–40.   [112] BAK R 73 Nr 169 Rassenforschung.

Viernstein were leaders in this area, it opened the door to Rüdin's participation in Fischer's survey. Criminological research by Lange and Vogt was also supported.[113] Rüdin was allocated five districts where he would study 'hereditary psychopathic signs'. In 1932 the survey was extended to encompass sixty-three districts. Fischer also undertook animal experiments on the forces determining skull shape. Kallius and Münter researched the hereditary disposition to TB. Siemens worked on Dutch anthropology, and Thilenius combined physical anthropology with cultural ethnology. Scheidt worked on twenty-one of the districts; by 1932 he had collected material on 250,000 people on 464,100 cards.[114] His aim was a survey of the genetics of talent and degeneracy in the population.

The comprehensiveness of the survey indicates the extent to which biologists were taking on the role of total surveillance of human populations. Details of a family's health, school record, ancestry, fertility and police records were all to be correlated. Medical officers, welfare administrators, parish priests and school teachers were mobilized for the survey. The use of official records meant that the survey cemented bonds between eugenicists and the state. Fischer was able to co-ordinate and extend what had in the early 1920s been only pilot projects. The work complemented the criminal biological indices of Bavaria, Prussia and Saxony, and surveys of psychiatric abnormalities. The end product was to be a population index that could be used for such practical eugenic measures as sterilization and subsidies for such elite groups as the police.[115] The preparation of a medical and demographic data base was subject only to minimal public scrutiny. Eugenic data banks were of potentially high value to the authorities. The biological sciences thus prospered at a time of national economic crisis.

NORDIC HEALTH

As the welfare state, starved of funds, looked set to wither away, a new force arose in German politics. The early 1930s saw a broad-based alliance coalesce under the banner of Hitler's Nazi Party. Agrarian interest groups, Nordic idealists, middle-class professionals hit by the slump, farmers and workers in rural areas rebelling against low prices and high interest rates, and, above all, the lower middle class came together to overthrow the democracy that had failed them. With doctors and scientists yearning for a strong state that would support their work, right-wing extremism became acceptable among the professions. While some doctors responded positively to Nazi propaganda, many others moved to the right as a result of concerns and conflicts internal to the medical profession.

Nazism meant many different things to regionally and socially diverse groups.

---

[113] BAK R 73 Nr 169 Rassenforschung, Rüdin to Schmidt-Ott 20 January; 22 February 1930 Besprechung über Rassenforschung.
[114] ZSTA P 15.01 Nr 9421 Menschliche Vererbungslehre und Rassenkunde.
[115] Roth, *Erfassung*, pp. 58–62; BAK R86 Nr 2370 22 January and 5 May 1931 on hereditary surveys of police.

Anti-semitism, anti-capitalism and anti-socialism were invoked opportunistically; athough having a powerful emotional appeal, their slogans kept a deliberate vagueness. What was attractive in Nazism and what it meant varied according to region, religion, economic circumstances and gender. It has been assumed that at the heart of Nazism lay undisputed convictions about racial purity and anti-semitism. The anatomy of these racial concepts merits scrutiny as there were distinct varieties of racist nationalism, which served to mobilize different groups in support of Nazism. As factions within Nazism plundered scientific and *völkisch* varieties (e.g. occult, anti-semitic or populist Pan-Germanic) of racial thought, Nazi racial ideology came to have an eclectic character. Scientific racial hygiene and eugenics were appropriated by Nazis as appealing to professional classes and as offering the basis for selective welfare policies. But as eugenics itself encompassed a wide range of intellectual variations, certain positions were difficult to reconcile with Nazism. An ambivalent relationship developed between the Nazis and the eugenicists. On the one hand there was an affinity between Nazi and eugenic ideas of struggle, the healthy family as the basis of national unity, rural settlement and hostility to Marxism and radical sexual reform; on the other there was competition for leadership of such a key group as the medical profession. The eugenicists sought to inculcate the profession with the belief that it could assume a leadership role in national regeneration. The Nazis were also keen to mobilize the medical and scientific communities and attempted to win converts among the eugenicists. Nazism was to some extent parasitic on an already well organized and socially sensitized scientific community and medical profession.

While scientists could provide authoritative proof of eugenic differentials among Germans, they could also disprove vague and wild uses of racial concepts. This double-edged feature of scientific objectivity was to cause much embarrassment in the Third Reich and to be the basis of conflicts between Aryan ideologues and medical technocrats. It was a conflict that had its roots in Weimar eugenics. The racializing of science and medicine between 1919 and 1924 had resulted in two broad groups of eugenicists. On the one hand, there were the eugenic experts of the Weimar welfare state, building up a modernist edifice of science-based civilization. On the other, there were those who, while fragmented and differing in their ideas, were united in common opposition to the Weimar state. They accused Weimar politicians of having betrayed German ideals at Versailles. From their perspective 'racial hygiene' was neutralized as 'eugenic' by 'Jewish-democratic and clerical circles'. But at the margins of both groups were those who wished to keep on the winning side. They could opportunely switch allegiances when the Weimar edifice crumbled with the economic crisis and onslaught of the right. Pacts were formed between state-sanctioned eugenics and the right in response to the dissolution of the republic.

In the mid-twenties fragmented groups of racial enthusiasts were out in the wilderness. Anti-democratic thought took varied forms in groups ranging from monarchists to revolutionary 'national bolsheviks'. Opposition groups calling for a

Führer were associated with the army, heavy industry (for example Fritz Thyssen was inspired by the hierarchical theories of Othmar Spann) and Junkers. The slogans of blood, health and race continued to exert a powerful unifying appeal. Among the opponents of democracy were Nordic racists and ideologues of peasant life and rural settlements.[116] *Völkisch* prophets of a regenerated race were isolated figures who survived on publishers' advances and royalties. Examples were Moeller van den Bruck (the prophet of 'the Third Reich' in 1923) and Spengler. Lehmann gave financial support and some loose coherence to widely scattered and mutually antagonistic *völkisch* propagandists: Günther was in Sweden until the economic crisis forced him to return, Clauss spent years in Palestine, Liek resided in the Free City of Danzig, before his death in 1927, and Schemann hovered on the fringes of Freiburg academic life. Chamberlain was decrepit and ailing. Hentschel was an obscure eccentric with his *Mittgart* plans for breeding colonies. Ploetz soldiered on with his scientific research on alcoholism and heredity. Boeters waged a single-handed campaign to drum up support for sterilization. The racial hygienists were in disarray. At the Munich Hygiene Institute Lenz and Kaup were locked in bitter controversy. The well-connected and reputable scientist, Baur, fell foul of the authorities when he slandered certain rural settlements at a meeting of the Prussian Health Council. The racial side to racial hygiene was fragmented and fissiparous.

The Lehmann circle

The most powerful force for ideological unity among right-wing racist culture was Lehmann, the publisher. His achievement was to flood Germany with racial literature. He combined dual interests in medical publishing and in *völkisch* propaganda to support racial hygiene. He did much to create a climate of opinion that blurred science and *völkisch* nationalism. Medical journals and textbooks for students and doctors poured from Lehmann's publishing house. These were at one level strictly scientific. But at another they served to racialize medical science. Lehmann tried to break the links between social hygiene and the Weimar social order. Much of what Lehmann disliked was symbolized by Grotjahn, who attacked racial hygiene as one-sided in its links to Aryanism, total reliance on Darwinism and its aim of breeding elite families which amounted to 'aristogenics' rather than 'eugenics for all'.[117] In Lehmann's *Münchener Medizinische Wochenschrift* Lenz denounced Grotjahn's social hygiene as *Sozial – (demokratische) Hygiene*, and urged that biology be the basis of social policy.[118] Kaup agitated in the same journal for welfare benefits for the 'child rich'.[119] There were many levels

---

[116] E. Sontheimer, *Antidemokratisches Denken in der Weimarer Republik* (Munich, 1962 reprinted 1978).
[117] A. Grotjahn, *Die Hygiene der menschlichen Fortpflanzung* (Berlin and Vienna, 1926), pp. 152–3.
[118] Lenz, review of Grotjahn, *Hygiene der menschlichen Fortpflanzung, MMW*, (1926) 1760–1; for Fischer's disapproval of Lenz's tactics Schemann papers, Fischer to Schemann 15 June 1929.
[119] Kaup, *MMW*, (1928) 359, (1929) 409, 443.

of Lehmann's activities in the combining of racism and medicine: the popularization of Günther's racial anthropology, the launching of a popular journal for racial hygiene, the publishing of Ploetz's eugenic journal, and the attack on social insurance by Liek. Doctors were drawn towards the racial right by Lehmann's sponsorship of racist biology. Lehmann continued to publish a stream of works by Günther. He persuaded Günther to expand short essays into books such as *Rasse und Stil* (Race and Style) in 1926 and *Der nordische Gedanke* (The Nordic Idea). By 1926 Günther was earning 12,000 marks in royalties. Eight titles were published between 1924 and 1929. It is estimated that by 1945, 500,000 copies of his works were sold. Antipathy to Günther from the academic community was overcome by Lehmann's efforts in winning Lenz, Ploetz and Fischer to Günther's side.

A kindred Nordic spirit, who was spotted by Lehmann, was the Freiburg racial psychologist, Ludwig Ferdinand Clauss. He used photographs and an impressionistic style to conjure up the sense of *Die nordische Seele* (Nordic Soul) and of *Rasse und Seele* (Race and Soul) as his books of 1923 and 1926 were entitled. Lehmann also recruited Schemann, the Gobineau expert. He promised to provide Schemann with some of the 2,000 racial illustrations which he had collected. Schemann had to accept the offer because of Lehmann's virtual monopoly on publishing racial works. The first volume appeared in 1927. The relationship with Lehmann was clouded when Schemann began to criticize Günther as a superficial popularist. Lehmann's enthusiasm for Schemann was rekindled by the storm over the Emergency Fund grant in 1929, and Lehmann financed Schemann for a third and final volume on *Die Rassenfrage im Schrifttum der Neuzeit* (The Racial Question in Literature).[120]

Lehmann was able to give an institutional backbone to the right-wing of the racial hygiene movement when he launched the popular journal, *Volk und Rasse* in 1926. It was in competition with the state-supported journal *Eugenik* of the League for Regeneration, which Lehmann loathed.[121] Lehmann's journal achieved a circulation of 1,000. It linked the fragmented Nordic groups and provided a channel of communication to academics in the racial hygiene movement. Lehmann offered cash prizes for photographs of Nordic racial types, for compiling pictorial family trees to show the inheritance of facial features, and for essays on German customs. He involved organizations such as the Nordic Ring and the Young Nordic League. Subscriptions to the journal involved membership of a *Werkbund* for Germanic *Volk* Character and Racial Research. The aim of this association was to link scientific and popular racial research. Plans were mounted for travelling exhibitions, collections of genealogies, photographs of outstanding men and women, descendants of long-established families and occupational groups, and editions of *Heimat* culture.[122]

Lehmann had connections with psychiatrists and researchers on constitutional or

[120] Stark, *Entrepreneurs*, pp. 198–9.
[121] Rüdin papers, Luxenburger correspondence, Luxenburger to Muckermann, 2 March 1932.
[122] *Volk und Rasse*, vol. 1 (1926).

hereditary diseases. Anthropologists participated most actively in Lehmann's scheme for broadening the social basis of racial studies. The journal, *Volk und Rasse*, was edited in 1926 by Scheidt, the rising star in racial anthropology. His study of the Elbe island, Finkenwerder, was distributed to the *Werkbund*. The editorship was handed over in 1927 to Reche, the serologist, and Zeiss, the bacteriologist. A supplement was produced by Boerries Freiherr von Münchhausen, a Nordic poet. In 1931 Bruno Kurt Schultz, an NSDAP and SS convert, took over from Zeiss who returned to research on Russian Germans in the Soviet Union. The list of associate editors included as many academics as Lehmann could muster. From 1926 this included Fischer and Thurnwald as distinguished anthropologists and Schultze-Naumburg, the Nordic enthusiast and architect. Among the contributors were a number of right-wing ideologues such as Darré and Julius Langbehn. The Munich racial hygienists were conspicuously absent until Lenz and Ploetz contributed articles in 1931.

Lehmann continued to publish medical works on racial hygiene. Most authoritative in linking genetics and medicine with racial hygiene was the Baur-Fischer-Lenz textbook. The 1917 work on heredity by the dermatologist Hermann Werner Siemens remained in print and by 1940 55,000 copies were sold. In 1929 Otto Kankeleit's work on sterilization was published, to be followed in 1932 by a work on racial welfare in the *völkisch* state.[123] A torrent of publications gave a racial interpretation to all aspects of culture: art, music, jokes, religion and facial expression. Lehmann's aims were a racial hygiene programme, a dictatorship, anti-semitic and anti-Catholic discrimination, and a racial Germanic culture.[124] In 1932 Lehmann joined the NSDAP; until then, he had wished to retain a 'broad church' approach to the right allowing contact with old friends such as Hugenberg of the DNVP.[125] Lehmann's endeavour to racialize medical values and mobilize the profession against the welfare state won support when he published works by Liek, a Danzig practitioner. In a book called *Der Arzt und seine Sendung* (The Mission of a Doctor), first published in 1925, Liek attacked liberal values for corrupting medicine. He contrasted the science of medicine, which he stigmatized as degenerate, with the humanity of the doctor. His argument that the doctor had a mission to serve the nation included a eulogy of the achievements of the Munich Society for Racial Hygiene, and he supported demands for coercive racial hygiene legislation.[126] He attacked social insurance as a symptom of a decadent socialist society, impeding the ability to work hard and save, and causing a 'proletarianiza-tion' of the medical profession. He wrote diatribes against leading Jewish medical scientists; with echoes of the Försters in the 1880s, he accused German medical science as having fallen prey to a 'Jewish spirit'. By 1940, 50,000 copies of Liek's book had been sold. He followed this up with an attack on surgical treatment of

---

[123] O. Kankeleit, *Die Unfruchtbarmachung aus rassenhygienischen und sozialen Gründen* (Munich, 1924).
[124] Stark, *Entrepreneurs*, p. 207.
[125] M. Lehmann, *Verleger J.F. Lehmann*, pp. 265–6; Thomann, 'Weg', pp. 177–8.
[126] E. Liek, *Der Arzt und seine Sendung* (Munich, 1929), pp. 96–114.

cancer. Liek's success did much to racialize medical ethics and professional attitudes.[127]

Lehmann's publicizing of their ideas created a *völkisch* climate of medical thought, but he did not tie this to any one single organization or political party. This had the advantage that the ideas of Liek, the medical criticisms of the liberal heritage of localist pathology and of an overly rational and calculating approach to disease, and the glorification of popular folk movements in medicine from Paracelsus to the nature therapists, could be synthesized. Constitutional medicine incorporated hereditarian, psychosomatic and nature therapists' approaches. Doctors made an effort to gain popular support for constitutional medicine as an antidote to the current crisis of medicine.[128] The broadened constitutional medicine bridged the rift between scientific medicine and nature therapy. At the same time this opened the door to *völkisch* theories and racial ideology in medicine. It was when a tightly knit and dynamic party organization was fused with *völkisch* racism that the anti-democratic attack on the Weimar welfare state would triumph.

The Nordic ring

The emergence of the Nazis, from a political *Freikorps* of street violence to becoming a mass party political force that could transform the German state and society, necessitated organizing a party capable of winning votes and implementing policies. For electoral success Hitler had to create internal bureaucracies and the party had to police its violent SA storm troops. This was the opening for the building up of an internal police-force, the *Schutzstaffel*[129] or SS, over which Himmler emerged supreme. This required a series of transformations: not only the imposition of officer elites and military drill, police discipline, and bureaucratic procedures, but also a reformulation of racial ideology in modern scientific terms. Himmler recruited a staff of biological and medical experts, who combined Nordic idealism, agricultural economics and Mendelian hereditary biology to aid his task.

In May 1926 there was an attempt to weld the disparate Nordic idealists into unity. Konopacki-Konopath, a Ministry of Reconstruction civil servant, founded the Nordic Ring as a league of Nordic groups. Other leading lights of the Ring were the architect Schultze-Naumburg, who led opposition to Bauhaus architecture as disfiguring the nation's racial physiognomy, and the animal breeding expert Darré.[130] They met to rekindle the spirit of sagas, to interpret runes and to revive old customs. They organized propaganda and rallies on behalf of what they feared was the dying peasantry. Eugenics was a moot issue. Among the founders were the

[127] *Fünfzig Jahre J.F. Lehmann Verlag 1890–1940* (Munich, 1940), pp. 30–6.
[128] B. Aschner, *Die Krise der Medizin* (Stuttgart, 1931).
[129] guard squadron.
[130] Miller Lane, *Architecture and Politics*, pp. 136–7; P. Schultze-Naumburg, *Kunst und Rasse* (Munich, 1928).

Swedish geneticist Nilsson-Ehle, the hygienist Philaletes Kuhn and the Berlin eugenicist Christian. The Ring was at loggerheads with the cantankerous Kaup. Other Nordic-minded racial hygienists such as Lenz and Ploetz were conspicuously absent, although Konopacki-Konopath tried to woo them.[131] The Nordic idealists feld uneasy about the stereotype of the calculating and rational scientist. When Darré recommended several potential sympathizers in 'racial science', Konopacki-Konopath refused to contact them; he dismissed mere racial hygienists as not always on their side, 'because Professor Poll of Hamburg, although a racial hygienist, was half-Jewish'.[132] Science was mechanistic and unwholesome for such back-to-nature idealists. But they nonetheless saw the need to cultivate a Germanic science. Konopacki-Konopath urged the compilation of family genealogies (or *Ahnentafeln*) to show ancestry and the prevalance of diseases and causes of death. Genealogical societies were to be mobilized to compile a racial hygienic national census. Indeed, he hoped that the Racial Hygiene Society and League for Regeneration would support his Nordic biological crusade.[133]

Whereas Konopacki-Konopath remained a dilettante amateur, Darré fused Nordic ideals with the practicalities of agrarian economics and eugenics. Darré was a product of a generation of war service followed by *Freikorps* violence, loss of family wealth in the 1923 inflation, and membership of a radical right-wing party, the DVFP; he was an enthusiast for *Lebensreform*, nudism, Darwinism and *völkisch* ideas. He studied agriculture from 1923 to 1925, and by 1927 had published fourteen articles on animal breeding as well as articles on inner colonization and the racial views of Rathenau. After years of economic insecurity he wrote his eugenic tract on 'The Peasantry as the Living Source of the Nordic Race',[134] which was published by Lehmann in 1927. This was followed in 1930 by the seminal text of the blood and soil ideology, called 'A New Aristocracy from Blood and Soil'.[135] Darré blended Nordic racism with human genetics derived from study of the Baur-Fischer-Lenz textbook and Gobineau.[136] His dissertation on the domestication of the pig pointed to how the degenerative effects of domestication were comparable to civilized human society. It led to a doctrine of racial hygiene based on breeding an aristocracy from uncorrupted peasant stock. The racial nobility would replace the worn-out ruling class, and have superior capacities of will-power, bravery, health and intelligence. Advances in Mendelian genetics would enable national laws of heredity to be codified. He recommended that the state appoint a scientific body of experts on human reproduction. They should inspect all young males to check their racial suitability for marriage. The woman's main role was for child-bearing. Darré drew up proposals for tying peasants with a proven German ancestry dating back to 1800 to their farms. Once a breeding pool

[131] Ploetz papers, Konopacki to Ploetz, 12 November 1927.
[132] A. Bramwell, *Blood and Soil*, (Abbotsbrook, 1985), pp. 48–9.
[133] H. Konopacki-Konopath, 'Biologische Ahnentafeln mit Bildern', *Die Sonne*, vol. 5 no. 5 (1928), 22–30.   [134] *Das Bauerntum als Lebensquell der nordischen Rasse.*
[135] *Neuadel aus Blut und Boden.*   [136] Schemann papers, Schemann to Darré, 24 August 1929.

of Nordic peasants was established, leaders were expected to emerge. This idea of the *Hegehof* was the basis for a set of laws on peasant property and settlement which were enacted during the Third Reich. Others regarded Darré's master plan as too utilitarian. Günther tempered admiration for Darré with criticism that his breeding plans emanated from a 'chicken farm mentality'.[137]

During the late 1920s Darré forged links with Nazi activists in Thuringia, the fabled heartland of German life. He spearheaded an alliance between the Nordics with the Nazis. The publisher Lehmann dissuaded Darré from working through the DNVP to realize his agrarian master plan. Instead, Darré joined the NSDAP in July 1930 with the promise of a leading role in the party's rural organization and policies. Lehmann contributed to Darré's salary. The Nazis were not making the hoped-for headway in rural areas where there was a severe economic crisis with bankruptcies and foreclosures. Darré turned the tide, establishing an effective agricultural organization for the NSDAP. This was a semi-autonomous network of farmers and peasants, promoting discussions of land reform and land tenure.[138] In 1931 Darré inspired Himmler with the vision of an impregnable ring of 200 million Nordic farmers, who would form a bastion against the bolshevik enemy of the Nordic race.[139]

Darré's influence was brought to bear on Himmler's SS. While Darré had scant sympathy for the occult and esoteric Aryan philosophy, he formed a bond with Himmler. They both had agricultural qualifications, and believed in Nordic settlements and in elite breeding. They represented a politically radicalized form of Baur's agrarian eugenics. In December 1931 Darré assisted Himmler in drawing up a code requiring SS approval for marriage. Himmler appointed Darré head of an SS Racial Office. By vetting all SS men's marriages, the SS could become the kernel of a Nordic aristocracy. There was to be a health inspection; genealogies were to prove sound breeding and good 'racial' qualities.[140] The ultimate aim was that these supermen should take over farms and populate garden cities. The combination of agricultural expertise and racial biology gave birth to the distinctive Nazi ideology of 'blood and soil'.[141]

The marriage code corresponded to the racial hygienic health certificate, and was much praised by eugenicists like Lenz. He had been a member of the DNVP in 1924–26 and had, despite pessimism as to the implementing of eugenics, taken great interest in Mussolini's pro-natalist measures.[142] The International Federation of Eugenics Organizations held a meeting in Rome in 1929, which gave Lenz and Fischer the opportunity to admire Mussolini's population policy. The Duce was hailed as saviour of the races of the Western world for implementing exemplary

[137] W.L. Heinrich, 'Richard Walther Darré und der Hegehofgedanke', med. Diss., University of Mainz, 1980; Lutzhöft, *Der Nordische Gedanke*, p. 53; Bramwell, *Blood*. pp, 48, 52, 69.
[138] Bramwell, *Blood*, pp. 76–85.   [139] R.L. Koehl, *The Black Corps* (Wisconsin, 1983), pp. 48–9.
[140] Bramwell, *Blood*, p. 90.   [141] Koehl, *Black Corps*, p. 51.
[142] Lenz papers, Lenz to Verschuer, 20 September 1929 on Mussolini; Schemann papers, Fischer to Schemann, 15 June 1929 on Lenz and Mussolini.

eugenic policies. Lenz greatly admired the Duce's taxation policies that benefited large families.[143] In 1931 Lenz wrote in Ploetz's *Archiv* of the positive strengths of Hitler's programme for racial hygiene. Lenz saw an affinity between the anti-parliamentarian position of the NSDAP and the eugenicists' own depoliticized stance. He praised the Nazis as the first political party to have made racial hygiene central to its programme. He pointed out that Hitler had appropriated ideas from the Baur-Fischer-Lenz textbook. He stressed the importance of the Führer's support for sterilization and for a rural settlement as a basis of population policy, although at the same time he was concerned about Hitler's exaggerated fears of racial interbreeding and the rabble-rousing oratory that generated support among lower orders in which psychopathy was prevalent. Lenz's informant about the SS's breeding rules was Darré.[144] While Lenz did not join the Nazi Party until 1937, his article showed that there was sympathy for the Nazis among the hitherto aloof racial hygienists. But this appreciation of positive qualities of the Nazi programme should not be confused with whole-hearted support. Indeed, Lenz's article attempted to impose racial hygiene and demographic science on Hitler's very different racial and anti-semitic concepts. Nowhere did Hitler mention the Nordic race or 'racial hygiene', and Lenz was embarrassed by Hitler's racial anti-semitism, which he blamed on pseudo-scientific ideologues such as Chamberlain and Fritsch. Lenz could present Hitler as an advocate of racial hygiene only by omissions and distortions in his reading of *Mein Kampf*. He disliked the Nazis' party political authoritarianism, as he felt that biology should be supreme. He complained to Verschuer in December 1931 that the Nazis regarded themselves as infallible as the Pope.[145] The continuing gulf between the Nazis and the eugenicists was made clear by Verschuer's comment to Lenz in February 1931 about a course for pastors in Spandau:

The interest of the 180 participants was so intense that I succeeded in conveying the great significance of eugenics for pastors. It was not so simple as among many pastors strongly National Socialist tendencies prevailed, making them convinced that the Jewish problem was the central problem. At the end of the course a pastor pronounced to the approval of those present that heredity and eugenics should be included in the second theological examination.[146]

This distinction between eugenics and Nazism suggests that on the German right there were competing ideologies of anti-semitism and racial hygiene which were to be fused under the pressure of political circumstances. For the moment eugenics and Nazism could remain distinct.

From the 1930s, other Nordicists attempted to fuse Nazism and racial hygiene

---

[143] F. Lenz, 'Ueber Möglichkeiten und Grenzen eines Ausgleichs der Familienlasten durch Steuerreform', *ARGB*, vol. 24 (1930), 376–98; Thomann, '*Weg*', pp. 153–5.
[144] Personal communication from Anna Bramwell on Lenz-Darré correspondence; F. Lenz, 'Die Stellung des Nationalsozialismus zur Rassenhygiene', *ARGB*, vol. 25 (1931), 300–8.
[145] Lenz papers, Lenz to Verschuer, 30 December 1931.
[146] Lenz papers, Verschuer to Lenz, 11 February 1931.

with varying degrees of success. A lucky Nazi win in the Thuringian elections meant that the Nazi Minister of the Interior, Wilhelm Frick, could impose *völkisch* culture. He banned jazz and the anti-war film 'All Quiet on the Western Front'; he promoted Schultze-Naumburg to director of the Art Academy at Weimar, and Günther to a chair of social anthropology at the University of Jena. Günther was not yet a member of the NSDAP. He owed his appointment to the recommendation of a *völkisch* publicist, Robert Gestenhauer, and support came from Plate, Lenz and Ploetz.[147] The appointment of Günther encountered staunch resistance from many professors at Jena, despite the approval by Plate, the anti-semitic professor of zoology and racial hygienist. Autodidact racial prophets, however much their views were in line with nationalism, were still regarded as intruders by university academics, although certain biologists stretched out a welcoming hand.

Konopacki-Konopath, the founder of the Nordic Ring, had high hopes of the Nazis. He became a member of the Race and Culture Department of the NSDAP, and expected to be the party's future Minister of Culture. By June 1930 he was in contact with Darré, Josef Goebbels, Frick, Hermann Göring, Rosenberg, Baldur von Schirach and Günther. For a time Darré became an ally with Konopacki-Konopath against Goebbels, who was seen as someone lacking understanding of 'scientific-racial concepts', and Darré warned Konopacki-Konopath about Himmler: 'Many people laugh at him but his influence over Hitler is greater than is often thought'.[148] But Konopacki's Nordic Marriage Ring offended Himmler, perhaps because it rivalled the SS, and personal slurs were made over a sexual indiscretion. Darré discarded Schultze-Naumburg and then Konopacki-Konopath, whose journal *Die Sonne* was suspected of freemasonry. In 1931 Konopacki-Konopath was expelled from the Nordic Ring, which contained budding Nazis such as the lawyer Falk Ruttke. The Ring itself was disbanded by the Nazis in 1934 and even the use of Norse names for months was banned.[149] Instead Darré built up the Race Office with Bruno Kurt Schultz and the veterinary expert Horst Rechenbach. They worked with Darré from 1930 but they joined the SS only in 1932, and developed the Race and Settlement Office from 1934.[150]

The Nazification of medicine

In 1932 Himmler began to wield power through a series of bureaucratic and policing offices. Darré headed Section V as the Racial Office. The SS retained an elite character with its stringent racial qualifications for entry and for marriage. Himmler's turning to professional experts in 1931–32 was paralleled by other developments in Nazism. By July 1931 the National Socialist Student League had captured a leading position in national student associations. The Nazi strategy of

---

[147] Lutzhöft, *Nordische Gedanke*, pp. 38–9.   [148] Bramwell, *Blood*, pp. 84–5.
[149] BDC Konopacki-Konopath to Himmler, 29 Sept 1931, Günther to Himmler, 1 June 1932.
[150] Koehl, *Black Corps*, p. 83.

establishing corporate organizations (which had led to the meteoric rise of Darré as Reich Peasant Führer) was also evident in law, medicine, architecture and engineering. The Nazi Doctors' League extended the party's electoral support, while linking Nazism with professional interests and discussions of racial hygiene. A comprehensive health and welfare policy was formulated. Until then the Nazis had been content with borrowing slogans on 'child riches' and with the impromptu support of women giving first aid to their menfolk after street violence. But in the later 1920s the NSDAP realized that mass propaganda had to be reinforced by capturing the allegiance of strategic elites, one of which was the medical profession. On 3 August 1929 the National Socialist German Doctors' League (NSDÄB) was founded at the Nuremberg rally. The chairman was Ludwig Liebl (a surgeon and gynaecologist), the vice-chairman was Theo Lang (a psychiatrist in Rüdin's institute) and the treasurer was Gerhard Wagner (a general practitioner) who led a nucleus of fifty founders. Doctors and pharmacists feared falling earnings and the further socialization of medicine.[151]

From the outset there was a conflict over the purpose of the organization. Lang, who was assistant at Rüdin's Genealogical-Demographic Department of the German Psychiatric Institute, supported the idea that the league's aim was primarily educational. It was to spread scientific knowledge and ideas of 'national biology' among the profession and the public, so ensuring acceptance of Nazi and racial hygienic values. Martin Staemmler, the Chemnitz doctor and advocate of sterilization, was especially active in promoting the fusion of scientific racial hygiene with Nazism. He demanded family welfare measures in support of the 'child rich' and the peasantry. These were a continuous strand in Nazism, appearing in the programme of 1920, but also advocated by many other groupings on the right. The 1930 conference of the league was held on the theme of 'maintaining and racially improving the nation's health'. The league supported 'national biology', public health and extending the powers of the medical profession.

In September 1930 the Nazi electoral success meant that the league became important for Nazi propaganda as well as functioning as a professional organization. Its purpose was to give expert advice to the party on all issues of health and racial biology. It promoted racial ethics in medicine. Anti-semitism in the form of removing Jews from the medical profession figured among the league's aims.[152] This marked a response to the profession's economic grievances during the depression. By 1932 Nazi and professional aims replaced those of racial hygienic propaganda. Membership had been disappointing, and the league sought to make this up by admitting dental and veterinary surgeons, and apothecaries. There was emphasis on Nazi ideology and anti-semitism combined with professional opposition to nature therapists and insurance controls. Lang and Liebl were replaced in a process of a complete turnover in the league's leadership from March

[151] M.H. Kater, *The Nazi Party* (Oxford, 1983), pp. 67–8.
[152] G. Lilienthal, 'Der Nationalsozialistische Deutsche Ärztebund (1929 bis 1943/5): Wege zur Gleichschaltung und Führung der deutschen Ärzteschaft', in Kudlien, *Ärzte*, pp. 105–7.

1931, although Lang continued to expect a senior position with the imminent Third Reich.[153] The culmination came in September 1932 when Wagner ousted Liebl as chairman. Wagner, along with Conti, Erhard Hamann and Eugen Stähle, took a key role in the *Gleichschaltung* of the medical profession and in the imposition of Nazi racial policies. Membership rose: whereas 300 attended the first meeting in 1930, over 1,000 attended the third rally in September 1932. By January 1933 there were 2,786 members and 344 associates who were not NSDAP members. This exceeded the 1,500 in the Association of Socialist Doctors.[154]

Professional aims meant that women were excluded from taking on medical functions in the party. In 1931 Conti denounced the *Deutschen Frauenorden*, whose members sewed torn stormtrooper uniforms and patched up their menfolk after violent clashes. Conti accused these 'sisters' of lacking even nursing qualifications. He successfully forced the party to establish a women's organization, the *NS-Frauenschaft*, in which women would be drilled in the duties of 'mothers' service'.[155] The case of the National Socialist Doctors' League suggests that the fusing of Nazism with racial hygiene was a difficult manoeuvre; many stumbling-blocks due to conflicting interest groups within Nazism and the medical profession had to be overcome. Given the high degree of scientific and medical interest in racial hygiene, there were inevitably those who regarded race as primarily a scientific and cultural matter. This was the position of Liebl and Lang. Other like-minded activists were medical scientists such as Reiter, the professor of hygiene who was elected to the Mecklenburg assembly in 1932, and the psychiatrist Wilhelm Holzmann, who represented the Nazis in Hamburg in 1931. Among those who signed an electoral petition of university professors for Hitler in 1932 were about a dozen medical professors. The powerful impetus of Nazi allegiance to Hitler, the party, and racial purity confronted medical scientists with conflicts which never were to be resolved.

RESISTANCE TO RACIAL HYGIENE

The links between Nazism and racial hygiene became stronger after 1930. Although eugenic and racial assumptions had taken root in biology, medicine and welfare, remarkably there was virtually no opposition to the totality of racial and eugenic thought. Opponents singled out specific issues. The coercive powers of the state and medical profession were contentious with regard to sterilization, birth control and abortion. There were disagreements over scientific evidence for the inheritance of diseases and behavioural anomalies. Opinions differed over the relations of heredity to politics and legislation. It was more a question of clashes between varieties and types of eugenic and sociobiological thought, than a

---

[153] Rüdin papers, Luxenburger correspondence, Luxenburger to Verschuer, 18 April and 12 December 1932, pointing out that Rüdin was unaware of Lang's NSDAP membership as 'er kümmert sich um Politik überhaupt nicht'.   [154] Lilienthal, 'Ärztebunde', pp. 108–9.
[155] J. Stephenson, *The Nazi Organization of Women* (London, 1981), p. 47.

wholesale rejection of their validity. As Nazism gained in popularity, critics of racial hygiene shifted their attack to the supposed links between racial hygiene and anti-semitism.

The greatest barriers to eugenics were those of legal rights, guaranteeing individual freedoms, Christian ethics and socialism. Yet all of these were flawed by organicist biology and philosophy. Although political rights were further extended by the Weimar constitution, such legal guarantees were no match for the extension of professional powers by state welfare experts and by professional interest groups. Law could not control science and medicine, which were rapidly advancing and making inroads into the spheres of welfare provision and the family. Legal and ethical theories were subject to biological interpretations as shown by organicist theories of natural law. Binding's legal positivism justified the superior claims of corporate interests. Justice officials were a bulwark against the advance of eugenics, but legal guarantees could seem weak when faced by the claims of society as a whole, of future generations, or of immutable scientific truth. Judicial criticisms were important in moderating proposals on compulsory sterilization in the Criminal Code reform of 1928. The vestiges of liberal values in thinking on health and welfare were threatened not only by the rise of Nazism but also by scientifically based social philosophies. The latter remained uncontroversial at a time of political polarization between the extremes of Nazism and communism.

A reversal occurred in the relations between biological and social values. Whereas in the nineteenth century biology spearheaded the movement for liberal reforms, by the 1920s biological values were claimed as the basis for authoritarian political and social convictions. Biologists felt that they were guardians of a deeper and greater truth than politicians. There was a weakness to most biological critics of Social Darwinism and eugenics in that they sought to substitute one form of biological authority for another. This can be seen in the case of Oscar Hertwig's 'Critique of Ethical, Social and Political Darwinism', which was written in the context of the debate on Pan-Germanist militarism during 1918. While Hertwig's views were organicist, anti-Darwinian and anti-socialist, more advanced social thinkers developed concepts of the 'human economy' and of society as an organism that were in keeping with Weimar modernism. The widespread distrust of mechanistic values meant that non-eugenic sociological thought drew on biological concepts. There was a vast body of social thought on elites, selection, the community, *Volk* and living space which could be appropriated and racialized by the Nazis. Organicism was rife in sociology, even while it remained controversial. Statistical demography endowed organicism with innovative research techniques and offered the state new social technologies.[156]

Leading psychologists rejected Gobineau and racial hygiene, but they remained within the organicist paradigm of the cell state and of the social and mental

[156] W. Bergmann *et al.*, *Soziologie im Faschismus 1933–1945* (Köln, 1981); O. Rammstedt, *Deutsche Soziologie, 1933–1945* (Frankfurt-on-Main, 1986).

organisms. This characterized the views of the liberal politician and psychologist, Willy Hellpach, who was the Democratic Party's presidential candidate in 1925. In 1928 he rejected the idea of a racial essence peculiar to the German character. There were too many ethnic types in Germany for the nation to be identified with a single race or blood type. He predicted that while castration laws or a genocidal blood bath might eliminate small and dark-haired people, it would be impossible to sustain a single physical type. The findings of Franz Boas on physical changes in US immigrants contradicted the fixed types of Ammon, Günther and Eugen Fischer. Such issues were a corrective to German political dogmas of the need to rejuvenate and reinvigorate the race.[157] At the same time Hellpach regretted the decline of self-help that resulted from the growth of the welfare state.[158] The future lay in organicist social co-operation. He advised Jews that the best way to end anti-semitism was through intermarriage.[159]

Eugenics was taken up and developed by sexual reformers, pacifists, socialists and Jewish scientists as keenly as by right-wing intellectuals and politicians. Most scientists and doctors regarded constitutional, genetic and hereditarian theories of disease as uncontentious. The rise of Nazism caused some unease among the scientific leaders of racial hygiene who feared that socialist and Jewish eugenicists would become alienated. The Berlin Racial Hygiene Society proposed in 1930 to abandon the term 'racial hygiene' for 'eugenics'. Ploetz responded to Eugen Fischer's support for the change by pointing out that the term racial hygiene attracted public and academic interest in the Munich society. He cited the cases of many Jews and socialists who had supported racial hygiene. These included Julius Schwalbe, the editor of the *Deutsche medizinische Wochenschrift*, Crzellitzer, Auerbach and Weinberg. Socialists and Jews included Tandler, Eduard David and Viktor Adler, the leader of the Austrian socialists. Other Austrian socialists were Rudolf Wlassak and Fröhlich.[160] Many eugenic radicals including Blaschko, Chajes, Hirschfeld and Löwenstein, were of Jewish origins. They favoured a type of social eugenics, or *Volkseugenik*, in conjunction with a planned economy and greater social justice.[161] Other notable advocates of social hygiene who came from Jewish families were Gottstein, Martin Hahn and Max Hirsch. Poll and Alfons Fischer each had one Jewish parent. Among the many Jews in such fringe disciplines as dermatology and sexual science, traces of eugenic thought abounded. Some advocates of social hygiene were vigilant in their opposition to authoritarianism and anti-semitism, whereas other eugenicists condoned the fusion of hereditary biology, anthropology and social hygiene. Their position can be compared with that of such 'reform eugenicists' as the communist sympathizers,

---

[157] W. Hellpach, *Politische Prognose für Deutschland* (Berlin, 1928), pp. 1–17, 243.
[158] Hellpach, *Prognose*, pp. 302–10.
[159] D.L. Niewyk, *The Jews in Weimar Germany* (Manchester, 1980), pp. 97–8.
[160] Ploetz papers, Ploetz to Fischer, 9 March 1930.
[161] M. Hirschfeld, *Race* (London, 1938), p. 173; for biographies see Hansen, *Verschüttete Alternativen*, pp. 148–9, 192.

H.J. Muller in the USA and J.B.S. Haldane in Britain. There was also a more neutral expert body of eugenicists, who did not politicize their position but acted as state advisers or welfare administrators. Doctors and scientists asserted intellectual and social leadership, and had scant regard for democratic procedures.[162] There were leading Jewish doctors and eugenicists such as Goldschmidt and Lubarsch who had conservative sympathies. The Jewish editor of the Munich journal, *Süddeutsche Monatshefte*, initiated a vein of conservative and *völkisch* publicity that drew on ideas of racial hygiene.[163] On left and right these eugenicists did not perceive themselves as Jews but as dispassionate scientific experts, who patriotically prescribed solutions to social problems. Goldschmidt was openly in favour of sterilization legislation. That the Jewish Welfare Organization's delegate to the Prussian conference on sterilization of 1932 did not venture to speak signified a lack of perception that sterilization of the hereditarily ill could lead to racial persecution. Eugenics was regarded as a technocratic means to control social deviants and eradicate inherited disease. This accounts for the support by James Loeb, the expatriate American-Jewish banker, for psychiatric research. The Jewish eugenicists did not perceive that once anti-semitism became institutionalized in the apparatus of welfare eugenics and hereditarian research, they could fall victims to the system which they had helped to construct. Chajes, Goldschmidt, Hirsch, Marcuse and Tandler were among those who succeeded in emigrating, whereas Poll failed to secure a scientific post. Crzellitzer, Moses and the communist doctor Georg Benjamin were to die in concentration camps.[164]

Roman Catholic eugenicists such as Eugen Fischer, Luxenburger and Muckermann found themselves caught between the forces of the Catholic Church, which demanded allegiance to the *casti-conubii* encyclical, and the shift to right-wing politics. Under this strain the Catholic bloc broke down in disorder and disunity. Church-goers and theologians could oppose racial hygiene on a sporadic basis or, as with the *casti-conubii* encyclical, condemn a key issue such as abortion. On the Protestant side, eugenicists such as Verschuer welcomed the shift to the right. The churches did not present an organized and coherent alternative to racial hygiene; many churchmen, in fact, succumbed to Nazism.

Eugenics was losing its capacity to act as a basis for social integration in an expanding state welfare system. By the late 1920s the Soviet Union was becoming hostile to genetics and eugenics, and Nazism posed a threat to the independence of the scientific community which gave eugenics authority. Socialist biologists such as Schaxel were a rare breed in Germany, and the socialist welfare eugenicists found themselves under pressure from both left and right. Liberal geneticists such as Paula and Günther Hertwig, and psychiatrists such as Kretschmer voiced opposition to right-wing opportunists, but could not prevent their work from being appropriated for Nazi racial ends. Pacifist and republican sympathizers like Driesch the

[162] H. Döring, *Der Weimarer Kreis* (Meisenheim, 1975), p. 249.
[163] Niewyk, *Jews*, p. 99; Thomann, 'Weg', pp. 88–97.
[164] Labisch and Tennstedt, *GVG*, II, 390–1, 395.

embryologist, and Tönnies the sociologist also suffered the fate of seeing their ideas used in the Nazi creed of an organic folk community.

While science tended to bolster up an authoritarian social structure, it was inherently unstable. This is shown by those racial anthropologists who were critical of Nordic and Aryan racism. The complexity of racial hygiene is indicated by the example of Ploetz who did not allow personal anti-semitic prejudice to intrude into his publications. The geneticist Plate complained in 1930 that Ploetz was much too mild in his opinions on the Jewish question and that he ought to raise the issue in the Racial Hygiene Society.[165] Eugen Fischer attempted to please all sides, as he continued to regard Schemann, the Gobineau publicist, as an outstanding anthropologist and 'geistiger Führer'.[166] But others were more determined to defend scientific standards. The Nordic racial concept had many empirical defects. The Kiel anthropologist, Karl Saller, wrote a thesis in 1926 attacking the concept of a Nordic race. (He was included in Fischer's national racial survey until 1933).[167] Anthropologists had many objections to Günther's suggestion of a contrast between the 'Nordic' and 'Ostic' (Slav) races, and politically the view of Germany as a racial mixture was unsettling. It meant that there could only be a few surviving pockets of pure Nordic racial types, and the very existence of a 'Nordic type' with superior psychological and physical characteristics was controversial. The Kiel botanist Fritz Merkenschlager wrote a critical review ironically entitled 'Gods, Heroes and Günther', debunking Günther's assertions as 'un-German'. Merkenschlager and Saller combined to suggest a 'dynamic' theory of race, with the complication that there were Slavic elements in Germany. The idea of Nordic racial purity was absurd.[168] Scientific criticisms of Nordic racial theory retained a high degree of patriotic fervour.[169] The only substantial criticism by a non-scientist was by the economist Friedrich Hertz who had made a timely move from the Austrian civil service to the University of Halle in 1930. His attack on Günther's racial doctrines analyzed *völkisch* ideology as a means of suppressing the proletariat. He condemned the 'zoological world view' as lacking in humanity, individuality and a sense of social responsibility, and opposed the role of scientific nationalism in *völkisch* thought.[170] Whereas most critics wished to separate scientific from non-scientific eugenics, Hertz's social analysis grasped the totality of racial theories by subsuming the eugenicists in Günther's categories. The problem was that as many racial anthropologists and biologists were critical of Günther as unscientific, the critique by Hertz left the views of more scientific eugenicists intact.

[165] Ploetz papers, Plate to Ploetz, 13 February 1930; Niewyk, *Jews*, p. 65.
[166] Schemann papers, Fischer to Schemann, 22 June 1931.
[167] K. Saller, *Die Entstehung der "nordischen" Rasse* (Kiel, 1926).
[168] Lutzhöft, *Nordische Gedanke*, p. 20.
[169] F. Merkenschlager, *Götter, Helden und Günther. Eine Abwehr der Güntherschen Rassenkunde*, (Nürnberg, nd); Mühlen, *Rassenideologien*, pp. 249–66.
[170] L. Meyer, Gesundheitspolitik im Vorwärts, med. Diss. Berlin 1986, p. 231; F. Hertz, *Hans Günther als Rassenforscher*, (Berlin, 1930).

Human experiments

The doctor and socialist, Julius Moses, attempted to distinguish unscientific racial prejudice from legitimate scientific eugenic and medical research. He prevented the use of public funds for continuing finance for the Gobineau edition of Schemann.[171] He insisted on the accountability of medical research to both the public and the individual patient. He opposed research carried out in children's and municipal hospitals without patients' consent. From 1928 he waged a relentless press and parliamentary campaign against human experiments. He focused on research on children suffering from rickets at the Kaiserin Auguste Viktoria Haus. He enraged Langstein, the Director of the KAVH (who was to be dismissed by the Nazis) with an article entitled '100 Rats and 20 Children. Workers' Children as Guinea Pigs'.[172] Moses insisted that individual consent had to be given by the patient, and that the prime duty of the doctor was that of therapy. Research was a matter of public interest, as it occurred in state institutions and was financed by public funds. He accused scientists of being 'progress-crazed', and of claiming an unwarranted position as commanding military officers who justified the sacrifice of life in the battle against disease. In such a situation the poor and the dying were especially vulnerable. Controls were all the more necessary because of the quickening pace of medical research.[173] While it was an argument that had echoes of the anti-vivisectionist accusations of 'human guinea pigs' of the 1890s, Moses was in favour not of rejecting such research wholesale but of hedging it with mechanisms of public accountability.

The socialist attack on 'experiment mania' resulted in state guidelines for clinical research. Moses stood for a compromise between science and the public interest. Eugenics was legitimate provided that it was scientific and benefited the welfare of the patient and society. As a result of Moses' campaign, the Reich Health Council agreed guidelines for human experiments on 14 March 1930. This council was composed of university professors, doctors and medical officers. A number were moderate eugenicists such as Drigalski and Gottstein. Thus the position of the state was determined by professional scientists. They agreed that experiments should not be carried out on the dying, and that children required special protection. Moses claimed that asking for the doctor to behave as if he was experimenting on his family, was no more that what had been demanded by the veteran eugenicist Abderhalden or the anti-socialist Liek.[174] The Council reduced a political problem

---

171 Schemann papers, Fischer to Schemann, 22 June and 19 December 1931, 12 December 1929; Nemitz, 'Antisemitismus'.
172 J. Moses, '100 Ratten und 20 Kinder', *Der Kassenarzt*, vol. 5 no. 10 (10 March 1928) 1–2; Moses, 'Meine Erwiderung an Herrn Prof Langstein', *Der Kassenarzt*, vol. 5 (14 April 1928) 1–2.
173 J. Moses, 'Arzt und Experiment', *Der Kassenarzt*, vol. 5 (21 April 1928) 1–2; Moses, 'Der Kampf gegen das Menschenexperiment', *Der Vorpommer. Organ der Sozialdemokratischen Partei*, vol. 9 no. 178 (1 August 1928). I am grateful to Herr Nemitz for items from the Moses papers, Bremen.
174 ZSTA P 15.01 Nr. 26226 Missbrauch medizinischer Eingriffe 1928–1933; ZSTA M Rep 76 Va Sekt 1 Tit X B1 59, 124–6 Ärztliche Versuche an Menschen 1928–1931; E. Abderhalden, 'Versuche an Menschen', *Ethik*, vol. 5 no. 1 (1928), 13–16; reply by Liek in *Ethik*, vol. 5 no. 1 (1928), 19–26.

to one of professional ethics. As long as these ethics remained consistent with democracy then there were safeguards, but the unforeseen risk was that the ethical basis of medicine was vulnerable to change. The only addition made by the state was to indicate that the reformed legal code would remove medical operations from coming under the law of assault. Legal barriers to uncontrolled medical intervention were thus eroded.

Opposition to eugenics and racial hygiene has to be distinguished from opposition to Nazism and to the Führer. Gruber's observation that Hitler was a psychopath and had the physiognomy of a *Mischling* was taken up by socialist critics of Nazism such as Käte Frankenthal. Hirschfeld cited Gruber's criticism of Nordic racial character. The accusation that Hitler was a psychopath was quietly nurtured among eugenicists, as it reinforced the eugenicists' sense of expert superiority. It was often pointed out that Hitler was anything but Nordic.[175] Most racial hygienists remained aloof from the NSDAP, while prepared to exploit its rising power to support research and to boost their social prestige. This is shown by the fact that only thirteen out of fifty-one medically qualified members of the Munich Racial Hygiene Society in January 1933 were members of the Nazi Doctors' League.[176] Baur, Fischer, Lenz, Ploetz, Rüdin and Verschuer had not yet joined the NSDAP, even though they opportunistically attempted to benefit from its rise to power by improving their academic status and influencing policies.

Medical critics of racial hygiene protested against its racism, and scientific errors, but few rejected the principle of eugenics. In 1925 Georg Benjamin, a communist doctor, published a tract entitled 'Death of the Weak?'[177] He attacked the bourgeois critics of welfare and the racial hygiene of such as Boeters as damaging to the body politic, and demanded welfare for the proletariat and its offspring. While Benjamin differed from 'bourgeois' social hygienists such as Grotjahn, he was also concerned with the declining birth rate and the welfare of 'future generations'. With other socialist doctors he demanded 'a population policy in the interests of the proletariat'.[178] Most socialists accepted the desirability of a buoyant birth rate. There were few socialist critics of theories of the dangers of depopulation.

Chajes, an SPD *Landtag* representative and Grotjahn's successor in Berlin, considered that such a radical measure as eugenic sterilization could be broadly applied and that eugenic birth control and incarceration could ensure progressive improvement in the people's quality.[179] Socialists accepted scientific proof that many mental illnesses were inherited, and that heredity was a priority in combating TB and VD. After the Nazi electoral success in September 1930, Moses denounced Nazism as a threat to medical welfare and humanitarianism. In July 1932 he warned that the lives of incurable patients were at risk.[180] A lone article in

[175] Hirschfeld, *Race*, p. 41.
[176] Staatsarchiv München, Pol-Dir Mü 6848 Nationalsozialistischer Deutscher Ärzte Bund 21 November 1932.   [177] *Tod den Schwachen?* (Berlin, 1925).
[178] H. Benjamin, *Georg Benjamin* (Leipzig, 1977), pp. 72–5, 84–5.
[179] B. Chajes, *Kompendium der sozialen Hygiene* (Leipzig, 1931), pp. 144–9.
[180] Nadav, *Moses*, pp. 88, 300–2; Moses 'Seltsame Ärzte', *Arbeiterwohlfahrt*, vol. 7 (1932), 664–7.

the SPD journal *Vorwärts* in April 1932 predicted that the Nazis would exterminate the sick and infirm.[181] One of the few groups to launch a concerted attack on racial hygiene as Nazi was the Socialist Doctors' Association after 1930.[182] Their journal, speeches and rallies as in Berlin and Chemnitz in July 1932 included a good deal of sharp criticism of Nazi racism. The hostility of Nazism to sickness insurance, and the acceptance of 'euthanasia' by such as Staemmler and by NSDAP ideologues was pointed out. Frankenthal declared that a visit to a doctor would prompt the diagnostic question, 'are you a degenerate or of noble quality [*Edeling*]?' Therapy would follow on the basis of kill or cure.[183] Her verdict on Hitler was that his weak physical constitution meant that he would not have survived one of his racial tribunals.[184] Even more radical was Friedrich Wolf who rejected all professional medicine as coercive, and took one of the most individualistic and anti-authoritarian positions at that time. Yet this socialist onslaught was too little and too late. The opposition to eugenics failed to achieve an institutional basis comparable to that of Lancelot Hogben's Department for Social Biology at the London School of Economics. German socialists had been so involved in eugenics that many in social hygiene could not be drawn into this campaign. Issues such as birth control and abortion remained contentious. Socialists were politically divided between the SPD and KPD and too prone to mutual recriminations for the critique of Nazi racism to have much impact.[185]

Anti-medical groups such as the feminists and lay sexual reformers, nature therapists and psychotherapists were prone to organicist views. While they were at daggers drawn with the medical profession, some opponents of the profession also looked to the NSDAP for support for their demands. For their part the Nazis could exploit and appropriate a politically, professionally and socially highly varied organicism that was widely disseminated. Nature therapy and psychotherapy were to find protected niches in the Nazi social system. From 1930 Nazism was attractive to many groups who felt that they had been betrayed by the republic. A situation arose that the more powerful the NSDAP became, the more apparently necessary it became to support this rising power in German politics for the gains it might bring. Few doctors or biologists thought that Nazism's extreme authoritarianism, anti-semitism and militarism would result in subordination of the profession to the NSDAP, loss of status, emigration or extermination.

---

[181] L. Meyer, 'Gesundheitspolitik', pp. 261–2.   [182] Thomann, 'Weg', pp. 160–4.
[183] Kudlien, *Ärzte*, p. 41; K. Frankenthal, 'Ärzteschaft und Faschismus', *Der sozialistische Arzt*, vol. 8 no. 6 (1932), 101–7, reprinted in Leibfried and Tennstedt, *Berufsverbote*, pp. 203–9, and Bromberger and Mausbach, 'Widerstand', pp. 323–30.   [184] Frankenthal, *Der dreifache Fluch*, pp. 182–6.
[185] Leibfried and Tennstedt, *Berufsverbote*, pp. 106–28.

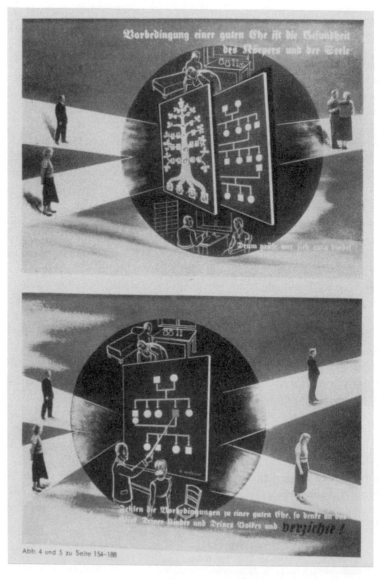

8 Publicity for hereditary health examinations. Reproduced from M. Elster and F. Rott, *Liebe und Ehe* (Dresden 1941). Hereditary screening prior to marriage had been a priority of the eugenicists since the early years of the racial hygiene movement. Rott was a leading paediatrician associated with the infant welfare institution, the Kaiserin Auguste Viktoria-Haus.

8

Nazi racial hygiene

IDEOLOGUES AND TECHNOCRATS: THE SCIENTISTS' STRUGGLE

Racial hygienists had great expectations that National Socialism would allow medical experts to impose scientific solutions to social problems. The Nazi destruction of the fledgling democratic institutions of the Weimar Republic was welcomed as clearing the way for eugenic legislation to solve the problems of the anti-social, degenerate and chronically sick. Racial hygienists nurtured ambitions of extending their influence over health and population policy, for which Nazism was to provide a conducive atmosphere and the political machinery. Racial hygienists expected to be able to lead Germany towards better health and morals, and to boost the numbers and quality of future generations. The Nazis rapaciously plundered elements from pre-existing movements for motherhood, family welfare, and national health, and incorporated these into their distinctive ideology of racial purity. This looked promising for incorporating positive eugenics as the basis of public health. Propaganda depicted the Führer as a shining example of a non-smoker and abstainer from alcohol, a hard worker, an animal lover and an enthusiast for national and racial biology. Yet privately the racial hygienists suspected that he had psychopathic traits, and classified him as an un-Nordic East Slav, at the same time underestimating the ruthless authoritarianism of his regime.[1]

Health and race were values central to Nazi Germany.[2] Hitler, leading Nazis, and those doctors and scientists who became fervent converts believed that a racialized concept of health justified anti-semitism and their plans for territorial expansion of the nation. This marked a break between welfare-minded eugenicists and the Nazi activists in medicine, resulting in contrasting visions of the aims, organization and methods of racialized medicine. Nazi concepts of health meant that Jews, gypsies and homosexuals were stigmatized as 'alien parasites' or as

---

[1] Lenz, 'Die Stellung des Nationalsozialismus zur Rassenhygiene' can be interpreted as expressing these manipulative expectations and criticisms of Nazism.

[2] W. Wuttke-Groneberg, *Medizin im Nationalsozialismus. Ein Arbeitsbuch* (Tübingen, 1980); G. Baader and U. Schultz (eds.), *Medizin und Nationalsozialismus. Tabuisierte Vergangenheit – Ungebrochene Tradition* (Berlin West, 1980).

'cancerous growths' in the German body politic. Health care was selectively to promote a Nordic elite, which would lead a purged but a fitter and healthier nation to military victories. Physical capacity (*Leistung*) and mental vigour were the criteria for a hierarchical and functional reorganizing of society. Medical institutions, propaganda programmes and policies had to serve the aims of selectionist, racial ideology. Nazis were determined to uproot every liberal value and replace these with National Socialist ideology. Frick, the Reich Interior Minister at the first meeting of the Council for Population and Race Politics in June 1933, denounced the costs of welfare as 'a system of exaggerated care for the single individual'. Having children was to be a matter of racial duty rather than personal choice. Hereditary defectives were to be eliminated from procreation, and miscegenation had to cease. Nordic blood had to be united to the soil in a policy favouring large peasant families.[3] Yet these pro-natalist and agrarian expectations were to be disappointed as the war economy requiring women industrial workers and male military service gathered momentum.

The Führer's eugenics

Although Hitler's *Mein Kampf* was a product of the post-war crisis, its ideas retained authoritative status. Its relevance for family life in the new Germany was indicated by its presentation to newly weds. Hitler elaborated his distinctive National Socialist ideology of a *völkisch* state based on purity of blood and race. The racial hygienists were naive in believing that they had formulated a eugenic programme which Hitler would enact out of respect for their scientific objectivity and professional expertise. The illuminating passages on the social role of science and medicine in *Mein Kampf* marked a reaction against liberal concepts of science and of the professions. All human culture, art and civilization were the achievements of the 'culture-bearing' Aryan race. The *völkisch* state had race as its central value. It was essential to maintain racial purity, because interbreeding between races caused degeneration of the higher race. Only the healthy should be allowed to have children, and medical controls should be imposed on the degenerate to prevent them from reproducing.[4] Hitler praised the American immigration laws that excluded undesirables on the basis of illness and race. He opposed the liberal view that the nation was a civic association as debasing the nation to the level of 'an automobile club'.[5] After military service, every citizen should receive a citizen's diploma and a health certificate confirming the man's physical health for marriage.[6] He hoped that 'A prevention of the faculty and opportunity to procreate on the part of the physically degenerate and mentally sick, over a period of only six hundred years, would not only free humanity from an immeasurable misfortune but would lead to a recovery which today scarcely

---

[3] 'German Population and Race Politics', *Eugenical News*, vol. 19 (1934), 33–8.
[4] A. Hitler, *Mein Kampf*, with an introduction by D.C. Watt (London, 1974), p. 354.
[5] Hitler, *Mein Kampf*, p. 400.   [6] Hitler, *Mein Kampf*, p. 376.

seems conceivable'. In addition to marriage controls for all, there were to be measures to secure border colonies of exemplary racial purity: 'specially constituted racial commissions must issue settlement certificates to individuals.'[7] While Lenz suggested on the basis of these proposals that racial hygienic schemes were integral to the National Socialist vision, Nazi concepts of race, science and society were distinctive.[8]

On the one hand Hitler expressed faith in racial science, but on the other he despised liberal scientific education and professions as decadent symptoms of materialism. He gave science a racial rather than a liberal pedigree. Human thought and invention were to serve man's struggle for existence. The function of 'the most brilliant scientific knowledge of the present era' was 'to alleviate mankind's struggle for existence and to forge its weapons for the struggle of the future'.[9] He attacked the German higher educational system as training not '*men*' but 'officials, engineers, technicians, chemists, jurists, journalists, and to keep those intellectuals from dying out, professors.'[10] Hitler rejected science as based on mass education with 'endless schooling' and examinations. This led to materialist culture which he associated with Jews and Marxists.[11] It was a mistake to believe that civil society had transcended the limitations of nature and biology to which primitive societies were subject.

Hitler found himself in the midst of a contradiction similar to that of the socialists during the 1920s: reliant on the techniques of science and yet wishing to undermine its basis in liberal institutions. For their part, scientists favoured a system of national government by experts. This vision of a ruling technocratic elite should be contrasted with Hitler's plan to divide the *völkisch* state into political and professional chambers. This social system would breed an elite of leaders.[12] Hitler viewed scientists as a subordinate group, whose expertise was of value in realizing the *völkisch* state. Hitler escaped from the contradiction of subordination and leadership requirements by extolling science as something advanced by the leadership of creative minds endowed with superior personalities. In practice Hitler recognized that the support of the middle classes and of the professions was an essential precondition for the Nazi takeover. From around 1930 doctors and scientists were welcomed into the ranks of National Socialism. After 1933 the state's need for a functioning technocracy was to be greater than ever.

The tensions between academic science and *völkisch* politics were evident in Hitler's concept of race. His view of blending heredity was out of step with Mendelism, and the theories of an Aryan and Germanic race were scorned by anthropologists. Hitler recognized that German nationality was no longer based on 'a unified racial nucleus'. A 'blending process' had corrupted the purity of

---

7 Hitler, *Mein Kampf*, p. 368.
8 Lenz, 'Die Stellung des Nationalsozialismus zur Rassenhygiene', 300–8.
9 Hitler, *Mein Kampf*, p. 405.   10 Hitler, *Mein Kampf*, p. 373.
11 Hitler, *Mein Kampf*, pp. 407–8.
12 Hitler, *Mein Kampf*, pp. 409–10.   13 Hitler, *Mein Kampf*, pp. 358–61.

Germanic-Aryan blood. Unmixed stocks of Aryan-Germanic blood should be regarded as 'the most precious treasure for our future'.[13] Race as based on a theory of blending heredity, derived not from biologists but from racial philosophers such as Gobineau to be reformulated by such *völkisch* ideologues as Chamberlain. Hitler might have read a copy of the textbook of human genetics written by the eugenicists Baur, Fischer and Lenz, but he showed no understanding of Mendelism and particulate inheritance. Those racial hygienists inclined to Nazism and the SS advocated abandoning the concept of an inclusive Germanic-Aryan race for a rigorous selectivity to bring the Nordic racial qualities to the fore. This raises a key problem of how the separate strands of racist ideology and advances in medicine and biology could be welded into some sort of unity after 1933.

The image of the Führer was of a superhumanly healthy and hardworking man. Hitler did not endorse a single type of medicine or system of health care. As in politics and administration he allowed competing systems to develop, and occasionally intervened to radicalize measures and ensure that no one group, or type of science and medicine gained supremacy. Hitler was vegetarian (from 1931 or 1932) and teetotal. This outlook coincided with a distrust of scientific medicine and a preference for natural therapies. Behaviour traits that doctors were inclined to interpret as signs of a diseased psyche might have been little more than evidence of sharing a widespread popular antipathy to medical science.[14] Hitler apparently never allowed a doctor to see him naked for a whole-body check-up, and this reluctance not to concede authority to the professional gaze was shared by many contemporaries.[15] The pluralism within Nazi biology and medicine was reflected in Hitler's choice of medical practitioners. He used a great variety of medicines, even dosing himself with one based on gun-cleaning fluid as a tried remedy for stomach upsets in the First World War. He continually experimented with new doctors and treatments, and was distrustful when radical surgery was threatened. His medical preferences ranged from the impeccable scientific credentials of his personal physician from 1934 until 1944, Karl Brandt, to the fashionable hormones, vitamins and glucose treatments administered by Theo Morell from October 1936. Brandt was a product of the medical establishment having trained under the eminent surgeon Sauerbruch. He retained a high professional reputation, and was a dedicated servant of Hitler in initiating the 'euthanasia' measures.[16] There was immense rivalry between Brandt and the preventive nutritional therapies of Morell, who felt that the Führer was burning up his energy as if in the tropics, and that to replace it such patent medicines as his *Vitamultin* were necessary.[17] Hitler's dealings with his personal doctors show a mixture of credulity and scepticism towards medical science.

[14] L.E. Hoffmann, 'Psychoanalytic Interpretations of Adolf Hitler and Nazism, 1939–1945: A Prelude to Psychohistory', *Psychohistory Review*, vol. 11 (1982), 68–87.
[15] N. Bromberg and V.V. Small, *Hitler's Psychopathology* (New York, 1983); W. Langer, *The Mind of Adolf Hitler. The Secret Wartime Report* (London, 1973).
[16] Lifton, *Nazi Doctors*, pp. 114–17.
[17] D. Irving, *Adolf Hitler. The Medical Diaries* (London, 1983).

Racial hygiene and professional leadership

Inherent in the de-politicized authoritarianism of the ultra-right was a contradiction between a leadership cult boosted by propaganda about virtually superhuman powers as opposed to reliance on professionalism. On the one hand, the Führer was to be an 'iron-surgeon' to cure 'national ills'. The national leader was to renew and regenerate a decaying and disintegrating nation, conceptualized as a 'social organism'. Radical political interventions against opponents, who were stigmatized as biological degenerates, were to regenerate the body politic. A medical mystique, drawing on the supernatural powers of traditional healers, boosted the leadership cult and sanctioned the blood-letting of political violence. On the other hand, like other dictators Hitler wished to modernize political structures while avoiding politicization in directions other than National Socialism. Concepts of a 'social pathology' were helpful in transposing economic and political problems into naturalistic terms that were amenable to scientific solutions. Hitler and kindred fascist dictatorships felt obliged to promote the welfare of workers, soldiers and their families on a selective basis in order to realize grandiose military and economic schemes. Modern administrative and medical systems were necessary to maintain an efficient war economy. While the Nazi state was to be placed on a biological basis, it was to be a racial and nazified vision of biology rather than one which drew on the conventional types of science. Technocrats found themselves in a perilously unstable situation, despite being tempted to direct the implementation of biologically based programmes of social regeneration.[18]

Racism and anti-semitism have often been depicted as simple and homogeneous categories. Yet there were many strands in their illiberal rejection of humanitarianism and tolerance. While Hitler's blend of Aryan glorification and violent anti-semitism had great influence, other biological, medical and anthropological variants of racism influenced Nazi health and social policies, which were responses to social processes of urban and industrial growth, professionalization of health and welfare, and the emergence of a scientific technocracy. Racial concepts of public health were a means of social control and of promoting social integration in terms of both ideology and everyday habits. There resulted conflicting social interests, concepts and aims in the eugenics and racial hygiene movement, as well as rifts between scientific racial hygiene and anti-semitism. Racial hygiene had to undergo a series of transformations so that it could be adapted to Nazism. The long-term shift from the radicalism of the *Lebensreformer* and from liberal individualism to corporate and biologized social values made racial hygiene ripe for further metamorphosis. The term 'eugenics', associated with the welfare programme of the 1920s, was abandoned. The serologist Reche argued that racial hygiene should not degenerate into a welfare-oriented eugenics that promoted health without

---

[18] P.J. Weindling, 'Fascism and Population Policies in Comparative European, Perspective', in M. Teitelbaum and J. Winter (eds.), *Population, Resources and the Environment: The Interplay of Science, Ideology and Intellectual Traditions* (Cambridge, 1989).

regard to racial origins.[19] A process of renegotiation and reformulation of racial hygiene was unleashed after 1933. The leaders of racial hygiene made pacts with their political masters by offering ideological racial programmes in such areas as health education and technical skills in racial classification and health promotion. The Nazis needed this support. As racial hygienists were influential in academic and professional spheres, they could mobilize doctors, nurses and other medical personnel to disseminate racial values. The Nazis needed the skills of anthropologists, demographers, psychiatrists and public health experts to identify and 'solve' the problems of the antisocial and the racially degenerate. Just as the Nazis had to compromise with other sectors of society such as the churches and the army, so a functioning, normal science was tolerated, even in spheres such as psychology and psychotherapy where the premises about the mind-body relations were individualistic and rationalist. But tensions persisted between scientists and the Nazi social system.[20]

The Nazi social system inherited a eugenics movement which was itself riven by conflicts. Competing power blocs and rival biological theories among the racial hygienists were overshadowed by power struggles among Nazi leadership groups. Scientific racial hygiene and public health were broken into splinter groups by rifts within Nazism. There was a growing rivalry between Nazi ideologists, seeking a populist type of national revival on the basis of widespread anti-semitism, violence and propaganda and Nazi technocratic elites, especially among the SS and state officials whose elitist cadres deployed policing and scientific technologies. At the same time economic factors, war and territorial expansion, settlement and racial policies contributed to the further fragmentation and polarization of racial hygiene. In 1933 racial hygienists hoped that they would be given enlarged financial resources, and privileged social status. They would be dictators of social policy, moving from the position of advisors to executors of power. The fragmentary eugenic experiments of the Weimar Republic would be uniformly implemented throughout society. The spheres of health and race would be extended into the economic, financial and political dimensions. These hopes were the outcome of a fusion of authoritarian nationalism and scientific elitism. The publisher Lehmann typified this position with his burning ambition of a national front, combining a range of nationalist forces from monarchism to Nazism. Medical and scientific expertise was central to this vision. He wrote to the Empress Hermine praising Baur's agricultural research on vines, potatoes and lupins as providing Germany with natural resources in the event of war. He pleaded that the Nazis might be personally uncouth, but they were dedicated and effective in removing divisive political elements.[21] Most scientists, providing they were not Jewish, felt that the authoritarian social values paralleled their belief in the primacy

---

[19] Saller, *Rassenlehre*, p. 61.
[20] U. Geuter, *Die Professionalisierung der Psychologie im Nationalsozialismus* (Frankfurt-on-Main, 1984); G. Cocks, *Psychotherapy in the Third Reich, The Göring Institute* (New York and Oxford, 1985).   [21] J.F. Lehmann papers, Lehmann to Empress Hermine, 30 June 1933.

of natural forces. The geneticist Goldschmidt (a Jew) felt that Nazism was better than Bolshevism. Otto Warburg, who was half-Jewish, informed the Rockefeller Foundation that the regime would not last longer than 1934, and other scientists perceived Hitler as a moderating force. Many professors hoped that their privileged social status in which they had basked in Wilhelmine Germany would be restored.[22] The petty bourgeois insecurities as to financial position and hostility to socialism were shared by most academics. The popularity of Nazism among students was a hopeful sign. The vulgarity and lack of education of the mass of the NSDAP aroused the hope that leading academic lights would increase in brilliance and power.

There was an affinity of intellectual structures of science with authoritarian politics. The two areas were linked by further developments of professionalization. Science-based professions hoped for corporate privileges from an authoritarian political structure. The liquidation of socialism was welcomed by those professions such as engineering which depended on an industrial up-swing. The nationalist stress on self-sufficiency offered opportunities for developing synthetic substitutes for oils, fibres and foodstuffs. The managing of the human resources of the nation could justify the medical profession's demands for exclusive privileges and an extension of powers. Nazism swept away the autonomy of sickness insurance funds and municipalities that threatened to develop socialized medicine. Practitioners expected that controls would be imposed on nature therapists and 'quackery'. The removal of Jewish practitioners would provide lucrative opportunities for practice, and relieve pressure in an overcrowded profession. Doctors found immense opportunities in the NSDAP, SS, army and industry in addition to private, hospital and insurance practice. The funding and scope for research in all these spheres was increased. Research and medical practice were often combined. In 1939 the military authorities welcomed the development that military medical officers were more frequently gaining the habilitation qualifications for lectureships.[23] Nazism boosted professional status, prestige and earning capacity.[24] It was hoped that racial hygiene would take a central role in placing medicine on a sound basis of nationalist values, and in enhancing professional powers. Medical students were to be inculcated with scientific principles of heredity and race. Medicine was to be transformed from being a liberal profession serving the individual patient to one in which the doctor would become the Führer of the people. He should supervise all aspects of family life such as diet and child care, and promote a reformed national lifestyle. Racial hygiene could thus advance professional powers and promote social integration.

Most accounts of Nazi medicine focus on the extreme forms of medical killing and concentration camp experiments that subjected human victims to extremes of cold, low pressure and sea water just as embryologists had subjected animal

---

[22] Weindling, 'Rockefeller Funding', pp. 119–40.
[23] BA Militärarchiv Freiburg 420/480 Heeressanitätsinspektion, 10 June 1939.
[24] Leibfried and Tennstedt, *Berufsverbote*, pp. 2–18.

embryos to injury experiments during the 1890s. Little is known about daily medical practice, health conditions and the expectations of patients. Nazi eugenics is revealing of ultimate intentions and novel routines in a wide spectrum of medical and biological contexts. In certain respects expectations of the Nazi authorities were fulfilled. Racial values were given a privileged place in all aspects of education, NSDAP propaganda and policy-making. A series of racial laws had a strongly medical and hereditarian component. Public health was reorganized on a racial basis. The medical profession was purged of 'alien' Jewish and socialist elements, and given increased opportunities and powers. University chairs, research institutes and courses were established in racial hygiene. The German Racial Hygiene Society began to expand under the direction of leading medical scientists and public health experts.

Yet there were many points of tension between eugenicists and racial ideologues. There were intellectual discrepancies between the Nazis' simple and popular glorification of a pure Aryan and German race, and anthropologists' views on the complex racial composition of the German population. Professionals and academics often found it difficult to accept the dictates of autodidact party ideologues. 'Unscientific' aspects of anti-semitism, as promoted by Nazi Jew-baiters such as Julius Streicher, could only be reconciled to objective science by subordination to the Führer, party and *Volk*. The Nazi system could not allow academics a privileged position unless they submitted to the controls of party-political organizations such as the Racial Political Office of the NSDAP or SS. Factions within the party were hostile to antiquated academic privileges and promoted new forms of applied scientific research and practice.

A power struggle to control racial hygiene occurred. The rivalry was initially between the party allied to the Nazi Doctors' League, and public health officials allied to those racial hygienists advocating compulsory sterilization and segregation of the anti-social. By 1937 the SS emerged as a major force seeking to unify anti-semitism with the technocratic machinery of public health. The Nazi system of power was based on competing hierarchies which proliferated due to the Führer's divide and rule policy and because of the need to reconcile a diversity of social interests. Hitler was skilled in the manipulation of his entourage, their associated power blocs and public opinion. Moreover, there were elements of sheer anarchy in a system based on brute power rather than legitimate status or scientific excellence. As racial hygiene became caught up in Nazi power politics, its aims, institutions and active leadership were transformed.

The Nazis were able to play on inherent divisions within the racial hygiene movement, especially the tensions between those eugenicists, who were more state- and science-oriented, and the more radical right-wing party activists who were motivated by *völkisch* anti-semitism. There emerged two factions. One was party dominated. This consisted of ideologues such as Alfred Rosenberg and the Racial Political Office of Walter Gross (a protégé of Rudolf Hess), the National Socialist Welfare League (*NSV*), and the Nazi Doctors' League under Gerhard

Wagner. They emphasized the role of the family doctor as fundamental in promoting primary health care. The alliance was held together by a high degree of ideological motivation to the party and to Aryan racial ideals, and benefited from the party infrastructure. The rival faction was more technocratic and elitist. This consisted of public health administrators, medical researchers, and the SS and its daughter racial organizations, the *Ahnenerbe* and *Lebensborn* which had racial hygienic programmes. Himmler emerged as the controlling power. He envisaged a German-dominated Europe, led by a Nordic elite. He advocated harsh policies of Germanization and elimination of other ethnic groups. These policies required medical expertise for sterilization, segregation, and mass killing, as well as for health-promoting and breeding policies. For their part, the scientists had fatal flaws in their beliefs. In many cases, the more scientific their outlook, the more politically naive they were. The more scientists tried to maintain authority and status, the more concessions had to be made to Nazism. The racial hygienists made a Faustian pact with Nazism. Its powerful forces and organizations had aims that went far beyond the racial hygienists' nationalism, and professionalized control over health care. Instead of leading a national revival to a healthy society, the racial hygienists became subordinate to forces leading to war and mass killings.

THE REMNANTS OF RACIAL HYGIENE

Selective integration

Ideologues and technocrats projected alternative views of the past history of racial and eugenic thought. Those working to link racial hygiene with popular anti-semitism and a mass party glorified the *völkisch* tradition. This looked back to nineteenth-century critics of liberalism, and linked biological racism, the cultural racism of Gobineau, and the cultural pessimists like Lagarde. All were hailed as *Vorkämpfer* – as apostles of Germanic nationalism and as laying the foundations for Nazism. This interpretation highlighted the Aryanism and anti-semitism of racial hygiene. Some, such as Schemann who was awarded the Goethe medal in 1937, accepted this role.[25] Others such as Günther shifted attention to questions of the family, the birth rate and the promotion of peasant life.[26] Prophets of national renewal such as Spengler and Arthur Moeller van den Bruck (the author of *The Third Reich*) recoiled into 'inner emigration'. The intellectual crusade for a racially based social order was broader and more diverse than that encompassed by Nazism.

The unresolved tensions between racial hygiene and national socialism resulted in conflicting historical accounts of racial hygiene. Whereas the party ideologues argued that racial hygiene had been a vital inspiration to those in the vanguard of Nazism, there were those who preferred racial measures to be imposed by an expert

---

[25] F. Ruttke, 'Ludwig Schemann: ein deutscher Gelehrter', *Volk und Rasse*, vol. 13 (1938), 66–8.
[26] H.F.K. Günther, *Volk und Staat in ihrer Stellung zu Vererbung und Auslese* (Munich, nd); Lutzhöft, *Der Nordische Gedanke*, p. 42.

elite, and subjected the history of racial hygiene to more critical scrutiny. A group of SS racial hygienists headed by Astel in Jena (which was situated in what they felt was the German peasant heartland of Thuringia), carefully considered the legacy of Haeckel, Darwinism and racial hygiene. They gathered archives of pioneers of eugenics. The human geneticist, Lothar Stengel von Rutkowski, built up an archive for the history of racial ideas[27] at Jena in Thuringia. He collected the papers of Schallmayer, and was planning to incorporate archives of Ploetz and Rüdin.[28] The SS historians came to the conclusion that there had been close connections between socialism and racial hygiene, and that Darwinism had contributed much to socialism. Those who had integrated Aryanism and socialism were suspect: for example, it was considered whether Woltmann was Jewish, and the Haeckel archives were vetted for Jewish and masonic monists.[29] The works of Darwin, Haeckel and the early racial hygienists could not be accepted as precursors of Nazism. But they distinguished between natural selection as consistent with 'Nordic Germanic Science', and other types of liberal, mechanistic and Marxist science. A new biology, dynamic enough to be consistent with Nazism, was called for. An Ernst Haeckel Society was founded in January 1942 under the patronage of the Thuringian Gauleiter, Fritz Sauckel.[30] The Haeckel Society stressed that it in no way shared the aims of the now disbanded Monist League, which had support from materialists and socialists.[31]

A careful process of sifting through the inherited legacy of scientific theories resulted in diametrically opposed types of biology and medicine. The Gross-Wagner 'ideologue' faction was holistic and environmentalist. Gross sought to depose SS-oriented medical officers such as Astel, who enjoyed Himmler's confidence. Astel and his academic colleagues offered the SS the prospect of a public health system which integrated the racial sciences of anthropology, biology and medicine with the SS's plans to promote the Nordic racial heritage. These SS-oriented researchers stressed the need for a vigorously Darwinist and selectionist type of science.[32] The integration of the selectionist academic camp into the process of formulating a racial policy for Eastern Europe meant that the SS offered a powerful fusion of science and the ruthless pursuit of racial political aims. While many racial hygienists were cold-shouldered by the SS and other racial political authorities, it is important to recognize that there were scientific advisors and executors of racial policies, and that certain key SS or party figures had a sound grasp of genetics, demography and anthropology. That there were anthropologists such as Scheidt in Hamburg who sought to disengage their institutes from the racial

---

[27] 'eine grosse Sammelstätte aller für die Geschichte der Rassenidee bedeutungsvollen Dokumente'.
[28] Ploetz papers, Stengel von Rutkowski to Anita Ploetz, 7 January 1941.
[29] F. Lenz, 'War Ludwig Woltmann ein Jude?', *ARGB*, vol. 27 (1933), 112; Saller, *Rassenlehre*, pp. 12–14.
[30] V. Franz, *Das heutige geschichtliche Bild von Ernst Haeckel* (Jena, 1934); H. Bruecher, *Ernst Haeckels Bluts- und Geisteserbe*, (Munich, 1936).
[31] 'Ernst-Haeckel-Gesellschaft', *ARGB*, vol. 35 (1942), 503–4.
[32] BAK NS 19 Nr 838, Gerlach to Himmler, 15 January 1938.

political policy-making and adjudication does not cancel out the selective integration of other academics in population and racial policies. The view that there were autonomous groups of scientific anthropologists and racial hygienists, and that these were distinct from fanatical and ignorant racists in the state, party and SS is not tenable.[33]

The marginality of racial hygiene

As the power of the SS grew, that of the Racial Hygiene Society diminished. Given its problematic historical legacy, the Nazis were in fact highly selective in the elements that they chose from racial hygiene. Racial hygiene had to be purged and reconstituted. This transformation resulted in a reorganization of the German Society for Racial Hygiene, a reallocation of university teaching posts, and far-reaching changes in the administration and structure of public health. The Racial Hygiene Society grew in size but it lost its autonomy and its importance as a scientific and educational forum.

Membership of the Racial Hygiene Society[34]

Date	Local Groups	Numbers
1930	16	1300
1931	13	1085
June 1933	12	950
Jan. 1934	19	1300
Jan. 1935	44	2400
Jan. 1936	54	3250
Dec. 1936	56	3700

In June 1933 the society was subjected to reorganization as part of the general process of *Gleichschaltung*. This removed the autonomy of all educational, scientific and welfare organizations, so marking an end to the liberal values once enshrined in German educational, professional and scientific associations. Local groups of the Racial Hygiene Society like that in Munich were dissolved. They were refounded with a membership purged of Jews and others unacceptable to the new order. On 10 June 1935 the national society met to have its fate decided on in the new Germany. Members had to be 'Germans of Aryan origins'. Virtually no local group survived with its membership intact. The society lost about 500 members, suggesting that about one-third of eugenicists were out of favour with Nazism. The Racial Hygiene Society became a part of the Reich Committee for Public Health of the Reich Ministry of the Interior.[35] This completed the long-term process of the Society's incorporation into the public health administration.

---

[33] Such a distinction has been made by Saller, *Rassenlehre*; compare G. Lilienthal, 'Zum Anteil der Anthropologie an der NS-Rassenpolitik', *Medizinhistorisches Journal*, vol. 19 (1984), 154.
[34] E. Fischer, 'Aus der Geschichte der Deutschen Gesellschaft für Rassenhygiene', *ARGB*, vol. 24 (1930) 1–5; *Volk und Rasse*, vol. 11 (1936), 299.   [35] *Reichsausschuss für Volksgesundheit.*

The final blow was delivered to the League for Regeneration. It had decided to unite with the Racial Hygiene Society on 5 December 1932. Its glossy monthly journal *Eugenik* ceased publication after June 1933. Its editor, Ostermann, was dismissed from the Prussian Ministry of the Interior, and its other supporters, like Muckermann, were eased out of office. The funds went into the coffers of the Racial Hygiene Society.[36] The journals *Archiv für Rassen- und Gesellschaftsbiologie* and *Volk und Rasse* were recognized as official journals of the society and of the Reich Committee for Public Health. That Ploetz remained editor of the *Archiv* and was joined by Rüdin in 1936, might be taken as a sign of continuity. But their editorial board included new men such as Gross of the Racial Political Office, Gütt of the Ministry of the Interior, and the Nazi lawyer and racial legislator Falk Ruttke. They symbolized the controls to which the *Archiv* was subject. It was permitted to include only scientific articles, and had to exclude anything touching on racial and population policy. Its scope was limited to human genetics; another scientific journal, *Zeitschrift für induktive Abstammungs- und Vererbungslehre*, was deemed more appropriate for articles on plants and animals. The *Archiv* was vulnerable to official criticism whenever a party functionary took offence to an article. Himmler was outraged when articles (by Lenz and Siegfried Tzschucke) stigmatized illegitimate children as degenerate.[37] This conflicted with the *Lebensborn* welfare scheme for the offspring of unmarried mothers.[38] For this, Rüdin as editor was sharply reprimanded. Scientists became subject to intrusive controls.[39] The *Archiv* leavened its scientific content with articles on Nazi leaders such as Frick and Gütt, and fulsome praise of Nazi policies. These demonstrated the bonds between racial hygiene and Nazism. Such articles can be seen as having a dual function. On the one hand they served to integrate racial hygiene with the NSDAP. On the other, such articles can be interpreted as formal tokens of allegiance, necessary to guarantee a measure of autonomy to racial hygienists.[40]

The popular journal, *Volk und Rasse*, was even less of a platform for the eugenicists. Before 1933 it had been edited by Bruno K. Schultz and the serologist Reche. In 1933 it was promptly taken over by the SS. Schultz, who was an SS officer, became sole editor. He used the journal to popularize such racial theories as that of Nordic superiority. The editorial board was joined by Himmler and SS men such as Astel, Darré and Gütt. The journal became more and more a mouthpiece for Himmler's Nordic programme. The circulation rose from 1,000 to 12,000. In

[36] Landesarchiv Berlin, Vereinsakten. Rep 42/Acc 1743 Nr 9018.
[37] F. Lenz, 'Gedanken zur Rassenhygiene (Eugenik)', *ARGB*, vol. 37 (1943), 84–109.
[38] G. Lilienthal, *Der 'Lebensborn e.V.' Ein Instrument nationalsozialistischer Rassenpolitik* (Stuttgart, 1985).
[39] BDC, Rüdin file; Ploetz papers, Lenz to Rüdin 28 April 1936, Lenz to Wettstein 28 April 1936, Wettstein to Lenz 27 April 1936.
[40] A. Ploetz and E. Rüdin, 'Zur Entwicklung des Deutschen Reichs seit der Machtübernahme unseres Führers am 30. Januar 1933', *ARGB*, vol. 32 (1938), 185–186; Ploetz and Rüdin, 'Die Vollendung Grossdeutschlands', *ARGB*, vol. 32 (1938), 186.
[41] ZSTA P 15.01 Nr 26243 Bl. 127. Ploetz to Reichskanzler 6 April 1933.

1933 the activities of the Racial Hygiene Society were given glowing reports; that by 1935 coverage ceased was a sign that the Racial Hygiene Society was losing its importance.

Many of the founders of racial hygiene were too elderly to participate actively in the Third Reich. Ploetz wrote to Hitler as Reich Chancellor in April 1933 explaining that his age and his still incomplete theoretical treatise prevented practical co-operation, but he honoured 'the man who had the will to implement racial hygiene'.[41] Ploetz was showered with honours such as the Pettenkofer Prize in 1934, the title *Professor* in 1936, and, through Abderhalden, election to the Leopoldina academy of sciences.[42] He was venerated as the founder of racial hygiene. The authorities allowed his beloved brainchild, the *Archiv*, to continue. In return he could give legitimacy to Nazi policies and theories among scientists and the medical profession. Ploetz supported the fusion of Nazi sterilization and welfare policies with racial hygiene. After years of isolation during the Weimar period, Ploetz at last enjoyed academic recognition, and even hoped for a Nobel Peace Prize in 1936.[43]

Ploetz was invited to join a state committee on racial hygiene policy in June 1933 and was courted by the Nazi Minister of the Interior, Frick. Ploetz was on friendly terms with Gütt, and was ready to co-operate with the racializing of public health.[44] He regaled Gross, the *Leiter* of the Racial Political Office, with tales of how the Hauptmanns and himself had planned a racial colony.[45] Ploetz hoped that by attempting to link the utopian youthful escapades with an embryonic spirit of racial purification, he could improve his own and Gerhart Hauptmann's standing with the Nazis, as Hauptmann's democratic commitments of the 1920s were resented. Bluhm and Rüdin were also congratulated for their pioneering contributions to racial hygiene. Bluhm's eightieth birthday in 1942[46] and Rüdin's seventieth birthday in 1944 were much celebrated, but the age of these figure-heads indicated that a younger generation had gained control.[47] Racial hygienists reinterpreted their past, overlooking their support for the welfare measures of the 1920s, in an attempt to ingratiate themselves with the authorities.[48]

The Racial Hygiene Society was subject to conflicting forces of professional autonomy, and National Socialist control. As long as racial hygienists could secure autonomy by offering the Nazi state services, then a working compromise was maintained. But whenever the state or another Nazi organization wished to interfere in the internal running of the society, there was a threat to the position of racial hygiene and its exponents. The society remained dominated by the medical profession. Virtually every *Leiter* of a local branch was a medical officer, or

---

[42] Ploetz papers, diary, 26 June 1937. [43] Saller, *Rassenlehre*, pp. 72–5.
[44] Ploetz papers, Gütt to Anita Ploetz, 23 March 1940.
[45] Gerhart Hauptmann papers, Ploetz to Hauptmann, 13 November 1936.
[46] G. Just, 'Agnes Bluhm und ihr Lebenswerk', *Die Ärztin*, vol. 17, (1942), 516–26; A. Bluhm, 'Dank an meine Studienzeit', *Die Ärztin*, vol. 17 (1942), 527–35. [47] *ARGB*, vol. 37 (1944), 160–2.
[48] 'Alfred Ploetz zum Gedächtnis', *ARGB*, vol. 34 (1940), 1–8.

qualified in a medical specialism such as hygiene or psychiatry. There were exceptional cases only in more remote areas, as when a branch established in Marienwerder in 1934 was headed by a teacher. The society's constitution was revised. The society continued to aim to disseminate racial hygienic ideas and practices, and to encourage research. It was 'to support the government in the realization of racial hygiene aims'. Only German nationals of Aryan descent could be members. These statutes came into force in April 1934. Yet as long as Ploetz, Lenz and Rüdin were not NSDAP members, the Racial Hygiene Society was peripheral to Nazi racial policy.[49] The society retained dual functions as a scientific and educational organization with teachers being encouraged to join. Meetings were addressed by local public health officials, newly schooled in racial hygiene, or by leading scientists. For example on 22 October 1936 Fischer and Verschuer lectured on racial research to an audience of over 1,000 at the University of Cologne. Rüdin, Luxenburger and Lenz continued to hold large numbers of lectures until 1937. In the latter six months of 1936, there were forty-five evenings of lectures in the society on medicine and heredity.[50]

From 1937 the Racial Hygiene Society's importance was eroded as it was caught up in a conflict between the Racial Political Office of Gross, and the SS, which had ambitions to take control of public health and university sciences. Rüdin initially enjoyed considerable prestige: he had an international scientific reputation, and from 1935 he was head of the Society of Neurologists and Psychiatrists. He sought to maintain the hegemony of medically qualified psychiatrists over psychotherapy, stressing the scientific importance of biology and the professional status of medicine.[51] He took a leading role in the drawing up and implementing of compulsory sterilization legislation. As long as he could offer the regime expertise and recognition, his position – and the Racial Hygiene Society's – was secure. But the more the Racial Political Office vied with the SS for control of education and propaganda in racial hygiene and of psychiatric and medical research, the more insecure became the Racial Hygiene Society and Rüdin's position. That the SS officer Schultz became secretary of the Racial Hygiene Society in 1938 indicated the challenge which the SS issued to Rüdin's scientific leadership.

In 1933 Gross, a physician and NSDAP member since 1925, founded the Reich Office for Education on Population Policy and Racial Welfare.[52] Its purpose was to educate the nation, especially youth, on the need to have a racial conscience and duty to the family. In 1934 this was incorporated into the Racial Policy Department of the NSDAP. Gross had strong links with Hess and with Wagner of the Nazi Doctors' League, with Rosenberg (the theorist of racial purity) and the fanatical anti-semite, Streicher. Gross was a racial ideologist and public propagandist in the causes of Nazism and anti-semitism. Armed with the massive resources of the party for racial education, Gross's power overshadowed that of the

[49] For NSDAP membership, see below p. 512 and fn. 95.
[50] *Volk und Rasse*, vol. 13 (1937), 299.
[51] Cocks, *Psychotherapy*, pp. 105–9, 193–4.   [52] BDC file Gross.

Racial Hygiene Society. The Racial Hygiene Society needed a protector. Rüdin required the support of the public health official, Gütt of the Reich Ministry of the Interior, to maintain the autonomy of the Racial Hygiene Society under the protection of the state health administration. Yet, the published reports on the society suggest that after 1936 the level of activity declined. This coincided with mounting pressure on the public health administration by rival factions in the party and the SS.

The Racial Hygiene Society was challenged by the Racial Political Office under Gross, and by the growing power of the SS, which exerted influence on archaeology through the *Ahnenerbe* and on physical anthropology. In September 1937 the Society for Physical Anthropology was reconstituted as the German Society for Racial Research.[53] In deference to the past, Ploetz was elected an honorary member. But the organization was dominated by those in the vanguard of Nazi racial research. The society was directed by B. K. Schultz and the Tübingen anthropologist Gieseler (both with strong SS links), and a committee of Reche, Verschuer and Lothar Loeffler, a party activist. SS-oriented researchers such as Reche, Heberer and the anatomist Robert Wetzel regaled the society with accounts of archaeological research carried out in conjunction with the SS's organization for racial culture, the *Ahnenerbe*.[54] In 1942 the influence of this society was offset by a Society for Constitutional Research, founded by the psychiatrist Kretschmer, in which social hygienists like Rott and Coerper and human geneticists were active. This society sought to defend the biological concept of an integrated constitution on an academic rather than party political basis.[55]

International tensions

The Racial Hygiene Society under Rüdin initially served to boost the international prestige of Nazi legislation such as the sterilization laws. Rüdin was Swiss, and had many international contacts. Yet within the international eugenics movement there was increasing polarization that resulted in the isolation of German eugenics. Certain contacts were maintained. Attempts were made to continue the German–Soviet Racial Research Laboratory in Moscow for diplomatic reasons during 1933 and 1934.[56] German serologists and population geneticists valued their Soviet contacts, but as genetics came under pressure from Stalin, eugenics was out of favour with the Soviet authorities. The Germans organized a series of international congresses, such as the one on demography in Berlin in 1935. As German racial hygiene became isolated internationally, its prestige in domestic politics also diminished. Racial hygienists such as Reche, who had once cultivated international contacts, turned to the army and SS with plans for the 'removal' of 'inferior'

[53] *Deutsche Gesellschaft für Rassenforschung.*   [54] *ARGB*, vol. 32 (1938), 83–6.
[55] G. Koch, *Die Gesellschaft für Konstitutionsforschung* (Erlangen, 1985).
[56] BAK R86 Nr 74 Prof Dr Heinrich Zeiss; R73 Nr 229 Russisch-Deutsches Laboratorium 1933–35.

504 *Nazi racial hygiene*

populations of the East. Internationalism gave way to a devotion to German military power.

Nazism polarized extreme racist versus reformist tensions among eugenicists in other countries. There were conflicts of opinion over the virtues and vices of Nazi racial hygiene. For example, in Britain Blacker's reform eugenics, based on human genetics and social science, gained the upper hand over the more racist and imperialist views of such as Cora Hodson and the demographer George Pitt-Rivers, who was associated with the pro-Nordic and Nazi propagandist Lord Lymington.[57] Blacker strenuously attempted to dissociate the Eugenic Society's campaign for voluntary sterilization from Nazism. He stressed that anti-semitism and eugenics fundamentally differed.[58] Although there was a wave of sterilization legislation in Northern Europe after the Danish law of 1929, opinions divided over the German sterilization measures.[59] In Norway, the racist Mjöen was opposed by the advocates of the sterilization law which was passed in 1934.[60] In Sweden, where a sterilization law came into force in 1935, Nordic idealists such as Lundborg were opposed by the geneticist, Gunnar Dahlberg.[61] In the United States, the Eugenics Record Office (ERO) of Davenport and Harry Laughlin – advocates of immigration controls and sterilization – retained warm contacts with Rüdin and supported the German hardline views of compulsory sterilization.[62] The ERO cultivated cultural ties with Germany and a native US Nazi movement.[63] The ERO was subjected to scrutiny by human geneticists who condemned its data as useless because of the large amount of qualitative information on character and emotions. In 1939 the ERO was closed and Laughlin was asked to retire; global population control became a new object of concern. There was a shift in international scientific circles away from eugenics to a more rigorous human and population genetics and demography.

These tensions came to a head in the International Federation of Eugenics Organizations. Rüdin retained his presidency with US and Scandinavian support. In 1934 an international congress was held in Zürich with delegations from Germany, Denmark, Britain, British Borneo, France, Holland, Dutch East Indies, Austria, Poland, Switzerland and Czechoslovakia. Eugenicists such as Fetscher

[57] R. Griffiths, *Fellow Travellers of the Right. British Enthusiasts for Nazi Germany 1933–39* (Oxford, 1983), pp. 317–29.

[58] C.P. Blacker, in *The Lancet*, (3 June 1933), 1203–4, (10 June 1933), 1265–6; Blacker, 'Eugenics in Germany', *Eugenics Review*, vol. 25 (1933), 157–9.

[59] Critics included Aubrey Lewis, 'German Eugenic Legislation', *Eugenics Review*, vol. 26 (1934), 183–91.

[60] N. Roll-Hansen, 'Eugenics before World War II, the Case of Norway', *History and Philosophy of the Life Sciences*, vol. 2 (1980), 269–98.

[61] G. Dahlberg, translated by L. Hogben, *Race, Reason and Rubbish* (London, 1943).

[62] 'A Letter from Dr Ploetz', *Eugenical News*, vol. 19 (September–October 1934), 129; C.G. Campbell, 'The German Racial Policy', *Eugenical News*, vol. 21 (March–April 1936), 25–9; Kevles, *Eugenics*, p. 347.

[63] G.E. Allen, 'The Eugenics Record Office at Cold Spring Harbor, 1910–1940', *Osiris*, ser.2 vol. 2 (1986), 225–64, pp. 251–3; M.D. Miller, *Wunderlich's Salute* (New York, 1985).

were excluded by the Nazi authorities.[64] Rüdin presided and Ploetz opened the congress with a resolution against war as eugenically destructive.[65] The climate of internationalism changed, as the Nazi academic system became self-reliant and disengaged from international scientific circles. Criticism of German racial hygiene increased, as a result of Nazi anti-semitism and the persecution of Jewish scientists. The fourth 'international' congress of eugenics was held in Vienna in 1940. The German Racial Hygiene Society under the patronage of Frick, the Minister of the Interior, organized a gathering of Axis intellectuals imbued with military and racial fanaticism.[66] To international observers German racial hygiene was a monolithic ideology that was united with Nazism; but judged from within the complex of national socialist Germany, the Racial Hygiene Society indicated the diminishing influence of the pioneers of racial hygiene.

SCIENTIFIC FAILURE

The defeat of racial hygiene as a public organization was paralleled by its failure as a scientific discipline. The pattern was similar: growth of academic posts and institutes until 1935 was followed by stagnation and decay. There were a number of signs that racial hygienists were under pressure. A series of conflicts between scientists and Aryan ideologues during the 1930s signified that academics had become subject to the dictates of party, state and the SS. Bureaucratic functions and service duties became immense burdens to researchers. The SS and Racial Political Office sought direct control of university departments, so that during the war the activities of racial hygienists were subordinate to Nazi racial and military aims.

In 1933 biology and racial hygiene seemed poised for a bright future. Proclamations that national socialism was politically applied biology gave biology a privileged place among the sciences. Yet the Nazis were discriminating in the elements that they chose from biology and philosophy when constructing their *Weltanschauung*. While many biologists had holistic sympathies, it was important to choose the right type of theoretician. The vitalism of the embryologist and philosopher Driesch was condemned. When the work of another biologist, Bernhard Dürken, was approved by the party, Astel's Jena group remained opposed to holistic theories that they saw as linked to Roman Catholicism. They similarly criticized Spann's corporatist theories, and were implacably opposed to Muckermann and his Weimar associates. The older generation of scientists were reluctant to sacrifice scientific commitments to Nazism. The embryologist, Spemann, whose theory of the organizer was in many ways compatible with authoritarian values, warned the younger generation of zoologists that they would have to abide by the rock-hard values of scientific truth.[67] Although biological concepts of unity had long been associated with one another, the creation of a

---

[64] Fetscher papers, Rüdin to Fetscher, 24 June 1934, preventing Fetscher's lecture on criminal families.
[65] *Volk und Rasse*, vol. 9 (1934), 297.   [66] BHSTA M Inn 79477 Rassenhygiene.
[67] Horder and Weindling, 'Hans Spemann and the Organizer', pp. 207–9.

distinctively Nazi biology was a protracted task of imposing controls on and incentives for the scientific community to adopt racial values.[68]

Much effort went into the making of national socialist biology. It was to be dynamic and action-oriented. Biology was a valuable resource for Nazism in that it was meant to provide objective proof for racial ideology. At the same time there were scientific innovations in the fields of heredity, animal behaviour studies and ecology. Animal and human populations were resources that could be cultivated, improved on, and from which worthless elements could be weeded out.[69] Human genetics was to serve the needs of 'hereditary pathology'. This concept linked research in human and population genetics to the eradication of malformations and hereditary diseases. The geneticists, Fritz von Wettstein (of Austrian origin and director of the Kaiser Wilhelm Institute for Biology), Alfred Kühn and Verschuer were in the vanguard of this action-oriented approach, which included being official advisers on sterilization and genealogy.[70] Animal behaviour studies typify the action-oriented new biology. Biological concepts such as 'survival', 'formative powers' and 'will' were deemed to be in keeping with Nazi ideology. Jakob von Uexküll, the theorist of the *Umwelt*, linked animal behaviour with environmental adaptation. He had long-standing *völkisch* commitments, being an admirer of Houston Stewart Chamberlain, and enjoying an honoured position in Nazi Germany.[71] Karl von Frisch, another biologist of Austrian origin in Munich who was famous for his interpretation of 'the language of bees' typified the readiness of academic biologists to support the ideological aims of the Nazis. Biologists urged human selection as a means of ridding the nation of hereditary defects and the degenerative diseases of civilization. Frisch's popularization of evolutionary biology benefited the Goebbel's Military Fund.[72]

There were casualties even among dedicated Nazis. Wettstein was outraged that the botanist Ernst Lehmann had attacked his *Plasmon* theory of inheritance through the protoplasm. Lehmann had organized the nationalist *Deutschen Biologen Verband* in 1931. Günther was furious when Lehmann attacked his racial theory. The wounded pride of Günther and Wettstein coupled with suspicions of Lehmann's Freemasonry account for why this pioneer National Socialist biologist was ousted from the party and university. Lehmann was expelled from the *Biologen Verband* in October 1938. The *Verband* was taken over by the *Ahnenerbe* of the SS with support of geneticists such as Wettstein, the SS biologists W. Greite and Martin Riedel, and

[68] E. Lehmann, *Irrweg der Biologie* (Stuttgart, 1946).

[69] *Science and Salvage. From the German 'Verwertung des Wertlosen'*, editor: Claus Ungewitter (London, 1944); A. Bramwell, *Blood and Soil. Walther Darré and Hitler's 'Green Party'* (Abbotsbrook, 1985).

[70] A. Kühn, M. Staemmler and F. Burgdörfer, *Erbkunde, Rassenpflege, Bevölkerungspolitik* (Leipzig, 1935); A. Gütt, E. Rüdin and F. Ruttke, *Gesetz zur Verhütung erbkranken Nachwuchses* (Munich, 1934), p. 7.

[71] J. Schmidt, 'Jakob von Uexküll und Houston Stewart Chamberlain. Ein Briefwechsel in Auszügen', *Medizinhistorisches Journal*, vol. 10 (1975), 121–9; J. v. Uexküll (ed.), *H.S. Chamberlain. Natur und Leben* (Munich, 1928); F. Brock, 'Die Grundlagen der Umweltforschung Jacob von Uexkülls und seiner Schule', *Verhandlungen der Deutschen Zoologischen Gesellschaft*, vol. 41 (1939), 16–68.

[72] K.v. Frisch, *Du und das Leben* (Berlin: Dr Goebbels-Spende für die Deutsche Wehrmacht, 1936).

by the anthropologist Reche. The SS thus exploited scientific disputes to extend their control over academic institutions.[73]

Konrad Lorenz, the Austrian biologist, exemplified how the Nazi social system opened career opportunities and intellectual horizons to those researching on heredity. He undertook studies of animal behaviour which confirmed the degenerative effects of civilization. He interpreted changes in instinctive animal behaviour resulting from domestication as a process of degeneration. He compared domesticated animals to civilized humans, and observed that changes due to domestication were similar to those resulting from diseases in wild animals. He was influenced by the view of his father, a distinguished orthopaedic surgeon, that patients suffering from hereditary defects should not be treated. He also cited the view of racial hygienists such as Fischer that urbanization was a degenerative process, and co-operated with the SS-anthropologist Heberer. Lorenz urged racial hygiene should eliminate inferior characteristics so as to replace the selective effects of the natural environment. Lorenz felt alienated from an Austrian social system that did not support his work, and sought academic contacts and finance in Germany. Wettstein praised his research in German Research Fund applications. Lorenz backed von Frisch and Uexküll in the founding of a Society for Animal Behaviour in 1936. After Austria was incorporated into Germany in 1938, Lorenz joined the Nazi Party.[74] He was active on behalf of the Racial Political Office, taking an interest in the *Lebensraum* question, and was rewarded with the directorship of an Institute for Comparative Psychology in Königsberg in 1940.[75]

The shift from static morphological categories to dynamic, action-oriented research also overtook racial hygiene. Here the lead was taken by Verschuer's concept of 'hereditary pathology' (*Erbpathologie*). It marked the culmination of the transition from the descriptive approach of physical anthropology to a hereditarian and biological understanding of the process of human variation and heredity. This led to efforts to control and eliminate pathological defects. Verschuer came to blend human genetics with evangelical devotion to Nazi ideology. His outline of hereditary pathology, written for doctors in 1934, stressed the racial duties of the *Erbarzt* in the *völkisch* state.[76] His 1941 textbook on racial hygiene began with the reflection that while he could not serve in the infantry as in the 1914–18 war, his book was to be a Führer in scientific combat. Verschuer praised Hitler as the saviour of the Nordic race, and linked genetics with anti-semitism and the eradication of hereditary diseases and psychoses.[77] Hereditary pathology was to link genetic research with the screening of the health and racial quality of populations.

---

[73] IFZ Fa Copy of Amtsgericht Akten Charlottenburg, Deutscher Biologen Verband Berlin 1931–1944; BDC Lehmann file.

[74] T.J. Kalikow, 'Die ethologische Theorie von Konrad Lorenz', in H. Mehrtens and S. Richter (eds.), *Naturwissenschaft, Technik und NS-Ideologie* (Frankfurt-on-Main, 1980), pp. 189–214.

[75] T.J. Kalikow, 'Konrad Lorenz's Ethological Theory: Explanation and Ideology, 1938–1943', *Journal of the History of Biology*, vol. 16 (1983), 39–73.

[76] O. v. Verschuer, *Erbpathologie. Ein Lehrbuch für Ärzte* (Dresden and Leipzig, 1934).

[77] Saller, *Rassenlehre*, p. 140; O. v. Verschuer, *Leitfaden der Rassenhygiene* (Leipzig, 1941), p. 6.

Reorganizing racial hygiene

Initially, the authorities treated racial hygiene with care. A priority was to separate and isolate the Berlin group of Fischer from their strong Catholic contacts through Muckermann and their links with non-Nazi officials such as Ostermann. Given the inherent Berlin–Munich tensions in the Racial Hygiene Society, this was easily done by arranging a shift of power towards the more authoritarian and Nazi-oriented Munich group, and the isolation of Fischer. During 1933 Fischer adopted a strongly nationalist but explicitly non-Nazi stance. His speech on 1 February 1933 to the Kaiser Wilhelm Gesellschaft made critical comments on national socialism. In May 1933 he spoke on human hereditary science as the basis of eugenic population policy, with a healthy peasantry as a priority. He warned that leaders could have few children, and demanded that the Nazi state subsidize eugenics and support measures for indirect coercion such as sterilization.[78]

There was a concerted effort by the politically more right-wing Munich racial hygienists to break the power of Fischer, Muckermann and Verschuer. On 29 May 1933 Astel and B.K. Schultz, both SS members of the Munich Racial Hygiene Society publicly denounced Fischer, Muckermann and Ostermann as relics of the Weimar Republic. But Fischer continued his rearguard action in support of Muckermann. An assistant was induced to testify that Muckermann had referred to the Führer as 'an idiot' (a particularly galling remark to any eugenicist who favoured sterilization for the mentally subnormal). A directive came from the Prussian Ministry of the Interior that Fischer should be watched by assistants who ought to be exclusively party members. Fischer was forced to cede control of the German Racial Hygiene Society to Rüdin, and the society was transferred back to Munich. Fischer's name was temporarily struck off the list of editors of Ploetz's *Archiv*.[79] This marked the end of the Weimar coalition of eugenicists.

Fischer was elected Rector of Berlin University on 29 July 1933, beating a national socialist rival. But Fischer now showed that he was prepared to compromise with the new order. At his inaugural speech, he praised the Nazis for being able to see and think biologically. This speech revealed Fischer as a turncoat, but it was also an attempt to maintain the supremacy of biologists on issues of social policy. Fischer remained out of favour for some time. An indication is provided in a letter by the publisher Lehmann on 12 January 1934. Lehmann appreciated that Fischer was the first anthropologist to praise the racial popularizations of Günther, but Fischer's support of Muckermann as a Jesuit during the 1920s had placed an insuperable barrier between them. Lehmann offered to publish a popularization of racial anthropology so as to tempt Fischer to resume work for the Fatherland.[80]

Fischer responded positively to such invitations to support the new Germany. As

---

[78] E. Fischer, 'Die Fortschritte der menschlichen Erblehre als Grundlage eugenischer Bevölkerungs-politik', *Deutsche Forschungen*, no. 20 (1933), 55–71.

[79] ZSTA P 15.01 Nr 26243 Bl. 289, 348.

[80] J.F. Lehmann papers, Lehmann to Fischer, 12 January 1934.

early as 5 July 1933 the Reich Ministry of the Interior requested the support of Fischer, along with Rüdin, Baur and Verschuer, in the rapid implementation of sterilization legislation.[81] Fischer complied with the request to serve the *Volksstaat* and remained director of the Kaiser Wilhelm Institute for Anthropology, placing the institute's expertise at the service of the authorities.[82] The case of the plant geneticist Baur shows that right-wing scientific autocrats who had flourished under the Weimar Republic, which they had so despised, were now being challenged by the new breed of Nazi officials. In 1933 Baur clashed with Darré and the Ministry of Agriculture, and the strain was considered to have precipitated a fatal heart attack.[83] Goldschmidt's verdict was that Baur was 'a Nazi killed by super-Nazism'. Baur's assistant, Nachtsheim, clashed with Karl Vetter, an underling of Darré, over control of the Reich League of Rabbit Breeders.[84] That Nachtsheim resorted to the protection of Frick of the Ministry of the Interior shows that scientific technocrats still had a niche because of their value in hereditary health policies.[85]

Positive enthusiasm for the Nazi order was shown by Verschuer. Officials felt that he too should be separated from his mentor, Fischer. Their verdict, that he was prepared to co-operate but did not understand the extent of national socialist aims, was revealing as to the disparate aims of many who collaborated with Nazism.[86] Verschuer was dispatched to Frankfurt-on-Main to open an institute for racial hygiene. Verschuer's academic position in the Kaiser Wilhelm Gesellschaft was filled by Lenz from Munich. Lenz's chair in racial hygiene combined responsibilities in human heredity with public health, that made him in effect also the successor of the social hygienists, Grotjahn and Chajes. Muckermann was forced into retirement, and his journal, *Das kommende Geschlecht*, ceased publication in 1934. But he continued to pontificate on family welfare and was sporadically criticized by Nazi ideologues. Ploetz and Fischer sought to improve their positions by denouncing ex-collaborators with Muckermann. The Nazis effectively had broken the old system of welfare-oriented eugenics by 1934.[87]

A failed ideologue: the Tirala case

Subordination of universities opened them up to the power struggles and factionalism of the Nazis. The conflict of ideology and technocracy can be illustrated by the appointment of a professor of racial hygiene in Munich. With the move of Lenz to Berlin, and the rise in prestige of Munich in the Nazi social system, a full chair of racial hygiene was regarded as essential. An academy of public health

[81] ZSTA P 15.01 Nr 26244 Bl. 12, Fischer to Minister.
[82] MPG Generalverwaltung Nr 2413 Finanzierung 1932–1941 Bl. 18.
[83] Goldschmidt, *Ivory Tower*, p. 272; L.G. Tirala, 'Nachruf zum Tode Erwin Baurs', *Volk und Rasse*, vol. 9 (1934), 2–5; *Völkischer Beobachter*, (6 December 1933).
[84] H.H. Scheffler, *Karl Vetter*, (Berlin, nd).
[85] MPG Dahlem, Nachtsheim papers, deposition for US Intelligence Service, 26 March 1946.
[86] ZSTA P 15.01 Nr 26244 Bl. 81–2, Gross to Gütt, July 1933.
[87] Ploetz papers, Bluhm to Ploetz, 24 February 1938, on links between Muckermann and Lenz.

was established in Munich, requiring the training of medical officers in racial hygiene and social medicine. The candidate supported by *völkisch* and party circles was a Sudeten German physician, Lothar Tirala. In August 1933 he was recommended as an outstanding scientist by Chamberlain's wife, Eva Wagner (daughter of the composer), Lehmann and the Nazi physicist Philipp Lenard. Tirala had trained in experimental zoology in Vienna, and had collaborated with the environmental biologist, von Uexküll, who was also a Chamberlain protégé. From 1918 he gave occasional lectures in eugenics and racial hygiene. In 1925 he worked as a urologist under Kroiss, the chairman of an early Nazi Doctors' League. In 1927 he attempted to gain a teaching post with the Mendelian, Tschermak, in Prague, but encountered political opposition. Tirala's highly eccentric views on the laws of heredity exposed him to criticism from Mendelians such as Rüdin.

The racial hygienists were antagonistic to Tirala whom they regarded as an unqualified ideologue. Ploetz, Lenz and Rüdin were asked to comment on his suitability for the Munich chair of racial hygiene. Ploetz dismissed Tirala as a superficial popularist and unsuited for a prestigious post at Munich. His only achievement had been to expose Muckermann's vacillation over sterilization. Lenz condemned Tirala as a propagandist rather than a scientist, who lacked an elementary grounding in hygiene. Lenz interpreted Tirala's ambition to have a chair as pathological egoism. Rüdin, politically more astute, praised Tirala's writings on eugenics and settlement as 'fresh and lively'. However, he expressed a preference for the bacteriologist, Ernst Rodenwaldt, as an excellent 'Führer, teacher and organizer', and as scientifically better qualified. Ploetz also supported Rodenwaldt as having long been associated with Nazism and as having worked for expatriate Germans in the East Indies. Ploetz was silent about Rodenwaldt's son being his son-in-law. But Rodenwaldt was disliked by the head of the public health services in Bavaria, owing to an internal feud within the party, and the chair was offered to Tirala on 14 October 1933.[88]

Trouble quickly flared up owing to hostility to the flamboyant ideologist. On 6 February 1934 the German consulate in Brünn objected that Tirala's main earnings had been from abortions; that he had been prosecuted for a patient's death; that he had worked in conjunction with Jewish doctors and lawyers; and that he had been opposed by Nazi students at Brünn because of his dishonourable conduct. Although Tirala brushed the accusations to one side as 'the lies of Jews and Freemasons', the accusations continued to be made against him. In 1934 and 1935 there were student demonstrations, and doctoral students and assistants left because of Tirala's inadequate research and practice. The Racial Political Office also came to regard Tirala as an unreliable propagandist. The Faculty and lecturers agreed that Tirala was unfit to serve as examiner. On 18 April 1936 he lost his position as a Bavarian official and his duties were taken over by Rüdin and Luxenburger. It seemed that scientifically orthodox racial hygiene had triumphed.[89]

[88] BHSTA MK 39596, Ordinarius für Rassenhygiene; MK 34604 Institut.
[89] BDC Tirala files.

In 1935 the Munich university Institute for Racial Hygiene was transferred to Rüdin's Kaiser Wilhelm Institute. It provided a convenient niche for the employment of two of Rüdin's assistants, Albert Harrasser and Ernst Longo. Both were Austrians. Longo had organized a Nazi cell in the Vienna General Hospital in 1932, and the local SA doctors in 1935. In 1936 Tirala enraged Rüdin when he criticized Mendelism at the Munich Racial Hygiene Society. Tirala advocated a theory of hereditary rhythms rather than genes. Rüdin felt it was his responsibility as *Leiter* of the society to prevent further lectures by Tirala. Gross of the Racial Political Office joined the attack on Tirala as incompetent.[90]

Yet Tirala found support from Winifred Wagner and Streicher, who pointed out that the Führer liked autodidacts. This touched on a weak point of all academics that made them vulnerable to attack from party ideologues. Luxenburger ventured some academic criticisms of Tirala, but he was humiliated when Tirala's high-ranking allies forced him to withdraw the accusations.[91] Streicher urged that the German Research Fund support Tirala's racial biological research in a new institute in Nuremberg. By March 1940 Tirala built up an adequate private medical practice. Discussion continued until 1944 over whether Tirala had been wrongfully dismissed or ill-treated. But by this time it was Rüdin whose position was vulnerable. The Tirala case shows the tensions between medical expertise and party-oriented ideology.[92] The party and the SS were later to be more astute in their choice of loyal academic personnel. The tension between Tirala and his scientific critics shows how eugenicists could be out of step with Nazi racial ideology. Tirala's critic, Luxenburger, found himself in difficulties and was unable to gain a chair. In 1940 he was forced to leave the Munich Institute and serve in the army. Verschuer felt that Luxenburger should be supported on scientific grounds as there were so very few racial hygienists. But the consensus was that Luxenburger's position was untenable.[93] The forcing out of one of the most active eugenicists was symptomatic of the weakening power of the old guard.

A failed discipline

Despite the regime's racial priorities and centralized university administration, establishing racial hygiene as a university discipline remained dependent on local circumstances and interests. An uneven pattern resulted, due partly to local resistance, but also to the power struggle between the SS and the Racial Political Office. Leading members of the old guard of racial hygienists were slow to join the Nazi Party. Lenz, Ploetz and Rüdin all became party members in 1937, joining at the recommendation of Gütt.[94] Verschuer joined in September 1941, and Fischer

[90] L. Tirala, 'Medizin und Biologie', *Ziel und Weg* (1935), 136–138.
[91] Luxenburger papers, 12 February 1935 NSDAP Ärztebund.   [92] BDC Tirala, Personal file.
[93] Lenz papers, Verschuer to Lenz, 26 June 40, Lenz to Verschuer, 26 July 1940.
[94] Nachtsheim papers, Lenz to Nachtsheim, 11 August 1946, Nachtsheim to Gütt, 21 August 1946. Lenz claimed that hostility to anti-semitism and to international scientific contacts distanced him from the NSDAP.

also in 1941.[95] Himmler commented that it was a political necessity that Lenz and Fischer join the party as one could not use their theories to reinforce party policies while rejecting them as individuals.[96] Kaup never joined. Although some of the old guard of racial hygienists had *völkisch* and Nordic sympathies, they were overtaken by a younger generation more committed to the Nazi Party. But this meant that problems arose over the lack of scientific achievements of the more youthful ideologues. When Ploetz died in 1940 he was venerated from all sides – by Gütt, by Astel and the SS, and by the Wagner faction. All laid claim to having realized his ideas.[97]

Professorial elitism remained a barrier to the development of scientific disciplines. Racial hygiene was no exception. The University of Halle shows how it was possible for vested professorial interests to evade the establishing of an institute for racial hygiene. Most medical professors were nationalist but not Nazi, as exemplified by the biochemist Abderhalden who had long been active in social welfare matters. Before 1933 only a few medical men on the fringe of university life were Nazis. These included the chest specialist, Karl Heinz Blümel who ran the TB dispensary; the professor of general medicine, Heinz Kürten; and the municipal medical officer, Schnell. In June 1933 Kürten was given the teaching post in human heredity and racial hygiene, but by 1934 he had been promoted to Munich. Schnell was rewarded with a lectureship in hygiene, and finally a chair in population policy, heredity and racial studies. That he was appointed to the Technical University of Hanover in 1935 meant that racial hygiene at Halle suffered a setback. He directed the Racial Office in Halle and the Racial Political Office of the local Nazi *Gau* (or region). Kürten led a Committee for the Implementation of the National Revolution, which attacked Abderhalden for having had Jewish students, and found support among the state authorities. Jewish professors were dismissed, and liberal professors such as Theodor Brugsch, and the psychiatrist Alfred Hauptmann were forced out of office between 1934 and 1937. The hygiene lecturer, Joachim Mrugowsky, took over teaching in racial hygiene in 1935. He was a convinced Nazi ideologue, with a deep interest in the history of medicine in the age of Goethe and in holistic medicine. He also became head of the Hygiene Institute of the Waffen SS, SS Oberführer, and undertook 'research' in Auschwitz and Sachsenhausen.[98] The plan for an institute for racial hygiene at Halle was allowed to lapse. The priorities of the SS became more important than university matters.[99] The best solution was co-operation between the old guard, given jobs as rewards for loyalty during the *Kampfzeit* and yet scientifically incompetent, and a

[95] BDC files, Rüdin joined 1 May 1937, party number 5773608; Lenz joined 1 May 1937 and was no. 3833993; Fischer applied 28 December 1939, membership from 1 January 1940, no. 7383062; Verschuer, no. 8140376.
[96] BDC Fischer file, Himmler to Stellvertreter des Führers, 17 August 1938.
[97] Ploetz papers, Gütt to Anita Ploetz, 23 March 1940; Stengel von Rutkowski, 7 January 1941.
[98] He was to be hanged in 1947.
[99] W. Kaiser and A. Völker, 'Die faschistischen Strömungen an der Medizinischen Fakultät der Universität Halle', in Thom and Spaar, *Medizin im Faschismus*, pp. 68–76.

younger generation of experts seeking opportunities and support. Such symbiosis developed between the Giessen professor of racial hygiene, Heinrich Wilhelm Kranz, and the medical statistician, Siegfried Koller, who in 1931 held a Rockefeller grant for developing the statistics of coronary heart disease. Kranz had been a veteran of the *Freikorps* and Kapp Putsch, and had joined the NSDAP in 1930 and advanced in the racial political office of *Gau* Hessen. Koller worked on the statistics of hereditary defects and of anti-social characteristics.[100] His Giessen index became a national model for medical statistics in 1941. Kranz drew on Koller's investigations for publicizing the concept of euthanasia for the 'anti-social'.

Four universities – Danzig, Jena, Frankfurt and Tübingen – had institutes for racial hygiene which also functioned as NSDAP Racial Political Offices for the local *Gau*. Such an identification of party political functions was the exception rather than the rule, although many institutes for anthropology and hygiene adjudicated on race and paternity. Between 1933 and 1939 racial hygiene institutes were founded only at Frankfurt, Jena and Königsberg. The universities of Giessen, Hamburg, Leipzig and Tübingen converted existing anthropological institutes.[101] Other universities extended the responsibilities of teachers in hygiene or psychiatry. By 1945 under half of the universities in the Reich had a special institute for racial hygiene or human heredity. This meant that despite immense political pressures, the institutional development of racial hygiene was slow.[102] It became difficult to fill vacant teaching posts. The Berlin psychiatrist, Max de Crinis, who had a ministerial responsibility for medical appointments, voiced his concern over the lack of suitably qualified younger staff in racial hygiene, hygiene and psychiatry on many occasions during the 1940s. There was dismay early in 1944 that no one could be found to fill the chairs at Munich and Königsberg. The ideological role of these subjects and the gruesome 'research' carried out were deterrents.[103]

From a teaching point of view racial hygiene was of fundamental importance in the racializing of medicine. The aim of the reformed medical curriculum was to transform the doctor from having a sense of duty to the individual to being a 'national physician'. Lenz complained that most universities merely gave a perfunctory lecture on hereditary pathology as part of a general course on pathology, instead of a special course on human heredity.[104] In 1936 the discipline became part of the medical teaching curriculum, and students were examined in those universities with a chair in the subject. In 1938 Verschuer urged that professors of racial hygiene band together in order to lobby the Education Ministry

[100] G. Aly and K.H. Roth, *Die restlose Erfassung, Volkzählen, Identifizieren, Aussondern im Nationalsozialismus* (Berlin, 1984), pp. 98–109; BDC file on Kranz.
[101] For the resistance of the medical faculty at Leipzig see STA Dresden Rassenpflege Nr 10209/48 on Reche's improved position at the Grassi Museum.
[102] H.W. Kranz, 'Zur Entwicklung der Rassenhygienischen Institute an unseren Hochschulen', *Ziel und Weg* vol. 9 (1939), 286–90.
[103] BDC Astel to Rector of Strasburg, 1 September 1941; De Crinis to Kuhnert, 15 February 1944; Zeiss to De Crinis, 31 August 1942.
[104] F. Lenz, 'Der rassenhygienische Unterricht für Mediziner', *Ziel und Weg*, vol. 4 (1934), 246–9.

as a group. But neither Lenz nor Rüdin wished to have the honour of convening such a meeting, vehemently denying that they were the longest serving racial hygienists.[105] The racial hygienists could neither engineer the situation so that all universities would have a chair in the subject, nor could they dictate the curriculum. In the general reform of medical education, implemented on 1 April 1939, pre-clinical students were taught hereditary science and racial studies in their second semester for three hours per week, and population policy for one hour in the third semester. Clinical students were taught human heredity for three hours per week in the ninth semester, and two hours of racial hygiene in the tenth semester. The arrangements remained controversial. Professors of racial hygiene wanted to extend the hours allocated to their subject whereas the demands of a practical medical education in wartime meant that ministerial officials wished to shorten the curriculum. Revised arrangements were made in spring 1944 for a single pre-clinical course on human heredity in the fourth semester and for a clinical course on hereditary pathology, racial hygiene and population policy in the tenth semester. This aroused such protest that in the autumn of 1944 the Reichsgesundheitsführer Conti obtained a doubling of the hours taught. That medical students were given a shortened course of training so that they could quickly be drafted into service as military doctors shows the depth of ideological commitment to racial values.[106]

Innovation in racial hygiene must be seen in the context of the institutional power structure of Nazi Germany. Some racial hygienists encountered difficulties which limited the role they could have as 'experts' on racial, health and settlement policies. Others such as Verschuer were drawn into the party political power structure. These changes occurred in the context of a weakening of the power of technocrats such as Rüdin and Gütt oriented to the public health administration, and a strengthening of groups in the SS and party for radical solutions to the Jewish and *Lebensraum* 'problems'. Political and strategic considerations overrode the scientific demands of the eugenicists. It is necessary to turn to the broader social context of the reorganizing of health care to understand the forces that restructured racial hygiene and embedded it in the terrain of the state, party and SS.

RACIAL HEALTH CARE

Racial hygiene was subordinated to the needs of the Nazi system of medicine. The aim of integrating racial hygiene, population policy and health care was to achieve total control over the body of every citizen. In certain respects the Nazi aims of a fit work force and a buoyant birth rate were in line with those of public health services in other countries. But Nazi leaders regarded the elimination of Jews and social deviants as a precondition for achieving a healthy people. Nazification of the 300,000 doctors, nurses, midwives, pharmacists, disinfectors, nursery nurses,

---

[105] Lenz papers, 22 December 1938, Lenz to Verschuer, 19 December 1938.
[106] BDC Lenz to De Crinis, 1942; De Crinis to Astel, 9 June 1944.

Table 8. *The growth of racial hygiene*

1 University institutes

Year/Institution	Appointee	Position	NSDAP/SS (Year)
1923–33 Munich	Lenz	aoP Rassenhygiene, Doz (1918)	NS (1937)
1927–45 Leipzig	Reche	oP Rassenkunde (Grassi-Museum)	NS (1937)/SS
1927–41 Berlin	E. Fischer	oP Anthropologie	NS (1939)
1933–45 Berlin	Lenz	oP Inst. für Rassenhygiene	NS (1937)
1933 Halle	Kürten	Lehrauftrag	NS
1933–45 Hamburg	Scheidt	Dir. Inst. für Rassen- und Kulturbiologie	none
1933–36 Munich	Tirala	oP Rassenhygiene	NS (1934)
1933–42 Greifswald	Just	oP Menschliche Erblehre und Eugenik	NS (1934)
1933–43 Graz	Reichel	oP Bevölkerungspolitik und Rassenhygiene Vorstand des Hygienischen Instituts	NS (1933)
1934–45 Jena	Astel	oP Inst. für Menschliche Erbforschung und Rassenpolitik RPolA	NS (1930) SS (1934) SS
1934–45 Tübingen	Gieseler	aoP, oP (1938) Dir.	
1934 Halle	Schnell	Lehrauftrag aoP (1935), aplUP (1939)	
1934–42 Königsberg	Loeffler	Dir. Rassenbiologisches Instituts	NS (1932)
1934–40 Düsseldorf	Haag	aoP	
1935 Halle	Mrugowsky	Doz. Lehrauftrag	NS/SS
1935–42 Frankfurt/M.	Verschuer	oP Dir. Inst. für Erbbiologie und Rassenhygiene	NS (1941)
1935–55 Kiel	Weinert	oP Dir. Anthropol Inst.	
1936–45 Hamburg	Weitz	oP Abteilung für Erb- und Zwillingsforschung an der II. Medizinische Universitätsklinik	
1936–45 Cologne	Claussen	aoP (1939) Inst. für Erbbiologie und Rassenhygiene kommissarischer Dir. Inst. für Rassenhygiene	NS (1937)
1936–44 Munich	Rüdin		NS
1937–42 Giessen	Kranz	aoP, oP (40) Erb und Rassenforschung. RPolA	NS (1937)
1937–45 Bonn	Panse	Doz., aoP (44). Rheinisches Inst. für psychiatrisch-neurologische Erbforschung	NS (1937)
1937–41 Würzburg	Schmidt-Kehl	aoP, Dir. Inst. für Vererbungswissenschaft und Rassenforschung. RPolA	NS

Table 8 (*cont.*)

Year/Institution	Appointee	Position	NSDAP/SS (Year)
1939 Graz	Polland	apl UP, Lehramt für Rassenhygiene	SS
1939 Breslau	W. Lehmann	Doz. Menschliche Erblehre und Rassenhygiene	
1939 Posen	Ponsold	Rassenkunde AoP	
1939 Strasburg		Rassenkunde	
1939–45 Innsbruck	Stumpfl	Inst. für Erb- und Rassenbiologie	
1940–45 Prague	Thums	aoP, Dir. Erbbiologie und Rassenhygiene	
1941–45 Strasburg	Neureiter	aoP, Dir. Inst. für gerichtliche Medizin und Kriminalistik	
1942–45 Berlin	Abel	oP Inst. für Rassenbiologie	SS
1942–45 Prague	B.K. Schultz	oP Inst. für Rassenbiologie	NS (1932)/SS
1942 Prague	K.V. Müller	Inst. für Sozialanthropologie	
1942–45 Berlin	Verschuer	oP menschliche Erblehre	NS (1941)
1942–45 Greifswald	Steiniger	oP Inst für menschliche Erblehre und Eugenik	
1942–45 Danzig	Grossmann	Lehrstuhl für Erbbiologie und Rassenhygiene	
1942–45 Königsberg	Duis	Rassenbiologisches Inst.	
1942–45 Vienna	Loeffler	oP Rassenbiologie und Rassenhygiene	NS
1942–45 Frankfurt/M.	Kranz	oP Erbbiologie und Rassenhygiene	NS
1943–45 Strasburg	W. Lehmann	aoP Rassenkunde	SS
1943–45 Würzburg	Just	Dir. Inst. für Rassenbiologie	NS
1943–45 Giessen	Boehm	oP Erb- und Rassenforschung	NS
1944 Rostock	Grebe	Dir. Inst. für Erbbiologie und Rassenhygiene	NS

2 Non-university institutes

Year	Location	Director	Institution	NS
1919	Munich	Rüdin	Deutsche Forschungsanstalt für Psychiatrie, Dir. Genealogisch-demographische Abteilung (from 1933, Inst. für Genealogie und Demographie), Dir. of Forschungsanstalt from 1928.	NS (1937)
1927–41	Berlin	Fischer	Dir. Kaiser Wilhelm Inst. für Anthropologie	NS (1939)
1934–	Berlin	Schütt	Doz. Staatsakademie des öffentlichen Gesundheitsdienstes	NS (1930)
1935–42	Alt-Rehse	Boehm	Erbbiologisches Forschungsinstitut	NS
1936–45	Berlin	Ritter	Reichsgesundheitsamt: Leiter d Rassenhygienischen und Bevölkerungsbiologischen Forschungsstelle	none
1937–42	Berlin	Just	Reichsgesundheitsamt: Leiter d Erbwissenschaftlichen Forschungsstelle	NS
1938–41	Berlin	Neureiter	Reichsgesundheitsamt: Dir. Kriminalbiologische Forschungsstelle	NS
1942–45	Berlin	Verschuer	Dir. Kaiser Wilhelm Inst. für Anthropologie	NS (1941)
1934	Berlin	Schütt	Poliklinik für Erb-u. Rassenpflege KAVH	NS (1930)

Note: Universities without an institute for anthropology or racial hygiene were Bonn, Düsseldorf, Erlangen, Göttingen, Halle, Marburg, Münster.
oP = Ordentlicher Professor, aoP = ausserordentlicher Professor, apl UP = ausserplanmässiger Universitätsprofessor, Dir. = Direktor, Doz. = Privatdozent, Inst. = Institut, NS = NSDAP member, SS = SS member, numbers in brackets denote year, RPolA = Rassenpolitisches Amt.
Sources: BDC; ARGB; Volk und Rasse; Koch, Gesellschaft für Konstitutionsforschung; Kürschners Gelehrtenlexikon (various edns); Proctor, Racial Hygiene, pp. 327–9.

welfare workers, statisticians, and university academics was a priority. A perceptive report by the British Foreign Office commented that each health worker was to be drilled and trained in the use of the latest and best weapons of science, so as to attack health problems. A massive army of volunteers also assisted in welfare work. Health meant not merely freedom from diseases, but positive measures to promote the health and fertility of elite racial groups to ensure racial progress towards Nazi social ideals.[107]

The fragmented eugenic initiatives of the Weimar welfare services were incorporated into the Nazi system of public health. New laws gave immense powers to public health officials. In 1933 came the law for compulsory sterilization, in 1934 the law for the unification of municipal and state health administrations, and in 1935 a marriage law accompanying the 'Nuremberg Laws' for the purity of the German blood. Their administrative machinery enabled 'total' morbidity, demographic and eugenic surveys to be built into public health procedures. Laws, as for midwifery reform, which had been planned but not implemented during the 1920s, were enacted. Authoritarian controls were imposed, where it was felt that the individual posed a threat to the health of the social order. Measures to control VD were intensified. Abortion and contraception were to be removed from the realm of individual choice. To compensate there were positive inducements of marriage grants and child allowances as part of a campaign to promote child rich families. Individualistic concepts of health were condemned as outmoded. Reichsgesundheitsführer Conti stated that no one had the right to regard health as a personal private matter, which could be disposed of according to individualistic preference.[108] Therapy had to be administered in the interests of the race and society rather than of the sick individual.

These innovations were countered by the deterioration since 1934 in rates of mortality and morbidity. Stricter enforcement of the registration of diseases meant that morbidity rates rose. The reality was difficult to determine, but worst of all was the increase in the diphtheria death rate. In 1933 there were 77,340 cases; in 1937 the number had risen to 146,733. An indictment of Nazi health care – *Heil Hunger* – reported upward trends for scarlet fever, spinal meningitis, infantile paralysis, typhoid and paratyphoid, although infant and TB mortality rates were falling as in France and Britain. There was also a growth in industrial accidents owing to the priorities of preparations for war.[109] The greater the hazards, the greater was the necessity for medical intervention. This can be illustrated by industrial health, an area in which cadres of industrial medical officers were recruited from 1936. Their function was not so much to diagnose sickness in the individual, but to raise

---

[107] Foreign Office and Ministry of Economic Warfare, *The Nazi System of Medicine and Public Health Organization* (London, 1944).

[108] Conti, quoted in M.H. Kater, 'Die Gesundheitsführung des Deutschen Volkes', *Medizinhistorisches Journal*, vol. 18 (1983), 349–75.

[109] R.M. Titmuss, review of M. Gumpert, *Heil Hunger!* (London, 1940), *Eugenics Review*, vol. 32 (1940), 63–4.

productivity by minimizing absenteeism due to illness.[110] Fitness and health were to be achieved on a selective basis that involved positive measures for physical regeneration (*Aufartung*) and the elimination of the degenerate. Social hygiene continued to be a priority, with particular interest in early diagnosis in matters such as TB among youth, and efficient use was made of the new technology of mobile X-ray units.[111] Deteriorating health intensified the resolve of eugenicists to conserve human population resources and to expand health and welfare services.

There was a coherence in the medical aims of Nazi leaders such as Himmler and the Reichsgesundheitsführer Conti during the 1940s. But the system did not evolve smoothly. Competing strategies resulted in conflicting eugenic policies. Power blocs within the state, party and SS had differing aims, and they were supported by rival factions among the medical profession and racial hygiene experts. The lack of unity among racial hygienists resulted in vacillations in legislation, and in unstable administrative and professional structures. The medical profession lost autonomy. Whereas during the 1920s medical police had been virtually replaced by professionalized welfare, after 1933 public health became an arm of policing powers. The Reich Ministry of the Interior ensured co-ordination between public health and the police. As the medical authorities became subject to the SS, the racial aims of extermination, conquest and raising hereditary quality became priorities. Policing measures required centralization, which was achieved at a number of levels. The Bismarckian balance between autonomous chambers of doctors and sickness funds was ended in 1933 by the law unifying the sickness funds. At the same time the profession was nazified.[112] In April and June 1933 'non Aryans' were excluded from sickness insurance practice. This was enforced by doctors' organizations of the NSDAP. It was a hasty and violent process administered by the henchmen of Reichsärzteführer Wagner and professional leaders such as Haedenkamp. The medical dictators came into conflict with the Reich Ministry of Labour which temporarily gained control of the sickness insurance system.[113] Each provincial *Gau* had a medical commissioner in the Reich Ministry of the Interior during 1933. Conti was representative for *Gau* Gross-Berlin, Blome for Mecklenburg, Walther Schultze for Bavaria, Carl Oskar Klipp for Thuringia, and Stähle for Württemberg-Hohenzollern. These medical *Gauleiters* had been party activists since the 1920s, and were to have a powerful role in implementing Nazi racial policies.[114] The health commissioners unified the

110 D. Milles, 'Tendenzen und Konsequenzen. Arbeit und Krankheit unter Einfluss nationalsozialistischer Sozialpolitik', in Milles and R. Müller (eds.), *Berufsarbeit und Krankheit* (Frankfurt-on-Main, 1983), pp. 111–26.
111 M. Stahl, 'Krankheit und Politik am Beispiel der Tuberkulose', *Volk und Gesundheit*, pp. 85–100.
112 M.H. Kater, 'Medizin und Mediziner im Dritten Reich. Eine Bestandsaufnahme', *Historische Zeitschrift*, vol. 244 (1987), 249–352.
113 S. Leibfried and F. Tennstedt, 'Sozialpolitik und Berufsverbote im Jahre 1933', *Zeitschrift für Sozialreform*, vol. 25 (1979); (reprinted Bremen, 1981).
114 BDC, Stähle joined the NSDAP on 8 August 1927, Nr. 65877.

medical administration. Whereas in many states health had been subordinate to other ministries, centralized administrative bodies for health were established in every province. That the health commissioners were doctors represented the fulfilling of the long-cherished professional dream of a central health administration under medical control. Health commissioners had authoritarian powers, and could override the legal structures that had posed barriers to implementation of medical measures.

The National Socialist Doctors' League enhanced the unity of the profession, while placing it at the service of the Nazi Party. Wagner sought to obtain guarantees that the medical profession was a 'free profession', and that nature therapists should cease to have the right to practise. At the same time he obtained control over medical representative associations so giving the profession greater internal cohesion.[115] Nazism initiated a phase of professional power based on co-ordination and unity. In spring 1936 a *Reichsärztekammer* was established. A power struggle occurred for control of health care between state and party. Each allied with factions in the profession. Wagner wished to unify professional and public health administration under the auspices of the party *Gauleiter*. This failed in Berlin where Conti had only a Prussian and not the Reich post. Gütt took over on 19 February 1934 as *Leiter* of the Reich Ministry Department of Health. Gütt used his position to strengthen a centralized state structure of public health, limiting the power of Wagner's populist party organization. In Thuringia Klipp, supported by Gross of the NSDAP's Racial Political Office, was challenged by the racial hygienist Astel, who was protected by Himmler and the SS. In Munich the powers of the local *Gau* representative were checked by Staatskommissar Schultze.[116] Party ideologues were challenged by state public health administrators.

Wagner's power base in the National Socialist Doctors' League steadily grew. Its membership rose from 2,786 in January 1933 to 11,000 in October and by 1942 there were 42,000 (including an unknown proportion of dentists, veterinary surgeons and pharmacists). This represented a complete *Gleichschaltung* of the profession, and meant that doctors were strongly represented in the Nazi Party. Wagner was a party animal in contrast to Gütt who was a state creature. Wagner was close friends with Martin Bormann, who as head of the party chancellery ensured links with the central party machinery as well as with the Führer, to whom he acted as private secretary. This covered Wagner in his expansive policy to extend health care on a racial basis.[117]

Racial hygiene retained an influence on key medical officials. For example, Gütt and Astel had been thoroughly schooled in eugenics before 1933, and continued to cultivate links with Ploetz and Rüdin. But they came into conflict with racial ideologues when Wagner tried to establish institutions for public health and racial hygiene. In April 1933 a Propaganda Office for Population Policy and Racial

[115] G. Lilienthal, 'Der Nationalsozialistische Deutsche Ärztebund (1929–1943/1945)', in F. Kudlien (ed.), *Ärzte im Nationalsozialismus* (Cologne, 1985), pp. 109–114.
[116] Lilienthal, 'Ärztebund', pp. 115–16; BDC Astel file.
[117] Lilienthal, 'Ärztebund', pp. 116–19; Labisch and Tennstedt, *GVG*, I, pp. 266–78.

Welfare[118] was inaugurated. Rudolf Hess decreed in November 1933 that all racial questions in the party were to be submitted to this office.[119] In May 1934 this became the Racial Political Office of the NSDAP under Gross, and assumed responsibility for racial ideology. Rivalling these initiatives of the party was the Expert Committee for Population and Racial Policy,[120] which was established in May 1933 by Gütt on behalf of the Reich Ministry of the Interior. This was on the pattern of previous expert committees such as that for population policy during the First World War. Its members included veteran racial hygienists such as Lenz, Ploetz and Rüdin, medical leaders of welfare organizations such as Bodo Spiethoff of the Society to Prevent Venereal Diseases, and ideologues such as Baldur von Schirach, Darré, Günther and Schultze-Naumburg. But it was dominated by Nazi medical reformers such as Bartels, Gütt, Lösener, Ruttke and Wagner. It was divided into three sections. The first was for finance, taxation, statistics, social policy and settlement, with the aim of introducing family welfare benefits as in France and Italy. The second *Arbeitsgemeinschaft* was for racial hygiene and racial policy. This was to oversee research in the Kaiser Wilhelm Gesellschaft and universities, and the training of public health and other medical personnel. It was to scrutinize the organization and costs of public health services, and to suggest how biological research in racial hygiene could be applied, particularly in sterilization measures. It was also to develop propaganda in racial hygiene for the general public, and to transform the registry offices into 'family offices'. Gütt was appointed with Himmler's approval as head of the second section and with orders to ensure unified precepts for racial hygiene policies. The third section was for women's and maternal health and welfare.[121] It represented an attempt by the Ministry of the Interior to incorporate such organizations as the Reich League for Child Rich Families. The committee was initially dominated by such racial hygienists as Rüdin when it held its first sitting on 28 June 1933 on the birth rate. Political figures such as Himmler wrote of their interest in the discussions.[122] This committee was too large and disparate to be a real policy-making body; regular meetings ceased after 1936 and it had fallen into abeyance by 1939 as Gütt's influence was also on the wane.[123]

Although the committee system was too unwieldy for health and population policy, attempts to create streamlined administrative hierarchies resulted in conflicts between and within party and state. Gütt avoided using the Reich Health Office as an advisory body so as not to create a competing authority. Later, this resulted in a dispute within the SS and between Reiter of the Health Office and

---

[118] *Aufklärungsamt für Bevölkerungspolitik und Rassenpflege.*

[119] ZSTA P 15.01 Nr 26297.

[120] *Sachverständigen Beirat für Bevölkerungs- und Rassenpolitik im Reichsinnenministerium.*

[121] BAK R73 Nr 170 Reichsinnenministerium, 4 November 1933; BHSTA MF 68015 Medizinalwesen 1931–40.

[122] ZSTA P 15.01 Nr 26228/1 Sachverständigen Beirat June 1933–February 1934, Himmler 27 September and 27 October 1933; Bock, *Zwangssterilisation*, pp. 85, 95.

[123] H. Kaupen-Haas, 'Die Bevölkerungsplaner im sachverständigen Beirat für Bevölkerungs- und Rassenpolitik', in Kaupen-Haas (ed.), *Der Griff nach der Bevölkerung*, pp. 103–120.

[124] BAK NS 19/1063 Reiter to Gütt, 25 September 1939.

Gütt.[124] In August 1933 a committee of health experts was founded with Wagner at its head. This became the party's health office[125] in May 1936, with powers to ensure Nazi priorities in all aspects of health care. It meant that the Nazi party became the controlling body in racial and health questions, rather than the Doctors' League. The latter was a subordinate component of the Nazi machinery. Wagner continued to strive for a central health organization controlled by the party and not by state ministries.[126] The Ministry of the Interior lost the battle to control medical organizations and policies for the 'child rich'. Hess argued that the League for the Child Rich was an ideological organization, which ought to be taken under the wing of the party and of Gross' Racial Political Office.[127] These developments amounted to a weakening of the status and influence of medically qualified experts in racial hygiene.

Wagner's idea was to nazify medicine by a reformed system of primary care. He spoke of the need to return to 'the family doctor system of the good old days'. He established a medical training centre for school doctors. Instead of considering single diseases, the Nazi doctor should concentrate on the 'racial and *völkisch* diseases of the body politic'. Nature and dietary therapies should be incorporated into medicine in order to bring the doctor closer to the *Volk* and a mythical pedigree of the doctor as folk hero and Paracelsian magician was conjured up. In Dresden the Rudolf Hess Hospital developed a synthesis of medicine based on science, racial hygiene and folk remedies. The nutritional department was placed under a Swedish chemist, Ragnar Berg, and attempts were made to appoint Bircher-Brenner, the muesli discoverer (and once an associate of Ploetz) from Switzerland. Wagner opposed narrowly scientific medicine and the extension of hospitals. Plans were made to replace hospitals by 'Health Houses' where work therapy and health education were priorities. Hohenlychen, an orthopaedic hospital opened by the Waffen SS surgeon Karl Gebhardt, was a model.[128] (Gebhardt was Himmler's personal doctor.) It suggests that Wagner was competing with SS-sponsored innovations. Wagner's aims denied a privileged expert role to racial hygiene, and rejected its scientific methodology. His *völkisch* appropriation of nature therapy accounts for the intense hostility to academic racial hygiene which appeared by the mid-1930s.

STERILIZATION AND RACIAL SURVEYS

Drafting the law

The Law to Prevent Hereditarily Sick Offspring[129] by compulsory sterilization was rapidly drafted and decreed during 1933. The law drew on the protracted

---

[125] Amt für Volksgesundheit der NSDAP.   [126] Lilienthal, 'Ärztebund', pp. 118–21.

[127] J. Stephenson, '"Reichsbund der Kinderreichen": the League of Large Families in the Population Policy of Nazi Germany', *European Studies Review*, vol. 9 (1979), 350–75.

[128] A. Haug, 'Pläne für ein Gesundheitshaus der deutschen Ärzteschaft', in Kudlien (ed.), *Ärzte*, pp. 139, 147–9.   [129] *Gesetz zur Verhütung erbkranken Nachwuchses.*

discussions during the Weimar Republic; its swift implementation and the switch from voluntary to compulsory sterilization resulted from pressure by Nazi medical officials who saw sterilization as part of racial and population policy. Racial hygiene and Nazism were a potent combination. Weimar democracy limited the authority of scientific experts, whereas Nazism initially enhanced their powers. Hitherto, only the closed world of medical institutions offered scope for unbridled pursuit of the scientific laws of hereditary pathology. Certain asylums and clinics had conducted secret sterilizations. Indeed, Paul Nitsche, the veteran racial hygienist who took a key role in the T4 medical killing programme, testified that secret 'euthanasia' had occurred before 1933. The time had come to extend the authority of experts in medical genetics over the totality of society, as if it were one vast closed institution.

The pressures for sterilization legislation that had built up during 1932 were interrupted by the Nazi seizure of power on 31 January 1933 and by the dissolution of the Reichstag. Papen suggested a decree as the most economic and effective way of implementing sterilization laws. In March 1933 the Prussian Minister of the Interior, Hermann Göring, transferred the draft law that had been prepared in 1932, to the Reich Ministries of the Interior and Justice. The aim was to add compulsory clauses. In April 1933 Sauckel, the *Gauleiter* of Thuringia, suggested that no time be lost in implementing sterilization. This should be done by the existing public health authorities, and university anthropological institutes. All that was needed was a law on the basis of the Enabling Law of 24 March. Sauckel showed how readily the existing administrative and academic structures could be turned to racial purposes. In May 1933 this long-term aim of racial hygienists was achieved, simply by legalizing sterilization by a clause in the revised criminal code: this declared that sterilization did not constitute assault.[130]

The Nazis required a system that would locate and refer people to the authorities for sterilization. Procedures restricted to individuals requesting sterilization as a means of contraception were anathema. Sterilization had to serve the collective interests of society and the race, and not the individual. This was to be achieved by extending the scope and powers of public health officials and by reorganizing public health on a racial basis. The measures were the responsibility of Gütt, a medical officer, whom the Nazis promoted to the Reich Ministry of the Interior in May 1933. Gütt had joined the Nazi Party in July 1932, having previously organized a cell of the *Nationalsozialistische Freiheitspartei* after the Hitler Putsch of 1923. In 1926 he had been appointed medical officer under the Prussian official Krohne. In September 1932 he addressed the Congress of German Medical Officials on the need to reorganize public health on the basis of hereditary science, racial hygiene and population policy. In February 1933 Gütt sent a memorandum on 'state population policy' to the *Gauleiter* of the *Ostmark* with the request that the plans be brought to the attention of Frick and Göring.[131] Gütt won the support of

---

[130] ZSTA P 15.01 Nr 26248.
[131] U.D. Adam, *Judenpolitik im Dritten Reich* (Düsseldorf, 1979), pp. 31–3.

Frick, the Reich Minister of the Interior (and earlier the patron of Günther in Thuringia), for a fusion of state and municipal health offices.[132] State health officials were to be responsible for a hereditary biological census, sterilization, hereditary health, and a racial population policy. Sterilization was thus part of a powerful institutional network, and was a component of health and racial policies. Emigration of high value German racial stocks was to be prevented, whereas the emigration of such racial degenerates as Jews was encouraged. Gütt's memorandum urged the subordination of every facet of social life to racial hygienic priorities of improving the quantity and quality of the German people. His attack on individualism was similar to that of the scientific racial hygienists – even voting should be on a family basis. In many ways his views – such as hostility to alcohol and tobacco – can be seen to derive from broader eugenic currents. Yet what was novel was his insistence on centralization of health administration and on an interventive state with powers to segregate, sterilize and decree abortions. He coined the term for hereditary and racial welfare, *Erb- und Rassenpflege*. He supported settlement policies in the East to remedy urban degeneration and to fulfil the German national mission. Gütt's manifesto reveals influence of Darré's idealization of the German peasant and of Nordic racism. It shows the racist premisses of the planned system of health care and sterilization.[133]

Gütt owed his appointment to medical qualifications in public health, zeal in promoting racial hygiene and population policy, and contacts in the National Socialist Doctors' League. Although his energy in the pursuit of sterilization resulted in his admission to the SS in 1933, his policies were state and professionally oriented. He described this as pursuing a pragmatic middle way between academic racial hygiene and the wilder fantasies of party political racists.[134] He recruited competent experts to assist him. Between May and July 1933 Gütt worked feverishly on the sterilization law with the able lawyer, Ruttke, who had previously represented the meat traders' association.[135] He relied on the psychiatrist and racial hygienist, Rüdin, to secure rigorously scientific legislation that would be acceptable to both academics and the medical profession.[136] They planned measures to promote positive health and to solve the problem of 'hereditary crime' by sterilization or castration of criminals. But the Reich Justice Minister objected to having hereditary diseases and crime in the same law. Eugenic abortion was shelved for political reasons.

The law was presented to the cabinet on 14 July 1933. Papen objected that some of the diseases were curable and that the Catholic Church could not allow the state to usurp control over reproduction. The law was supported by Hitler, and after

---

[132] On the centrality of Gütt to Nazi public health see Labisch and Tennstedt, *GVG*, I, pp. 236–78.
[133] BDC Gütt file, 'Staatliche Bevölkerungspolitik'; Gütt, *Dienst an der Rasse als Aufgabe der Politik* (Berlin, 1934); W. Frick and Gütt, *Nordisches Gedankengut im Dritten Reich* (Munich: Lehmann, 1936).   [134] BDC Gütt file, 21 June 1944.
[135] BDC Ruttke file NSDAP member from 1 May 1932 Nr 1097130.
[136] A. Ploetz and E. Rüdin, 'Ministerialdirektor Dr Gütt 5 Jahre Leiter der Abteilung für Volksgesundheit im Reichs- und Preussischen Ministeriums des Inneren', *ARGB*, vol. 33 (1939), 89.

waiting for the Catholic concordat on 20 July, it was published on 26 July, so as to come into force on 1 January 1934.[137] A Law Against Compulsive Criminality[138] was passed in November 1933, enabling preventive detention and castration. These laws were regarded by Gütt, Rüdin and Ruttke as demonstrating that liberal and Christian humanitarian solutions to disease and crime were outmoded. Hereditary defects were to be eliminated by medical intervention so that future generations would be free from crime and disease.[139]

The sterilization law shows how professional powers and state authority reinforced one another. Nine 'diseases' were selected: hereditary feeble-mindedness, schizophrenia, manic-depression, hereditary epilepsy, Huntington's chorea, hereditary blindness, hereditary deafness, hereditary malformations, and (indicating the historical roots of the law) severe alcoholism. A system of hereditary courts was established; each tribunal was composed of a lawyer, a medical officer and a doctor with specialist training in racial hygiene. The medical officer could initiate proceedings as well as adjudicate, and doctors were in the majority. The state established primacy over reproduction, but left the operating of the controls to the medical profession. Such professionalism benefited from state decrees rather than cumbersome parliamentary procedures.

Racial hygiene and state health services

The passing of the law needed the support of the Nazi state and was designed to reinforce its authority. The law was more than just a 'strictly medical' measure. It provided the opportunity for a massive state publicity campaign on racial hygiene. Gross' Racial Political Office competed with Ruttke's Reich Committee for Health Education. This campaign emphasized the cost of institutional care, and the need for healthy, vigorous families, so looking forward to other 'reforms'. Publicity was drummed up by radio talks, the drama *Erbstrom*, the film 'Sins of the Father', and the exhibition 'Hereditary Health − Hereditary Disease'.[140] The publicity techniques developed during the 1920s welfare campaigns served Nazi ideological ends.[141]

The medical profession and especially psychiatrists benefited greatly from the drive for sterilization. They had responsibilities in training, administering and adjudicating on the law in 250 tribunals. These enhanced status and also income, since the work paid well. Racial hygienists such as Fischer, Rüdin and Verschuer took a leading role in organizing the tribunals. The institutes for social hygiene were expanded. These were to provide courses for medical officers and psychiatrists, adjudication on problematic cases, and further research on inherited

[137] GSTA Dahlem Rep 84a Nr 871 Bl. 23–45.
[138] *Gesetz gegen gefährliche Gewohnheitsverbrecher.*
[139] A. Gütt, E. Rüdin and F. Ruttke, *Gesetz zur Verhütung erbkranken Nachwuchses vom 14. Juli 1933* (Munich: Lehmann, 1934), p. 6. [140] *Erbgesund-Erbkrank.*
[141] Bock, *Zwangssterilisation*, pp. 90–3.

diseases. Certain welfare experts working for the churches, such as Harmsen, fervently supported the laws. Police, civil servants and social workers had to be alerted as to their duty to notify the authorities of cases of hereditary diseases. The laws enlarged the responsibilities of a wide range of authorities, and of medical and academic institutions.

Many of the eugenicists who in the 1920s had supported a welfare-oriented and voluntaristic approach became converts to the principle of compulsion. Behr-Pinnow praised the compulsory law, illustrating his transition from being a staunch opponent of birth control while in the retinue of the Empress, to becoming a positive eugenicist during the 1920s as president of the League for Regeneration. He wrote that although he had been active in eugenics since 1909, twenty-five years ago one hardly could speak of eugenic sterilization.[142] Some of those active in the Weimar Marriage and Sexual Advice Clinics also used their position as medical officers to demand sterilization of the proletariat.[143] Not all racial hygienists were satisfied. For Boeters, the sterilization campaigner and NSDAP member since 1930, the laws were too moderate.[144] To others, the principle of compulsion was unwarranted. Luxenburger and Lenz dissented. They were aware that once scientists were compelled to refer patients for sterilization, popular hostility would impede research in human genetics. Rudolf Kraemer (significantly a lawyer and himself blind), went further by denouncing the whole law and the concept of degeneracy in May 1933.[145] He argued that hereditary biologists such as 'Lenzmann, Mucker and Fischbauer' confused heredity in animals and man, and that only 3.85 per cent of blindness was inherited. Such radical condemnation was a rarity. Other organizations for the blind welcomed the 'peace and order' of national socialism and accepted compulsory sterilization. Kraemer also acquiesced in voluntary sterilization.[146]

The laws were backed up by extensive institutional machinery, geared to hereditary censuses and surveys. From 1 April 1935, clinics for hereditary and racial care were instituted.[147] These were to use standardized genealogical forms and card indices for research on patients' families, ancestry and health over four generations. A second copy was to be sent to the health office at the place of birth 'as the basis for a hereditary biological survey of the total population'. The cards were colour coded for gender, and had further codings for categories including criminals, hereditary diseases, and non-Aryan races. A single centralized data bank was to be established at each health office. The clinics were to have the co-operation of state and party organizations, doctors, hospitals and medical institutions,

[142] ZSTA P 15.01 Nr 26248 Bl. 246 Behr-Pinnow to Reich Minister des Inneren, 29 May 1933.
[143] Bock, *Zwangssterilisation*, pp. 185–6.
[144] ZSTA P 15.01 Nr 26248 Bl. 362; BDC Boeters file NSDAP member from 1 December 1930, Nr 381455.   [145] ZSTA P 15.01 Nr 26248 Bl. 42–3, 263–5.
[146] Bock, *Zwangssterilisation*, pp. 279–80; R. Kraemer, *Kritik der Eugenik vom Standpunkt des Betroffenen* (Berlin, 1933); G. Richter, *Blindheit und Eugenik (1918–1945)* (Freiburg i.B., 1986); ZSTA P 15.01 Nr 26248 reply to Kraemer, 8 June 1933, by Zeiss.
[147] *Beratungsstellen für Erb- und Rassenpflege*.

genealogists, and, hopefully, patients' relatives. Doctors were to advise 'burdened families' on how to 'revive their ancestries', and healthy families on how they could be best kept in good form.[148]

The state and party gained control of racial hygiene and genealogy. Diverse genealogical societies were collected together into a *Reichsverein für Sippenforschung* (Reich Association for Family Research) by Achim Gercke, a party activist who in February 1933 was appointed as an expert on racial research to the Prussian Ministry of the Interior. In 1935 he headed a *Reichsstelle für Sippenforschung* (Reich Office for Family Research) where ancestries were gathered together from the *völkisch* movement. For example, one million cards were included from parish registers in Berlin from 1800 to 1850. Stormtroopers, doctors and teachers (of the *Sturmabteilungen* or SA) collected genealogies of 300,000 Jews. The aim was to register every German in a *Sippenkartei* (an index of family ancestry) including details of hereditary health. This Reich Office was responsible for certificates of Aryan ancestry and adjudication in dubious cases.[149] By 1937 half a million cards were collected by the Thuringian Health Office, and by 1936 300,000 cards were prepared for psychiatric and neurological research in the Rhineland. In Hamburg there was an extensive 'health passport' system, and a hereditary index combined records from sickness funds, police, welfare offices and institutions. Over one million cards were collected by 1939, but there was a backlog of 750,000 records. Hamburg was remarkable for its efficient administration, but low degree of ideological Nazism. It was no coincidence that here were the greatest numbers of sterilizations, and compulsory labour camps for the 'antisocial'.[150]

By way of contrast the health office of Thuringia under Astel showed a high degree of racial motivation in its pursuit of the elimination of the antisocial and the promotion of peasant health. Both Hamburg and Thuringia were indebted to developments in racial hygiene and population policy before 1933. The state could profit from the welfare work of the 1920s. The card indices of the SPD and sickness funds supporting Berlin health centres were taken over by the Nazis. From two million cards, several thousand hereditarily ill were selected.[151] In Saxony Fetscher's criminal biological survey was used.[152] Although Fetscher pressed for a stronger law, he was deprived of his professorship and was banned from lecturing and publishing by the Saxon health commissioner.[153] (After a brief period of research on the pesticide Zyklon for IG-Farben, he opened a general practice; he

[148] Bock, *Zwangssterilisation*, pp. 283–6.
[149] Roth, 'Bestandsaufnahme', pp. 63–64.
[150] A. Ebbinghaus, H. Kaupen-Haas and K-H. Roth, *Heilen und Vernichten im Mustergau Hamburg. Bevölkerungs- und Gesundheitspolitik im Dritten Reich* (Hamburg, 1984).
[151] Hansen, *Verschüttete Alternativen*, p. 468 on health centre records; Roth, 'Bestandsaufnahme', p. 65; W. Tourne, 'Erfahrungen bei der erbbiologischen Bestandsaufnahme in der Erbbiologischen Zentrale des Verbandes der Krankenkassen in Berlin', *Der Erbarzt*, no. 1 (1935), 9.
[152] R. Fetscher, *Rassenhygiene, eine erste Einführung für Lehrer* (Leipzig, 1933).
[153] Fetscher papers, Rüdin to Fetscher, 24 June and 2 July 1934; E. Reinhardt Verlag to Fetscher, 3 November 1937; Rektor der Technischen Hochschule to Fetscher, 12 November 1936; Bock, *Zwangssterilisation*, p. 94.

became a major figure in a largely communist resistance group, which used his surgery as a cover for illegal contacts.) Surveys were made of patients in mental hospitals, special schools, alcoholic rehabilitation centres, and homes for those with disabilities. Paul Nitsche led a research group in the German Psychiatric Association.[154] These surveys were a precondition for extermination.

Sharpening up procedures

Racial hygienists had an important role in compiling and organizing hereditary data banks. In January 1934 Rüdin presided over a conference on 'Heredity and racial hygiene in the *völkisch* state', attended by the elite of geneticists, directors of hospitals, NSDAP racial experts and state officials.[155] Division of labour was agreed with the *Reichsstelle für Sippenforschung*. Plans were laid to co-ordinate census taking and hereditary biological research for the total population as a basis for hereditary health legislation.[156] This initiated co-ordination and planning of the medical surveys. The conference coincided with the implementation of hereditary health tribunals, and paved the way for clinics for heredity and racial health.

Behind the efforts of the racial hygienists to promote surveillance lay the expansive plans of Gütt and the Reich Ministry of the Interior. Gütt co-ordinated the Hereditary Biology Department of the Reich Health Office, and the Health Department of the Reich Ministry of the Interior. Gütt insisted on standardization of medical examinations and records, the main aim being to evaluate families. The model was the criminal biological survey of Rüdin and Viernstein that had been operating for over ten years but had extended its documentation with records from the NSV Mother and Child welfare organization. The Hereditary Biological Commission of the German municipalities[157] (representing municipal health authorities) joined forces with these efforts from June 1935.[158] Procedures were laid down in a decree of 8 February 1936 by the Reich Ministry of the Interior. The *Gemeindetag* (supportive of local health authorities) initiated a national survey of hospitals and welfare institutions in September 1935, and results were ready for Bavaria within a year. It was carried out by Wilhelm Stemmler (previously director of the Hereditary and Racial office of Hessen Nassau) of Wiesbaden.[159] The national survey completed in 1939, formed the basis of the T4 medical killing programme, as it provided medical and statistical information on 'incurables', and there was continuity of personnel. The committee convened in June 1935 included not only the veteran eugenicist Rüdin, but also psychiatrists such as Nitsche, Rodenberg and Hans Roemer and the medical administrator with Reich responsibility for hospitals, Herbert Linden. Although not all members of the

[154] Roth, 'Bestandsaufnahme', pp. 64–5; L. Schmidt-Kehl, 'Praktische Bevölkerungspolitik an der Rhön', *ARGB*, vol. 30 (1936), 392.
[155] E. Rüdin (ed.), *Erblehre und Rassenhygiene im völkischen Staat* (München, 1934).
[156] Roth, 'Bestandsaufnahme', p. 67.   [157] *Deutscher Gemeindetag*.
[158] BHSTA M Inn 79478 Erbbiologische Bestandsaufnahme.
[159] Roth, 'Bestandsaufnahme', pp. 78–80.

committee were involved in medical killing – indeed Roemer resigned as asylum director in protest – the committee and its statistical survey formed the nucleus of later Reich commissions designed to liquidate asylum patients.[160]

There were model schemes to racialize public health on Nazi lines. Astel in Thuringia set to work to build up a public health structure that was to combine a high degree of ideological commitment to Nazism and the SS with genetic screening of the population.[161] In 1937 Astel elaborated to Himmler his policing aims that included a preventive death penalty for would-be murderers.[162] He set to work to build up a data bank of index cards by means of which he could sift out the 'antisocial' and 'pathologically degenerate' from the supposedly racially valuable elements of the population. He hunted for homosexuals, criminals and the mentally subnormal, while praising the value of the peasant stock for the regeneration of the Volk.[163] He sought a favourable rate of differential fertility to achieve these ends.[164] He established an institute for racial policy and human heredity at the university of Jena, where he was renowned for enforcing his hatred of tobacco as a racial poison by striking cigarettes from students' mouths.

Demographers were enthusiastic supporters for combining policing with racial and health measures. The director of the Reich Statistical Office, Burgdörfer, was on good terms with Astel, Gütt and Rüdin. They formed a powerful alliance. Burgdörfer developed statistics for those of 'high' and 'low' hereditary worth, and analyzed the age-structure of the population. He masterminded the national censuses of 1933 and 1939. He supported compulsory registration of the population in January 1938,[165] identity cards (in 1939) and identity numbers. Pro-natalist and racial hygienic statisticians provided a technology of registration and analysis, and categories for investigation of the family, race, heredity and cultural identity. Hollerith punch-cards were automatically sorted. Cohort analyses were made of fertility in the 1939 census of the population as relevant to marriage loans and to long-term planning for military recruitment, as well as for ascertaining the statistics of religions and races. Demographers provided the regime with technologies of surveillance and control. Whereas Burgdörfer was a state technocrat, Richard Korherr was recruited by Himmler as an SS statistician. Korherr had dedicated his study on the declining birth rate to Spengler, and it attracted praise from Mussolini and Himmler. From 1940 his duties were to provide the statistical basis for 'resettlement' policies in the East by providing military and racial statistics.[166] Heydrich, the chief of the security services, criminal police and Gestapo, greatly valued systematic demographic statistics. They were of

[160] BHSTA M Inn 79478 *Erbbiologische Bestandsaufnahme in den Heil- und Pflegeanstalten, Deutscher Gemeindetag, 1939.*   [161] K. Astel, *Die Aufgabe* (Jena, 1937).

[162] BDC Astel file, 14 April 1937, Astel to Himmler.

[163] BDC Astel file, *Bericht über die Tätigkeit des Thüringischen Landesamtes für Rassewesen seit Gründung der Behörde 15 Juli bis 22 November 1933.*

[164] K. Astel and Erna Weber, *Die unterschiedliche Fortpflanzung. Untersuchung über die Fortpflanzung von 14000 Handwerkern Mittelthüringens* (Munich, 1939).   [165] *Reichsmeldeordnung.*

[166] Aly and Roth, *Restlose Erfassung,* pp. 32–5; R. Korherr, *Geburtenrückgang. Mahnruf an das Deutsche Volk mit einem Geleitwort des Reichsführers SS Heinrich Himmler* (Munich, 1935).

value for policies of Germanization and for Nazi racial measures. Medical statistics were an important component of the racial programme. The statistician, Siegfried Koller planned to sterilize not only the sufferers, but also the carriers of diseases. He calculated the possibilities of inheriting a wide range of hereditary conditions.[167] He researched on the inheritance of 'antisocial' characteristics and estimated that there were 1.6 million such undesirables in Germany. In 1941 Koller was appointed director of a Biostatistical Institute under Conti in Berlin. He supported a 'final solution' of the problem of the 'antisocial'.

The centralized state demographic, medical, and racial hygienic machinery functioned poorly. The task was greater than could ever be achieved. The compilation and processing of the statistics was left to the erratic quality of the regional health offices, hence the uneven implementation of the sterilization legislation. Problematic cases were referred for adjudication to experts in racial hygiene who often had more cases than they could cope with, although financial incentives were provided for rapid decisions. The sterilization law encountered hostility within the regime because it was not primarily anti-semitic in its conception or procedures. Aimed at the mentally ill and socially deviant, it enhanced the powers of Nazi state technocrats. Party ideologues such as Gross and Wagner actually condemned the law for its lack of anti-semitism. They loathed the *Ostjuden* as especially degenerate, and mass sterilization was later considered as a means of solving the 'Jewish question'. The technocrat lobby was constrained by the legalistic framework that it had erected. A meeting in March 1935 of the Reich Council for Population and Racial Policy, presided over by Rüdin and *Ministerialdirektor* Gütt, discussed sterilization of mulattos among whom were included 600 children born after the Rhineland occupation. Lenz and Rüdin urged enforced emigration of the mulattos, and Rüdin advised against plans for X-ray sterilization currently being discussed in the party. Gross and Wagner demanded secret and compulsory sterilization, and insisted that the Führer decide the issue. By 1937 Wagner's course of action was followed, and the human geneticists Fischer and Abel of the Kaiser Wilhelm Institute for Anthropology in Berlin were among the medical adjudicators. The rift between the racial hygienists was evident in the dispute with Rüdin who was allied to the state technocrat lobby of Gütt, and with Fischer who complied with Wagner's party-oriented racial policies. These sterilizations were technically illegal, in that they were carried out in secret, and were for purely racial rather than for hereditary biological reasons, in violation of the sterilization law.[168]

The Nuremberg and marriage laws

Wagner pressed for radicalization of the sterilization law. In September 1934 he decreed that abortion for degenerate parents was free of prosecution. Gütt

[167] Aly and Roth, *Restlose Erfassung*, pp. 96–101.
[168] Pommerin, *Rheinlandbastarde*, pp. 71–9; Bock, *Zwangssterilisation*, pp. 104–16.

attempted to convince the Führer that this was a mistake, although Hitler sided with Wagner. The law was extended to other supposedly deviant groups. In June 1935 castration was decreed for homosexuals. In February 1936 sterilization of women over thirty-six was to be undertaken by X-rays, so as to reduce mortality from the operation. From 1933 Wagner was urging a racial definition of citizenship. Wagner, Gross and Bartels (all medical ideologues of the NSDAP) urged a strong law to eliminate Jews from German life. The result was the infamous Nuremberg laws of 15 September 1935, to 'Protect German Blood and Honour'. A citizenship law went with a law forbidding marriage and sexual intercourse between Jews and gentiles. On 18 October 1935 marriages of the hereditarily ill with the healthy were forbidden. The state hesitated over comprehensive health certificates as a precondition for marriage for all citizens. Instead, registry officials were empowered to refer those whom they suspected of genetic inadequacies to health offices. Here, they were vetted for fitness and, if 'unfit', for sterilization.[169] The Nuremberg laws and the marriage laws reflected the dichotomy in Nazi health policies. The Nuremberg laws were the result of pressure from anti-semitic ideologues, and the marriage laws from the technocrat, public health lobby. They drew on racial hygienic precedents for marriage certificates, and were to be part of the extended structure of the *Gesundheitsämter*. Reichsärzteführer Wagner had pressured bureaucrats of the Ministry of the Interior for radical anti-semitic measures.[170] The tone and terminology of the two sets of laws differed. The Nuremberg laws stressed purity of 'blood', and the marriage laws were to 'protect hereditary health'.[171]

The Nuremberg laws attempted to settle an argument between hard-line eugenicists and more moderate Reich Ministry of the Interior officials over the fate of those of half and quarter Jewish ancestry. They erected categories based on ancestry of Jews, and racial hybrids or *Mischlinge*. Those who were half or quarter Jewish were a problematic group. Mendelian laws of heredity were taken seriously, as they suggested that Jewish characteristics might be recessive and emerge only after generations. 'Jewishness' could never be bred out of a population unless there was strict segregation. Despite marriage restrictions, half and quarter Jews remained tolerated in economic life and in the army.[172] The laws were also cautious with regard to whether there was a German or Aryan race. The term 'Aryan' was not mentioned. It was emphasized that there was no single 'German race', but that Germany was constituted from different racial elements. Of these the Nordic race was acknowledged as superior. This reflected the influence of racial anthropologists. Despite these concessions to science, the public health and racial hygiene technocrats were unhappy with the Nuremberg laws. They regarded these as based

---

[169] Bock, *Zwangssterilisation*, pp. 100–3.   [170] Adam, *Judenpolitik*, pp. 129–30.
[171] A. Gütt, H. Linden and F. Massfeller, *Blutschutz- und Ehegesundheitsgesetz*, (Munich, 1936).
[172] J. Noakes, 'Wohin gehören die 'Judenmischlinge'? Die Entstehung der ersten Durchführungsverordnungen zu den Nürnberger Gesetzen', in U. Büttner (ed.), *Das Unrechtsregime* (Hamburg, 1986).

on erroneous scientific principles. The anti-semitic ideologue, Streicher, contended that once a gentile had had sexual intercourse with a Jew, then all progeny – even if resulting from a different sexual partner – would be Jewish. This justification for segregation was criticized by the eugenicists. Others were unhappy with the regulations for the *Mischlinge*. Astel suggested that if cut off from sexual relations with other groups, the Jewish race would die out in a few generations, as their fertility was relatively low. Astel complained to Himmler that the Führer was wrongly advised in the laws, and gained the impression that Himmler supported the criticisms made against these ideological racists.[173]

The overall aim of the marriage laws was a 'healthy marriage' to benefit the state. No mention was made of racial categories such as Jewish or Aryan. This was taken care of by the Nuremberg laws, preventing marriage if there was a threat to the purity of the blood of future generations. Medical officers were charged with policing the marriage laws and with the issue of health certificates. The laws built on the administrative structure of the 1933 sterilization law and of the 1934 public health law, uniting state and municipal health services. The health offices were also to build up comprehensive data on heredity. The offices were responsible for educating the public as to the national need for large families. Complaints were to be brought before the hereditary tribunals which administered the sterilization laws. Those who were sterilized were banned from marriage unless this was with another infertile person. Also banned were those suffering from 'psychopathy' or compulsive criminality. Further provisions defined the laws as including chronic diseases such as TB and VD, but not epidemic infectious diseases subject to international regulations on quarantine and isolation. Latent TB posed especial problems, as the symptoms might only' be coughing and loss of weight. The commentary on the law assumed an inherited disposition to TB. As it was estimated that three-quarters of a million Germans had latent VD, the health offices had to collect information from doctors and clinics, to take blood-serum and urine tests, and to establish whether a treated case was really 'cured'. Alcoholics and psychopaths were also included. It was admitted that diagnosis was difficult as these were broad-ranging categories; medical officers were urged to make specially careful investigation of family background, ancestry, and to take into account the overall need of the state for a healthy population. A growing list of diseases was being compiled which were held to diminish working capacity and so harm the family; these included diabetes, obesity and blood diseases such as leukemia. Other diseases such as asthma were a threat to the family because of 'inherited disposition'. Racial categories were built into diagnoses. The form asked for details of 'physique and racial type', and for whether there were signs of non-German or racially non-related blood. That Kretschmer's categories of physique and psyche continued to be used indicated how non-Nazi categories became components of the racial machinery.[174]

[173] BAK NS 19 Nr 176 Astel to Himmler, 8 October 1935; J. Ackermann, *Heinrich Himmler als Ideologe* (Göttingen, 1970), p. 161.   [174] Gütt, *Blutschutz- und Ehegesundheitsgesetz*.

The running down of sterilization

Between 1934 and 1945 an estimated 360,000 persons were sterilized under the law. This amounted to 1 per cent of the population.[175] Certain localities had a higher rate of sterilization, notably Baden and Hamburg.[176] An unknown number of foreign workers, and ethnic groups such as gypsies, mulattos and Jews were illegally sterilized. Eugenicists estimated that 1.2 million Germans should be sterilized. But after 1937 numbers began to decline, because of the emptying of the reservoir in mental hospitals, public resistance, and the preparation of more extreme measures.[177] Most sterilizations were for 'hereditary feeble-mindedness', and over one-quarter were for schizophrenia.[178] The problematic and vague definition of 'feeble-mindedness' as a diagnosis suggests that even in strictly medical terms there must have been cases of doubt.[179] It also suggests that referrals were made for deviant 'antisocial' behaviour. Medical definitions of feeble-mindedness could include lying, querulousness, laziness and susceptibility to influence. 'Moral weakness' meant that criminals, vagabonds and single mothers could be sterilized. The priority was the person's value to the social organism and the law should be regarded as a policing measure to enforce order, hard work, sobriety and a healthy family life.[180]

There was resistance from individual patriots, families, a few doctors and above all the Catholic Church.[181] A key group who resisted were those members of the NSDAP and SA, who were found to be mentally deficient.[182] This situation illustrates how the technocracy of scientific racial hygiene could be at odds with Nazi ideology. Reichsärzteführer Wagner and Martin Bormann studied the party members' protests. In June 1937 Wagner criticized the impressionistic manner of diagnosis and the unpopularity of the law. He attacked Gütt, Rüdin and the state bureaucracy for depriving Germany of millions of children.[183] At the same time there was pressure from the SS for it to have an active role in public health. In 1937 Hitler gained recognition for SS medical officials to be recognized as public health officials.

Himmler had to adjudicate in the clash between the technocrat, Gütt, and the ideologue, Wagner. Gütt defended his state apparatus by arguing that abuses were limited. Wagner tried to subordinate the public health machinery to the party. He planned that the *Gauleiter* and party should have the right to intervene in

---

[175] Bock, *Zwangssterilisation*, p. 238.
[176] Over 1934–45, 20,000 were sterilized in Hamburg. If this rate applied to Germany, 1 million would have been sterilized.   [177] Bock, *Zwangssterilisation*, p. 241.
[178] H-G. Güse and W. Schmacke, *Zwangssterilisiert – verleugnet – vergessen. Zur Geschichte der nationalsozialistischen Rassenhygiene am Beispiel Bremens* (Bremen, 1984), p. 87.
[179] O. Bach, 'Zur Zwangssterilisierung in der Zeit des Faschismus im Bereich der Gesundheitsämter Leipzig und Grimma', in Thom and Spaar (eds.), *Medizin im Faschismus*, pp. 188–94.
[180] Bock, *Zwangssterilisation*, pp. 324–5.   [181] Bock, *Zwangssterilisation*, pp. 295–7.
[182] eg HSTA Stuttgart E 151 KVII Nr 1020 Bd 2 Rassenhygiene, to G. Wagner, 24 March 1936.
[183] Bock, *Zwangssterilisation*, pp. 341–5.

sterilization proceedings. At the same time, policies were initiated leading to the secret 'euthanasia' measures. There was also to be unification of state and party health services. In 1939 Wagner died, and Gütt retired, disappointed at the undermining of the state technocracy. His successor was Conti, who worked closely with Himmler on medical and racial policies.[184] A new phase of Nazi health measures was to begin.

SS MEDICINE

The SS represented the ultimate extreme of Nazi medicine, with the polarity of positive eugenic selection and negative eugenic extermination. The tentacles of the SS tightened their stranglehold not only on the population through Himmler's control of the police, but also on the scientific community. A type of ruthless racial hygienist, so well typified by Mengele, can be seen to emerge. In the SS there were a multiplicity of medical functions. The criteria of Nordic racial purity meant strict controls on the genealogy, physique and health of recruits. Health examination prior to marriage, to ensure the quality of the proposed spouse, was necessary. SS doctors had to have extensive training in racial theory and racial hygiene, and were imbued with the ideals and methods of population policy. Links were established with university institutes to provide this training, and there was a medical academy of the SS in Graz. The SS made racial biology the basis of their social policy and military strategy.

The rising prestige of the SS and its growing membership meant that its Race Office had to be expanded. In 1933 it became the Race and Settlement Office, and was directed by Darré until 1938. The SS applied anthropological criteria to itself with detailed physical measurements and genealogies of recruits. Racial experts supervised physical examinations for marriage. Special education offices provided courses on racial hygiene. Family welfare and settlement plans were developed. Racial hygiene thus took a part in shaping the SS state.[185] Every section of the SS had a *Rassereferent*.[186] The Race Office initially drew on outside experts who held an honorary rank (such as the Munich professor of hygiene, Kisskalt), and on courses provided by university academics. But from 1936 the SS relied on its own professional experts.[187]

The SS spawned a varied series of medical institutions. Ernst Grawitz was the chief doctor of the SS; at the same time he had an influential social position as president of the German Red Cross and for a time was Hitler's personal physician. Like Mrugowsky he looked to medical history for holistic alternatives to orthodox medicine. His second-in-command was Karl Gebhardt, who was also Himmler's personal doctor. Other doctors supervised recruitment (Berndt), the health of the security services (Werner Kirchert and Hans Ehlich), racial and settlement policies

---

[184] Bock, *Zwangssterilisation*, p. 348.
[185] R.L. Koehl, *The Black Corps; the Structure and Power Struggles of the Nazi SS* (Wisconsin, 1983), pp. 82–4.   [186] *Oberabschnitt.*   [187] Koehl, *Black Corps*, p. 117.

(Helmut Poppendick), police (Albert Döderlein), administration (Ernst Lolling) which was responsible for hygiene in the concentration camps, the *Ahnenerbe* and *Lebensborn* (under Ebner), and the Waffen SS (Karl Genzken and Mrugowsky from 1943).[188] Some doctors could use their expertise to transfer opportunistically from one power bloc to another. For example, Wilhelm Martin Kinkelin, a country doctor, moved from the SA in 1937 to the SS Racial Office and in 1941 to state and party service, and had an office for *Blutpflege und Rassenkultur* in the Agricultural Office of the NSDAP.[189]

The glorification of Nordic superiority and of the German peasantry had conceptual similarities to the convictions of many experts in racial hygiene. But the SS was highly selective of those racial hygienists with whom they chose to collaborate. The Nordic Society and the use of Nordic racial ideology were strictly controlled. Nordic groups were patronized by the less powerful Rosenberg, Günther was brushed aside, and Nordic ideology fell into disuse after the declaration of war.[190] Kaup tried in vain to rehabilitate himself with rural welfare schemes after he was retired in 1935.[191] Lenz and Rüdin of the 'old guard' of racial hygiene attempted to gain SS support. Lenz disapproved of Astel's policing methods, although Rüdin was on better terms with him as an intermediary between Munich racial hygiene and the SS. Both Lenz and Rüdin were distrusted by Himmler, even though Lenz was a veteran Nordic enthusiast. In 1937 Himmler sought Lenz's advice on how homosexuality worsened the demographic problem of excessive numbers of women.[192] Himmler favoured polygamy to ensure that women of racially high quality should have as many children as possible so as to make up for war losses. But Lenz incurred the anger of Himmler over his view that 'illegitimate' children were of below average genetic value and intelligence.[193] Lenz's view was closer to that of Gross, who warned that illegitimacy was a sign of degeneracy in marriage and the family.[194] When Lenz proposed collaboration with the Race and Settlement Office in 1940 and 1941, his participation was not welcome. Lenz advised against Nordic settlement in the Crimea in 1941 on climatic grounds. Fischer's influence was also limited in that his ties were closer to the relatively impotent *Ostministerium* of Rosenberg.[195] The old guard of racial hygiene, Fischer, Lenz and Rüdin, were brushed to one side by the SS.

The SS established a strong caucus at the University of Jena with the backing of the Thuringian Gauleiter, Sauckel. Astel was appointed to the Racial Political Office in Thuringia in 1933; he joined the SS in 1934 and was appointed to a chair in

---

[188] Y. Ternon and S. Helman, *Histoire de la Médecine SS* (np, 1969); B. Bromberger and H. Mausbach, 'Die Tätigkeit von Ärzten in der SS und in Konzentrationslagern', in Bromberger, Mausbach and K.-D. Thomann (eds.), *Medizin, Faschismus und Widerstand* (Cologne, 1985), p. 213.

[189] E. Stockhorst, *5000 Köpfe* (Kiel, 1985), p. 233.

[190] BAK NS 3 Nr 41 on reactivation of the Nordic Society; Lutzhöft, *Der Nordische Gedanke*, pp. 370–83. [191] BDC Report on Kaup, 2 July 1942, by NSDAP Gau Tirol.

[192] BAK NS 2 Nr 41 Bl. 62–73.

[193] F. Lenz, 'Zur Frage der unehelichen Kinder', *Volk und Rasse*, vol. 12 (1937), 91–5.

[194] G. Lilienthal, *Der 'Lebensborn e.V.'* (Stuttgart, 1985), pp. 25–6; Lutzhöft, *Der Nordische Gedanke*, pp. 383–9. [195] Müller-Hill, *Tödliche Wissenschaft*, p. 53.

racial biology.[196] At this stage he was on good terms with Gütt and Rüdin, as well as with the SS. Astel built up a ruthlessly efficient public health administration. He was resisted by Gross of the Racial Political Office who pressed for his removal in 1935. Himmler and Sauckel were important in maintaining his position. The Jena scientists drew on Haeckel's monism, in an anti-Christian crusade in line with the SS's pantheistic Nordic creed. In 1935 Astel wrote to Himmler that he felt it was his mission to give the people a new code of life. The caucus of SS scientists was based at the SS Mannschaftshaus at the University. They wished to link theory and national socialist practice. Astel's assistant Stengel von Rutkowski was a human geneticist, public health expert and pioneer historian of racial hygiene. The anthropologists Reimer Schulz and Heberer developed racial programmes on the basis of genetics. Heberer, an SS Sturmführer, came from Göttingen in 1938 and built up an institute for general biology and anthropology.[197] Ruttke was appointed professor for law and race in 1935 and took over SS training on race in occupied Poland.[198] Others included Brücher (the botanist and biographer of Haeckel), Walther Haupt and Heinrich Jörg (both gynaecologists), Gerlach (the pathological anatomist and Dean of the Medical Faculty), Goertler (the professor of veterinary medicine), and, from 1936, Johann von Leers, the racist historian of peasant life (also an SS officer). Astel was appointed Rector of Jena University in 1939, advocating that Jena was to be built up into the leading German university by the SS.[199] In 1935 Astel encouraged Himmler to mastermind a takeover of university posts in racial hygiene by the SS. Astel believed that Nazism's significance was the recognition that the laws of nature were the basis of state and society. Only by ridding society of the burden of weak, infirm, criminal and alien types could the healthy elements in the *Volk* fully realize their powers.[200] Jena was to provide academics for the Reich universities that were founded in the wake of German military expansion. The University of Strasburg was to engage in ideological combat with Western materialism and individualism, and the universities of Posen, Breslau and Prague were to form an eastern bulwark of German culture.

The power struggle between the SS-led group of scientific technocrats, and the Wagner-Streicher ideologues can be further illustrated with the controversy over the appointment of Karl Kötschau to a chair of nature therapy in June 1934. Kötschau attempted to develop an alternative type of 'biological medicine'. Reichsärzteführer Wagner appointed him as director of a Reich 'Working Group for a New German Therapy'[201] in 1935, which was a direct challenge to conventional scientific medicine. This aroused the opposition of leaders of the medical profession, and of a group within the party, who attacked holism as synonymous with clericalism and individualism. Racial values conflicted with

---

[196] BDC Astel file, joined SS on 16 February 1934.
[197] Saller, *Rassenlehre*, pp. 57–8.   [198] Saller, *Rassenlehre*, p. 58.
[199] BDC Astel file, Astel to Himmler, 8 May 1935; Abel file, Sauckel to Rust, 10 March 1943.
[200] *Volk und Gesundheit*, p. 39.   [201] *Reichsarbeitsgemeinschaft für eine Neue Deutsche Heilkunde.*

ideas of the 'totality of the individual'. Astel led a campaign for the dismissal of Kötschau from the University of Jena. Like another ideologue, Tirala, Kötschau found refuge with Streicher in Nuremberg.[202] The attack on holism was aimed at a wide range of Catholic and other academics such as the disciples of Spann, and at Gestalt psychology. The SS was determined to purge organicist thought of values and thinkers other than their own.[203] Himmler established a balance between scientific and holistic medicine. He personally favoured dietary therapies and massage.[204] He cultivated anthropologists for the insight that they could provide into his German ancestors, and he believed that he was the reincarnation of Frederick Barbarossa. He encouraged research on herbal remedies. A plantation for herbal medicines was established at the Dachau concentration camp. Karl Fahrenkamp, a cardiologist, researched on life-enhancing elixirs. Nature therapy was developed at the SS sanatorium of Hohenlychen.[205]

The attack on racial hygiene

The SS had a foothold at the University of Munich with the university administrator, Walter Wüst, an ambitious young philologist who had furthered his career by joining the SS.[206] The SS planned to remove Rüdin, who had lost an important supporter when Gütt's attempt to form a unified state public health administration as the basis of Nazi health care was challenged by rival groups within the party and SS. In 1937 Gütt was given control of the *Sippenamt*, or Genealogical Section, of the Race and Settlement Office of the SS. He combined this with administrative responsibility for population policy and racial hygiene. Gütt was increasingly at loggerheads with Himmler. The overlapping responsibilities provided the SS with opportunities to intervene in Gütt's eugenic and public health empire.[207] From 1938 Rüdin's grandiose research plans were in jeopardy. He had been supported by the Rockefeller and Loeb foundations. Rockefeller money ceased for genealogical and demographic research in 1935. Loeb money continued to be paid until 1940. As the Loeb family was Jewish, this was an unreliable source. Rüdin expected that money would cease to be paid after the Nuremburg laws of 1935. This did not happen, and Loeb funds continued to finance criminal biology. It illustrates the perception that eugenics was to provide a solution to the problem of social deviancy rather than racial impurity.[208] Other sources of funds such as from the Bavarian Ministry of the Interior, the Prussian

[202] A. Haug, 'Der Lehrstuhl für Biologische Medizin in Jena', in Kudlien (ed.), *Ärzte*, pp. 130–138; M. Stürzbecher, 'Aus der Vorgeschichte des Heilpraktikergesetzes vom 17.2.1939', *Medizinische Monatsschrift*, no. 7 (1967), 313–20.   [203] *Volk und Gesundheit*, pp. 41–3.
[204] F. Kersten, *The Kersten Memoirs 1940–1945* (London, 1956).
[205] W. Wuttke-Groneberg, 'Leistung, Vernichtung, Verwertung', *Volk und Gesundheit*, pp. 48–53.
[206] M.H. Kater, *Das 'Ahnenerbe' der SS 1935–1945. Ein Beitrag zur Kulturpolitik des Dritten Reiches* (Stuttgart, 1974).
[207] Koehl, *Black Corps*, p. 325; BAK NS Nr 38, 28 June 1935 Gütt-Klumm Besprechung; Labisch and Tennstedt, *GVG*, vol. 2, pp. 332–9.   [208] Loeb papers, Max-Planck-Institut für Psychiatrie.

provinces, and certain districts and municipalities were in danger of drying up due to the threat of war.

SS control of research funds meant a weakening of the position of scientists. During the 1920s scientists had dispensed research funds on the basis of a self-reviewing peer group system. The German Research Fund (DFG)[209] was subjected to control of the SS through its president, SS Brigadeführer Rudolf Mentzel, who considered that Fischer and Verschuer could conduct the research more economically, and that Rüdin's demands were extravagant. Rüdin's collecting of patient records from psychiatric institutions and hospitals had led to the need for a small army of clerical and research staff to process the data. Mentzel felt that Rüdin's use of motor cars for his researchers meant that he spread the net of his hereditary demographic surveys too widely, and that they were trespassing on the territory of Verschuer and Fischer. In 1939 Rüdin found that he could no longer rely on Loeb funds, or on the DFG. In September 1939 Rüdin applied for funding to the *Ahnenerbe*, the cultural and scientific organization of the SS. The response of the *Ahnenerbe* was that although Rüdin was unsuitable as not in sympathy with the SS, Himmler considered that it was strategically important to take control of his institute. In October 1939 Oberführer Professor Wüst urged that Rüdin be granted research funds on condition that Wüst be placed on the governing committee of the institute. Control of Rüdin's institute was regarded as opportune by the SS as just at this time the reorganization of public health under Conti's direction was under way.[210]

For his part Rüdin offered to open up ideologically relevant areas of research. Instead of looking at degenerate characters, he decided to make positive racial qualities a research target. Projects on genius and heredity, and on the prospects for the breeding of social elites were established. (In fact research on genius and heredity had begun by 1926.) Rüdin concluded what amounted to a Faustian pact with the *Ahnenerbe*. In November 1939 the *Ahnenerbe* agreed to pay 30,000 marks from the funds of Heydrich's security police. Later money came from the *Ahnenerbe*. Heydrich's interest in hereditary biology for policing and racial purposes was decisive. The SS funded three assistants, Fräulein Hell (researching on the work-shy, the antisocial and prostitution), Riedel (researching on the inheritance of criminality and homosexuality), and Erwin Schroeter (a Waffen SS doctor researching on the biological value of the illegitimate). Schroeter conducted his research while based at the SS hospital at Dachau from 1940 until 1943.[211] They began to agitate against Rüdin's other assistants including the devout Catholic Luxenburger, who had to be drafted into the army, and against Rüdin himself as director. They were joined in May 1939 by SS Hauptsturmführer Dr Greite researching on adopted children. Greite and Riedel had already succeeded in ousting Lehmann from the *Biologen-Verband*. The university curator of Munich University, Wüst, allied himself with the assistants in their attempt to force

---

[209] *Deutsche Forschungsgemeinschaft.*   [210] BDC Rüdin file.   [211] BDC file.

Rüdin's resignation from the institute and from the presidency of the Racial Hygiene Society.[212] In 1941 Himmler and the *Ahnenerbe* reaffirmed the financial support for the institute as part of their strategy of taking control.[213] The situation between Rüdin and the SS was tense as he sought to regain the initiative in the management of his institute.

The clash between the SS and the Racial Political Office of the NSDAP is shown by the difference of opinion over the eugenic value of 'illegitimate' children. Himmler wished to provide special homes for illegitimate children and their mothers as he regarded these children as having a potential racial value. Gross of the Racial Political Office condemned illegitimacy as a sign of degeneracy in marriage and the family. In December 1935 Himmler established an organization to care for the illegitimate, called the *Lebensborn* (or Well of Life). It was administered by Gregor Ebner, Himmler's physician and a long-standing member of the Munich Racial Hygiene Society. The *Lebensborn* established maternity homes and child care institutions. The offspring, if from single mothers, could be adopted and were considered future material for the SS. Himmler's organization rivalled the 'Mother and Child' organization of the National Socialist Welfare League, which was allied to the party. While the Nazis never went quite as far as planned breeding, there was some sympathy for 'giving the Führer a child' through extra-marital relations with a party member or SS officer. Ultimately, the Nazis aimed to supplant such Christian institutions as marriage with their own ceremonies and moral norms.[214]

The SS not only became self-sufficient with regard to medical and welfare matters, but it also sought control in the state and scientific institutions. In 1938–39, Darré, Gütt and Rüdin were all under pressure from the SS. This meant that the generation of experts, who had emerged around 1932, had dominated racial policy for about five years. The technocratic policies of the SS incurred the distaste of Günther and Darré during the 1940s. They condemned the new 'mass society' and its economic, welfare measures and settlement policies as mechanistic and lacking in concern for the peasantry and for the natural environment. Darré found refuge in organic farming, and Günther withdrew from Berlin to Freiburg. Günther and Darré hated the primacy of mechanistic science and industry because of the needs of the war economy. They too were disenchanted ideologues.[215]

Territorial expansion

With the invasion of Poland came a major opportunity for racial hygienic supporters of German *Lebensraum*. Policies for replacing Poles, Slavs and Jews by German settlers were initiated and endorsed by racial hygienists. After Darré's departure in 1938, the Race and Settlement Office of the SS continued under SS

[212] BDC Rüdin file, Wüst to Mentzel, 29 September 1939.
[213] BDC Rüdin file, notes of US interrogation.   [214] Lilienthal, *Lebensborn*, pp. 35–53.
[215] Lutzhöft, *Der Nordische Gedanke*; BDC Günther file, Günther to Darré 17 October 1938, 13 September 1942.

Gruppenführer Günther Pancke. The *Sippenamt* was transferred to the medical section of the SS. Pancke, a *Freikorps* veteran and SS administrator, continued to base policies on scientific expertise. In 1937 the office had been joined by the Breslau professor of pathology and racial hygienist, Martin Staemmler. The invasion of Poland unleashed a surge of ambition among racial researchers to be at the forefront of policy-making on repopulating the East. Medical and anthropological experts took part in formulating and executing the SS's population policy. ˙Comprehensive recommendations for deportation of occupied populations, the Germanization of selected groups, and major resettlement from Germany were drawn up by Gross of the NSDAP Racial Political Office and submitted to Himmler in autumn 1939. These plans included the screening of ancestry by racial experts and the medical supervision of orphans. In October 1939 Hitler gave Himmler authority to undertake a massive policy of resettlement in the East. When Himmler drew up his plans for population engineering of 28 May 1940 they were based on those Gross had outlined, and the result of extensive consultation with health, population and race experts.[216]

There was much interaction between racial hygienists and the executors of racial policy.[217] Gross, a physician by training, had close contacts with Lenz and Fischer of the Kaiser Wilhelm Institute for Anthropology. Lenz suggested that there be a Reich commissioner for population policy, responsible for evaluating the racial quality of German ethnic groups in the East.[218] Yet it was the anthropologist Reche, rather than Lenz, who made headway with the SS. Reche exemplifies how racial research contributed to the formulating of the SS's population engineering in the East. During the 1920s and 1930s he made the transition from ethnology to human hereditary biology by studies of serology and of twin schoolchildren in Leipzig.[219] He was keen to move from academic to policy-oriented studies, when war brought an opportunity for resettlement in the East.[220] In October 1939 Reche, armed with the experience of blood group surveys in the Soviet Union during the 1920s, proclaimed himself to the SS as the ideal expert for the East and for the solution of how to settle Germans and remove the 'Polish lice'.[221] He aimed to produce a warrior caste based in rural settlements. Himmler approved of him. Reche in 1939 urged comprehensive resettlement of Germans and removal of the Jews to Madagascar and the Poles further to the East.[222] Reche also recommended an assistant, Hesch, to work in Prague to assess the racial value of Czech Germans.[223] The SS required racial evaluation of the existing ethnic groups of

---

[216] R.L. Koehl, *RKFDV: German Resettlement and Population Policy* (Cambridge, Mass., 1957), pp. 65–7, 77.

[217] A. Ploetz and E. Rüdin, 'Die völkische Umsiedlung ins grossdeutsche Vaterland', *ARGB*, vol. 33 (1939), 527–8.   [218] BDC Lenz file, 31 March 1941, for Himmler's verdict on Lenz.

[219] STA Dresden Nr 10209/49 Zwillingsforschung. Institut für Rassen- und Völkerkunde der Universität Leipzig 1934–37.

[220] A. Harrasser, 'Prof. Dr O. Reche 60 Jahre alt', *ARGB*, vol. 33 (1939), 374–5.

[221] BDC Reche file, Reche to Pancke, 2 October 1939.

[222] BDC Reche file, 21 December 1939, May 1940.

[223] BDC Reche file, 22 December 1940, 12 December 1940, 8 January 1941.

Germans in the East. These *Volksdeutschen* were to be returned to Germany for a Nazi education prior to resettlement. Reche regretted that war meant that the best German settlers were in the army.[224] Reche had heard that settlers were being recruited from Baden in south west Germany. He warned that these were the least Nordic Germans.[225] Reche offered the SS training in fingerprinting and other anthropological techniques, and specialist literature and advice on Eastern European ethnic groups. Reche's role as anthropological specialist enhanced the importance of his institute in wartime, when he might otherwise have expected to lose assistants and funds.[226] Reche's views suited the Commissariat for Strengthening Germandom, the RKFDV, headed by Himmler. Advisors on racial questions found further opportunities after the invasion of the Soviet Union. Anthropologists such as Abel worked for the *Volksdeutsche Mittelstelle*, which evaluated the racial quality of ethnic Germans in the Eastern territories, and the geneticist Wettstein advised on the appropriation of Soviet plant-breeding stations. Race and settlement officers with six weeks' biological training sifted the Nordic elite from the inferior races, who were earmarked for death. The SS planned a medical dystopia: midwives were to be abortionists, there were to be mass sterilizations and encouragement of high infant mortality, and all family allowances and welfare services were to be scrapped.[227] For inferior races the racial programme of the SS represented the negation of the ideals of health and welfare.

THE NEGATION OF HEALTH CARE

Extermination of mental disease

War provided the opportunity for dictatorial centralization of health services and for accelerating the imposition of racial measures. On 20 April 1939, Conti was appointed *Reichsgesundheitsführer* (Reich Health Leader). This was a new title, as Wagner had been *Reichsärzteführer* (Reich Doctors' Leader) owing to his power base among family doctors. Conti's title symbolized his power in the state public health machinery. Conti united several functions as *Leiter* of the NSDAP Office for Public Health and Secretary of State in the Reich Ministry of the Interior. This unification of powers ended deep rooted divisions in the administration of health care, dating back to the liberal structure of Imperial Germany. It needed an authoritarian state to remove obstacles to this centralization; administrative autonomy, unregulated medical practice and individual rights had to be eradicated. Conti was more a state technocrat than a party ideologue. He had made a career in the health administration in Berlin, owing his appointment in the Prussian Ministry of the Interior to Göring and to having joined the SS in 1930.[228] He had

---

[224] BDC Reche file, Pancke to Reche, 27 December 1939.
[225] BDC Reche file, Reche to Pancke, 10 January 1939.
[226] BDC Reche file, Reche to Pancke, 14 November 1939.
[227] H. Heiber, 'Der Generalplan Ost', *Vierteljahreshefte für Zeitgeschichte*, vol. 6 (1958), 280–323.
[228] BDC Conti file.

little contact with the Munich power base of the Nazi party. That he was to be assisted by Wagner's deputy, Kurt Blome, was a sign of the attempt to fuse the state public health and professional power blocs in 1939.[229]

In August 1939 Conti managed to depose Gütt as secretary of state. Gütt had opposed Himmler's incursions in the sphere of state public health. Although Gütt was an SS officer, he insisted that doctors should not be subject to orders from _Stabsführer_ who were not medically qualified. Resentment of professional autocrats was shown when the SS feared domination of their _Sippenamt_ by an _Ärzte Clique_. During 1937 Himmler took a lenient view of Gütt, who had conceded that the SS could take on responsibilities for welfare and population policy.[230] While training for the sport qualification of the SS in the summer of 1937 Gütt suffered a heart attack, and from then on deteriorating health and a hunting accident (which might have been an attempted assassination) weakened his position. In June 1938 Gütt had a frank discussion with Himmler in which he criticized the Race and Settlement Office of the SS for exaggerating racial over health issues, for being unscientific and encouraging the birth of children out of wedlock. Gütt confided that Hitler was suffering from paranoia. It marked the beginning of the end for Gütt's time in office, and for his medical officer-based approach to health care.[231]

Conti intended to unify health care administration with the welfare responsibilities in the Reich Ministry of Labour. In January 1941 he sought the support of Robert Ley, the Labour Minister, for a 'socialization of the medical profession'. While the doctors were off at the front, occupational health, sickness insurance, welfare and medical care were to be directed by a single ministry. The patient was to be registered with a family doctor, who would receive a capitation fee rather than be paid for each item of service. At the same time the doctor was to be 'the soul of the factory'. The plan ran into difficulties with Conti accused of placing the interests of the medical profession above those of the party.[232] Conti's aspirations for attaining a unified system of welfare controlled by the medical profession – a long-standing professional demand – resulted in a further power struggle with Conti pitted against Blome and Bormann. Between 1941 and 1943 Conti attempted but failed to realize his vision of socialized health care. In September 1943 Brandt, who was Hitler's personal physician, was appointed _Reichskommissar für das Sanitäts- und Gesundheitswesen_ (Reich Commissioner for Sanitation and Health). Conti's power was eroded when in January 1943 the National Socialist Doctors' League was suspended.[233] That Brandt took a leading role in medical killing suggests the key role of 'euthanasia' in the Nazi system of medicine.

The transition from medicine as care for the individual to the welfare of society and future generations attained the most extreme and brutal realization in the

---

[229] K. Blome, _Arzt im Kampf_ (Leipzig, 1942).   [230] BAK NS 2 Nr 41 Bl. 99, 108, 143.
[231] M. Stürzbecher, in _Jahrbuch für die Geschichte Mittel- und Ostdeutschlands_, vol. 16/17 (1968), 398–400; Labisch and Tennstedt, _GVG_, vol. 2, pp. 345–7.
[232] M.-L. Recker, _Nationalsozialistische Sozialpolitik im Zweiten Weltkrieg_ (Munich, 1985), pp. 121–8.
[233] Lilienthal, 'Ärztebund', pp. 120–1.

killing of the sick and disabled.[234] While 'euthanasia' of the supposedly incurable was supported and legitimated by Hitler, and overseen by his Chancellery, medical experts took a crucial role in its administration. The SS had only a subordinate role with the provision of personnel, as the killing was meant to be administered in a strictly 'medical' manner.[235] Terms like 'euthanasia' and 'the incurable' were a euphemistic medicalized camouflage with connotations of relief of the individual suffering of the terminally ill. The victims were primarily children under three years of age, diagnosed as mentally retarded or congenitally malformed, and the mentally ill. Heydrich intervened on behalf of the SS to suggest that social deviants[236] be included.[237] In practice those of 'lesser races' were also victims. The procedures were painful and violent. Many patients met their death with resignation and dignity. Those who resisted were subjected to brutal force. Measures that were originally meant to be reserved for the most serious cases became practised on a random, haphazard and widespread scale.

During 1938 Hitler and medical authorities decided to exterminate the newborn and those young children who suffered from congenital diseases which made their lives 'valueless'.[238] In August 1939 the medical sacrifice of babies' lives for the health of the race was bureaucratized with a system of medical registration of all newborn crippled children by doctors, medical officers or midwives. These procedures resulted from discussions from February until May 1939 between the Führer's Chancellery and a group of selected professors of medicine. This was under the auspices of Philipp Bouhler and Hans Hefelmann (of the Führer's Chancellery), Victor Brack (Hitler's personal physician), the ophthalmologist Hellmuth Unger (Wagner's subordinate), the paediatricians Ernst Wentzler (recommended by Conti) and Werner Catel, and Linden of the Reich Ministry of the Interior. This group initiated the medical killing of children under cover of the 'Reich Committee for the Scientific Registration of Serious Hereditary and Congenital Illnesses'.[239] Shortly before the war, on 18 August 1939, they issued a secret decree in the name of the Ministry of the Interior for registration by doctors and midwives with the health offices of all 'idiots', 'mongols', spastics and malformed births.[240] Medical officers were to register and check all details. The centralized structure of public health was to feed victims into the new machinery.

Towards the end of October 1939 Hitler empowered Bouhler and Brandt to administer *Gnadentod* (mercy killing) to those patients judged incurable 'by critical

---

[234] E. Klee, '*Euthanasie' im NS-Staat. Die Vernichtung lebensunwerten Lebens* (Frankfurt-on-Main, 1983); R.S. Lifton, *The Nazi Doctors* (New York, 1986), pp. 45–79; for a controversial overview, H.W. Schmuhl, *Rassenhygiene, Nationalsozialismus, Euthanasie*, (Göttingen, 1987).
[235] Lifton suggests the term 'medical killing' instead of euthanasia.
[236] *Gemeinschaftsfremde*.
[237] K.H. Roth and G. Aly, 'Das "Gesetz über Sterbehilfe bei unheilbare Kranken"', in Roth, *Erfassung*, pp. 101–179.   [238] Klee, *Euthanasie*, pp. 78–80.
[239] *Reichsausschuss zur wissenschaftlichen Erfassung von erb- und anlagebedingten schweren Leiden.*
[240] Klee, *Euthanasie*, pp. 77–81.

evaluation of their sickness'. The order was symbolically back-dated to 1 September 1939, when Poland was invaded. This was an order relying not on law – the Führer rejected any legislation – but on the supreme power of the Führer as legitimating medical authority over life and death. Measures for adult 'mercy killing' were initiated. By July 1939 Hitler had empowered Conti with implementing 'euthanasia'. Conti's centralization of administrative and medical powers made him an appropriate choice. However, his power aroused the jealous opposition of Brack, who began to intrigue against Conti. As a result Bouhler and Brack gained control over the medical killing. Reliable helpers were recruited from the ranks of psychiatrists who had a scientific reputation for clinical research on the causes of diseases and were concerned with the costs and administrative rationalization of institutions. These reformers included the Heidelberg psychiatrist Carl Schneider, Berthold Kihn of Jena, and the Nazi *Altkämpfer* Werner Heyde of Würzburg. The 'euthanasia' of children was charged to Wentzler, Unger, Heinze, Pfannmüller and Bender (the latter three coming from child care institutions). Heyde took a central role in overseeing the organization. The psychiatric reformer and veteran racial hygienist, Nitsche, director of a mental hospital at Sonnenstein near Pirna in Saxony and advocate of psychiatric therapies as insulin and electric shock, later joined the team.[241]

The planning for euthanasia provided psychiatrists with the opportunity for pursuing professional ambitions, and resolving internal power struggles between state, party and army-oriented groups. A major demand was the ending of church-controlled asylums, often staffed by lay personnel and coping with vulnerable long-stay patients, as a state system offered the greatest prospect for professional controls. This was a long-standing professional demand, advocated by such as Kraepelin at the turn of the century. The intricate web of links of psychiatrists with state health administrations and the army provided the background and crucial impetus towards the euthanasia programme. Many professors of psychiatry including Nitsche and de Crinis held office as military medical advisers. Military reservists included Bonhoeffer, Gaupp, Hoche and Rüdin.[242] Psychiatrists were aware that the First World War had caused the deaths of many mental hospital patients. The immediate circumstances – and camouflage – for the killing of the adult mentally ill were those of mobilization for war. It was explained that hospitals and medical personnel were needed for the army. In December 1939 Jewish and Polish patients from Meseritz-Obrawalde in the province of Posen were killed in nearby woods after being injected with a strong sedative. The method of killing was debated. Brandt recommended lethal injection as a more medical approach. In January 1940 Brandt and Conti carried out the first killings by injection, on behalf of the administrative cover, code-named 'T4'. This name derived from the address Tiergartenstrasse 4, where the administrative office was located. That the staff were

[241] Klee, *Euthanasie*, p. 83; G. Aly, 'Der saubere und der schmutzige Fortschritt', *Beiträge zur Nationalsozialistische Gesundheits- und Sozialpolitik*, vol. 2 (1985), 9–78.
[242] BA Militärarchiv Freiburg H 20/ 483 (b).

included on lists for medical conferences suggests that their function was known to professional colleagues. The staff experimented with gassing patients, and concluded that this was a more effective method. Gas killings in lorries were also used in January 1940 on Polish patients. From April 1940 an inventory of Jewish patients was undertaken, and in June the first gassings of Jewish mental patients took place.[243] The 'euthanasia' programme was meant to be a depersonalized and technically a relatively efficient form of killing. Gas chambers were a technology suited to mass extermination under secure conditions. After the invasion of the Soviet Union on 22 June 1941, the SS found that their 'cleansing operations' on Poles and Russians by mass shooting were laborious and a psychological strain. Himmler's witnessing of mass shootings made him realize that a more efficient means of extermination was necessary. On 31 July 1941 Göring commanded Heydrich to undertake the 'final solution' of the 'Jewish question'. Heydrich transferred the 'euthanasia' technology to the killing of Jews. In autumn 1941 Zyklon B was used experimentally in Auschwitz on Soviet prisoners of war. The results showed that it was appropriate for mass killing. 'T4' specialists such as Wirth were transferred to setting up gas chambers in concentration camps.[244] The policies represented a declaration of war on inherited diseases and disabilities with doctors as heroic warriors defending the health of future generations. Although the war provided circumstances for imposing policies of medical killing for the incurable and degenerate, demands for medical killing had a complex although obscure prehistory in power struggles among psychiatrists and racial hygienists with racial ideologues.

The origins of medical killing

In 1928 Hitler wrote of his admiration for how the Spartans killed newborn weaklings. He associated selective killing with the type of Spartan military prowess that was needed to wage a war for *Lebensraum*.[245] Thus war and the killing of the hereditarily weak were linked by Hitler whose subsequent speeches threatened extermination of the mentally ill.[246] At the Nuremberg Party rally of 1929 Hitler denounced those welfare measures which meant that Germany was breeding the weak and killing off the strong, and considered the possibility of ridding the nation of a million incurably sick 'burdensome lives'.[247] After 1933 there were many occasions when dark threats were made of a radical solution to the problem of the antisocial, mentally ill and disabled. The cost of institutional care was drummed into the population. Schoolchildren calculated such costs in mathematics lessons,

---

[243] Klee, *Euthanasie*, p. 105.   [244] Müller-Hill, *Tödliche Wissenschaft*, p. 49.
[245] G.L. Weinberg, *Hitlers Zweites Buch* (Stuttgart, 1961), pp. 56–7.
[246] Bock, *Zwangssterilisation*, p. 349.
[247] *Ballastexistenzen*: according to Ploetz, diary 3 July 1911, the term *erbliche Belastung* dated from 1899. J. Noakes and G. Pridham (eds.), *Nazism 1919–1945. A Documentary Reader* vol. 3 (Exeter, 1988), p. 1002.

and biology classes inspected asylums, so as to write essays on racial degeneration and its economic burdens.[248] Yet what these radical solutions were to be remained, as with the 'Jewish question', imprecise and open to many alternatives. Concentration camps were proclaimed by Schultze, the Bavarian health commissioner, as the best way of ridding the state of worthless psychopaths and the feeble-minded. In 1937 Himmler ordered 2,000 'moral and hereditary criminals' to be sent to concentration camps. From 1938 police rounded up gypsies, vagabonds, beggars and criminals, and packed these off to concentration camps. The official propaganda excused this as 're-education into the discipline of work'. Such violence was a means of terrorizing the rest of the population into good behaviour. Isolation, segregation and 'preventive detention' retained a value for public order and racial hygiene.

Mass killing of the mentally and physically disabled, as well as infirm patients of 'inferior races', had long been intended by certain national socialist doctors. Although the radicalization of sterilization led to medical killing, not all who had been fervent sterilizers favoured medical killing. Indeed, certain racial hygienists who had a vested interest in the sterilization programme were passive onlookers rather than active perpetrators of medical killing. In 1933 the Prussian Ministry of Justice produced a memorandum on the admissibility of sterilization, eugenic abortion and 'the extermination of valueless life' in the cases of 'incurable mental diseases'. The legalized killing of the incurable was initially critically received by doctors in psychiatric institutions, but from 1935 there was renewed discussion, and in 1937 a change of medical opinion on euthanasia was noted by officials.[249] The *Deutscher Gemeindetag* committee which conducted a national survey of the numbers, types and costs of patients in hospitals and welfare institutions between 1935 and 1939 marked a turning point in providing a rationale as well as personnel for medical killing.[250] The major force for radicalization of measures against the biologically degenerate was the party-based group of Wagner, the Reich Doctors' leader, who was able to exert crucial influence on Hitler. The Gütt-Wagner compromise of 1939 enabled extension of sterilization to ethnic and antisocial minorities, and a radicalization of sterilization into euthanasia policies. When on 18 August 1939 the Reich Ministry of the Interior considered a change in the sterilization law, they also decreed the registration of children under three years of age by doctors, midwives and medical officers with a tribunal for the registration of hereditary diseases.[251] While it initially seemed as if this was to function as a Reich Hereditary Health Tribunal[252] and possibly an advisory committee on racial research, it in fact selected 5,000 children, many with Down's Syndrome, for extermination.[253] This committee became a key link between the Führer's

---

[248] Klee, *Euthanasie*, p. 76.   [249] Bock, *Zwangssterilisation*, p. 349.
[250] BHSTA M Inn 79478 Erbbiologische Bestandsaufnahme.
[251] Reichsausschuss zur wissenschaftlichen Erfassung erb- und anlagebedingter schwerer Leiden.
[252] 'Reichserbgesundheitsgericht'.   [253] Aly and Roth, 'Gesetz', pp. 104–5, 118.

Chancellery and the Reich health administration at a time when the Führer's Chancellery was actively discussing 'euthanasia'.[254]

Wagner, the Reich Doctors' leader, took a lead in the change of emphasis from sterilization to medical killing. He was a link between Hitler, the wresting of control of sterilization from Gütt and Rüdin, and the new Reich committee. Hitler is reported to have secretly informed Wagner of the intention to implement 'euthanasia' in 1935.[255] In 1936 Wagner encouraged discussion of 'euthanasia'. An ophthalmologist on his staff, Hellmuth Unger, wrote the novel 'Mission and Conscience' to give the issue greater public acceptability.[256] Party members drummed up a broad public debate, which culminated in the 1941 feature film 'Ich klage an'.[257] Schools visited asylums in order to be shown the degenerate, and be convinced of the need for radical solutions. A turning-point came towards the end of 1938: a petition from a family for the killing of their crippled child in a Leipzig children's clinic was sent to the Führer. Hitler then authorized killing of such children. This staged justification of euthanasia shows how the Führer's image was strengthened by the image of his benignly responding to pressure from the people.[258] In fact, policies were drawn up by an elite of Nazi doctors who sought to make them publicly acceptable.

That Reichsärzteführer Wagner and his associates supported 'euthanasia' but were critical of the lack of racism in sterilization, suggests that for dedicated Nazis, sterilization led to 'euthanasia'. But for racial hygienists the situation was more complex. The interests of those in authority over sterilization procedures could be undermined by the forced 'euthanasia' measures. There were advocates of sterilization, and even of mass sterilization of the racially inferior, who objected by varying degrees to medical killing. Clear differences can be seen among psychiatrists. In July and August 1939 an attempt failed to organize a collective protest by professors of psychiatry against 'euthanasia'. Only Gottfried Ewald of Göttingen protested. While in sympathy with Nazi politics, he argued for biological bonds of mothers for infirm children to be respected, and considered that the sterilized could still enjoy life.[259] Bonhoeffer exemplifies how a psychiatrist could favour eugenic sterilization but oppose medical killing, and generally disapprove of Nazism.[260] Rüdin, who had taken the lead in formulating and implementing the sterilization law, was apparently not consulted by the authorities on the initial planning of euthanasia as by 1939 he was out of favour. Officials

---

[254] Aly and Roth, 'Gesetz', p. 104, date the committee from 1937, whereas Bock, *Zwangssterilisation*, p. 349 and Klee, *Euthanasie*, pp. 79–80, date it from early 1939.

[255] Klee, *Euthanasie*, p. 52.   [256] H. Unger, *Sendung und Gewissen* (Berlin, 1936).

[257] A title with ironic echoes of Zola's defence of Dreyfus. K.H. Roth, 'Filmpropaganda für Vernichtung der Geisteskranken und Behinderten im "Dritten Reich"', *Beiträge zur Nationalsozialistischen Gesundheits- und Sozialpolitik*, vol. 2 (1985), 125–93.

[258] Klee, *Euthanasie*, pp. 78–9 suggests that in 1938 the state deported patients from church asylums with the intention of killing them.   [259] Lifton, *Nazi Doctors*, p. 84.

[260] Klee, *Euthanasie*, p. 83.

expected him to be unsympathetic, and in 1940 Rüdin sought to establish a collective professional decision by psychiatrists on euthanasia. However, that Rüdin acquiesced in 'euthanasia' is shown by a memorandum on the implications of 'euthanasia' for psychiatry of 1942 which he drafted with Nitsche, Heinze and de Crinis. They expected public acceptance of 'euthanasia', once psychiatrists could convince the public that in each case every possibility of cure and therapy had been tried, and when legislation had been enacted.[261] This was a vain hope. Psychiatry was losing credibility among patients and the public. An authoritarian state, medical authority, closed institutions, and subterfuge could not shield medicine from public pressures. A distinction, based on contrasting forms of the organization of state and professional powers, is necessary between sterilization policies as a public procedure based on expert tribunals, and the covert 'euthanasia' methods and institutions. Both Gütt and Rüdin were prepared to initiate research on the concentration camp internees; but Gütt had no personal involvement in 'euthanasia', and Rüdin was a fringe and subordinate figure in the context of 'euthanasia' policies.[262] Yet Gütt laid the foundations of a centralized bureaucracy, and selected ruthless personnel. For example, in 1936 Heyde, a psychiatrist was recommended by Gütt to the SS medical officer, Grawitz. Heyde was given responsibility for hereditary research on criminals and prostitutes in concentration camps. For Heyde, this was a stepping stone to taking charge in 1939 of the selection of 'euthanasia' patients.[263] The situation was complex owing to the divergent aims of medical personnel, but nevertheless evolving towards Hitler's goal of a Spartan warrior race, maintaining fitness by killing the sick and weak.

Euthanasia and public health

The T4 'euthanasia' organization was designed to be efficient and secret. Sterilization had a basis in law, and was overseen by tribunals and public health officials. But 'euthanasia' was implemented as a strictly medical measure justified by racial biology. During the autumn of 1940 a law legalizing euthanasia was discussed by psychiatrists, the racial hygienist Lenz, and senior health officials, but it was never implemented. Significantly the SS was represented by Heydrich, who wished to extend killing of the incurable to the antisocial and unproductive.[264] The SS pressed to extend racial policy so that Jews, gypsies and social problem groups could be subjected to the lethal measures of deportation, forced labour and extermination.[265] Medical killing became a pilot scheme for the holocaust. Medical powers were so extensive that they provided techniques of coercion, control and killing.

[261] Müller-Hill, *Tödliche Wissenschaft*, pp. 45–6.
[262] No evidence is cited by Schmuhl that Rüdin was a *Euthanasieplaner*; Schmuhl, *Rassenhygiene*, pp. 178, 267. For a contrasting interpretation see P.J. Weindling, 'Compulsory Sterilisation in National Socialist Germany', *German History*, no. 5 (1987), 10–24.
[263] Klee, *Euthanasie*, p. 60.   [264] Aly and Roth, 'Gesetz', pp. 101–20.
[265] D. Peukert, *Volksgenossen und Gemeinschaftsfremde* (Cologne, 1982), pp. 246–79.

The medical rhetoric and organizational forms of welfare and closed medical institutions concealed the 'euthanasia' killings. For the complex organization of surveys, deportation of patients and resource allocation, the support of public health officials was indispensable. Some like Otto Mauthe (an ex-Centre Party member) in Württemberg were long-serving public health administrators; others such as Stähle and Walther Schultze were doctors who were dedicated Nazis since the 1920s.[266] Medical procedures and the euphemisms of 'special treatment', 'disinfection' and 'cleansing the body politic' provided elaborate forms of subterfuge. These were reinforced by medical confidentiality, security and authority, which combined to protect the Führer's Chancellery and Hitler personally from being implicated in the procedures they had authorized. The operation was concealed by cover names, giving the appearance that this was just one more welfare programme. The overall cover was provided by the 'Community Foundation for Institutional Care'.[267] Transport was by the 'Charitable Corporation for the Transport of the Sick'.[268] The killing institutes were administered by the 'Reich Association for Hospitals'.[269] That Linden was delegated from the Reich Ministry of the Interior made these organizations look as if they were state-sponsored welfare organizations, which were part of the normal machinery of public health. The medical mystique that cloaked the killings enabled doctors to participate and procedures to be effective.[270]

Selection of patients for killing was meant to be rigorously medical. The racial hygienist Lenz objected that at least photographs of patients were necessary. Other psychiatrists were confident that they could judge on case histories sent in by institutions to a central panel of adjudicators. The criteria were scientifically elaborate, and there were to be a number of exempt groups such as First World War veterans; but in practice many were killed who should have been exempt, as well as those who were simply old, infirm or querulous. That large quantities of records were filled out often under pressure of time, and cursorily adjudicated meant that the scientificity of the procedures degenerated into routine orders for deportation and death. Statistical analyses of the records of those killed suggest that of those from state hospitals, most were diagnosed as schizophrenics, which was the most frequent reason for sterilization. Of patients from the longer-stay church-run psychiatric institutions, most were diagnosed as 'feeble-minded', 'idiots' or 'epileptics'.[271] False causes of death such as carbuncles and typhus were invented. Epidemics had the advantage of justifying cremation and enabling post-mortem requests to be avoided. Each euthanasia institution had a registry office to issue the false certificates, and a fictitious registry office of Cholm (a Polish town) was

[266] E. Klee, *Was sie taten – was sie wurden* (Frankfurt-on-Main, 1986), pp. 84–93.
[267] *Die gemeinnützige Stiftung für Anstaltpflege.*
[268] *Die gemeinnützige Kranken-Transport GmbH* – abbreviated to *Gekrat.*
[269] *Die Reichsarbeitsgemeinschaft Heil- und Pflegeanstalten.*
[270] Lifton, *Nazi Doctors*; Noakes and Pridham, *Nazism*, III, pp. 996–1048.
[271] Klee, *Euthanasie*, pp. 100–23.

invented for the deaths of Jews killed in the Brandenburg institution. Added to this came false reasons for re-location (to dupe the patients, relatives and health care personnel). That the gas chambers were disguised as tiled shower facilities exploited compliance with notions of hygiene.[272] Nazism manipulated expectations of medicine as something cleansing and curative. The coercive and isolating aspects of medical institutions served Nazi ends. Medical powers over life and death became subordinate to ulterior racial and political purposes.

Yet euthanasia also revealed limitations to medical powers. Medicine was a double-edged weapon, as it allowed for residual defence mechanisms by patients, carers and relatives. Health care personnel had emotional attachments to patients. Many institutions relied on the labour of relatively fit patients who might otherwise have been discharged. Families were concerned about their relatives being removed and mysteriously dying. There were cases when relatives tried to visit the sealed-off institutions, or when a patient was notified as having died on a date before having been seen alive. Protests began to mount. Death notices were placed in papers in such a way as to alert a broader public that many had died on one day from the same unexpected cause at a certain institution. The churches, already sensitized to sterilization, began to protest with sermons against euthanasia. Protests were registered with the Reich Ministry of Justice, which dutifully began to investigate the legal basis for the killings until it was informed that they were on the Führer's order. Inhabitants living around the killing institution soon discovered what was going on.

There was an inherent diversity and instability in the 'euthanasia' measures. The separate programme for the killing of sick and disabled children was administered by paediatricians and medical authorities. There were thirty 'special children's departments' in which 6,000 were killed. In Autumn 1941 the T4 programme was 'ended' due to public pressure. This was, however, a further deception as new organizations for killing were used. Sick concentration camp inmates were killed by procedures similar to those inflicted on the mentally ill. What was known as 'Aktion 14 f 13' offered a connection between the T4 programme and the Final Solution. T4 personnel were transferred to the death camps, and helped to build the gas chambers at Belzec, Sobibor and Treblinka from autumn 1941. From 1942 Jews and mixed race children were killed. In the face of mounting opposition to the use of Grafeneck asylum, a stage of decentralized 'wild euthanasia' was initiated. Patients were killed by starvation, exhaustion through work, fatal medicines and injection. More were killed in this way than in the T4 programme, and there was a greater integration with the normal structures of medical 'care'. In occupied Poland and the Soviet Union, SS X-ray units sought out the tubercular, who were then shot. It is estimated that 100,000 died in this way. From 1942 a variety of racially undesirable, sick or 'antisocial' foreign workers, orphans, and youth 'delinquents' were killed. While the T4 programme resulted in the deaths of

[272] G. Fleming, *Hitler and the Final Solution* (Oxford, 1986), pp. 25–7.

between 70,000 and 95,000 persons, these other programmes resulted in considerably more deaths. This phase of medical killing was integrated into normal medical practices, procedures and institutions.[273]

Infertility treatment

'Euthanasia' was an extreme form of negative racial hygiene. At the same time certain patients deemed to have curable diseases, and those from racially elite groups received medical care of high quality. There was a radical pursuit of positive eugenic methods for raising the fertility of selected populations. In 1936 infertility became recognized as a condition for which free medical treatment was available, provided that the offspring were in the interests of the *Volk*. The close link with medical killing can be shown in the case of Württemberg. Here the health official, Stähle, organized a central data bank on the infertile, and took a lead in organizing medical killing. While wanting to prevent reproduction of the antisocial, he loathed contraceptives that threatened the rural birth rate. He instigated an *Arbeitsgemeinschaft* for the cure of lack of children, which was referred to as 'child poverty'. Health offices were to provide examinations, therapy and counselling for the infertile.[274] Much attention was paid to the shape, vigour and number of sperm. Here there was a burgeoning scientific literature.[275] The male was to be examined for libido, the quality of erection, orgasm and ejaculation. A weak erection was taken as a sign of diabetes, kidney disease, alcoholism, nicotine abuse or drug abuse. The female was to have a complete medical history and physical examination of reproductive organs. There was also to be education on the basic rules of a healthy lifestyle. The health offices were to compile a *Sippenkartei* of all childless or 'child poor' couples. In May 1943 this endeavour was suspended for the duration of the war as offensive to public sensibilities.[276] Other welfare measures such as the SS's *Lebensborn* represented the positive eugenic side of racial policy: medical killing and the combating of infertility provide extreme examples of the fusion of medicine and population policy.

The 'euthanasia' measures were both the culmination of, and a break with, earlier eugenic measures. There was continuity in diagnostic categories, but the mode of implementation was different. Sterilization was a mass procedure, with a tribunal system. The medical killing was intended to be rigorously secret. That the draft law was scrapped meant that medical killing depended on the Führer's authority. Racial hygienists were divided over their support for Nazi measures. Some considered that the distinctive combination of a racial warrior elite and

---

[273] Lifton, *Nazi Doctors*, pp. 96–102.
[274] F.H. Bardenheuer, *Die Unfruchtbarkeit der Frau* (Munich, 1942).
[275] Stiasny, 'Untersuchungsmethode und Therapie der Sterilität beim Manne', *Zentralblatt für Gynäkologie*, no. 27 (1941). Stiasny, 'Feststellung und Beurteilung der Männlichen Unfruchtbarkeit', *MMW*, vol. 90 (1943), 653.
[276] HStA Stuttgart, E 151 K VI Hilfe beim Kinderlosigkeit; E 151 X 1015 II 1921–45 Massregeln zur Hebung der Volkskraft, Stähle to Linden, 9 December 1942.

extermination of the degenerate went beyond the scientific measures necessary for the salvation of the race. Others were swept away by enthusiasm for Nazi militarism and racism. 'Euthanasia' was the culmination of a deadly combination of subordination to the Führer, a war economy, and professionalism taken to an extreme of scientific authoritarianism.

FROM RACIAL RESEARCH TO HUMAN GENETICS

The conflict between ideology and technocracy in the attempt to realize racial policies was never resolved. As well as requiring a functional medical science, the SS indulged in Nordic mystic rites, and built up its mythology of symbols and rituals. Anthropologists were necessary for formulating racial policies and for adjudicating on individual cases and racial groups. Medical personnel was needed in concentration camps. Doctors trained in racial hygiene selected those that were to be worked to death by forced labour, and those that were sent straight to the gas chambers. They became used to screening the forced labour contingents for those so sick and exhausted that they too were killed. Epidemics such as dysentery and typhus had to be controlled. Medical and dental services for the SS personnel were needed. Medicine was integral to the final solution. While the SS needed to have a subordinate and compliant medical corps, the concentration camps offered opportunities to doctors keen to advance their careers by undertaking medical research. Some of the research was carried out by special units for military or racial purposes. Other projects were initiated by the universities or the Kaiser Wilhelm institutes. Even in the most lethal, regimented and racialized forms of medicine, there was a plurality of ideas, interests and allegiances.

Racial hygienists and biologists were in an inherently conflict-ridden and unstable situation. The case of the Kaiser Wilhelm Institute for Anthropology under Fischer and then Verschuer may be taken as a representative case-study of the attempt to apply science to realize racial aims, for the Institute kept up with the latest work in human genetics, while cultivating Nazi authorities in the party and state. Research on disparate medical, biological and psychological problems was conducted in locations varying from children's holiday camps for the racial elite to Mengele's block in Auschwitz for the killing of humans for scientific purposes. There was, however, a coherent rationale of hereditary pathology.

The Racial Political Office of the NSDAP under Gross appreciated the utility of Fischer and Verschuer as allies. Fischer could claim appropriate ideological credentials with his early links with Günther, and with Schemann's Gobineau cult. Both Fischer and Verschuer became concerned with 'the Jewish problem'. It was overlooked that before 1933 Fischer had advocated racial intermarriage as a healthy regenerative process. After 1933 he condemned miscegenation as degenerate, and with Verschuer praised the Nuremburg laws for segregating Jews from Germans. Lenz continued to value the Jewish spirit as culturally and intellectually creative, but an edition in 1936 of the Baur-Fischer-Lenz text book contrasted the Jewish and

Germanic aspirations for power. He pointed to a range of positive Jewish characteristics such as intellectual creativity and abstinence from alcohol. He compared Jewish and German statistics for crimes, indicating that Jews were less deceitful, and less prone to physical violence just as the Nordic Hamburgers were better in commerce. His aim was to outline the strengths of the adversary of the German race, so heightening the struggle between Germans and Jews. He pointed out that the term 'anti-semitism' was pseudo-scientific as there was no semitic race as such, and that the Nazi concept of race was unscientific. However, Nazism was valuable in creating the mental climate to reinculcate a 'will' in the German race to adopt selective processes that could restore their racial qualities. Lenz laid stress on the superiority of the scientific approach to the racial question.[277] The institute's attempt to dominate hereditary biology could be seen when Fischer joined forces with Gross in condemning the Nordic ideologist Ludwig Ferdinand Clauss for philo-semitism.[278] Fischer's attack on Clauss was that of a human geneticist on an impressionistic psychologist. Academic vendettas found convenient party political channels.

The university institutes for racial hygiene expanded on the basis of offering services to the state. Courses in racial pathology were provided for SS, NSDAP and public health officials. Bureaucratic functions accumulated with adjudication of cases for sterilization and for racial categorization. The Nuremberg and marriage laws meant that additional assistantships were necessary. Among Verschuer's assistants at Frankfurt was Mengele, who refereed on prosecutions under the Nuremberg laws.[279] The Kaiser Wilhelm Institute for Anthropology, its personnel and research aims became attuned to the requirements of Nazism. Just as Fischer and Verschuer successfully served the social welfare aims of the Centre Party and SPD in the 1920s, so now they offered their new masters a number of services. Verschuer, while in Frankfurt, and Fischer in Berlin provided training for SS personnel, and research expertise for racial surveys. Informal contacts were maintained with doctors who were thoroughly schooled in human genetics and had scientific credentials in racial anthropology. Routine adjudications of racial ancestry in controversial cases were part of the Anthropological Institute's functions. Although it was possible for racial adjudicators to adopt a benevolent attitude to cases, Fischer insisted that racial evaluations be rigorously carried out.[280] The painstaking exactness with which these tasks were executed raises the question of whether they were formal tokens of allegiance, offered up so as to shield the fundamental research work of the institute, or whether they were generated by racial convictions of science that was placed in the service of Nazism.

Verschuer's move to Frankfurt in 1935 gave him the opportunity to develop 'hereditary biology and racial hygiene' as an integrated discipline. He endeavoured

277 Müller-Hill, *Tödliche Wissenschaft*, p. 38; Baur, Fischer, Lenz, *Menschliche Erblehre*, pp. 746–73.
278 BDC Gross file.   279 Müller-Hill, *Tödliche Wissenschaft*, p. 39.
280 H. Seidler and A. Rett, *Das Reichssippenamt entscheidet. Rassenbiologie in Nationalsozialismus* (Vienna and Munich, 1982) pp. 274–81.

to combine clinical practice, demographic surveys and research into a unified science of human heredity. He signalled his intention by establishing a periodical, *Der Erbarzt*, which was initially a supplement of the *Deutsches Ärzteblatt* which had the aim of indoctrinating the medical profession with racial science. After 1939 Verschuer was scientifically more assertive and *Der Erbarzt* became the leading periodical for human genetics. Verschuer's institute for hereditary research was installed in ultra-modern premises, which had been a municipal *Haus der Volksgesundheit* opened in 1928.[281] Racial hygienists organized family surveys and the registration of total populations, which pointed to the persistence of diseases and characteristics over long periods. The inheritance of diseases such as schizophrenia and cancer was studied in twins. In 1938 'crossing over' of hereditary factors in a human population was observed, using cases of red–green colour blindness.[282] Mengele, as Verschuer's assistant, claimed that cleft lip, jaw and palate were inherited through attenuated forms as the result of a dominant gene.[283] Verschuer succeeded in building up a talented research team of human geneticists which included Ferdinand Claussen and Hans Grebe, both of whom quickly gained university chairs. Their researches continued to be co-ordinated by Verschuer.[284] When he was appointed director of the Kaiser Wilhelm Institute for Anthropology he was able to take his Frankfurt team with him, and hoped eventually to appoint Mengele.[285]

In 1936 Verschuer proposed a large-scale research project on *erbklinische Forschungen* (clinical research on heredity). It comprised clinical investigations into 'heredity and racial qualities', hereditary diseases in twins, and cancer as an inherited disease, as well as animal experiments in hereditary pathology. The *Deutsche Forschungsgemeinschaft* supported this research.[286] Further grants extended the research programme. Courses were given to medical students, doctors and to the SS and Nazi organizations in Frankfurt and Berlin. These activities ensured that Verschuer had positive support from the authorities, as well as the academic blessing of such senior figures as Fischer. Verschuer developed an enthusiasm for work on the 'Jewish problem'. In May 1937 he went to Munich where he advised on the registration of Jews and *Mischlinge*. Fischer and Verschuer were determined to give racial policies an objective and scientific basis.[287]

To understand the social position of leading racial hygienists such as Fischer and Verschuer it is necessary to locate them in the polycratic power-bloc structure of

[281] K.-D. Thomann, 'Rassenhygiene und Anthropologie: Die zwei Karrieren des Prof. Verschuer', *Frankfurter Rundschau*, no. 116 (21 May 1985).

[282] Bruno Rath, 'Rotgrünblindheit in der Calmbacher Blutersippe, Nachweis des Faktorenaustausches beim Menschen', *ARGB*, vol. 32 (1938).

[283] J. Mengele, 'Sippenuntersuchungen bei Lippen-Kiefer-Gaumenspalte', *Zeitschrift für menschliche Vererbungs- und Konstitutionslehre*, vol. 23 (1939), 17–42.

[284] O. v. Verschuer, 'Vier Jahre Frankfurter Universitäts-Institut für Erbbiologie und Rassenhygiene', *Der Erbarzt*, (1934), 57–64.   [285] Verschuer papers, Verschuer to Lehmann, 11 June 1942.

[286] BDC Reichsforschungsrat cards; BAK R 73 Nr 15342 Bl. 125–35 Verschuer, Bericht, 1938.

[287] Verschuer papers, Verschuer to Fischer, 8 and 20 May, 5 November 1937.

Nazi Germany. The Berlin Institute made attempts to ingratiate itself with the Racial Political Office of Gross and Wolfgang Knorr. The orientation to the NSDAP was shown in links with Rosenberg and the National Socialist Welfare League, the NSV. From 1936 the NSV put its holiday colony programme for children at the disposal of researchers by collecting twins for a special 'twin camp'. Here the behaviour of twins could be observed in psychological tests, filmed, photographed and measured, particularly by Gottschaldt who was interested in the inheritance of intelligence.[288] Gross of the NSDAP Racial Political Office was invited on to the management committee of the Anthropological Institute, and Fischer joined conferences organized by the Racial Political Office.[289] Fischer found the support of the party more congenial than the interventionist tendencies of the SS. While Fischer's protectors did not have the power of the SS, they were more inclined to give scientists free rein to develop a functioning science.

Links with the SS were more distant, and it was difficult to resolve contradictions between racial ideology and science. The anthropologist Wolfgang Abel had joined the NSDAP in Vienna in June 1933 prior to transfer to the Kaiser Wilhelm Institute in 1934; he then joined the SS.[290] Abel's position in the SS was regarded by the *Ahnenerbe* as a valuable means for potential control of anthropology in Berlin. Once Fischer retired, there was a vacuum created for an anthropologist in Berlin. In 1942 the *Ahnenerbe* planned to support an independent Institute for Anthropology and Racial Biology. Given that Verschuer concentrated on genetics and racial pathology, Abel hoped that he could use contacts with the SS to secure an institute and professorial chair. He was on good personal terms with Sievers, the secretary of the SS, and with the SS police chief, Ernst Kaltenbrunner, a fellow Austrian. Abel's research on gypsies and bushmen would have fitted in well with both the 'hereditary pathology' research programme, and the racial policies of the SS. However, the plan was blocked at ministerial level.[291] Moreover, Abel's views were condemned as scientifically flawed. He became convinced of the common Indo-Germanic origins of Slavs and Germans. This led him to propose the Germanification rather than the extermination of Eastern stocks.[292]

During the 1940s the racial hygienists were not allocated the directing role in population policy that they hoped for. While Lenz and Fischer were involved in formulating the grandiose schemes for population engineering in the East, they remained peripheral figures. Fischer's patronage derived from Rosenberg and the *Ostministerium*. Although Lenz had offered his services to the SS's *Ahnenerbe* regarding settlement policy, he was a difficult figure to accommodate. Abel joined the criticisms of the SS's support for 'illegitimate' births, which Lenz regarded as the product of degeneracy. Lenz drafted articles to argue his point in the SS's

[288] K. Gottschaldt, 'NSV und Zwillingsforschung', *Wochen-Dienst. NSDAP. Gau Berlin Amt für Volkswohlfahrt*, vol. 3 no. 28 (11 July 1939), 335–59; Verschuer papers, Verschuer to Fischer, 4 May and 29 September 1944.   [289] Verschuer papers, Verschuer to Fischer, 25 April 1944.
[290] BDC Abel file.   [291] BDC Abel file, 6 June 1942.
[292] Müller-Hill, *Tödliche Wissenschaft*, pp. 135–48, Abel interview.

journal, *Der schwarze Korps*.[293] In June 1940 he expounded his views to the Race and Settlement Office of the SS.[294]

Fischer's cordial relations with the leading Nazi ideologist Rosenberg help to clarify the position of the Anthropological Institute. Fischer published under the auspices of Rosenberg's Office. Fischer by 1934 was offering up public statements on the need to build up a state based on 'blood and soil', folk customs, race and German spirit. He and Verschuer were keen to work on the 'Jewish problem'. In 1937 they co-operated on a memorandum on the anthropological distinction of Jews from mixed-race *Mischlinge*, which was deemed relevant to military call-up plans. They were concerned racial policies should be grounded in 'objective science'.[295] Verschuer co-operated with the Reich Institute for Historical Research on racial aspects of history. His writings became virulently hostile to Jews as degenerates. On 27 and 28 March 1941 Rosenberg organized a conference at his Frankfurt Institute for Research at which the 'total solution of the Jewish question' was discussed. Fischer suggested extermination through work. Rosenberg spoke of 'a cleansing biological revolution'. Fischer took on propaganda responsibilities, arguing for the degeneracy of the Jewish race.[296] From 1940 Fischer devoted his main energies to research on Jews as having constant racial characteristics. He sent an assistant to make observations and photographs on the Jews in the Litzmannstadt ghetto. He compared photographs with ancient pictures, using these in a book on Old Testament Jewry.[297] After the Germans invaded the Soviet Union in June 1941, Fischer pronounced Bolsheviks and Jews to be a distinct degenerate species.[298] Abel and Fischer advised the SS on the feasibility of 'Germanizing' Nordic elements in the Russian population.[299] In 1943 he urged mass sterilization of gypsies on the grounds that they were primitive and antisocial. When Rosenberg became Minister for the Occupied Territories, Fischer accepted an invitation to an anti-Jewish congress at Cracow in 1944.[300] Despite Rosenberg's interest in the Nazification of sciences such as physics, prehistory and *Volkskunde*, his lack of concern with racial biology has been regarded as an anomaly.[301] Fischer's institute contributed to Rosenberg's ideological and institutional powers. Gross and Rosenberg's administrative posts were weakened by the SS which used its policing powers to secure racial aims. Rosenberg's lack of effective power accounts for the Anthropological Institute's status: protected but not integrated into the police and racial policies of the SS. Fischer had hitherto been on good terms

---

[293] Lenz papers, Lenz to *Schwarze Korps*, 10 May 1940.

[294] Lenz papers, Lenz to Verschuer, 12 and 17 June 1940.

[295] Poliakov and Wulf, *Denker*, p. 104; Verschuer papers, Verschuer to Fischer, 8 May 1937, 20 May 1937, 5 November 1937.   [296] Müller-Hill, *Tödliche Wissenschaft*, p. 49.

[297] Müller-Hill, *Tödliche Wissenschaft*, p. 74.

[298] Poliakov and Wulf, *Denker*, pp. 79–80; Müller-Hill, *Tödliche Wissenschaft*, p. 49.

[299] Müller-Hill, *Tödliche Wissenschaft*, pp. 108–9.

[300] Müller-Hill, *Tödliche Wissenschaft*, pp. 80–1.

[301] R. Bollmus, *Das Amt Rosenberg und seine Gegner, Zum Machtkampf im national-sozialistischen Herrschaftssystem* (Stuttgart, 1970), p. 69.

with Gross and with Wagner, the Reich Doctors' leader.[302] The replacing of Wagner by Conti was to stand the Institute in good stead as Fischer valued Conti as a link with the state's medical and racial policies.[303] Verschuer found Conti to be a reliable supporter.[304] As Conti's power was also eroded, it helped to maintain the autonomy of the institute.

Hereditary pathology

The internal coherence of the Kaiser Wilhelm Institute for Anthropology was due more to its concerted research programme of 'racial pathology' than to party-political or administrative links. Of the institute's departmental directors in 1945, Abel, Lenz and Verschuer were party members, although they were all marginal figures. Gottschaldt and Nachtsheim were not in the party. Indeed, Gottschaldt, who had been appointed on 1 April 1935 by Fischer, was suspected of left-wing sympathies, since Clauss had counter-attacked against Fischer with accusations against Gottschaldt.[305] Some junior members of staff such as Karin Magnussen and Diehl had been party members for longer than the directors but their importance was slight and other staff were not in the NSDAP.[306] In contrast to, the lack of political uniformity, there was a unity of scientific purpose and method. The coherence of the institute's organization and activities derived not so much from external forces of the party, SS or *völkisch* racial interests, as from a systematic research strategy of hereditary pathology conceived by Fischer and developed by Verschuer. In March 1940 Fischer confided that he hoped Verschuer would succeed him, and organize a large-scale research project on human heredity. Lenz was criticized as too erratic and individualistic to direct the institute. Fischer considered that 'a large research institute must have an ambitious plan'. Lenz was working without planning and was unsystematic in allocating projects to students.[307] Lenz attempted to persuade the Education Ministry that racial hygiene must be maintained as a subject in which university teaching was linked with research, and that there should be an additional university institute for racial hygiene for clinical medical students as well as a university institute for racial anthropology.[308] Fischer intervened with the authorities against Lenz, arguing that Verschuer ought to be entrusted with the organizing of a major research project in hereditary pathology, whereas Lenz should be relegated to teaching duties.[309] Fischer insinuated that Lenz's dedication to racial hygiene as a Nordic and Platonic ideal made him

---

[302] MPG Nr 2403 Fischer to Gross, 14 June 1935.
[303] MPG Nr 2403 Fischer to Telschow, 18 March 1940.
[304] Verschuer papers, Verschuer to Fischer, 23 November 1942.
[305] Verschuer papers, Verschuer to Fischer, 30 September 1941, on the necessity of party membership; BDC Gross file. [306] BDC Magnussen had joined the NSDAP on 1 June 1931, Nr. 549763.
[307] Verschuer papers, Fischer to Verschuer, 8 March 1940.
[308] MPG Nr 2400 31 July 1941, Lenz to Reichsminister für Wissenschaft.
[309] MPG Institut für Anthropologie und Eugenik Hauptakten 4.12.1940–18.6.1945, Fischer to Kaiser Wilhelm Gesellschaft President 20 October 1941.

temperamentally unsuited to directing large-scale research. The grand scientific plan was to be realized by Verschuer. Fischer remained in close contact with him after retirement in 1941, and was felt to be a spiritual presence at the institute.[310]

The geneticist Nachtsheim exemplifies the continuities in German biology between the 1890s and 1950s. He originally wished to study with Haeckel, but as Haeckel was retiring he studied zoology under Richard Hertwig in Munich and assisted Doflein in Freiburg. The shock of the German defeat in 1918 convinced him that science was necessary to provide social cohesion. In 1921 he joined the plant geneticist (and vehement nationalist) Baur at the Agricultural University in Berlin. He researched on domestic animals with the aim of understanding inherited human diseases, characteristics such as lactation, and hair and eye colour, as well as nerve and blood diseases such as epilepsy, pellagra, and fetal erythroblastosis. His position as a leading figure in the German Rabbit Breeders' Association resulted in conflicts with the party, although it also made him a well-known biologist. He aligned his research with Verschuer's concept of hereditary pathology. In 1941 he joined the Kaiser Wilhelm Institute for Anthropology, and a post was established for him in the Department for Experimental Hereditary Pathology.[311]

In contrast to Verschuer, Lenz did not embark on a large-scale research programme. He lectured to a wide variety of organizations, ranging from the university to the Racial Office of the SS. He advised the state authorities on many issues, including the draft of the 'euthanasia' law. Perhaps because of his temperamental pessimism or as a result of a deliberate strategy of disengagement from the crumbling Reich, Lenz seems to have remained a theoretician, and an air of aloofness from the Nazi social system helped him to achieve a smooth transition to human genetics.[312] An 'inner emigration' into the secure realms of scientific certainties was to be an escape route for racial hygienists from the National Socialist power structure once the loss of the war became apparent. The Berlin institute had a prestigious and protected existence during the 1940s, as the pace of research accelerated.

Fischer's research programme was wide-ranging, but well integrated. He aimed to link the genetics of human racial variation with biochemical processes. In addition to the hereditary surveys of populations, he suggested an anatomical collection on human heredity for research on the genetics of development (phenogenetics). A department of hereditary pathology was to be established under Nachtsheim, who would switch from research on the genetics of fruit flies (*Drosophila*) to phenogenetics and use rabbit embryos to examine disease and heredity. Fischer hoped that Nachtsheim might replace the 'dated' Department of Racial Hygiene under Lenz.[313] Fischer and Verschuer were firm supporters of the

[310] Verschuer papers, Verschuer to Fischer, 20 September 1943.
[311] H. Grüneberg and W. Ulrich (eds.), *Moderne Biologie. Festschrift zum 60. Geburtstag von Hans Nachtsheim* (Berlin, 1950).
[312] Lenz papers, Tätigkeitsbericht Kaiser Wilhelm Institut für Eugenik.
[313] Verschuer papers, Fischer to Verschuer, 8 March 1940.

psychologist Gottschaldt. They regarded his methodology based on statistical genetics to be relevant for physiology and pathology.[314]

Fischer's fusion of genetics and physiological chemistry combined research on population genetics and biochemical theories of blood and cell protein. The biochemist, Abderhalden, regarded proteins as racial characters. He argued that proteins took a key role in heredity and attempted to explain genetic mutations by an interaction of proteins in the reproductive glands. He undertook experiments on different species of rabbit, and suggested research on twins with comparison of each twin's blood protein and injections to modify the protein structure. This research complemented the work of Nachtsheim on rabbit strains. Abderhalden's research was supported by the military medical authorities from 1943.[315] Between April 1943 and March 1944 Abderhalden co-operated with the Kaiser Wilhelm Institute for Anthropology for research on the racial specificity of proteins; it was reported that 'a special laboratory' was established for this.[316]

Fischer's imprint on the institute was indicated by its being renamed the *Eugen-Fischer-Institut* on the occasion of his seventieth birthday in 1944.[317] But it was Verschuer who implemented the integrated research programme on racial pathology. The German Research Fund approved Verschuer's various research projects in March 1943. There were some additions. Ströer, a Dutch embryologist, was included. He researched on growth anomalies using dwarf rabbits. Diehl, a tuberculosis researcher and NSDAP activist who had co-operated with Verschuer since 1928, was to research on pulmonary dust diseases. There was also to be research on still births and twins. Grebe worked on genetic diseases and the occurrence of hernias in families. Verschuer wished to research on physical anomalies and metabolic changes. For this research on physique, he recruited the school doctor Karin Magnussen, who was interested in the inheritance of eye-colour anomalies.[318] Her publications on educational matters suggest that a high degree of commitment to hereditary research was the basis of Nazi education.[319]

Verschuer was an enthusiastic supporter of the war. He extolled the enlarged *Grossdeutschland* as a reunification of German racial stocks. In January 1942 he wrote on how the war would see a 'final solution' to the 'Jewish problem'. The war provided opportunities for research into hereditary pathology.[320] Verschuer needed human specimens for research. In 1942 North African prisoners were used by Baader for research on bone structure.[321] Verschuer's favoured Frankfurt assistant, Mengele, was to take on a special role. In 1935 Mengele qualified in

314 Verschuer papers, Verschuer to Fischer, 23 November 1942.
315 BA Militärarchiv Freiburg H2o Nr 857.
316 Lenz papers, Tätigkeitsbericht KW Institut Eugenik, March 1944.
317 O. v. Verschuer, 'Eugen Fischer', *Der Erbarzt*, vol. 12 (1944), 57–9.
318 Lenz papers, KWI Tätigkeitsbericht April 1943–March 1944.
319 K. Magnussen, *Rassen- und bevölkerungspolitisches Rüstzeug: Statistik, Gesetzgebung und Kriegsaufgaben* (München, Berlin, 1939); Verschuer papers, Verschuer to Fischer, 12 July 1943.
320 O. v. Verschuer, 'Der Erbarzt an der Jahreswende', *Der Erbarzt*, vol. 10 (1942), 1–3.
321 *Guanchen-Gliedmassen Knochen.*

Table 9. *Reich Research Council: applications for research grants by Verschuer*

26.x.1934	heredity in twins
12.ix.1934	application to Fischer for referee's report
18.x.1934	application to Rüdin
6.xii.1934	application to Gütt
?.i.1934	application approved for 1920 M for 1 Electrocardiogram
11.ii.1934	application for clinical research on heredity
19.iii.1934	supported by Gütt
29.ii.1935	hereditary biological survey of the population supported by Gütt. 1,000 M approved
25.iii.1935	application for twin studies
	application for Dr Liebermann
	application for Dr Wehmeier
6.xi.1935	application withdrawn
xi.1936	application for clinical research on heredity
ii.1937	supported by Gütt
v.1937	15,000 M for hereditary biology
25.x.1936	twin research
v.1937	4,500 M granted
?.1937	1,200 M twin research
27.ii.1937	15,000 M
22.xii.1936	hereditary pathology, animal experiments
12.xii.1937	approved under 15,000 M grant
19.ii.1937	inheritance of cancer
7.vii.1937	3,000 M approved
21.xii.1937	subsidy of 31,500 M for hereditary biology
8.vi.1938	15,500 M granted for the district of 'Schwalm'
iii.1939	hereditary biology and racial welfare
?.1939	subsidy of 11,585 M
viii.1939	974 M for research support
24.iv.1939	2,800 M for hereditary biology
iii.1943	application for 40,000 M for the continuation of the work of professor Eugen Fischer on comparative hereditary pathology
24.v.1943	approval for 40,000 M
25.ii.1944	1,000 M clinical research on tuberculosis and heredity
6.iv.1944	1,000 M approved
iv.44	1 single lens reflex camera case
20.iii.1944	40,000 M for comparative hereditary pathology
16.v.1944	grant approved
18.viii.1944	joint research on hereditary pathology with Professor Nachtsheim
ii.1944	grant continued
18.viii.1944	tuberculosis research. Co-worker Dr Diehl
xi.1944	grant extended
18.vii.1943	protein research on spezifische Eiweisskörper
3.xi.1943	grant extended
7.ix.1943	eye colour
x.1944	report

Table 9 (*cont.*)

3.xi.1944	project extended
7.ix.1943	research application approved for twin camp (Zwillingslager)
4.x.1944	report
17.xi.1944	research project discontinued
7.ix.1943	research project on racial hygiene approved
3.xi.1944	project extended
7.ix.1943	hereditary biological racial survey
3.xi.1944	research project extended
7.ix.1943	research project on still births
14.x.1944	transfer of project to Dr Grebe, Rostock
7.ix.1944	pulmonary dust disease
14.x.1944	transfer of project to Dr Grebe

Note: M = Marks
Source: Berlin Document Centre, Reich Research Council records.

anthropology under Mollison in Munich, where he worked on the normal physical anthropology of the jaw. He had used skulls of Melanesian, ancient Egyptian, and European long- and short-headed races. He proved by a complex series of measurements on the alveolar region of the jaws of 122 skull specimens that variations were racially specific characteristics.[322] Verschuer's biological approach to anthropology enabled Mengele to complement the craniometrical approach with genetic and clinical investigations of cleft lip, jaw and palate, which were relevant to eugenic problems. Mengele was concerned that advances in the surgical treatment of cleft palates and hare lips would mean that these would continue to occur if they were inherited. He located 1,222 relatives of seventeen patients from the surgical clinic. He showed that there was a range of attenuated forms of jaw deformities, and he correlated these with other physical conditions such as heart weakness and mongolism. He applied genetic cross-over patterns to demonstrate inherited frequencies.[323] This research showed that Mengele was abreast of international trends in research on human genetics; indeed, the German work on the aetiology of cleft lip and palate won international recognition. But he greatly overestimated the extent that cleft palate and hare lip were genetically inherited; and correlations, as with inherited 'feeble-mindedness', and the collections of large pedigrees were the result of the paradigm of hereditary pathology.[324] Verschuer brought these researches to the attention of a wider academic audience in 1939.[325]

When Verschuer moved to Berlin, the intention was that Mengele's assistantship

[322] J. Mengele, 'Rassenmorphologische Untersuchung des vorderen Unterkieferabschnittes bei vier rassischen Gruppen', PhD thesis, University of Munich, 1937.
[323] Mengele, 'Sippenuntersuchungen', pp. 17–42.
[324] 'Die wissenschaftliche Normalität des Schlächters. Josef Mengele als Anthropologe 1937–1941', *Dokumentationsstelle zur NS-Sozialpolitik. Mitteilungen*, vol. 1 no. 2 (1 April 1985).
[325] Verschuer papers, Wolfgang Lehmann to Verschuer, 16 January 1939, 2 February 1939.

should be transferred. Mengele had joined the Stahlhelm in 1931, the SA for a period during 1934, the NSDAP in May 1937, and the SS in May 1938. From August 1940 he served as a doctor for three years in the Viking division of the Waffen SS, and was wounded at Stalingrad. Declared medically unfit for combat, he was appointed to the Racial and Settlement Office of the SS, and he returned to work with Verschuer at the Anthropological Institute from January 1943. Verschuer wrote with pride to Fischer of Mengele's endurance on the Eastern Front.[326] He was posted to Auschwitz as camp doctor from 30 May 1943. An SS report on Mengele in August 1944 makes it clear that his anthropological research was not part of his duties as camp doctor, but a voluntary activity conducted in off-duty hours.[327] His camp duties involved selections for the gas chambers and camp sanitation. While executing routine tasks, he remained dedicated to twin research, and unrelated children deceived him that they were twins.[328] That the research was conducted for the Kaiser Wilhelm Institute for Anthropology was attested to by Mengele's Jewish pathologist, Miklos Nyiszli, who assisted Mengele from May 1944. Because of his assiduous attention to routine and his success in containing a typhus epidemic Mengele was granted research facilities.[329] Mengele's scientific aims drew on Verschuer's method of twin research as the basis for hereditary pathology. Nyiszli related how experiments on living twins were complemented by pathological comparisons of healthy and diseased organs in twins, whom Mengele had killed for the purpose of simultaneous evaluation. Growth defects, reproductive biology resulting in twin births, variations like eye-colour in twins, and characteristics of racial degeneration such as endocrine and anatomical anomalies were of interest. Such killing was motivated by a calculated scientific logic.

Although the Reich Research Council records show that the 'twin camp' research (presumably of Gottschaldt) was no longer funded after 17 November 1944, Verschuer continued the research programme as long as it was possible. Fischer gave moral support, and Research Council officials regarded the programme as an urgent priority. The project on hereditary pathology was renewed in October 1944.[330] The work was seen as of lasting value in contrast to the crumbling Reich. For example, in January 1945 Blome, as deputy health leader, supported Nachtsheim's research on erythroblastosis in rabbits as offering parallels to human blood diseases, and efforts were made to evacuate Nachtsheim's rabbit stocks to Switzerland.[331]

A doctoral student of Fischer's, G. Wagner, had noticed eye-colour anomalies in

[326] Verschuer papers, Verschuer to Fischer, 25 January 1943, Fischer to Verschuer, 2 February 1943. I am grateful to W. Lenz for a critical evaluation of Mengele's research.
[327] BDC Mengele file.
[328] M. Weinreich, *Hitler's Professors. The Part of Scholarship in Germany's Crimes against the Jewish People* (New York, 1946), p. 198.
[329] M. Nyiszli, *Auschwitz: a Doctor's Eye Witness Account* (New York, 1960); BDC Mengele file.
[330] BDC Reichsforschungsrat; Verschuer papers, Verschuer to Fischer, 31 August 1944.
[331] Nachtsheim papers, Nachtsheim to Verschuer, 12 March 1945.

gypsies. At the Anthropological Institute, Magnussen compared the pathology of human and rabbit eyes regarding the overgrowth of corneas.[332] Magnussen was using Nachtsheim's rabbit stocks to study the genetics of eye pigmentation, a topic on which Nachtsheim had himself researched.[333] It has been suggested that she used the gypsy eyes obtained by Mengele from twins and a gypsy family, whom he had ordered to be killed for research on eye-colour anomalies as racial characteristics. The gypsy family had heterochromia of the eyes (with one brown and the other blue or potentially blue).[334] Her work was regarded as 'fundamental' by Verschuer.

The purity of science

Verschuer aimed at a grand synthesis of anthropology, genetics, biochemistry and immunology. Pointers had been given by the biochemist Abderhalden, who emphasized the racial specificity of proteins in blood plasma. In 1939 he suggested that reactions in the protein contained in organs of twins be studied.[335] Racial and hereditary characteristics could be found in the fine structure of cell and blood proteins which were generally constant over generations. Verschuer retreated into scientific work as in itself a battle for truth. He prided himself that his war-service strengthened his resolve to maintain a functioning institute in the midst of bombing. He made common cause with other Kaiser Wilhelm Institute directors such as Wettstein (the geneticist), Adolf Butenandt (the biochemist) and Heisenberg (the physicist) in the defence of their institutes and the Kaiser Wilhelm Gesellschaft.[336] In January 1945 Verschuer felt that he was on the verge of a breakthrough in connecting disease to blood plasma.[337] The research on protein involved over 200 racially mixed human samples. He was interested in studying differences in the blood serum in various races after infectious disease. It seems that Mengele provided specimens from over 200 persons, either of mixed race or twins. The plasma proteins were prepared with the help of Butenandt and the Kaiser Wilhelm Institute for Biochemistry. Nachtsheim's hereditary experiments on animals had certain similarities in aims and methods with Mengele's 'research' on humans. Nachtsheim worked on rabbit eyes, and on epilepsy in rabbits and on

---

[332] K. Magnussen, 'Über eine sichelformige Hornhautüberwachsung am Kaninchenauge und beim Menschen', Der Erbarzt, vol. 12 (1944), 60–2; Verschuer papers, Verschuer to Fischer, 28 October 1943, 13 November 1943.

[333] K. Magnussen, 'Die Einwirkung der Farbgene auf die Pigmententwicklung im Kaninchenauge', unpublished MS dated 20 February 1944; H. Nachtsheim, 'Die genetischen Beziehungen zwischen Körperfarbe und Augenfarbe beim Kaninchen', Biologisches Zentralblatt, vol. 52 (1933), 99–109.

[334] A paper was announced in 'Ueber die Beziehungen zwischen Irisfarbe, histologischer Pigmententwicklung und Pigmentierung des Bulbus beim menschlichen Auge', Zeitschrift für Morphologie und Anthropologie (1944).

[335] E. Abderhalden, 'Rasse und Vererbung vom Standpunkt der Feinstruktur von blut- und Zelleigenen Eiweisstoffen aus betrachtet', Nova Acta Leopoldina, n.s. vol. 7 no. 46 (1939), 59–79.

[336] Verschuer papers, Verschuer to Fischer, 25 August 1943.

[337] Verschuer papers, Verschuer to de Rudder, 4 October 1944 and 6 January 1945.

malformations. The same can be said of Ströer's research on dwarf rabbits, which were to serve as models for human pathology. Once gypsies and Jews were defined as a distinct degenerate species, like animals they could be used for experiments.[338] Many scientists (including Nachtsheim) had no moral qualms about using human specimens from concentration camps and prisons, on the grounds that the victims were to die in any case.

Verschuer's faith in science strengthened in the final year of the war. In April 1944 Verschuer wrote of consolation in the vigour of nature in the midst of human destruction.[339] He considered genes in a holistic context of a body's striving for unity, order and higher ideals of service to the state and *Volk*. A sick gene would only become apparent if the regulatory powers of an organism were defective. He drew from this the conclusion that because genes provided the basis of personality and culture, there was also a duty to serve a higher power.[340] The Reich Research Council continued to give energetic support for his research. In August 1944 Verschuer wrote of an uncertain fate, but that he was reassured by how his scientific colleagues found security in the objectivity of their work as providing firm values, in contrast to the transience of human life. Verschuer read the historian Jakob Burckhardt, who had praised the suprahuman values of intellectual creativity but had prophesied that demagogues would abuse science.[341] By November Verschuer felt 'we must maintain faith in miracles that it might be possible to have a national life after the war'.[342] It was only in February 1945 that Verschuer retreated to his estate at Solz bei Bebra, leaving Nachtsheim as acting director with orders to maintain normal functioning of the institute. Fischer began work on a treatise on the biological laws of racial policies – looking forward to helping with national reconstruction. The letters of Fischer and Verschuer suggest that in the final months of the Third Reich, science became linked with spiritual ideals, as well as being seen to have a 'truth' value which gave the research intrinsic worth. Science transcended a disintegrating society.

---

[338] Müller-Hill, *Tödliche Wissenschaft*, pp. 73–2; Tätigkeitsbericht April 1943–March 1944.
[339] Verschuer paper, Verschuer to Fischer, 25 April 1944.
[340] O. v. Verschuer, *Erbanlage als Schicksal und Aufgabe* (Berlin, 1944).
[341] Verschuer papers, Verschuer to Fischer, 31 August 1944.
[342] Verschuer papers, Verschuer to Fischer, 13 November 1944.

9

Eugenics and German politics

FINAL ACT

The defeat of Germany did not mean the defeat of eugenics or population policy. Although there was horror at Nazi atrocities, most academic and professional institutions survived unscathed, or were reconstituted in such a way that social interests were left intact. Generally, only party political activists lost their posts in public health and welfare administrations. The burden of guilt could be attributed to Nazi ideologues – to the extreme advocates of Germanic racial purity and of anti-semitism. The power struggles between ideologues and technocrats under National Socialism were reinterpreted as the persecution of objective scientists by Nazi fanatics. With varying degrees of justification the racial hygienists claimed that they had long disapproved of unscientific and political abuses of their science. These claims often had a hollow ring, as when Verschuer asserted that Mengele was an opponent of fascist cruelty.[1] The radicalization of policies with the shift from sterilization and racial screening to 'euthanasia' meant that supporters of compulsory sterilization could claim that they had disapproved of Nazi medical policies. The pressures for conformity during the Third Reich, with frequent denunciations and rivalries between competing authorities, provided valuable evidence of Nazi oppression. University professors and suspect doctors could plead that they had acted under pressure from state and party. Hereditary science was helped in that some compromised figures committed suicide before arrest – for example, Astel, de Crinis, Grawitz, Gross, Hirt, Kranz and Linden – or, as in the case of Conti, while being tried at Nuremberg. Others such as Eugen Fischer, Gütt, Reche and Rüdin had retired. Abderhalden enjoyed a brief spell as a biochemist and welfare expert in Switzerland.[2] There were remarkable continuities in the personnel and administrative structures of public health services, and many leading

---

[1] Nachtsheim papers, Nachtsheim to Lewinski, 17 September 1946.
[2] Nachtsheim papers, Fischer to Nachtsheim, 21 August 1946, Nachtsheim to Renner, 21 March 1946, Renner to Nachtsheim, 5 April 1946 on Astel's guilt, also on Franz and Heberer.

racial hygienists were reinstated between 1946 and the early 1950s as 'human geneticists', a concept which had been current in Britain and the USA since 1939.[3]

University teachers and researchers in racial hygiene were with rare exceptions back in office by the mid-1950s. While few were able to enjoy complete continuity, most experienced interruption of their careers for only three to five years. Even Panse who had adjudicated on 'euthanasia' had an academic post (in Düsseldorf) by 1955. Abel (the anthropologist) was one of the few racial hygienists who did not return to an academic life, and others like Thums took a position in clinical medicine.

The term 'racial hygiene' was jettisoned on account of its embarrassing ambiguity. The return to democracy meant a return to the voluntary eugenic plans of 1932 and to a pro-natalist population policy. The spectrum of opinions among eugenicists helped the survival of the movement, for at moments of political change hitherto marginal figures could assume leadership. Between 1945 and 1948 a power struggle for control of the eugenics movement erupted. The conflicts among the eugenicists demonstrate that the transition to a science which enshrined the values of free, objective and independent inquiry was not an instant result of liberation by the Allies. Instead it arose out of post-war political tensions between the Western powers and the Soviet Union. Science was only one minor flash-point, but political friction was necessary in order to rekindle the flame of scientific inquiry. This is illustrated by the case of the Kaiser Wilhelm Institute for Anthropology and its staff. Between 1945 and 1947 hereditary biology was suspected to be at the root of Nazi crimes. Americans said that anthropologists were 1,000 times more guilty than 'an idiotic SS man'.[4] A well-documented account of 'Hitler's professors' was published in 1946 by Max Weinreich in New York. This singled out Fischer and Verschuer for their complicity with the Final Solution.[5] As in many other aspects of German public and professional life, expectations of de-Nazification were disappointed.[6]

Eugenicists regrouped on the basis of professional allegiances, scientific priorities and a common sense of mission. Nachtsheim, who remained in Berlin, assumed the role of defender of the faith. Since he had not been a member of the Nazi Party, he was regarded with confidence by the Allies and continued as acting director of the Kaiser Wilhelm Institute for Anthropology. His position was further secured through professional allegiances among émigré geneticists such as Goldschmidt or Hans Gruneberg, who vouched for his integrity. Most of the Kaiser Wilhelm institutes were closed down and only the institutes for anthropology, international law, physical chemistry and silicate research were allowed to continue. Nachtsheim took a central role in the rehabilitation of biology and anthropology. Because the US authorities placed restrictions on research, he acquired a chair for hereditary

---

[3] Müller-Hill, *Tödliche Wissenschaft*, pp. 82–7.
[4] Nachtsheim papers, Nachtsheim to Lenz, 25 December 1947.
[5] M. Weinreich, *Hitler's Professors: The Part of Scholorship in Germany's Crimes Against the Jewish People* (New York, 1946).   [6] T. Bower, *Blind Eye to Murder* (London, 1981).

Table 10. *The re-appointment of racial hygienists, 1946–1955*

Name	Institution	Discipline	Year
Lenz	Göttingen	Human genetics	1946
Heberer	Göttingen	Anthropology	1947
Just	Tübingen	Anthropology	1948
W. Lehmann	Kiel	Human hereditary biology	1948
Verschuer	Münster	Human genetics	1951
Grebe	Marburg	Human genetics	1952
Loeffler	Hanover	Hereditary biology/social biology	1953
Schade	Münster	Human genetics	1954
Stumpfl	Innsbruck	Psychiatry	1954
Gieseler	Tübingen	Anthropology	1955
Panse	Düsseldorf	Psychiatry	1955

biology at the university and research facilities for comparative pathology with the Academy of Sciences, which were both in the Eastern (Soviet) zone. Initially the attitude of the Soviet authorities seemed benevolent. The scientific committee of the medical administration of the Eastern zone (under Major Karpov) adopted an indulgent attitude towards biology. The authorities wished to win over such leading figures in the academic community as the surgeon Sauerbruch and the internist Theodor Brugsch. On 3 January 1947 at the central office of the health administration for the Eastern zone a meeting was held to discuss the reactivation of the sterilization laws on the basis of the 1932 Prussian Health Council proposals. Nachtsheim re-established contact with Muckermann, who enjoyed prestige because of his rejection under the Third Reich.[7] Schopohl, the former ministerial director of the Prussian Health Department, attained the post of director of the Federal Health Office. Many of the SPD experts in social hygiene of the Weimar period did not return from emigration or being Jewish had been killed. Communist-inclined experts went to the Eastern Zone. The group that resurfaced in the West was dominated by the church-oriented bloc of such social hygienists as Harmsen and Muckermann. The old guard of the period 1929–32 was reinstated. Just as they had co-operated with the conservative right before 1933, so they were indulgent to medical and demographic experts who had occupied positions of power under Nazism.

Geneticists were faced by the problem of the legacy of their numerous links with the Nazi social system. Nachtsheim de-Nazified colleagues and sought to improve the international standing of German science. Lenz was the first of the old guard to attain a post in human genetics at Göttingen in 1946, although he was temporarily suspended during 1947 pending de-Nazification.[8] Privately, Nachtsheim regarded

[7] H. Nachtsheim, *Für und Wider die Sterilisierung aus Eugenischer Indikation* (Stuttgart, 1952).
[8] Nachtsheim papers, Nachtsheim to Saller, 28 July 1947.

Lenz as guilty in the rise of national socialism because of his long-standing devotion to Nordic racial ideals.[9] Nachtsheim was ready to vouch for Lenz as an opponent of anti-semitism, as he wished Lenz to assist in the re-activation of biological research. Nachtsheim provided a whitewashing *Persilschein* (Persil certificate i.e. a testimonial) stating that Lenz was neither a fanatic nor a party activist, and indeed had not endorsed Nazi anti-semitism.[10] Nachtsheim's major opportunity for the rehabilitation of German geneticists who had flourished under Nazism, such as Kühn and Hartmann, was the 8th International Congress of Genetics held in Stockholm in 1948.[11] Although the Swedish condition was that no eugenicists were to be invited who had either been NSDAP members, or had made any concessions to Nazism, Nachtsheim was broad-minded in his interpretation of these stipulations.[12]

Nachtsheim feared that Verschuer might resume his powers as director of the Kaiser Wilhelm Institute for Anthropology. Verschuer attempted to establish the anthropological institute on the basis of the facilities that he had built up in Frankfurt prior to his Berlin appointment in 1941. Between January and October 1946 Verschuer had the support of the municipal authorities and of the Americans for relocating the institute in Frankfurt. A major factor was the utility of his tuberculosis research. In March 1946 Nachtsheim was nervous about losing his pre-eminent position in genetics to Verschuer.[13] A de-Nazification tribunal classified Verschuer as a *Mitläufer* or nominal member of the NSDAP, for which he was fined a nominal 600 marks. In May 1946 accusations were made by the chemist Robert Havemann against Verschuer because of his involvement with Mengele.[14] Havemann had narrowly escaped execution for his role in the resistance, and was now director of the Kaiser Wilhelm Institute for Physical Chemistry. The accusations were supported by the psychologist, Gottschaldt, who adopted a pro-Soviet position. Nachtsheim considered that Verschuer would have known about the extermination of Jews through Mengele.[15] Nachtsheim joined in the denunciations for as long as it seemed that Verschuer might open the rival institute. On 5 November 1946 a committee of Gottschaldt, Havemann, Wolfgang Heubner, Nachtsheim and Warburg sat to consider Verschuer's guilt as a 'fanatical racist' and as having researched with blood samples that were criminally obtained. It was confirmed that the gypsy eyes originated from Auschwitz, but it was argued that the numbers were less than in the public accusations and that the purpose was 'scientific' rather than 'racial'. The commission of colleagues accepted that Verschuer acted as a scientist rather than as a racial fanatic. Verschuer admitted that

[9] Nachtsheim papers, Nachtsheim to Lenz, 25 December 1947.
[10] Nachtsheim papers, Lenz to Nachtsheim, 28 December 1945, 11 August 1946, 2 September 1946; Nachtsheim to Lenz, 21 August 1946.
[11] Nachtsheim papers, Nachtsheim to Stubbe, 27 July 1947.
[12] Bonnier to Nachtsheim 12 May 1947, Nachtsheim to Bonnier 12 June 1947.
[13] Nachtsheim papers, Nachtsheim to Curtius, 18 March 1946.
[14] Havemann in the *Neue Zeitung* of 3 May 1946; Nachtsheim papers, interview with Havemann, 9 May 1946.   [15] Nachtsheim papers, Nachtsheim to Lewinski, 7 November 1946.

blood samples came from Auschwitz, but this he equated with receiving samples from hospitals and he insisted that the purpose of his research on the Abderhalden ferment reaction was strictly scientific. The members of the commission felt that Verschuer knew of the mass extermination of gypsies and Jews, although Nachtsheim expressed sympathy for the view that use of human material was justified if a person was in any case to be killed. Muckermann added a note of condemnation of Verschuer's inhumane attitudes. Yet the commission accepted that Verschuer was not politically motivated but a dedicated scientist, who at most was guilty of having compromised scientific standards.[16] For the self-protection of the scientific community, a distinction between science and racial fanaticism was erected. However, the commission's verdict motivated the authorities in Hessen to ban Verschuer from taking office in any re-opened Kaiser Wilhelm Institute for Anthropology.[17]

Once Verschuer's plans were scuppered, Nachtsheim became more indulgent and supportive. At the same time Nachtsheim came under pressure from the Soviet authorities. A transition to overtly Stalinist policies was combined with the Lysenkoist onslaught against Mendelian genetics. Nachtsheim equated Lysenkoism with Nazi racism.[18] One year later Nachtsheim perceived Soviet controls as worse than the persecution of the Third Reich: he was outraged that publication of a dictionary of heredity written before 1945 was prevented.[19] The tightening of Soviet controls on scientists was important in establishing a British, American and French front in defence of the scientific community. The British took a lead in supporting a functioning science. Initially, only the British tolerated human genetics, as Lenz's position showed. Verschuer was appointed to a chair at Münster in 1951; this university typified how professors if left to themselves would reappoint leading figures from the Nazi era. The British educational officers were satisfied to hear from professors that Nazism was scientifically mistaken. With this the eugenicists could find acceptance for an argument that they had been making since 1933, and strengthened their position.[20] The British authorities did not adopt the same moralistic stance towards the medical atrocities as the Americans at the Nuremberg trials. Instead, Lord Moran presided over a commission to evaluate the scientific value of the Nazi research. This condemned the experiments as ill-designed and misconceived.[21] The British supported the continuation of the Kaiser Wilhelm Gesellschaft, which was re-christened and reorganized as the Max-Planck-Gesellschaft in Göttingen in 1947. These policies meant that the social ambitions of academics were left unscathed.

The founding of the Free University of Berlin in June 1948 symbolized the new

---

[16] Nachtsheim papers, Nachtsheim to Wolfgang Heubner, 5 November 1946.
[17] Thomann, 'Verschuer'.   [18] Nachtsheim papers, Nachtsheim to Lenz, 28 December 1947.
[19] Nachtsheim papers, Nachtsheim to Lenz, 16 October 1948.
[20] Bower, *Blind Eye*, chapter 8.
[21] C.P. Blacker, 'Eugenic Experiments Conducted by Nazis on Human Subjects', *Eugenics Review*, vol. 44 (1952), 9–19; Foreign Office, *Scientific Results of German Medical War Crimes* (London, 1949).

Western position on scientific freedom. The Americans were the major supporters of this anti-Soviet enterprise from August 1948. Nachtsheim gained a chair of human genetics in 1949 at the Free University; Muckermann had an appointment in anthropology at the Technical University and on 8 July 1949 was appointed director of a Max Planck Institute for Applied Anthropology. Thurnwald, one of the founders of the Racial Hygiene Society, held a chair in anthropology at the Free University. Nachtsheim attempted to reactivate the eugenics movement. He and other medical experts such as Harmsen argued that the sterilization laws were Nazi laws neither in their conception nor administration. Political abuse occurred only 'to a very insignificant extent'.[22] Nachtsheim preached the virtues of the 1932 draft law for voluntary sterilization on medical indications. Their argument that the sterilization policies were strictly medical and scientific was accepted by the authorities. They also urged marriage certificates and institutional commital of degenerates.[23]

Allied policies singled out extreme cases of crimes against humanity such as human experiments. That the spotlight fell on about 350 criminal doctors implied that the remainder of the profession had continued to uphold traditions of humane medical practice. Many coercive aspects of medical treatment inflicted on dissidents and non-conformists, as well as compulsory sterilization, went unprosecuted. The American staging of the Nuremberg Trials for doctors and scientists was something of a public show. Behind the scenes, 'operation paperclip' for the transfer to the USA of those engaged in rocket technology, such as Werner von Braun, included doctors who had participated in the human experiments on endurance of high altitudes and extremes of temperature. Human torture was valued for aviation and space medicine.[24] Social stabilization and strategic advantage were preferred to justice. The Cold War facilitated a retreat by the eugenicists into the hard factual bastions of medical and biological science. The attempt to superimpose scientific solutions on social problems was abandoned for the ideologies of 'freedom' and 'objectivity'. These principles protected academic empires that expanded with public funds but were shielded from public accountability and scrutiny.

Family policy and professional interests

While the Nazi political elite was removed, professional and administrative structures persisted. For purposes of de-Nazification – itself only partially implemented – a narrow political definition of Nazism was employed, leaving such key areas as health policy relatively unaffected. The medical profession illustrates the continuity which remained on the levels of personnel and institutions. De-Nazification of doctors was particularly haphazard as they were

[22] H. Harmsen, 'The German Sterilization Act of 1933', *Eugenics Review*, vol. 46 (1955), 227–32.
[23] H. Muckermann, *Zum Problem erblicher Belastung* (Berlin, 1951).
[24] T. Bower, *The Paper Clip Conspiracy* (London, 1987).

needed to cope with post-war health problems of epidemics and the still intractable problems of VD and TB. This was the case in all zones. For example, although in a highly racialized medical administration of Thuringia 80 per cent of medical practitioners had been NSDAP members, the Soviet authorities accepted that de-Nazification could not be rigorously enforced.[25] Prosecutions of the major figures in the T4 and child 'euthanasia' programmes were haphazard and partial. Of the involved psychiatrists, Nitsche was executed in the Soviet zone, but other leading perpetrators of euthanasia were given token fines or sentences, or were acquitted, as in the case of the Bavarian commissioner of health, Schultze, and the Hamburg paediatrician Werner Catel. It could be successfully claimed that the killing of those pronounced incurable was in accordance with prevailing medical and scientific standards. The public health officials who were central to the implementation of the medical killing were often treated with extreme leniency by the courts.[26] A brief account of the Nuremberg medical trials concerning human medical experiments was compiled by Alexander Mitscherlich and Fred Mielke.[27] It was received with hostility by the profession in 1948.[28] Heubner and Sauerbruch, who had moderated Havemann's attack on Verschuer, were among those leaders of the profession who were outraged by the publicity given by Mitscherlich to the Nuremberg medical trials.[29]

In the West the system of autonomous chambers of doctors was resurrected and the *Hartmannbund* representing the economic interests of the profession was outstandingly successful in its defence of the profession's economic interests. Professional leaders remained entrenched. An example was Haedenkamp: a DNVP representative in the 1920s, he continued in the *Reichsärztekammer* after 1933 and was an avid opponent of Jewish doctors in the Third Reich; he maintained an honoured position in the profession after 1945. The conservatism of the medical profession was expressed in hostility to socialized medicine as incipient communism. Whereas the Soviet authorities initiated a policlinic system as the basis of primary care, the West relied on the family doctor and independent specialist. Attempts to restore the insurance-based health centres failed in the West, and even group practices were highly suspect.[30] Cardinal principles of the insurance-based system of fee per service and differential benefits were maintained

---

[25] H. Domeinski, 'Zur Entnazifizierung der Ärzteschaft im Lande Thüringen', Thom and Spaar (eds.), *Medizin im Faschismus*, pp. 250–4.

[26] E. Klee, *Was sie taten – was sie wurden. Ärzte, Juristen und andere Beteiligte am Kranken- und Judenmord* (Frankfurt-on-Main, 1986).

[27] A. Mitscherlich and F. Mielke, *Medizin ohne Menschlichkeit*, (Frankfurt a.M., 1978); 1st edn as *Das Diktat der Menschenverachtung* (Heidelberg, 1947).

[28] H. Mausbach and B. Mausbach-Bromberger, 'Zur heutigen Stellung des antifaschistischen Widerstands der Ärzte im Bewusstsein und Traditionsverständnis der Bundesrepublik Deutschland', Thom and Spaar (eds.), *Medizin im Faschismus*, pp. 269–76.

[29] H. Hanauske-Abel, 'From Nazi Holocaust to Nuclear Holocaust: A Lesson to Learn?', *Lancet* (1986), 271–3.

[30] 'Die Konflikte um die Ambulatorien in Berlin 1947 bis 1953', Hansen, *Verschüttete Alternativen*, pp. 500–46.

in the two Germanies. The church-dominated private sector in the provision of hospitals and welfare institutions continued to flourish.

In public health, the 1934 law unifying state and municipal health services was not repealed. Although the umbilical cord linking the laws with racial ideology was cut, the bureaucratic structures became the basis of public health in the Federal Republic. The insurance and municipal system of preventive medicine, based on health centres, was not revived, which meant that professional advantage triumphed over academic accountability.[31] Links between medicine and population policy were not altogether severed, but reformulated in line with the conservative ethos of the early years of the Federal Republic. Leading health and welfare experts such as Harmsen, the instigator of the evangelical Union of Health and organizer of the German Mothers' Day, achieved great influence in public health and family planning. The sterilization legislation was neither repealed nor officially recognized as a Nazi measure. While the system of tribunals was allowed to lapse, this state of affairs meant that victims were denied compensation unless an abuse of procedures could be proven. Harmsen and Muckermann came out strongly in favour of a 'healthy and efficient family' in order to improve the quality of the population.[32] Homosexuals continued to be outside the law, and were denied compensation for Nazi persecution. There was no return to the laxity of the Weimar era, until legal reform was attained in 1969.[33] For their part eugenicists were reluctant to support coercive measures since they wished to maintain their distance from Nazism. Thus the post-war eugenicists supported a family-oriented welfare policy. The mood of the Adenauer administration was that of a moral defence of the family as the basis of social order.

Under the CDU/CSU administration the term 'population policy' was abandoned because of Nazi overtones, and replaced by 'family policy'. The structure of laws and welfare measures that amounted to a population policy persisted. The Nazi contraception laws of 1941 and 1943 continued to be operative in the Western zones. Hamburg was the first state to relax the laws on contraception in 1949 but insisted on medical controls over the distribution of contraceptives.[34] The abortion law was unreformed until the mid-1960s. After some liberalization in the Soviet zone, abortion was restricted in 1950 to parents suffering from a hereditary disease or to cases where there was a severe threat to the health of the mother. Advice on family planning remained under medical control. As before 1933, a few socialist-dominated insurance or administrative authorities, such as those in Berlin and Hessen supported the use of marriage guidance clinics for birth control advice. Radical birth control reformers were countered by the conservative pro-natalist ethos, tinged by eugenics, that lingered on in the standards set by the *Pro Familia* family planning association, which was

---

[31] Labisch and Tennstedt, *GVG*, vol. 2, pp. 352–74.
[32] H. Harmsen, 'The German Sterilization Act of 1933', *Eugenics Review*, vol. 46 (1955), 227–32.
[33] Stümke and Finkler, *Rosa Winkel*, pp. 340–51.
[34] V. Houghton, 'Birth Control in Germany', *Eugenics Review*, vol. 43 (1952), 185–7.

founded in 1952. Harmsen and Nachtsheim were leading members. The tendency was to consider contraception in medical and ethical terms of family health.[35] Leading demographers such as Burgdörfer, dismissed from Bavarian service in 1945, and Koller, continued to be venerated by their colleagues with academic positions and honours. A pro-natalist bias persisted along with discrimination against women in civil and economic spheres. Demography continued to be a focus for geneticists such as Nachtsheim and Verschuer, welfare experts such as Muckermann and statisticians such as Burgdörfer.[36]

The family ideology of the social policies of the Christian Democratic parties meant that the family remained an enclave of the patriarchal values with which it had been imbued by the population experts. The German situation can be compared to Italy where fascist-initiated organizations such as ONMI maintained their influence over maternal and infant welfare.[37] At the same time demographic threats to the nation were diminished. Ten million displaced Germans contributed to the population growth of the Federal Republic between 1945 and 1950, and the strong economy of the Federal Republic has required immigrants to boost the labour force. There was a mild baby boom between 1946 and 1948, and until the mid-60s there was a period of demographic stability. This meant that the demographic conditions militated against a nationalist ideology of a dying people, degeneration and invasion by alien cultures. However, from the mid-60s the birth rate entered into a phase of decline, which exacerbated such problems as prejudice against foreign workers, and led to a reassertion of nationalist ideology couched in demographic terms of the right of the 'German people' to maintain their identity.[38]

International associations for medical and demographic issues reassimilated the German eugenicists. Topics such as the population explosion were a common focus for international action. The mental hygiene movement, initiated at the crest of the biologistic wave in the late 1920s, lingered on. Biological approaches to mental disease were rehabilitated by the World Federation of Mental Health Organizations established in 1948. Given that British and US researchers shared hereditarian concerns in the mental hygiene movement, eugenic continuities in the medical sciences and of personnel in leading positions of those involved in the 'euthanasia' and sterilization programmes were regarded as unproblematic.[39]

Against the argument for continuity must be set changes in the scale and aims of the mental hygiene and eugenics movements.[40] Medical innovations meant that

[35] H. Kaupen-Haas, 'Eine deutsche Biographie – der Bevölkerungspolitiker Hans Harmsen', in Ebbinghaus *et al.* (eds.), *Heilen und Vernichten*, pp. 41–44; Klee, *Was sie taten*, pp. 150–1.
[36] H. Nachtsheim, 'Die Notwendigkeit einer aktiven Erbgesundheitspflege', *Gesundheitspolitik*, vol. 21 (1964), 321–39.
[37] L. Caldwell, 'Reproducers of the Nation: Women and the Family in Fascist Policy', in D. Forgacs (ed.), *Rethinking Italian Fascism* (London, 1986), 110–41.
[38] Heinsohn, *Bevölkerungslehre*, pp. 202–17; Marschalck, *Bevölkerungsgeschichte*, pp. 86–97.
[39] Schreiber, *Men Behind Hitler*, pp. 63–9, 79 accuses psychiatrists of wishing to erect a 'psychiatric slave state'.   [40] Jones, *Social Hygiene*, pp. 137–56.

antibiotics, anti-depressant drugs and the contraceptive pill replaced coercive eugenic measures for mental illness and sexually transmitted infections; antibiotics contributed to the final phase in the decline of TB mortality. The post-war boom in sociology, based on non-biological categories of status and economics, resulted in a transfer of professional competence away from the medical and biological. The professional expertise of technocrats was distrusted for its authoritarianism.[41] The exiled sociologists of the Frankfurt school – particularly Herbert Marcuse – developed a critique of technocracy and of scientific autonomy as inherently authoritarian and repressive. They suggested that science reduced wider pheno-mena of the natural and scientific environment to narrowly technical terms over which an elite had privileged access and control. The critical perceptions of medical authority that arose from the politically radical, feminist and Green movements have served to jolt the public into scrutinizing the heritage of racial thinking on the family and nature. It is a process that remains unfinished.

LOOKING BACKWARD

The demise of liberalism

Science and medicine, taken as indicators of liberal values and social structures, contribute to explanations for the decline and fall of the German Reich. Whereas initially biology and medicine were part of the liberal political discourse on unification, secularization and de-regulation, these sciences disengaged from liberal nationalism. The autonomous status claimed by biology and medicine could be used as a platform from which to adjudicate on political and social change, while augmenting the authority of expert groups. Wilhelmine Germany was notable for professorial demagogues who used their authority as scientists to pontificate on social issues in lectures, associations, journals and newspapers. The progress of urbanization and industrialization revealed liberalism to contain irreconcilable contradictions. Ideologically, there was a conflict between liberal individualism and organicist nationalism. There were tensions between political and economic accountability, and the bourgeois refuge in such privileged corporations as the universities and professions. As doctors became more concerned to gain a professional monopoly over health care, individual rights became threatened. At a micro-level this altered doctor-patient relations, shifting the emphasis from the doctor as responsible to the individual patient, to the doctor acting in the higher interests of hereditary health and the race. Health became increasingly a matter for expert advisors and professionally qualified bureaucrats, rather than for political parties formulating and implementing policies according to democratic principles of accountability and representational politics.

The attraction of biological sciences was that they offered solutions to social problems accompanying the modernization of Germany, and the prospect of the

41 L. Hogben, *Science in Authority* (London, 1963).

dawn of an age of health, prosperity and intellectual brilliance. Professional and welfare associations developed with great vigour, and shaped the welfare state that emerged from the Bismarckian insurance legislation of the 1880s. Power-hungry professionals assumed the position of scientific guardians of a social order based on healthy and fertile families. Expert groups formulated de-politicized social policies and publicized health as a means of integrating industrial populations. Organicist strategies for maintaining social cohesion under the direction of professional elites offer a gauge of the social position and influence of the academically educated middle class. Whereas liberal politics suffered a series of political crises and defeats, liberal culture, professionalism and ideas of a healthy and personally fulfilling lifestyle have persisted and established widespread norms in family and everyday life. Socialism and mass democracy were countered not only by political mobilization on the right, but also by a silent revolution in terms of promoting the health and welfare of families. Welfare services suggest that corporatist and authoritarian aspects of liberalism thrived at the expense of democratic individualism. Contemporary awareness of authoritarian and elitist implications of eugenic welfare policies resulted in political confrontations between left and right with feminists and sexual reformers against professionals, intra-professional rivalries such as those between doctors and social workers, and the shift from educational to biologically determinist approaches to health and behaviour.

It is customary to adopt a compartmentalized and restrictive analysis of German politics by concentrating on party membership and elections, without considering the impact of party politics on social policies, the actuality of welfare services, and the structuring of everyday life associated with housing, diet, exercise and the coping with sickness and children. As these areas of everyday life could themselves influence political attitudes (as over questions of poverty), it is necessary to arrive at a more balanced understanding of the interaction of politics with social life. Similarly, analysis of the professions has tended to be a rather static affair of charting the growth of professional qualifications and organizations, but ignoring broader socio-political dimensions. Because self-regulation is taken as a criterion of professional maturity, this has meant that a rather tame analysis of internal professional cohesion has resulted, ignoring the broader social manifestations of aggressive professional imperialism. By contrast, the present study has been based on evidence of the interaction of interest groups with state authorities. After a liberal phase of demands for de-regulation during the 1860s and 70s, the medical profession joined the scramble for power and social influence by the 1890s, and lobbied for a place in a system of national government. The biological and medical ideologies of the social organism as a human economy offered a way of deflecting attention away from economic issues, and shifted priorities to the health and welfare of the family. The activities of medical reformers can be compared to organizations of industrialists and landowners, and the mass patriotic associations, which were responses to the authoritarianism of a Bismarckian system that accorded only a limited role to elected and publicly accountable institutions.

Movements for social reform, in such cases as the prevention of the 'racial poisons' TB, VD and alcoholism, demonstrate the development of a strong alliance between state authorities and advocates of an enhanced social role for scientific medicine. Health and welfare policies became a means of social integration under professional leadership.

While German history is necessarily divided by generation gaps, regions, religion and social stratification, the attempts to impose integrating ideologies and institutions require attention. Biologically based politics represented a strategy of national unification and development at the level of the family and lifestyle. Science and medicine became involved in attempts to solve social and demographic problems regarded as a threat to national unity. Ideas of health, and its scientization through biology and medicine, took a part in creating the basis for a unified lifestyle and commitment to a range of national ethical and social values. Medicine and biology were prescriptive of moral and national codes of conduct. Doctors and scientists claimed that their expertise on medical issues could contribute to national salvation. The interaction of the state and population can be examined through intermediate social groups of welfare reformers and professional interests. In addition to the neglect of the intellectual assumptions related to the concept of the *Kulturstaat* as an integrated organism, political historians have found difficulties in accommodating the powerful influence of professionalization in the modernizing and restructuring of the *Bildungsbürgertum*. Professional expertise was in itself changing and contentious, as indicated by the transition from a free market with professions as competitive trades, to monopolistic demands for control of medical care. As a powerful lobby of technocratic experts penetrated state administrative authorities, conflicts erupted with legally educated officials who were more inclined to uphold civil rights; finance ministries were reluctant to support interventionist social welfare policies. Industrialization intensified contradictions inherent in liberalism: professional prescriptions for sobriety and order came into conflict with individual rights and the ground-rules of the non-interventionist state and the free-market economy.

Eugenics and welfare provide insight into administrative structures and their relations to party politics. Liberal ideas of the non-interventionist state resulted in a decentralized structure of public health left to the *Länder*, municipalities, sickness insurance and voluntary agencies. Yet this very decentralization meant that medical reformers and eugenicists could capture key administrative positions. The pace of change varied with different authorities. Prussia and Saxony took the lead in population policy and eugenics. By the 1920s there was a consensus in favour of social hygiene, although funds were lacking for more ambitious schemes such as family allowances. An internal administrative conflict occurred between public health officials with strong professional ties, and justice and financial officials who defended doctrines of non-interventionism. The erosion of these obstacles to comprehensive welfare enabled on the one hand the development of the complex structures of the welfare state, but on the other the removal of democratic barriers to negative eugenics. It was in the interests of a hard-pressed bourgeoisie to expand professional career opportunities through the welfare state during the 1920s. The depression at the end of the Weimar republic brought home to the bourgeoisie the high costs of the welfare state, and eugenics became viewed as a means of cutting the costs of welfare systems. The racial ideology of selective welfare and negative eugenics offered a means of resolving this contradiction.

The negation of welfare

Humanitarianism can be taken as one of the nobler qualities of liberalism, and a crucial value in medicine. The replacing of a humanitarian by a racial ethic was the result of political changes in Germany. Between the Kaiserreich and the Third Reich, biology and medicine show a continuity in building up professional and administrative structures, but also profound changes in aims and values. This can be seen if the schemes for midwifery reform under Althoff are compared with those of Gross and Himmler. Improving the distribution of midwives, their professional status and incomes remained state priorities. But the state changed from inclusive pro-natalism to racial selection. There was great pride in the education of Polish midwives in the decade after 1900 and a concern with extending the competence of the midwife as health educator and home visitor. By way of contrast, the population planners of Nazi Germany wished to use midwives for racial screening of the population for congenital disabilities; in the occupied East, midwives were to exterminate the newly born and to engender high infant mortality. Attempts dating from the 1880s to provide therapy for the tubercular and mentally ill, which resulted in the development of extensive networks of hospitals and clinics, also ended in policies of extermination with a racial rationale. In other fields of medicine there was a reversal of values in the imposition of schemes to boost the health and fertility of selected German population groups, and to segregate, starve, exhaust through forced labour and kill population groups deemed to be inferior. Whereas medicine was regarded in Imperial Germany as one of the highest achievements of the German intellect and as a distinctive national contribution to mankind, war, conquest, and racial service were deemed to be positively healthy during the Third Reich. The professional elite changed from the liberal political activism of the 1870s to demands for the profession to have a monopoly over all aspects of medical practice. The doctor was to be a Führer of the *Volk* to better personal and racial health.

The erosion of liberal values in education, law, science and medicine occurred as the result of a sequence of administrative, professional and political changes. The eugenics movement, born amidst the persecution of socialism in the 1880s, was integrated into welfare schemes of the 'one nation' ideology of the social liberal Naumann. Before 1914 it was not the *völkisch* Pan-Germanists who took positions of power, but more moderate public health and welfare experts who became dictators of social policy. The Naumannite fusion of science, humanitarian welfare and nationalism was a powerful force in re-shaping social policies designed to uphold the family and the social position of high value leadership groups of officials and professionals. During the First World War pro-natalism infused state welfare planning. It was only in the crisis of defeat that ideas of racial extermination came to motivate welfare schemes for social reconstruction in the Weimar welfare state. Eugenicists gained a high point of influence during the economic crisis between 1929 and 1932. Although such measures as sterilization were implemented during the Third Reich, racial hygienists came under considerable pressure once the initiative was taken by the NSDAP and SS. Not only was the development of eugenics dominated by the various phases of German political history between 1890 and 1950, but ideological tensions caused conflicts between eugenicists during each period, as well as intellectual, institutional and administrative discontinuities.

Professional experts felt responsible for moulding society in accordance with bourgeois predilections for sobriety and order, as well as with national values. The health of mothers and infants and of the future generations became national rallying cries that played on personal emotions and encouraged enjoyment of nature and the desire to resolve difficulties in securing decent employment, housing and income. Health and fertility became identified with German nationalism, and as a consequence changes in nationalism fed back into medicine and biology. While the present study has highlighted discontinuities and the myriad tensions between eugenicists, certain overall aims can be detected. There was a vision of a society in which individual interests should be sacrificed to higher ethical values of duty, hard work, a sober lifestyle and the health of future generations. It was a prescription for a type of biologically based collectivism. In the nineteenth century these aspirations were fuelled by a search for utopian alternatives to the state; but as science and medicine were developed these seemed to offer techniques for making the utopian vision a reality. This enhanced the prestige and authority of eugenically-minded demographic, medical and welfare experts, who appropriated the most valuable ideas of the radical *Lebensreformer* and deployed these for shoring up an authoritarian social structure. They pursued their aims as a cohesive elite who opportunistically co-operated or disengaged from party politics and state offices. A progression can be detected in terms of the extension of an institutional infrastructure of clinics and health visitors. There were direct lines of development from the TB clinics instituted in 1899 to the clinics for *Erb- und Rassenpflege* of the Nazi public health administration. At the same time there was intensive political and professional controversy over the scope and functions of 'semi-official welfare organizations'. The links between such public health officials as Krohne and the Racial Hygiene Society offer an instance of the penetration of eugenics in welfare and public health organizations.

Academic disciplines such as anatomy and anthropology underwent a transition from being enclaves of liberal radicalism in the mid-nineteenth century to being authoritarian arms of state social policy a century later. Anthropology changed from a public and participatory science to serving the state's requirements for racial classification of populations. The expectations of naturalistic academic disciplines as liberating and emancipatory gave way to authoritarian convictions of racial superiority. Ploetz metamorphosed from being an admirer of Kautsky to a supporter of Hitler. The physiologist, Abderhalden, provides a classic example of the transition of science from being a means of social emancipation to one of racial persecution with his commitments to temperance, family welfare and medical ethics, since he ultimately provided the scientific rationale for the human experiments by Mengele and Verschuer. The conviction that the survival of the German *Volk* as a specially endowed human group was at stake, and the ruthless pursuit of biological remedies to social problems, ended tragically in the placing of scientific research above individual lives. Eugenics as applied biology was a catalyst in bringing about an inversion of values.

The politics of population

Germany contrasts unfavourably with Britain and the USA in its lack of radical opponents to eugenics. German systems of professional education in medicine and of professional organization differed because of the high degree of involvement of universities and state authorities at a time when the German experience of industrialization and demographic development was exceptionally intense. These factors were compounded by the political and social upheavals in the wake of the First World War. Whereas before the war colonies had offered hopes for retaining 'surplus' population groups who otherwise were 'lost' through migration, the loss of overseas and European territories created the sense that application of racial hygiene to internal social policy was necessary. Biology and medicine became subsumed in debates on *Lebensraum* and the biological quality of the *Volk*. The experience of defeat and middle-class impoverishment was crucial to the strength of German racial sentiments. National isolation during the 1920s and 30s intensified the sense that certain populations were 'inferior' and parasitic burdens on the fit and healthy. Once financial resources were swept away by the economic crisis, and a preference for social structures as aggregate collectivities had replaced democratic individualism, those presumed to be racially inferior were in grave danger. With emigration and incarceration no longer safety valves during the Second World War, the persecution of social dissidents, the sick, and racial minorities resulted in the deaths of millions of supposedly 'surplus populations'.

Official statistics were political aggregates that were publicized in emotive and nationalist terms and concealed a wide range of social class, regional and urban/rural differentials. Germany's demographic and mortality statistics were compared to those of international rivals such as France (already in the grips of fertility decline) and Britain. The high fertility of Polish and Slav populations and the low fertility of Jewish families was regarded as a threat to the ideal of 'the German family'. Despite continuing population growth, alarmist predictions were made on the basis of the declining birth rate, conceptualized in terms of a pathological 'two child system'. The nationalist manner in which the population trends were analyzed between 1890 and 1945 suggests that the transition from the high birth and high mortality rates which characterized the pre-industrial era to modern social values was not a gradual trend that followed an even pace. The crucial features of the German experience were rapid industrialization and urban growth that concentrated a potentially revolutionary workforce in large cities. The responses to the 'social question' were alarmist and authoritarian.

The medical profession claimed success in the reduction of high mortality rates from infectious diseases. These claims must be regarded as suspect, given that diseases such as TB were greatly affected by social conditions of diet and housing. While the medical campaign for breast feeding and the advice given in infant health clinics coincided with the decline in infant mortality, the actual causes of the decline remain subject to debate. The eugenicists were the first group of medical experts to have focused on the problem of the chronic degenerative diseases which dominate the epidemiology of industrialized societies, but they exaggerated the role of heredity and made unwarranted extrapolations from chronic diseases to mental diseases such as 'feeble-mindedness' and 'psychopathy'. Physical disabilities such as blindness and diseases such as epilepsy were correlated with mental subnormality, and elaborate correlations between physique and psychology were suggested. Such widespread complaints as tooth decay and inability to breast feed were identified as indicators of degeneracy. An identikit picture was constructed of a degenerate constitution that was inherited from generation to generation. The objective basis of demographic and public health statistics was thus open to manipulation by nationalist and professional interests. Schemes for the total registration of diseases and health passports extended professional opportunities in school health and other public health services, and had authoritarian political implications.

The social ambitions of eugenicists exemplify the failure of the attempt to solve social problems by means of biology. Eugenicists presented a persuasive picture of an ageing and degenerating nation, which cannot be taken as corresponding with the reality of social and demographic conditions. Social, economic and cultural factors were reduced to categories of evolutionary biology. The actual reasons for the declining birth rate and decline in mortality rates have to be reconstructed from local studies, using indicators free from political and professional bias. The present study, however, has dealt with the *perceptions* of the declining birth rate and changing health conditions rather than their reality. The leaders of the medical profession took a reactionary stance against abortion and birth control. It was observed at the time that in practice, younger urban doctors were often sympathetic to patients' demands for abortions and contraceptives. The eugenic attempt to control medical practice had only limited success, and little is known of actual practice. Contraception spread like wildfire despite condemnation by the medical elite. Its value as a means of self-help in improving health and as a means of economic survival was well known. Claims for the effectiveness of eugenics in any sphere of health and welfare should be regarded with utmost scepticism. The actual conditions of medical practice and the determinants of demographic movements require different methods and sources than those employed in this study of the formulation of health policies.

The welfare state and the rise of the medical profession and social work have had strong eugenic inputs in most countries. Pro-natalist ideologies for welfare services have accompanied the demographic transition in most industrial societies, although the forms these have taken have been socially specific. Declining birth rates have become accepted as an inevitable feature of industrialization. The links between industrialization and fertility control are complex and vary in each society. The German fertility decline was analyzed and publicized as an indication of impending national disaster. Solutions were sought in plans for urban regeneration, inner colonization and ultimately of expanding *Lebensraum*. In fact German fertility rates were relatively high, and the processes of fertility decline affected different social sectors in a variety of ways. Aggregate statistics, notional predictions and emotive nationalism accompanied the analysis of the medical and social implications of demographic trends. Ideas of inculcating the 'will' to reproduce represented a nationalization of perceptions of the body and domesticity. Fertility control was associated with challenges to the ruling elite from cultural dissidents, feminists and socialists. There was political reluctance to accept the changes in family structure, class relations and the redistribution of wealth as unleashed by industrialization. Just as conservative moralists condemned the consumerism that was so important to the survival of industry and commerce, so they condemned fertility control despite its importance in maintaining personal health and prosperity, and in allowing women greater participation in social life. Self-determination of fertility was regarded as a legal and political right. By way of contrast, a buoyant birth rate meant that nationalists claimed that the unborn child was a matter of national biological importance.

Eugenicists sought to remove the techniques of fertility control, such as abortion, sterilization and the use of birth control appliances, from individual choice. They endeavoured to impose the authority of the medical profession and ancillary groups over all aspects of reproduction. While there were differences between voluntary and compulsory eugenic schemes, systems based on professional advice were often based on eugenic and authoritarian premises. Marriage certificates and the clinics for hereditary health (forerunners of modern genetic counselling) were the outcome of a strategy by professionals to promote larger families of better quality as being in the nation's military and economic interest. Fertility control represented the cutting edge of policies of intervention in the family. By placing medical and social services on a biological basis, the state and ruling elites were able to intervene in delicate areas of social life where policing was inappropriate. While health and life-expectancy were harmed by the stresses and strains of industrial and agricultural work, it was not in the labour process that the professional elite decided to operate. This would have been too de-stabilizing and would have undercut the financial and administrative resources required to maintain the authority of professionals. Instead, it was in the realms of everyday life, of the rhythms of birth, reproduction and death, of the daily patterns of eating, drinking and leisure, that the eugenicists attempted to impose hygienic standards that would promote the health of present and future generations. Eugenicists have left a legacy of clinics, social services and welfare benefits, even though the original eugenic rationale has been dissipated. The aura of expertise, professionalism and technical specialization in biology and medicine has obscured their political implications. By recreating the vanished ideologies of biological reform, insight can be gained into the political implications of social structures, values and policies associated with health and welfare. Past innovations in the medical sciences were accompanied by authoritarian political and social forces. As the post-war world dawned, it was burdened by this problematic legacy.

BIBLIOGRAPHY

MANUSCRIPTS AND ARCHIVES

State archives

Federal Republic of Germany
Berlin Document Centre
  Personal files of NSDAP and SS members, Ahnenerbe files, Reichsforschungsrat cards
Geheimes Staatsarchiv, Preusscher Kulturbesitz, Berlin-Dahlem
  Rep 77 Ministerium des Inneren
  Rep 84a Justiz-Ministerium
Landesarchiv Berlin
  Rep 42/Acc 1743 Nr 9018 Deutscher Bund für Volksaufartung
Staatsarchiv Bremen
  V2 Nr 1622 Arbeitsgemeinschaft für Volksgesundung
  4, 21 Bevölkerungspolitik, Eheberatung
Bundesarchiv Militärarchiv Freiburg
  H20 (Military Medicine in Nazi Germany)
Staatsarchiv Hamburg
  Medizinal-kollegium
Bundesarchiv, Koblenz
  R 73 Notgemeinschaft der Deutschen Wissenschaft
  R 86 Reichsgesundheitsamt
  NS 19
  Adele Schreiber papers
Bayerisches Hauptstaatsarchiv, Munich
  MA, MF Medizinalwesen
  Mk, MWi Kultusministerium
  MInn Ministerium des Inneren
  MJur Ministerium für Justiz
Staatsarchiv München
  Polizei-Direktion München, Vereinsakten
Hauptstaatsarchiv Stuttgart
  E 151 K VI Gesundheitswesen

German Democratic Republic
Stadtarchiv Berlin
  Rep 00, Rep 03 (Collections on Berlin Municipal Medicine)
Staatsarchiv Dresden
  Gesandtschaft Berlin
  Ministerium des Inneren
  Ministerium für Justiz
  Ministerium für Volksbildung
Zentrales Staatsarchiv Dienststelle Merseburg
  Rep 76 Kultusministerium
  Rep 76 viii B Medizinalabteilung
  Rep 151 Finanzministerium
  Althoff papers
Zentrales Staatsarchiv Dienststelle Potsdam
  15.01 Reichsinnenministerium
  30.01 Reichsjustizministerium

University, Academy and Institutional archives

Federal Republic of Germany
Staatsbibliothek Preussischer Kulturbesitz Berlin, Handschriftensammlung
  Gerhart Hauptmann papers
  Max Hirsch papers
  Luschan papers
Freie Universität Berlin, Universitätsbibliothek
  Roesle papers
  Rott papers
Max-Planck-Gesellschaft Archives, Berlin-Dahlem
  Bauakten, Generalverwaltung, Senatsakten concerning the Kaiser-Wilhelm-Institut für Anthropologie
  Nachtsheim papers
Technische Universität Berlin, Archives
  Muckermann autobiography
University of Freiburg Library
  Schemann papers
  Weismann papers
Schleswig-Holsteinische Landesbibliothek, Kiel
  Tönnies papers: correspondence with Grotjahn
Max-Planck-Institut für Psychiatrie, Munich
  Loeb Correspondence
University of Munich Archives
  Institute of Hygiene papers and personal files on Gruber, Hahn, Kaup, Kisskalt and Lenz
Institut für Zeitgeschichte Munich
  Deutscher Biologen Verband
  Wilhelm Hagen papers
University of Münster Archives
  Verschuer papers: correspondence with Eugen Fischer

University of Münster, Institute for History and Theory of Medicine
  Fischer and Verschuer offprints

German Democratic Republic
Literatur-Archiven der Akademie der Künste der DDR, Berlin
  Carl Hauptmann papers: correspondence with Ploetz
Humboldt University Berlin Archives
  Grotjahn papers
Hygiene Museum der DDR
  Library (Collection of exhibition catalogues and sources on Lingner)
University of Jena
  Haeckel papers: correspondence with Ploetz, Verworn, Woltmann, and H.E. Ziegler

Switzerland
University of Zürich, Institute for the History of Medicine
  Forel papers
  Gaule papers

United Kingdom
Cambridge University Library
  Darwin Letters
Eugenics Society, London
  Library and Offprint Collections
University College London
  Galton papers: correspondence with Ploetz
Wellcome Institute for the History of Medicine, Contemporary Medical Archives Centre,
  London
  Eugenics Society papers
History Faculty Library and Radcliffe Science Library, Oxford
  Books and periodicals deriving from Alfred Blaschko
Wellcome Unit for the History of Medicine, Oxford
  Martin Hahn papers

United States
Rockefeller Archive Center, Pocantico Hills, New York State
  Rockefeller Foundation papers

Private papers

Gunnar Broberg, Uppsala
  Lundborg papers, correspondence with Ploetz
Iring Fetscher, Frankfurt-on-Main
  Rainer Fetscher papers
Historisches Archiv Krupp, Essen
  Correspondence and drafts relating to 'Krupp' essay prize
Widukind Lenz, Münster
  Lenz papers – correspondence with Verschuer, papers of the Freiburg Society for Racial
    Hygiene, Kaiser Wilhelm Institut für Anthropologie reports

Kurt Nemitz, Bremen
  Julius Moses papers and publications
Wilfrid Ploetz, Herrsching
  Ploetz papers – diaries and correspondence
Otto Spatz, Munich
  J.F. Lehmann papers
Edith Zerbin-Rüdin, Munich
  Rüdin and Luxenburger papers

DISSERTATIONS

Baum, F., 'Über den praktischen Malthusianismus, Neo-Malthusianismus und Sozial Darwinismus', Diss., University of Munich, 1928.

Burgdörfer, F., 'Das Bevölkerungsproblem, seine Erfassung durch Familienstatistik und Familienpolitik', Diss., University of Munich, 1917.

Doeleke, W., 'Alfred Ploetz (1860–1940). Sozialdarwinist und Gesellschaftsbiologe', med. Diss., University of Mainz, 1975.

Engel, K., 'Der Gräfenberg Ring. Zu seiner Vorgeschichte, Entwicklung und frühen Rezeption', med. Diss., University of Erlangen-Nürnberg, 1979.

Gräbke, R., 'Wilhelm Liepmann als sozialer Gynäkologe', med, Diss., Free University of Berlin, 1969.

Grosch-Obenauer, D., 'Hermann Muckermann und die Eugenik seiner Zeit', med. Diss., University of Mainz, 1986.

Grossman, A., 'The New Woman, the New Family and the Rationalization of Sexuality. The Sex Reform Movement in Germany 1928–1933', PhD dissertation, Rutgers University, 1984.

Günther, M., 'Die Institutionalisierung der Rassenhygiene an den deutschen Hochschulen vor 1933', med. Diss., University of Mainz, 1982.

Hammer, W., 'Leben und Werk des Arztes und Sozialanthropologen Ludwig Woltmann', med. Diss., University of Mainz, 1979.

Heinrich, W.L., 'Richard Walther Darré und der Hegehofgedanke', med. Diss., University of Mainz, 1980.

Kintner, H.J., 'The Determinants of Infant Mortality in Germany from 1871 to 1933', PhD dissertation, University of Michigan, 1982.

Klasen, E.-M., 'Die Diskussion über eine "Krise" der Medizin in Deutschland zwischen 1925 und 1935', med. Diss., University of Mainz, 1984.

Kroll, J., 'Zur Entstehung und Institutionalisierung einer naturwissenschaftlichen und sozialpolitischen Bewegung: Die Entwicklung der Eugenik/ Rassenhygiene bis zum Jahre 1933', Doktor der Sozialwissenschaft, University of Tübingen, 1983.

Kröner, H.-P., 'Die Eugenik in Deutschland von 1891 bis 1934', med. Diss., University of Münster, 1980.

Lenmann, R.J.V., 'Censorship and Society in Munich 1890–1914', DPhil dissertation, Oxford University, 1975.

Lennig, M., 'Max Hirsch: Sozialgynäkologie und Frauenkunde', med. Diss., Free University of Berlin, 1977.

Löwenberg, D., 'Willibald Hentschel, seine Pläne zur Menschenzüchtung, sein Biologismus und Antisemitismus', med. Diss., University of Mainz, 1978.

Mattern, W., 'Gründung und erste Entwicklung des Deutschen Monistenbundes, 1906–1918', med. Diss., FU Berlin, 1983.

Meyer, L., 'Gesundheitspolitik im Vorwärts', med. Diss., FU Berlin, 1986.

Ortmann, V., 'Probleme der Geburtenregelung in Deutschland in den Jahren 1914–1932 besonders im Lichte der Protestantischen Anschauungen', med. Diss., University of Hamburg, 1963.

Riggelsen, H., 'Bremer Ärzte auf dem Wege zum Nationalsozialismus. Die Problematik der Rassenhygiene und Eugenik', Diplomarbeit, University of Bremen, 1982.

Saha, M.S., 'Carl Correns', PhD dissertation, University of Michigan, 1984.

Simon, F., 'Die Sexualität und ihre Erscheinungsweisen in der Natur. Versuch einer kritischen Erklärung', Diss., University of Jena, 1883.

Stürzbecher, M., 'Die Bekämpfung des Geburtenrückganges und der Säuglingssterblichkeit im Spiegel der Reichstagsdebatten 1900–1930. Ein Beitrag zur Geschichte der Bevölkerungspolitik', PhD Freie Universität Berlin, 1954.

Weindling, P.J., 'Darwinism and Cell Biology in Imperial Germany. The Contribution of Oscar Hertwig (1849–1922)', PhD dissertation, University of London, 1982.

Weiss, S.F., 'Race Hygiene and the Rational Management of National Efficiency: Wilhelm Schallmayer and the Origins of German Eugenics 1890–1920', PhD dissertation, Johns Hopkins University, 1983.

PUBLICATIONS

Abderhalden, E., 'Zum Abschied', *Ethik*, vol. 14 no. 6 (1938), 241–69.
   'Rasse und Vererbung vom Standpunkt der Feinstruktur von blut- und zelleigenen Eiweissstoffen aus betrachtet', *Nova Acta Leopoldina*, n.s. vol. 7 no. 46 (1939), 57–79.

Abrams, P., *The Origins of British Sociology 1834–1914* (Chicago, 1968).

Ackerknecht, E., *Rudolf Virchow, Doctor, Statesman and Anthropologist* (Madison, 1953).

Adam, U.D., *Judenpolitik im Dritten Reich* (Düsseldorf, 1979).

Adams, M.B., 'Science, Ideology and Structure: The Kol'tsov Institute 1900–1970', in L. Lubriano and S.G. Solomon (eds.), *The Social Context of Soviet Science* (Boulder and Folkestone, 1980).

Allen, G.E., 'The Eugenics Record Office at Cold Spring Harbor 1910–1940: An Essay in Institutional History', *Osiris*, ser. 2 vol. 2 (1986), 225–64.
   'The Misuse of Biological Hierarchies: The American Eugenics Movement, 1900–1940', *History and Philosophy of the Life Sciences*, vol. 5 (1983), 105–28.

Alvarez-Pelaez, R., 'Introduccion al estudio de la Eugenesia espanola (1900–1936)', *Quipu*, vol. 2 (1985), 95–122.

Aly, G. and K.H. Roth, *Die restlose Erfassung, Volkszählen, Identifizieren, Aussondern im Nationalsozialismus* (Berlin, 1984).

Ammon, O., *Der Darwinismus gegen die Sozialdemokratie* (Hamburg, 1891).

Andernach, N., *Der Einfluss der Parteien auf das Hochschulwesen in Preussen 1848–1918* (Göttingen, 1972).

Andree, C., 'Geschichte der Berliner Gesellschaft für Anthropologie, Ethnologie und Urgeschichte, 1869–1969', *Hundert Jahre Berliner Gesellschaft für Anthropologie, Ethnologie und Urgeschichte, 1869–1969* (Berlin, 1969), pp. 9–140.
   Rudolf Virchow als Prähistoriker, 2 vols. (Cologne and Vienna, 1976).

Anon., *Denkschrift über die Ursachen des Geburtenrückgangs und die bei der Bekämpfung desselbes in Betracht zu ziehenden Massnahmen* (Berlin, 1912).

Anon., *Die gesundheitlichen Einrichtungen der königl. Residenzstadt Charlottenburg, Festschrift gewidmet dem 3. internationalen Kongress für Säuglingsschutz* (Berlin, 1912).

Anon., 'Die wissenschaftliche Normalität des Schlächters. Josef Mengele als Anthropologe 1937–1941', *Dokumentationsstelle zur NS-Sozialpolitik. Mitteilungen*, vol. 1 no. 2 (1 April 1985).

Artelt, W., E. Heischkel, G. Mann and W. Rüegg, *Städte-, Wohnungs- und Kleidungshygiene des 19. Jahrhunderts in Deutschland* (Stuttgart, 1969).

Aschner, B., *Die Krise der Medizin* (Stuttgart, 1931).

Aschoff, L., *Pathologische Anatomie* (Jena, 1909).

Asmus, G. (ed.), *Hinterhof, Keller und Mansarde. Einblicke in Berliner Wohnungselend 1901–1920* (Reinbek bei Hamburg, 1982).

Astel, K., *Die Aufgabe* (Jena, 1937).

Astel, K., and E. Weber, *Die unterschiedliche Fortpflanzung. Untersuchung über die Fortpflanzung von 14000 Handwerkern Mittelthüringens* (Munich: Lehmann, 1939).

Auerbach, F., *Ernst Abbe* (Leipzig, 1922).

Baader, G., and U. Schultz (eds.), *Medizin und Nationalsozialismus. Tabuisierte Vergangenheit – Ungebrochene Tradition* (Berlin West, 1980).

Bach, O., 'Zur Zwangssterilisierung in der Zeit des Faschismus im Bereich der Gesundheitsämter Leipzig und Grimma', in Thom and Spaar (eds.), *Medizin im Faschismus*.

Baur, E., *Einführung in die experimentelle Vererbungslehre* (Berlin, 1911).

Baur, E., E. Fischer and F. Lenz, *Grundriss der menschlichen Erblichkeitslehre und Rassenhygiene* (Munich, 1921).

'Die biologische Bedeutung der Auswanderung für Deutschland', *Archiv für Frauenkunde und Eugenetik*, vol. 7 (1921), 206–8.

Bayer, H., *Über Vererbung und Rassenhygiene* (Jena, 1912).

Bayertz, K., 'Darwinism and Scientific Freedom. Political Aspects of the Reception of Darwinism in Germany 1863–1878', *Scientia*, vol. 118 (1983), 297–307.

Bebel, A., 'Das Reichs-Gesundheitsamt und sein Programm vom sozialistischen Standpunkt beleuchtet', *Die Zukunft*, vol. 1 (1878), 369–83.

Die Frau und der Sozialismus, (reprint of 1929 edition, Bonn-Bad Godesberg, 1977).

Behr-Pinnow, C. v., *Die Zukunft der menschlichen Rasse. Grundlagen und Forderungen der Vererbungslehre* (Berlin, 1925).

Behring, E., *Gesammelte Abhandlungen zur ätiologischen Therapie von ansteckenden Krankheiten* (Leipzig, 1893).

Beir, A., 'Arthur Ruppin: the Man and his Work', *Leo Baeck Institute. Year Book*, vol. 17 (1972), 117–42.

Beiträge zur Nationalsozialistischen Gesundheits- und Sozialpolitik, no. 1–4 (1985–7).

Benjamin, H., *Georg Benjamin* (Leipzig, 1977).

Berghahn, V., *Modern Germany* (Cambridge, 1982).

Bergmann, A., 'Frauen, Männer, Sexualität und Geburtenkontrolle. Zur "Gebärstreikdebatte" der SPD 1913', in K. Hausen (ed.), *Frauen suchen ihre Geschichte* (Munich, 1983), pp. 81–108.

Bergmann, K., *Agrarromantik und Grossstadtfeindschaft* (Meisenheim, 1970).

Bergmann, W. et al., *Soziologie im Faschismus 1933–1945* (Cologne, 1981).

Bernstein, E., *Der Geschlechtstrieb* (Berlin, 1910).

Biddiss, M.D., *Father of Racist Ideology. The Social and Political Thought of Count Gobineau* (London, 1970).

Biedert, P., *Die Kinderernährung im Säuglingsalter* (1880), 2nd edn (Stuttgart, 1893).

Binding, K. and A.E. Hoche, *Die Freigabe der Vernichtung Lebensunwerten Lebens. Ihr Mass und Ihre Form* (Leipzig, 1920).

Blackbourne, D. and Eley, G., *The Peculiarities of German History. Bourgeois Society and Politics in Nineteenth-Century Germany* (Oxford, 1984).

Blacker, C.P., 'Eugenic Experiments Conducted by Nazis on Human Subjects', *Eugenics Review*, vol. 44 (1952), 9–19.

Bl. (= Blaschko), Dr A., 'Bemerkungen zur Weismann'schen Theorie', *Die Neue Zeit*, vol. 13 (1894), 19–23.

Blaschko, A., 'Natürliche Auslese und Klassentheilung', *Die Neue Zeit*, vol. 13 (1894/5), 615–24.

Blasius, D., *Der verwaltete Wahnsinn* (Frankfurt-on-Main, 1980).

Bloch, I., *Das Sexualleben unserer Zeit* (Berlin, 1907).

Blome, K., *Arzt im Kampf* (Leipzig, 1942).

Blumel, K.H., *Handbuch der Tuberkulose-Fürsorge* (Munich, 1926).

Bock, G., *Zwangssterilisation im Nationalsozialismus* (Opladen, 1986).

Bollmus, R., *Das Amt Rosenberg und seine Gegner. Zum Machtkampf im national-sozialistischen Herrschaftssystem* (Stuttgart, 1970).

Bonhoeffer, K., 'Die Unfruchtbarmachung der geistig Minderwertigen', *Klinische Wochenschrift*, vol. 3 (1924), 798–801.

Bornträger, J., *Bewirkt die Geburtenbeschränkung eine Rassenverbesserung?* (Düsseldorf, 1913).

Bower, T., *Blind Eye to Murder* (London, 1981).

The Paper Clip Conspiracy (London, 1987).

Bowman, S.E. *et al.*, *Edward Bellamy Abroad* (New York, 1962).

Bradbury, S., *The Evolution of the Microscope* (Oxford, 1967).

Brady, R., *The Rationalization Movement in German Industry* (Berkeley, 1933).

Bramwell, A., *Blood and Soil. Walther Darré and Hitler's 'Green Party'* (Abbotsbrook, 1985).

Braun, L., review of L. Frank, Keiffer and L. Maingie, *L'Assurance Maternelle* (Paris, 1897), in *Archiv für soziale Gesetzgebung und Statistik*, vol. 11 (1897), 543–8.

Mutterschaftsversicherung und Krankenkassen (Berlin, 1906).

Bretschneider, H., *Der Streit um die Vivisektion im 19. Jahrhundert* (Stuttgart, 1962).

Breyer, H., *Max von Pettenkofer* (Leipzig, 1980).

Bridenthal, R., A. Grossmann, and M. Kaplan (eds.), *When Biology Became Destiny* (New York, 1984).

Bromberg, N. and V.V. Small, *Hitler's Psychopathology* (New York, 1983).

Bruch, R. vom, *Wissenschaft, Politik und öffentliche Meinung* (Husum, 1980).

Brücher, H., *Ernst Haeckels Bluts- und Geisteserbe* (Munich, 1936).

Bulferetti, L., *Cesare Lombroso* (Turin, 1975).

Bullivant, K. (ed.), *Culture and Society in the Weimar Republic* (Manchester, 1977).

Bulloch, W., *The History of Bacteriology* (London, 1938).

Bumke, O., *Über Nervöse Entartung* (Berlin, 1912).

Bumm, E., *Über das deutsche Bevölkerungsproblem. Rede zum Antritt des Rektorats* (Berlin, 1916).

Bumm, F., *Deutschlands Gesundheitsverhältnisse unter d. Einfluss d. Weltkrieges* (Stuttgart, 1928).

Burgdörfer, F., *Der Geburtenrückgang und seine Bekämpfung, die Lebensfrage des deutschen Volkes* (Berlin, 1929).

Familie und Volk, Sonderschau des Reichsbundes der Kinderreichen Deutschlands und zum Schutze der Familie, e.V. auf der Internationalen Hygiene Ausstellung Dresden 1930 (Berlin, 1930).

Burkhardt, H., *Der rassenhygienisch Gedanke und seine Grundlagen* (Munich, 1930).

Busch, A., 'The Vicissitudes of the *Privatdozent*: Breakdown and Adaptation in the Recruitment of German University Teachers', *Minerva*, vol. 9 (1962), 319–41.

Buttmann, G., *Friedrich Ratzel, Leben und Werk eines deutschen Geographen 1844–1904* (Stuttgart, 1977).

Calkins, K.R., 'The Uses of Utopianism: The Millenarian Dream in Central European Social Democracy Before 1914', *Central European History*, vol. 15 (1982), 124–48.

Castell-Rüdenhausen, Gräfin A. zu, 'Die Überwindung der Armenschulen, Schülerhygiene an den Hamburger öffentlichen Volksschulen im zweiten Kaiserreich', *Archiv für Sozialgeschichte*, vol. 22 (1982), 201–26.

Chajes, B., *Kompendium der sozialen Hygiene* (Leipzig, 1931).

Chamberlain, H.S., *Die Grundlagen des Neunzehnten Jahrhunderts* (Munich, 1899).

Briefe 1882–1924 und Briefwechsel mit Kaiser Wilhelm II (Munich, 1928).

Chamberlin, J.E. and S. Gilman (eds.), *Degeneration. The Dark Side of Progress* (New York, 1985).

Chickering, R., *We Men Who Feel Most German. A Cultural Study of the Pan-German League 1886–1914* (London, 1984).

Churchill, F., 'Weismann's Continuity of the Germ-Plasm in Historical Perspective', in K. Sander (ed.), 'August Weismann (1834–1914) und die theoretische Biologie des 19. Jahrhunderts', in *Freiburger Universitätsblätter*, nos. 87/88 (1985), 107–24.

Clark, L.L., *Social Darwinism in France* (Alabama, 1984).

Cocks, G., *Psychotherapy in the Third Reich, The Göring Institute* (New York and Oxford, 1985).

Coker, F.W., *Organismic Theories of the State* (New York, 1910).

Conrad-Martius, H., *Utopien der Menschenzüchtung* (Munich, 1955).

Corsi, P. and P.J. Weindling, 'Darwinism in Germany, France and Italy', in D. Kohn (ed.), *Images of Darwin* (Princeton, 1985), pp. 683–729.

Cowan, R.S., 'Nature and Nurture: the Interplay of Biology and Politics in the Thought of Francis Galton', *Studies in the History of Biology*, vol. 1 (1977), 133–208.

Crew, D.F., 'German Socialism, the State and Family Policy, 1918–33', *Continuity and Change*, vol. 1 (1986), 235–63.

Crook, D., *Benjamin Kidd* (Cambridge, 1984).

Cyankali von Friedrich Wolf. Eine Dokumentation (Berlin, 1978).

Dickinson, R.E., *The German Lebensraum* (Harmondsworth, 1943).

Dietl, H.-M. (ed.), *Eugenik. Entstehung und gesellschaftliche Bedingtheit* (Jena, 1984).

Dietrich, E., 'Fürsorgewesen für Säuglinge', *Bericht über den XIV. internationalen Kongress für Hygiene und Demographie. Berlin 23–29 September 1907*, vol. 2 (Berlin, 1908), pp. 393–427.

Doerner, K., *Madmen and the Bourgeoisie* (Oxford, 1981).

Donzelot, J., *The Policing of Families* (London, 1980).

Döring, H., *Der Weimarer Kreis* (Meisenheim, 1975).

Dowbiggin, I., 'Degeneration and Hereditarianism in French Mental Medicine 1840–1890: Psychiatric Theory as Ideological Adaptation', in W. Bynum, M. Shepherd and R. Porter (eds.), *The Anatomy of Madness* (London, 1985).

Druvins, U., 'Alternative Projekte um 1900', in H. Gnüg (ed.), *Literarische Utopie-Entwürfe* (Frankfurt-on-Main, 1982), pp. 236–49.

Duncan, D., *The Life and Letters of Herbert Spencer* (London, 1911).

Ebbinghaus, A., H. Kaupen-Haas and K.-H. Roth (eds.), *Heilen und Vernichten im Mustergau Hamburg. Bevölkerungs- und Gesundheitspolitik im Dritten Reich* (Hamburg, 1984).

Ebert, H., 'Hermann Muckermann', *Humanismus und Technik*, vol. 20 (1976), 29–40.

Ebstein, W., *Vererbbare celluläre Stoffwechselkrankheiten* (Stuttgart, 1902).

Eichholtz, D. and K. Grossweiler (eds.), *Faschismusforschung* (Berlin, 1980).

Eley, G., *Reshaping the German Right. Radical Nationalism and Political Change after Bismarck* (New Haven and London, 1980).

  From Unification to Nazism (London, 1986).

Elkeles, B., 'Medizinische Menschenversuche gegen Ende des 19. Jahrhunderts und der Fall Neisser', *Medizinhistorisches Journal*, vol. 20 (1985), 135–48.

Erlay, D., *Heinrich Vogeler* (Fischerhude, 1981).

Eulenberg, H., *Das Medizinalwesen in Preussen*, 3rd edn (Berlin, 1874).

Eulenburg, F., *Der 'akademische Nachwuchs'. Eine Untersuchung über die Lage und die Aufgaben der Extraordinarien und Privatdozenten* (Berlin and Leipzig, 1908).

Eulenburg-Hertefelde, P. zu, *Aus 50 Jahren*, 2nd edn (Berlin, 1925).

Euleutheropoulos, A., *Soziologie* (Jena, 1904).

Eulner, H.-H., *Die Entwicklung der medizinischen Spezialfächer an den Universitäten des deutschen Sprachgebietes* (Stuttgart, 1970).

Evans, R.J., *The Feminist Movement in Germany 1894–1933* (London and Beverley Hills, 1976).

  Death in Hamburg (Oxford, 1987).

Farrell, L.A., *The Origins and Growth of the English Eugenics Movement 1865–1925* (New York, 1985).

Fassbender, M., *Des deutschen Volkes Wille zum Leben. Bevölkerungspolitische und volkspädagogische Abhandlungen über Erhaltung und Förderung deutscher Volkskraft* (Freiburg, 1917).

Fetscher, R., 'Die Bewegung der Kinderreichen', *ARGB* vol. 14 (1922), 370–1.

  'Biologische Politik', *Dresdener Neueste Nachrichten*, (1 August 1924).

  'Eheberatung in Sachsen', *Eugenische Rundschau*, (1928), 60–8.

Field, G.C., *Evangelist of Race. The Germanic Vision of Houston Stewart Chamberlain* (New York, 1981).

Fischer, A., *Die Mutterschaftsversicherung in den europäischen Ländern* (Leipzig, 1911).

  Grundriss der sozialen Hygiene für Mediziner, Nationalökonomen, Verwaltungsbeamte und Sozialreformer (Berlin, 1913).

Fischer, E., *Sozialanthropologie und ihre Bedeutung für den Staat* (Freiburg, 1910).

  Die Rehobother Bastards und das Bastardierungsproblem beim Menschen (Jena, 1913).

  'Gustav Schwalbe', *Zeitschrift für Morphologie und Anthropologie*, vol. 20 (1917), i–viii.

  'Das Kaiser-Wilhlem-Institut für Anthropologie, menschliche Erblehre und Eugenik', *Zeitschrift für Morphologie und Anthropologie*, vol. 27 (1927), 147–52.

  'Aus der Geschichte der deutschen Gesellschaft für Rassenhygiene', *ARGB*, vol. 24 (1930), 1–5.

Fischer, H.C. and E.X. Dubois, *Sexual Life during the World War* (London, 1937).

Fletcher, R., *Revisionism and Empire. Socialist Imperialism in Germany 1897–1914* (London, 1984).

Fluegge, C., *Grundriss der Hygiene*, 5th edn (Leipzig, 1902).

Ford, H., *Das Grosse Heute und das Grössere Morgen* (Leipzig, 1926).

Foreign Office, *Scientific Results of German Medical War Crimes* (London, 1949).

Foreign Office and Ministry of Economic Warfare, *The Nazi System of Medicine and Public Health Organization* (London, 1944).

Forel, A., *Die sexuelle Frage* (Munich, 1905).

  Sexual Ethics (London, 1909).

Forman, P., 'Weimar Culture, Causality and Quantum Theory, 1918–1927', *Historical Studies in the Physical Sciences*, vol. 3 (1971), 1–111.

Frankenthal, K., 'Ärzteschaft und Faschismus', *Der Sozialistische Arzt*, vol. 8 no. 6 (1932), 101–7.

Der dreifache Fluch; Jüdin, Intellektuelle, Sozialistin (Frankfurt-on-Main, 1981).

Franz, V., *Das heutige geschichtliche Bild von Ernst Haeckel* (Jena, 1934).

Freeden, M., *The New Liberalism. An Ideology of Social Reform* (Oxford, 1978).

'Eugenics and Progressive Thought: a Study in Ideological Affinity', *The Historical Journal*, 22 (1979), 645–71.

Frevert, U., *Krankheit als politisches Problem 1770–1880* (Göttingen, 1984).

'The Civilizing Tendency of Hygiene. Working Class Women under Medical Control in Imperial Germany', in J.C. Fout (ed.), *German Women in the Nineteenth Century* (New York and London, 1984), pp. 320–44.

Frick, W. and A. Gütt, *Nordisches Gedankengut im Dritten Reich* (Munich; Lehmann, 1936).

Frisch, K.v., *Du und das Leben* (Berlin, 1936).

Führ, E. and D. Stemmrich, *'Nach gethaner Arbeit verbleibt im Kreise der Eurigen.' Bürgerliche Wohnrezepte für Arbeiter zur individuellen und sozialen Formierung im 19. Jahrhundert* (Wuppertal, 1985).

Fürth, H., *Die Regelung der Nachkommenschaft als eugenisches Problem* (Stuttgart, 1929).

Gall, L., 'Liberalismus und "Bürgerliche Gesellschaft": Zu Charakter und Entwicklung der Liberalen Bewegung in Deutschland', *Historische Zeitschrift*, vol. 220 (1975), 324–56.

Galton, F., 'A Theory of Heredity', *The Contemporary Review*, vol. 10 (1875), 80–95.

Gasman, D., *The Scientific Origins of National Socialism: Social Darwinism in Ernst Haeckel and the Monist League* (New York, 1971).

Georg, K., *Sociale Hygiene* (Berlin, 1890).

Geus, A., *Johannes Ranke (1836–1916). Physiologe, Anthropologe und Prähistoriker* (Marburg, 1987).

Geuter, U., *Die Professionalisierung der Psychologie im Nationalsozialismus* (Frankfurt-on-Main, 1984).

Glass, D.V., *Population Policies and Movements in Europe* (Oxford, 1940).

Introduction to Malthus (London, 1953).

Göbel, P. and H.E. Thormann, *Verlegt – Vernichtet – Vergessen . . .? Leidenswege von Menschen aus Hephaten im Dritten Reich* (Schwalmstadt-Treysa, 1985).

Gobineau, M.A. de, *Essai sur l'inégalité des races humaines*, 4 vols. (Paris, 1853–55).

Göckenjan, G., *Gesundheit und Staat machen* (Frankfurt-on-Main, 1985).

Goldscheid, R., *Höherentwicklung und Menschenökonomie – Grundlegung der Sozialbiologie* (Leipzig, 1911).

Goldschmidt, R.B., *Die Lehre von der Vererbung*, 2 vols. (Berlin, 1927).

In and Out of the Ivory Tower (Seattle, 1960).

Goldstein, W., *Carl Hauptmann, Eine Werkdeutung* (Breslau, 1931).

Gottstein, A., *Das Heilwesen der Gegenwart, Gesundheitslehre und Gesundheitspolitik* (Berlin, 1924).

Graeter, E., *Gustav von Bunge. Naturforscher und Menschenfreund* (Basle, nd).

Graham, L.R., 'Science and Values: the Eugenics Movement in Germany and Russia in the 1920s', *American Historical Review*, vol. 82 (1977), 1133–64.

Between Science and Values (New York, 1981).

Grant, M., *The Passing of the Great Race, or the Racial Basis of European History* (New York, 1916).

Gregory, F., *Scientific Materialism in Nineteenth Century Germany* (Dordrecht, 1977).

Griffiths, R., *Fellow Travellers of the Right. British Enthusiasts for Nazi Germany 1933–39* (Oxford, 1983).

Grossmann, A., 'Abortion and Economic Crisis: the 1931 Campaign against Paragraph 218', in Bridenthal *et al.* (eds.), *Biology*, pp. 66–86.

Grote, L.R. (ed.), *Die Medizin der Gegenwart in Selbstdarstellungen*, 5 vols. (Leipzig, 1923–28).

Grotjahn, A., *Der Alkoholismus nach Wesen, Wirkung und Verbreitung* (Leipzig, 1898).

Krankenhauswesen und Heilstättenbewegung im Lichte der sozialen Hygiene (Leipzig, 1908).

Soziale Pathologie (Berlin, 1912).

Geburtenrückgang und Geburtenregelung im Lichte der individuellen und sozialen Hygiene (Berlin, 1914).

Die hygienische Forderung (Königstein and Leipzig, 1921).

Die Hygiene der menschlichen Fortpflanzung (Berlin and Vienna, 1926).

Erlebtes und Erstrebtes. Erinnerungen eines sozialistischen Arztes (Berlin, 1932).

Grotjahn, A. and I. Kaup (eds.), *Handwörterbuch der Sozialhygiene* (Jena, 1912).

Gruber, M. v., 'Führt die Hygiene zur Entartung der Rasse?' *MMW*, vol. 50 (1903) 1713–8, 1781–5.

Mädchenerziehung und Rassenhygiene (Munich, 1910).

'Fürsorge für die schulentlassene Jugend', *Bayerisches ärztliches Correspondenzblatt*, vol. 13 (1910), 76–80.

'Organisation der Forschung und Sammlung von Materialien über die Entartungsfrage', *Concordia*, vol. 17 (1910), 225–8.

Hygiene des Geschlechtslebens (Stuttgart, 1917).

Gruber, M. v. (ed.), *Handbuch der Hygiene* (Leipzig, 1911).

Gruber, M. v. and E. Rüdin (eds.), *Fortpflanzung, Vererbung, Rassenhygiene. Katalog der Gruppe Rassenhygiene der Internationalen Hygiene-Ausstellung 1911 in Dresden* (Munich, 1911).

Grüneberg, H. and W. Ulrich, *Moderne Biologie. Festschrift zum 60. Geburtstag von Hans Nachtsheim* (Berlin, 1950).

Günther, H.F.K., *Ritter, Tod und Teufel. Eine Darstellung der Wesensart des nordischen Menschen* (Munich, 1920).

Rassenkunde des Deutschen Volkes (Munich, 1922).

Volk und Staat in ihrer Stellung zu Vererbung und Auslese (Munich, nd).

Güse, H.-G. and W. Schmacke, *Zwangssterilisierung – verleugnet – vergessen. Zur Geschichte der nationalsozialistischen Rassenhygiene am Beispiel Bremen* (Bremen, 1984).

Gütt, A., H. Linden and F. Massfeller, *Blutschutz- und Ehegesundheitsgesetz* (Munich, 1936).

Gütt, A., E. Rüdin and F. Ruttke, *Gesetz zur Verhütung erbkranken Nachwuchses vom 14. Juli 1933*, (Munich, 1934).

Guttstadt, A., *Krankenhaus – Lexicon für das Deutsche Reich* (Berlin, 1900).

Haberling, W., *Arthur Schlossmann, sein Leben und Werk* (Düsseldorf, 1927).

Haeckel, E., *Natürliche Schöpfungsgeschichte* (Berlin, 1868).

Prinzipien der Generellen Morphologie der Organismen (1866, reprinted Berlin, 1906).

Anthropogenie oder Entwicklungsgeschichte des Menschen (Leipzig, 1874).

'Die heutige Entwicklungslehre im Verhältnis zur Gesamtwissenschaft', *Amtlicher Bericht der 50. Versammlung Deutscher Naturforscher und Aerzte in München vom 17. bis 22. September 1877* (1877), 14–22.

Freie Wissenschaft und freie Lehre (Stuttgart, 1878).

Die Welträthsel (Bonn, 1899).

Kunstformen der Natur (Leipzig, 1899–1904).

Die Lebenswunder (Stuttgart, 1904).

Zellseelen und Seelenzellen. Vortrag gehalten am 22. März 1878 in der 'Concordia' zu Wien (Leipzig, 1920).

Haecker, V., *Allgemeine Vererbungslehre* (Braunschweig, 1921).

'Die Annahme einer erblichen Übertragung körperlicher Kriegsschäden', *Archiv für Frauenkunde*, vol. 4 (1920), 1–15.

Haecker, W., *Die ererbten Anlagen und die Bemessung ihres Werts für das politische Leben* (Jena, 1907).

Hahn, M., *Grenzen und Ziele der Sozialhygiene* (Freiburg, 1912).

Hahn, S., 'Positionen der Kommunistischen Partei Deutschlands zur lebensbewahrenden Aufgabe der Medizin in der Zeit der Weimarer Republik', *Zeitschrift für die gesamte Hygiene*, vol. 28 (1982), 468–71.

Haire, N. (ed.), *The Sexual Reform Congress* (London, 1930).

Hamburger, E., *Juden im öffentlichen Leben Deutschlands* (Tübingen, 1968).

Hamilton, D.N., *The Monkey Gland Affair* (London, 1986).

Hammond, M., 'Anthropology as a Weapon of Social Combat in the Late Nineteenth-century', *Journal of the History of the Behavioural Sciences*, vol. 16 (1980), 118–32.

Hanauske-Abel, H., 'From Nazi Holocaust to Nuclear Holocaust: A Lesson to Learn?', *Lancet* (1986), 271–3.

Hansen, E., M. Heissig, S. Leibfried and F. Tennstedt, *Seit über einem Jahrhundert . . .: Verschüttete Alternativen in der Sozialpolitik* (Köln, 1981).

Harmann, R. and J. Hermand, *Naturalismus* (Berlin, 1968).

Harmsen, H., *Praktische Bevölkerungspolitik* (Berlin, 1931).

'The German Sterilization Act of 1933', *Eugenics Review*, vol. 46 (1955), 227–32.

Hartmann, K., *Deutsche Gartenstadtbewegung: Kulturpolitik und Gesellschaftsreform* (Munich, 1976).

Hartung, K., 'Einhundert Jahre schulärztlicher Dienst – ein beinahe vergessenes Jubiläum', *Öffentliches Gesundheitswesen*, vol. 45 (1983), 615–17.

Harvey, E., 'Sozialdemokratische Jugendhilfereform in der Praxis: Walter Friedländer und das Bezirksjugendamt Berlin Prenzlauer Berg in der Weimarer Republik', *Theorie und Praxis der sozialen Arbeit* (1985), 218–29.

Youth Welfare and Social Democracy in Weimar Germany: the Work of Walter Friedländer (New Alyth, 1987).

Harvey, J., 'Evolutionism Transformed: Positivists and Materialists in the *Société d'Anthropologie de Paris* from Second Empire to Third Republic', in D. Oldroyd and J. Langham (eds.), *The Wider Domain of Evolutionary Thought* (Dordrecht, 1983), pp. 289–310.

Harwood, J., 'The Reception of Morgan's Chromosome Theory in Germany: Inter-war Debate over Cytoplasmic Inheritance', *Medizinhistorisches Journal*, vol. 19 (1984), 3–32.

'Geneticists and the Evolutionary Synthesis in Inter-war Germany', *Annals of Science*, vol. 42 (1985) 279–301.

Hauptmann, C., *Die Bedeutung der Keimblättertheorie für Individualitätslehre und den Generationswechsel* (Jena, 1883).

Hausen, K., 'Mütter zwischen Geschäftsinteressen und kultischer Verehrung, Der "Deutsche Muttertag" in der Weimarer Republik', in G. Huck (ed.), *Sozialgeschichte der Freizeit* (Wuppertal, 1980), pp. 249–80.

Haycraft, J.B., *Natürliche Auslese und Rassenverbesserung* (Leipzig, 1895).

Heberer, G. (ed.), *J. Walther, Im Banne Ernst Haeckels. Jena um die Jahrhundertwende* (Göttingen, 1953).

Hegar, A., *Der Zusammenhang der Geschlechtskrankheiten mit nervösen Leiden und die Castration bei Neurosen* (Stuttgart, 1885).

Der Geschlechtstrieb. Eine social-medizinische Studie (Stuttgart, 1894).
Alfred Hegar zum Gedächtnis (Freiburg, 1930).
Heiber, H., 'Der Generalplan Ost', *Vierteljahreshefte für Zeitgeschichte*, vol. 6 (1958), 280–323.
Heidel, C.P. and G. Heidel, 'Zu Carl Röses wissenschaftlichen Verdiensten um die Kariesätiologie und die soziale Zahnheilkunde', *Stomatologie DDR*, vol. 34 (1984), 173–9.
Heinemann, P.G., *Milk* (Philadelphia and London, 1919).
Heinson, G., R. Knieper and O. Steiger, *Menschenproduktion. Allgemeine Bevölkerungslehre der Neuzeit* (Frankfurt-on-Main, 1979).
Hellpach, W., *Politische Prognose für Deutschland* (Berlin, 1928).
Hentschel, W., *Varuna: eine Welt- und Geschichtsbetrachtung vom Standpunkt des Ariers* (Leipzig, 1901).
Mittgart, ein Weg zur Erneuerung der germanischen Rasse (Leipzig, 1904).
Herf, J., *Reactionary Modernism, Technology, Culture, and Politics in Weimar and the Third Reich* (Cambridge, 1984).
Hertwig, O., *Zur Abwehr des ethischen, des sozialen und des politischen Darwinismus* (Jena, 1918).
Der Staat als Organismus (Jena, 1922).
Hertz, F., 'Moderne Rassentheorieen', *Sozialistische Monatshefte*, vol. 6 (1902), 876–83.
'Die Rassentheorie des H. St. Chamberlain', *Sozialistische Monatshefte*, vol. 8 (1904), 310–15.
Hans Günther als Rassenforscher (Berlin, 1930).
Hertzka, T., *Freiland: Ein soziales Zukunftsbild* (Leipzig, 1890).
Hesse, A., *Natur und Gesellschaft* (Jena, 1904).
Heuss, T., *Anton Dohrn*, 2nd edn (Stuttgart and Tübingen, 1948).
Friedrich Naumann (Stuttgart and Tübingen, 1949).
Hinrichs, P., *Um die Seele des Arbeiters* (Cologne, 1981).
Hirsch, M., *Fruchtabtreibung und Präventivverkehr im Zusammenhang mit dem Geburtenrückgang* (Würzburg, 1914).
'Staatskinder. Ein Vorschlag zur Bevölkerungspolitik im neuen Deutschland', *Archiv für Frauenkunde*, vol. 4 (1919), 181–7.
Hirschfeld, M., *Die Verstaatlichung des Gesundheitswesens* (Berlin, 1919).
Race (London, 1938).
Sittengeschichte des Weltkriegs, 2 vols. (Leipzig and Vienna, nd).
Hirtsiefer, H., *Die staatliche Wohlfahrtspflege in Preussen 1919–1923* (Berlin, 1924).
His, W., *Die Front der Ärzte* (Bielefeld and Leipzig, 1931).
Hitler, A., *Mein Kampf* (Munich, 1925; trans. London, 1974).
Hoche, A.E., *Jahresringe* (Munich, 1935).
Hodann, M., 'Über Notwendigkeit und Aussichten der Eheberatung', *Die Neue Generation*, vol. 22 (1926), 337–9.
'Fürsorgestelle für Sexualberatung und Geburtenregelung in Berlin-Reinickendorf', *Die Neue Generation*, vol. 27 (1931), 117–18.
Hoeflmayr, L., 'Rassenhygiene in Theorie und Praxis', *Burschenschaftsblätter*, vol. 26 (1912), 186–8.
Hoffman, W., *Die deutschen Ärzte im Weltkriege* (Berlin, 1920).
Hoffmann, G. v., *Die Rassenhygiene in den Vereinigten Staaten von Nordamerika* (Munich, 1913).
Hohmann, J., *Sexualforschung und -aufklärung in der Weimarer Republik* (Berlin and Frankfurt, 1985).

Holmes, S.J., *A Bibliography of Eugenics* (Berkeley, 1924).

Hoppe, L. *Sexueller Bolschewismus und seine Abwehr* (Berlin, 1921).

Horder, T. and P.J. Weindling, 'Hans Spemann and the Organiser', in Horder, J. Witkowski and C. Wylie (eds.), *A History of Embryology* (Cambridge, 1986), pp. 183–242.

Hubenstorf, M., 'Sozialhygiene und industrielle Pathologie im späten Kaiserreich', in R. Müller *et al.* (eds.), *Industrielle Pathologie in historischer Sicht* (Bremen, 1985), pp. 82–107.

Hueppe, F., *Zur Rassen- und Sozialhygiene der Griechen im Altertum und in der Gegenwart* (Wiesbaden, 1897).

Hueppe, F. (ed.), *Handbuch der Hygiene* (Berlin, 1899).

Huerkamp, C., *Der Aufstieg der Ärzte* (Göttingen, 1985).

'A History of Smallpox Vaccination in Germany: A First Step in the Medicalization of the General Public', *Journal of Contemporary History*, vol. 20 (1985), 617–35.

Hull, I.V., *The Entourage of Kaiser Wilhelm II, 1888–1918* (Cambridge, 1982).

Irving, D., *Adolf Hitler. The Medical Diaries* (London, 1983).

Jaeger, G., *Seuchenfestigkeit und Konstitutionskraft* (Leipzig, 1878).

James, H., *The German Slump* (Oxford, 1986).

Jantzen, W., *Sozialgeschichte des Behindertenbetreuungswesens* (Munich, 1982).

Jarausch, K., *Students, Society and Politics in Imperial Germany* (Princeton, 1982).

Jaworski, M., *Ludwik Hirszfeld. Sein Beitrag zu Serologie und Immunologie* (Leipzig, 1980).

Jeschal, G., *Politik und Wissenschaft deutscher Ärzte im ersten Weltkrieg* (Pattensen, 1978).

Johnston, W.M., *The Austrian Mind* (Berkeley, 1983).

Jones, G., *Social Darwinism in English Thought* (Brighton, 1980).

'Eugenics and Social Policy between the Wars', *The Historical Journal*, vol. 25 (1982), 717–28.

Social Hygiene in Twentieth Century Britain (London, 1986).

Jost, A., *Das Recht auf den Tod. Soziale Studie* (Göttingen, 1895).

Just, G., 'Agnes Bluhm und ihr Lebenswerk', *Die Ärztin*, vol. 17 (1942), 516–26.

Kahle, M., *Das Gesundheitshaus. Einführung in das Aufgabengebiet der sozialen Hygiene unter besonderer Berücksichtigung der Gesundheitsfürsorge im Verwaltungsbezirk Kreuzberg der Stadt Berlin* (Berlin, 1925).

Kaiser, W. and A. Völker, 'Die faschistischen Strömungen an der Medizinischen Fakultät der Universität Halle', in Thom and Spaar (eds.), *Medizin im Faschismus*, pp. 68–76.

Kalikow, T.J., 'Konrad Lorenz's Ethological Theory: Explanation and Ideology, 1938–1943', *Journal of the History of Biology*, vol. 16 (1983), 39–73.

Kammerer, P., *Das Rätsel der Vererbung* (Berlin, 1925).

Kampe, N., 'Jews and Antisemites at Universities in Imperial Germany (II). The Friedrich-Wilhelms-Universität of Berlin: a Case Study on the Students' "Jewish Question"', *Leo Baeck Institute. Year Book*, vol. 32 (1987), 43–101.

Kankeleit, O., *Die Unfruchtbarmachung aus rassenhygienischen und sozialen Gründen* (Munich, 1924).

Kater, M.H., *The Nazi Party* (Oxford, 1983).

Das "Ahnenerbe" der SS 1935–1945. Ein Beitrag zur Kulturpolitik des Dritten Reiches (Stuttgart, 1974).

'Die Gesundheitsführung des Deutschen Volkes', *Medizinhistorisches Journal*, vol. 18 (1983), 349–75.

'Medizin und Mediziner im Dritten Reich. Eine Bestandsaufnahme', *Historische Zeitschrift*, vol. 244 (1987), 299–352.

'Physicians in Crisis at the End of the Weimar Republic', in P.D. Stachura (ed.), *Unemployment and the Great Depression in Weimar Germany* (Basingstoke, 1986), pp. 49–74.

Kaufmann, E., *Gustav Jaeger, 1832–1913. Arzt, Zoologe und Hygieniker* (Zürich, 1984).

Kaufmann, P., *Krieg, Geschlechtskrankheiten und Arbeiterversicherung* (Berlin, 1916).

Kaup, I., 'Was kosten die minderwertigen Elemente dem Staat und der Gesellschaft', *ARGB*, vol. 10 (1913), 723–48.

Frauenarbeit und Rassenhygiene (Hamburg, 1914).

Volkshygiene oder selektive Rassenhygiene? (Leipzig, 1922).

Kaup, I. and T. Fürst, *Körperverfassung und Leistungskraft Jugendlicher* (Munich and Berlin, 1930).

Kautsky, B. (ed.), *Karl Kautsky Erinnerungen und Eröterungen* (The Hague, 1960).

Kautsky, K., 'Medizinisches', *Die Neue Zeit*, vol. 10/1 (1891/2), 644–51.

Der Einfluss der Volksvermehrung auf den Fortschritt der Gesellschaft (Vienna, 1880).

Kautsky, K. jun (ed.), *August Bebels Briefwechsel mit Karl Kautsky* (Assen, 1971).

Kelly, A., *The Descent of Darwin* (Chapel Hill, 1981).

Kennedy, H.C., 'The "Third Sex" Theory of Karl Heinrich Ulrichs', *Journal of Homosexuality*, vol. 6 (1981), 103–11.

Kersten, F., *The Kersten Memoirs 1940–1945* (London, 1956).

Kevles, D.J., *In the Name of Eugenics* (Harmondsworth, 1986).

Kidd, B., *Soziale Evolution mit einem Vorwort von Professor Dr August Weismann* (Jena, 1895).

Kientopf, H., *The School Dentists' Society* (London, 1910).

Kirchner, M., *Hygiene und Seuchenbekämpfung. Gesammelte Abhandlungen* (Berlin, 1904).

Ärztliche Kriegs- und Friedensgedanken (Berlin, 1918).

Kisch, B., 'Forgotten Leaders in Modern Medicine: Valentin, Gruby, Remak and Auerbach', *Transactions of the American Philosophical Society*, vol. 44 (1954), 141–317.

Kittel, I.-W., 'Arthur Kronfeld (1886–1941)', *Psychologische Rundschau*, vol. 37 (1986), 41.

Klebs, E., *Die Allgemeine Pathologie* (Jena, 1887).

Klee, E., *"Euthanasie" im NS-Staat. Die Vernichtung lebensunwerten Lebens* (Frankfurt-on-Main, 1983).

Was sie taten – was sie wurden (Frankfurt-on-Main, 1986).

Knodel, J., *The Decline of Fertility in Germany* (Princeton, 1974).

Koch, G., *Euthanasie, Sterbehilfe. Eine dokumentierte Bibliographie* (Erlangen, 1984).

Die Gesellschaft für Konstitutionsforschung (Erlangen, 1985).

Koehl, R.L., *RKFDV: German Resettlement and Population Policy* (Cambridge, Mass., 1957).

The Black Corps; the Structure and Power Struggles of the Nazi SS (Wisconsin, 1983).

Kohler, R.E., 'A Policy for the Advancement of Science: The Rockefeller Foundation, 1924–29', *Minerva*, vol. 16 (1978), 480–515.

Kollwitz, K., *Ich sah die Welt mit liebevollen Blicken* (Wiesbaden, nd).

Kolney, F., *La grève des ventres* (Paris, 1908).

Körberle, K., 'Zur Kontroverse zwischen Schulmedizin und Naturheillehre vor dem Hintergrund der Entwicklung der Hydrotherapeutischen Anstalt der Universität Berlin', *Wissenschaftliche Zeitschrift der Humboldt-Universität zu Berlin*, mathematisch-naturwissenschaftliche Reihe, vol. 28 (1979), 309–15.

Krabbe, W., *Gesellschaftsveränderung durch Lebensreform* (Göttingen, 1974).

Kraemer, R., *Kritik der Eugenik vom Standpunkt des Betroffenen* (Berlin, 1933).

Krause, E., *Ernst Haeckel* (Leipzig, 1983).

Kretschmer, E., *Körperbau und Charakter*, 7th edn (Berlin, 1929).

Krohne, O., *Erziehungsanstalten für die verlassene, gefährdete und verwahrloste Jugend in Preussen* (Berlin, 1901).

Die Beurteilung des Geburtenrückganges vom volkshygienischen, sittlichen und nationalen Standpunkt (Leipzig, 1914).

Krutina, E., *Chronik eines guten Bundes* (Berlin, 1924).

Kudlien, F., 'Max von Gruber und die frühe Hitler-Bewegung', *Medizinhistorisches Journal*, vol. 17 (1982), 373–89.

Kudlien, F. (ed.), *Ärzte im Nationalsozialismus* (Cologne, 1985).

Kudlien, F. and C. Andree, 'Sauerbruch und der Nationalsozialismus', *Medizinhistorisches Journal*, vol. 15 (1980), 201–20.

Kühn, A. *et al.*, *Erbkunde, Rassenpflege, Bevölkerungspolitik* (Leipzig, 1935).

Kümmel, W.F., 'Die Ausschaltung rassisch und politisch missliebiger Ärzte', in Kudlien (ed.), *Ärzte*, pp. 56–81.

Labisch, A., 'Die gesundheitspolitischen Vorstellungen der deutschen Sozialdemokratie von ihrer Gründung bis zur Parteispaltung (1863–1917)', *Archiv für Sozialgeschichte*, vol. 16 (1976), 325–70.

'The Workingmen's Samaritan Federation (Arbeiter-Samariter-Bund) 1888–1933', *Journal of Contemporary History*, vol. 13 (1978), 297–322.

'Neue Quellen zum gesundheitspolitischen Program der MSPD von 1920/22', *IWK*, vol. 16 (1980), 231–47.

'Das Krankenhaus in der Gesundheitspolitik der deutschen Sozialdemokratie vor dem ersten Weltkrieg', *Medizinsoziologisches Jahrbuch*, vol. 1 (1981), 126–51.

'Selbsthilfe zwischen Auflehnung und Anpassung: Arbeiter-Sanitätskommission und Arbeiter-Samariterbund', *Argument-Sonderband*, vol. 77 (1983), 11–26.

'Doctors, Workers and the Scientific Cosmology of the Industrial World. The Social Construction of "Health" and of the "Homo Hygienicus"', *Journal of Contemporary History*, vol. 20 (1985), 599–615.

'"Hygiene ist Moral – Moral ist Hygiene" – Soziale Disziplinierung durch Ärzte und Medizin', in C. Sachsse and F. Tennstedt (eds.), *Soziale Sicherheit und soziale Disziplinierung* (Frankfurt-on-Main, 1986), pp. 265–85.

Labisch, A. and R. Spree (eds.), *Medizinische Deutungsmacht im sozialen Wandel. Der Beitrag der Medizin zur Prägung sozialer Rollen und gesellschaftlicher Randgruppen im 19. und frühen 20. Jahrhundert* (Bonn, 1989).

Labisch, A. and F. Tennstedt, *Der Weg zum 'Gesetz über die Vereinheitlichung des Gesundheitswesen'* (Düsseldorf, 1985).

Lacqueur, W., *Young Germany* (New York, 1962).

Landesgesundheitsamt Sachsen, *Einrichtungen auf dem Gebiete der Volksgesundheits- und Volkswohlfahrtspflege* (Dresden, 1922).

Landwehr, R. and R. Baron, *Geschichte der Sozialarbeit* (Weinheim and Basle, 1983).

Lange, A., *Berlin zur Zeit Bebels und Bismarcks* (Berlin, 1972).

Langer, W., *The Mind of Adolf Hitler. The Secret Wartime Report* (London, 1973).

Langstein, L. (ed.), *Beiträge zur Physiologie, Pathologie und sozialen Hygiene des Kindesalters* (Berlin, 1919).

Lee, W.R. (ed.), *European Demography and Economic Growth* (London, 1979).

Lee, W.R. and E. Rosenhaft (eds.), *The State and Social Change* (Oxford, in press).

Lehfeldt, H., 'Die Laienorganisationen für Geburtenregelung', *Archiv für Bevölkerungspolitik*, vol. 2 (1932), 63–87.

Lehmann, E., *Irrweg der Biologie* (Stuttgart, 1946).

Lehmann, E. and R. Beatus, 'Der Unterricht in der Vererbungswissenschaft an den deutschen Hochschulen', *Der Biologe*, vol. 1 (1931/2), 89–96.

Lehmann, M., *Verleger J.F. Lehmann. Ein Leben im Kampf für Deutschland* (Munich, 1935).

Leibfried, S. and F. Tennstedt, *Berufsverbote und Sozialpolitik 1933. Die Auswirkungen der nationalsozialistischen Machtergreifung auf die Krankenkassenverwaltung und die Kassenärzte*, 3rd edn (Bremen, 1981); also as 'Sozialpolitik und Berufsverbote im Jahre 1933', *Zeitschrift für Sozialreform*, vol. 25 (1979), 29–53, 211–38.

Leibfried, S. and F. Tennstedt (ed.), *Kommunale Gesundheitsfürsorge und sozialistische Ärztepolitik zwischen Kaiserreich und Nationalsozialismus – autobiographische, biographische und gesundheitspolitische Anmerkungen von Dr Georg Löwenstein* (Bremen, 1980).

Lenz, F., *Die Rasse als Wertprinzip, Zur Erneuerung der Ethik* (Munich: Lehmann, nd).

Über die krankhaften Erbanlagen des Mannes und die Bestimmung des Geschlechtes beim Menschen (Jena, 1912).

Menschliche Auslese und Rassenhygiene (Munich, 1921).

'Ein "Deutscher Bund für Volksaufartung und Erbkunde"', *ARGB*, vol. 17 (1925), 349–50.

'Das deutsche Forschungsinstitut für Anthropologie, menschliche Erblehre und Eugenik in Berlin-Dahlem', *MMW*, vol. 74 (1927), 1764.

'Ist Sterilisierung strafbar?', *ARGB*, vol. 25 (1931), 232–4.

'Die Stellung des Nationalsozialismus zur Rassenhygiene', *ARGB*, vol. 25 (1931), 300–8.

Lesky, E. (ed.), *Sozialmedizin. Entwicklung und Selbstverständnis* (Darmstadt, 1977).

Levy, R.S., *The Downfall of the Anti-Semitic Political Parties in Imperial Germany* (New Haven and London, 1975).

Lewis, J., *The Politics of Motherhood* (London, 1980).

Lichtheim, G., *Marxism* (London, 1964).

Liek, E., *Der Arzt und seine Sendung* (1925), 7th edn (Munich, 1929).

Lifton, R.J., *The Nazi Doctors. Medical Killing and the Psychology of Genocide* (New York, 1986).

Lilienthal, G., 'Rassenhygiene im Dritten Reich. Krise und Wende', *Medizinhistorisches Journal*, vol. 14 (1979), 114–34.

'"Rheinlandbastarde". Rassenhygiene und das Problem der rassenideologischen Kontinuität', *Medizinhistorisches Journal*, vol. 15 (1980), 426–36.

'Zum Anteil der Anthropologie an der NS-Rassenpolitik', *Medizinhistorisches Journal*, vol. 19 (1984), 148–60.

Der "Lebensborn" e.V. Ein Instrument nationalsozialistischer Rassenpolitik (Stuttgart, 1985).

'Max Taube, Ein Wegbereiter moderner Säuglings- und Jugendfürsorge', *Sozialpädiatrie in Praxis und Klinik*, vol. 8 (1986), 476–80.

'Der Nationalsozialistische Deutsche Ärztebund (1929–1943/1945)', in Kudlien (ed.), *Ärzte*, pp. 105–21.

'Paediatrics and Nationalism in Imperial Germany', *Bulletin of the Society for the Social History of Medicine*, no. 39 (1986), 64–70.

Linse, U., 'Arbeiterschaft und Geburtenkontrolle im Deutschen Kaiserreich von 1891 bis 1914', *Archiv für Sozialgeschichte*, vol. 12 (1972), 205–71.

Linse, U. (ed.), *Zurück o Mensch zur Mutter Erde. Landkommunen in Deutschland 1890–1933* (Munich, 1983).

Loeffler, L., 'Allgemeine ärztliche Studentenuntersuchungen', *Mitteilungen der Gesellschaft Deutscher Naturforscher und Ärzte*, vol. 3 (1926), 35–6.

Lohalm, U., *Völkischer Radikalismus. Die Geschichte des Deutschvölkischen Schutz- und Trutz Bundes 1919–1921* (Hamburg, 1970).

Lönne, K.-E., *PolitischerKatholizismus im 19. und 20. Jahrhundert* (Frankfurt-on-Main, 1986).

Lorenz, O., *Lehrbuch der gesammten wissenschaflichen Genealogie. Stammbaum und Ahnentafel in ihrer geschichtlichen, soziologischen und naturwissenschaftlichen Bedeutung* (Berlin, 1898).

Lubarsch, O., *Ein bewegtes Gelehrtenleben* (Berlin, 1931).

Luebbe, H., *Politische Philosophie in Deutschland* (Munich, 1974).

Lührs, W. (ed.), *Bremische Biographie 1912–1962* (Bremen, 1969).

Lundborg, H., *Medizinisch-biologische Familienforschungen innerhalb eines 2231 köpfigen Bauerngeschlechtes in Schweden (Provinz Blekinge)*, (Jena, 1913).

Lüthenau, F., *Darwin und der Staat. (Preisgekrönt in Jena, Krupp'sche Stiftung)* (Leipzig, 1905).

Lutzhöft, H.J., *Der Nordische Gedanke in Deutschland 1920–1940* (Stuttgart, 1972).

Lux, H., *Etienne Cabet und der Ikarische Kommunismus* (Stuttgart, 1896).

Magnussen, K., 'Ueber eine sichelförmige Hornhautüberwachsung am Kaninchenauge und beim Menschen', *Der Erbarzt*, vol. 12 (1944), 60–2.

Manchester, W., *The Arms of Krupp 1587–1968* (London, 1969).

Mann, E., *Die Erlösung der Menschheit vom Elend* (Weimar, 1922).

Mann, G., 'Medizinisch-biologische Ideen und Modelle in der Gesellschaftslehre des 19. Jahrhunderts', *Medizinhistorisches Journal*, vol. 4 (1969), 1–23.

'Ernst Haeckel und der Darwinismus: Popularisierung, Propaganda und Ideologisierung', *Medizinhistorisches Journal*, vol. 15 (1980), 269–83.

Mann, G. (ed.), *Biologismus im 19. Jahrhundert* (Stuttgart, 1973).

Mann, G. and R. Winau (eds.), *Medizin, Naturwissenschaft, Technik und des Zweite Kaiserreich* (Göttingen, 1977).

Manuel, F.E. and Manuel, F.P., *Utopian Thought in the Western World* (Oxford, 1979).

Marcuse, M., *Der Eheliche Präventivverkehr. Seine Verbreitung, Verursachung und Methodik. Dargestellt und beleuchtet an 300 Ehen* (Stuttgart, 1917).

Marks, S., 'Black Watch on the Rhine: A Study in Propaganda, Prejudice and Prurience', *European Studies Review*, vol. 13 (1983), 297–334.

Marschalck, P., *Bevölkerungsgeschichte Deutschlands im 19. und 20. Jahrhundert* (Frankfurt-on-Main, 1984).

Martin, J. and A. Nitschke (eds.), *Zur Sozialgeschichte der Kindheit* (Freiburg and Munich, 1986).

Martius, F., *Die Pathogenese Innerer Krankheiten* (Leipzig and Vienna, 1899).

Mason, T.W., *Sozialpolitik im Dritten Reich* (Opladen, 1977).

Matzat, H., *Philosophie der Anpassung* (Jena, 1903).

Mayer, A., *Alfred Hegar und der Gestaltwandel der Gynäkologie seit Hegar* (Freiburg, 1961).

McClelland, C.E., *State, Society and University in Germany 1700–1914* (Cambridge, 1980).

Medizinalabteilung, Preussische, *25 Jahre preussische Medizinalverwaltung seit Erlass des Kreisarztgesetzes, 1901–1926* (Berlin, 1927).

Mehrtens, H. and S. Richter (eds.), *Naturwissenschaft, Technik und NS-ideologie* (Frankfurt-on-Main, 1980).

Meier, R., *August Forel* (Zürich, 1986).

Mendelssohn-Bartholdy, A., *The War and German Society. The Testament of a Liberal* (New Haven, 1937).

Mensinga, W.P.J. (= C. Hasse, pseud.), *Facultative Sterilität*, 6th edn (Berlin and Neuwied, 1892).

Merckenschlager, F., *Götter, Helden und Günther. Ein Abwehr der Güntherschen Rassenkunde* (Nürnberg, nd).

Methner, A., *Organismen und Staaten* (Jena, 1906).

Michaelis, C., *Prinizipien der natürlichen und sozialen Entwicklungsgeschichte des Menschen* (Jena, 1905).

Miller, M.D., *Wunderlich's Salute* (New York, 1985).

Miller Lane, B., *Architecture and Politics in Germany, 1880–1940* (Cambridge, 1968).

Milles, D. and R. Müller (eds.), *Berufsarbeit und Krankheit* (Frankfurt-on-Main, 1985).

Mitscherlich, A. and F. Mielke, *Medizin ohne Menschlichkeit* (Frankfurt-on-Main, 1978); 1st edn as *Das Diktat der Menschenverachtung* (Heidelberg, 1947).

Mocek, R., *Wilhelm Roux-Hans Driesch* (Jena, 1974).

Möllers, B., *Robert Koch* (Hanover, 1950).

Mombert, P., *Studien zur Bevölkerungsbewegung in Deutschland in den letzten Dezennien* (Karlsruhe, 1907).

Mommsen, W., *Max Weber und die Deutsche Politik* (Tübingen, 1979).

Morel, B.A., *Traité des dégénérescences physiques, intellectuelles et morales de l'espèce humaine* (Paris, 1857).

Morgan, A.E., *Edward Bellamy* (New York, 1944).

Moses, J., *Arbeitslosigkeit. Ein Problem der Gesundheit* (Berlin, 1931).

Mosse, G.L., 'The Image of the Jew in German Popular Culture: Felix Dahn and Gustav Freytag', *Leo Baeck Institute YearBook*, vol. 2 (1957), 218–27.

The Crisis of German Ideology (New York, 1964).

Toward the Final Solution. A History of European Racism (London, 1978).

Nationalism and Sexuality. Respectability and Abnormal Sexuality in Modern Europe (New York, 1985).

Muckermann, H., 'Wesen der Eugenik und Aufgaben der Gegenwart', *Das kommende Geschlecht*, vol. 5 no. 1–2 (1929), 1–48.

Zum Problem erblicher Belastung (Berlin, 1951).

Mühlen, P. von zur, *Rassenideologien. Geschichte und Hintergründe* (Bonn, 1977).

Müller-Hill, B., *Tödliche Wissenschaft* (Reinbek bei Hamburg, 1984). English trans. by G. Fraser as: *Murderous Science. Elimination by Scientific Selection of Jews, Gypsies and Others: Germany 1933–1945* (Oxford, 1988).

Nachtsheim, H., 'Der V. Internationale Kongress für Vererbungswissenschaft', *Die Naturwissenschaften*, vol. 15 (1927), 989–95.

Für und Wider die Sterilisierung aus Eugenischer Indikation (Stuttgart, 1952).

'Die Notwendigkeit einer aktiven Erbgesundheitspflege', *Gesundheitspolitik*, vol. 21 (1964), 321–39.

Nadav, D.S., *Julius Moses und die Politik der Sozialhygiene in Deutschland* (Gerlingen, 1985).

Nemitz, K., 'Julius Moses und die Gebärstreik-Debatte 1913', *Jahrbuch des Instituts für Deutsche Geschichte*, vol. 2 (1978), 321–35.

'Antisemitismus in der Wissenschaftspolitik der Weimarer Republik. Der "Fall Ludwig Schemann"', *Jahrbuch des Instituts für Deutsche Geschichte*, vol. 12 (1983), 377–407.

Neuman, R.P., 'Working Class Birth Control in Wilhelmine Germany', *Comparative Studies in Social History*, vol. 20 (1975), 408–28.

Newman, E., *The Life of Richard Wagner*, 4 vols. (Cambridge, 1976).

Nieden-Rohwinkel, W. zur, 'Die Tuberkulosefürsorge in den Landkreisen der Rheinprovinz', *Schmollers Jahrbuch*, vol. 37 part 1 (1913), 103–18.

Niewyk, D.L., *The Jews in Weimar Germany* (Manchester, 1980).

Noakes, J., 'Nazism and Eugenics: the Background to the Nazi Sterilisation Law of 14 July 1933', in B.J. Bullen *et al.* (eds.), *Ideas into Politics* (London, 1984), pp. 75–94.

'Wohin gehören die "Judenmischlinge"? Die Entstehung der ersten Durchführungsverordnungen zu den Nürnberger Gesetzen', in U. Büttner (ed.), *Das Unrechtsregime* (Hamburg, 1986).

Noakes, J. and G. Pridham (ed.), *Nazism 1919–1945. A Documentary Reader* (Exeter, 1988), III.

Nordau, M., *Die conventionellen Lügen der Kulturmenschheit* (Leipzig, 1883).
  Degeneration (London, 1895).
Nossig, A., *Einführung in das Studium der Sozialen Hygiene* (Stuttgart, 1894).
Nowacki, B., *Der Bund für Mutterschutz. (1905–1933)* (Husum, 1983).
Nowak, K., *'Euthanasie' und Sterilisierung im 'Dritten Reich'*, 3rd edn (Göttingen, 1984).
Nyiszli, M., *Auschwitz: a Doctor's Eye Witness Account* (New York, 1960).
Oesterlen, F., *Handbuch der Hygeiene der privaten und öffentlichen* (Tübingen, 1851), (3rd edn, 1876/77).
Offenheimer, A., *Soziale Säuglings- und Jugendfürsorge* (Leipzig, 1912).
Olberg, O., 'Rassenhygiene und Sozialismus', *Die neue Zeit*, n.s. vol. 25 no. 1 (1907), 882–7.
Ostermann, O., 'Die Eugenik im Dienste der Volkswohlfahrt', *Eugenik, Erblehre, Erbpflege*, vol. 2 (1932), 241–53.
Parlow, S., 'Über einige kolonialistische und annexionistische Aspekte bei deutschen Ärzten von 1884 bis zum Ende des 1. Weltkrieges', *Wissenschaftliche Zeitschrift der Universität Rostock*, mathematisch-naturwissenschaftliche Reihe, vol. 15 (1964), 537–49.
Paulstich, T., *Sparsamkeit und Zweckmässigkeit in der Wohlfahrts- und Gesundheitsverwaltung* (Leipzig, 1932).
Pauly, P.J., 'The Political Structure of the Brain: Cerebral Localization in Bismarckian Germany', *International Journal of Neuroscience*, vol. 21 (1983), 145–50.
Peiper, A., *Chronik der Kinderheilkunde* (Leipzig, 1951).
Peukert, D., *Volksgenossen und Gemeinschaftsfremde* (Cologne, 1982).
Pfetsch, F.R., *Zur Entwicklung der Wissenschaftspolitik in Deutschland, 1750–1914* (Berlin, 1974).
Pick, D., 'The Faces of Anarchy: Lombroso and the Politics of Criminal Science in Post-Unification Italy', *History Workshop Journal*, issue 21 (1986), pp. 60–86.
Ploetz, A., 'Rassentüchtigkeit und Socialismus', *Neue Deutsche Rundschau. Frei Bühne*, vol. 5 no. 10 (October 1894), 989–97.
  Die Tüchtigkeit unsrer Rasse und der Schutz der Schwachen. Ein Versuch über Rassenhygiene und ihr Verhältnis zu den humanen Idealen, besonders zum Socialismus (Berlin, 1895).
  'Sozialpolitik und Rassenhygiene in ihrem prinzipiellen Verhältnis', *Archiv für soziale Gesetzgebung und Statistik*, vol. 17 (1902), 393–420.
  'Der Alkohol im Lebensprozess der Rasse', *Bericht über den 9. internationalen Kongress gegen den Alkoholismus* (Jena, 1903), 1–27.
  'Die Begriffe Rasse und Gesellschaft und die davon abgeleiteten Disciplinen', *ARGB*, vol. 1 (1904), 2–26.
  'Lebensdauern der Eltern und Kindersterblichkeit', *ARGB*, vol. 6 (1909), 33–44.
  'Die Begriffe Rasse und Gesellschaft' in *Verhandlungen des Ersten Deutschen Soziologentages* (Tübingen, 1912), pp. 111–136.
  'Die Bedeutung der Frühehe für die Volkserneuerung nach dem Kriege', *MMW*, vol. 65 (1918), 452.
Poliakov, L., *The Aryan Myth. A History of Racist and Nationalist Ideas in Europe* (London, 1974).
  The History of Anti-Semitism (Oxford, 1985).
Poliakov, L. and J. Wulf, *Das Dritte Reich und seine Denker* (Frankfurt-on-Main, 1983).
Pommerin, R., *Sterilisierung der Rheinlandsbastarde* (Cologne, 1979).
Poore, C., 'Der Krüppel in der Orthopädie der Weimarer Zeit. Medizinische Konzepte als Wegbereiter der Euthanasie', *Argument*, Sonderband 113 (1984), 67–78.
Prinzing, F., *Epidemics Resulting from Wars* (Oxford, 1916).
Proctor, R.N., *Racial Hygiene. Medicine Under the Nazis* (Cambridge, Mass., and London, 1988).

Pross, C. and R. Winau (eds.), *Nicht Misshandeln. Das Krankenhaus Moabit* (Berlin, 1984).

Puhle, H.-J., *Agrarische Interessenpolitik und preussischer Konservatismus im wilhelminischen Reich (1893–1914)* (Hanover, 1967).

Pütter, E., 'Wie ich dazu kam, vor 25 Jahren die erste Lungenfürsorgestelle in Halle a.S. zu begründen, und wie ich sie einrichtete', in K.H. Blümel (ed.), *Handbuch der Tuberkulose-Fürsorge* (Munich, 1926).

Rammstedt, O., *Deutsche Soziologie 1933–1945* (Frankfurt-on-Main, 1986).

Ratz, U., *Sozialreform und Arbeiterschaft. Die "Gesellschaft für soziale Reform" und die sozialdemokratische Arbeiterbewegung* (Berlin, 1980).

Recker, M.-L., *Nationalsozialistische Sozialpolitik im Zweiten Weltkrieg* (Munich, 1985).

Reclam, C., 'Die heutige Gesundheitspflege und ihre Aufgaben', *Deutsche Vierteljahrsschrift für öffentliche Gesundheitspflege*, vol. 1 (1869), 1–5.

Reibmayr, A., *Die Ehe Tuberculöser und ihre Folgen* (Vienna, 1894).

Reulecke, J., *Geschichte der Urbanisierung in Deutschland* (Frankfurt-on-Main, 1985).

Ribot, T., *Contemporary English Psychology* (London, 1873).

Heredity: A Psychological Study of Its Phenomena, Laws, Causes and Consequences (London, 1875).

Richter, G., *Blindheit und Eugenik (1918–1945)* (Freiburg, 1986).

Riffel, A., *Erblichkeit der Schwindsucht und tuberkulöser Prozesse* (Karlsruhe, 1891).

Ripley, W.S., *The Races of Europe: A Sociological Study* (New York, 1899).

Rissom, R., *Fritz Lenz und die Rassenhygiene* (Husum, 1983).

Roberts, J.S., *Drink, Temperance and the Working Class in Nineteenth-Century Germany* (Boston, 1984).

Rodriguez Ocana, E., 'La Academia de Higiene Social de Düsseldorf (1920–1933) y el Proceso de Constitucion de la Medicina Social como Especialidad en Alemania', *Dynamis*, vol. 3 (1983), 231–64.

Röhl, J.C.G., *Philipp Eulenburgs politische Korrespondenz* (Boppard, 1976).

Rohner, H., *Die ersten 30 Jahre des medizinischen Frauenstudiums an der Universität Zürich* (Zürich, 1972).

Roll-Hansen, N., 'Eugenics before World War II. The Case of Norway', *History and Philosophy of the Life Sciences*, vol. 2 (1980), 269–98.

Ronsin, F., *La grève des ventres* (Paris, 1978).

Rosen, G., *From Medical Police to Social Medicine* (New York, 1974).

Rosenbach, O., *Grundlagen, Aufgaben und Grenzen der Therapie* (Berlin, 1891).

Roth, K.-H. (ed.), *Erfassung zur Vernichtung. Von der Sozialhygiene zum "Gesetz über Sterbehilfe"* (Berlin, 1984).

Roth, K.-H. and G. Aly, 'Das "Gesetz über Sterbehilfe bei unheilbaren Kranken"', in Roth (ed.), *Erfassung*, pp. 109–79.

Rüdin, E., *Über die klinischen Formen der Gefängnispsychosen* (Berlin, 1901).

'Zur Rolle der Homosexuellen im Lebensprozess der Rasse', *ARGB*, vol. 1 no. 1 (1904), 99–109.

'Einige Wege und Ziele der Familienforschung mit Rücksicht auf die Psychiatrie', *Zeitschrift für die gesamte Neurologie und Psychiatrie*, vol. 7 (1911), 487–585.

Zur Vererbung und Neuentstehung geistiger Störungen (Jena, 1912).

'Psychiatrische Indikation zur Sterilisierung', *Das kommende Geschlecht*, vol. 5 no. 3 (1929), 1–19.

Rüdin, E. (ed.), *Erblehre und Rassenhygiene im völkischen Staat* (Munich, 1934).

Rüdin, P., *Beitrag zur Extrauteringravidität und deren Behandlung* (Zürich, 1890).

Runge, W., *Politik und Beamte im Parteienstaat* (Stuttgart, 1968).

Ruppin, A., *Darwinismus und Sozialwissenschaft* (Jena, 1903).

Rürup, R., 'Emancipation and Crisis. The "Jewish Question" in Germany 1850–1890', *Leo Baeck Institute Year Book*, vol. 20 (1975), 13–25.

Ruttgers, J., *Rassenverbesserung, Malthusianismus und Neo-malthusianismus* (Dresden and Leipzig, 1908).

Sablik, K., *Julius Tandler. Mediziner und Sozialreformer* (Vienna, 1983).

Sächsicher Landesgesundheitsrat, *Einrichtungen auf dem Gebiete der Volksgesundheits- und Volkswohlfahrtspflege* (Dresden, 1922).

Sachsse, C., *Mütterlichkeit als Beruf* (Frankfurt-on-Main, 1986).

Sachsse, C. and F. Tennstedt (eds.), *Soziale Sicherheit und soziale Disziplinierung* (Frankfurt-on-Main, 1986).

Saller, K., *Die Entstehung der 'nordische' Rasse* (Kiel, 1926).

Die Rassenlehre des Nationalsozialismus in Wissenschaft und Propaganda (Darmstadt, 1961).

Saul, K., 'Der Kampf um die Jugend zwischen Volksschule und Kaserne', *Militärgeschichtliche Mitteilungen*, vol. 10 (1971), 97–143.

Schalk, E., *Der Wettkampf der Völker mit besonderer Bezugnahme auf Deutschland und die Vereinigten Staaten von Nordamerika* (Jena, 1905).

Schallmayer, W., *Über die drohende physische Entartung der Culturvölker*, 2nd edn (Neuwied, 1895).

'Infektion als Morgengabe', *Zeitschrift für die Bekämpfung der Geschlechtskrankheiten*, vol. 2 (1904), 389–419.

'Selektive Gesichtspunkte zur generativen und kulturellen Völkerentwicklung' *Schmollers Jahrbuch*, vol. 30 (1906), 421–69.

Schaxel, J., *Entwicklung der Wissenschaft vom Leben* (Jena, 1924).

Scheele, I., *Von Lüben bis Schmeil. Die Entwicklung von der Schulnaturgeschichte zum Biologieunterricht zwischen 1830 und 1933* (Berlin, 1981).

Schemann, L., *Lebensfahrten eines Deutschen* (Leipzig, 1925).

Die Rasse in den Geisteswissenschaften, 3 vols. (Munich, 1928–32).

Scheumann, F.K., (with foreword by Krohne), *Eheberatung. Einrichtung, Betrieb und Bedeutung für die biologische Erwachsenenberatung* (Berlin, 1928).

Eheberatung als Aufgabe der Kommunen (Leipzig, 1932).

Schmidt, G., *Die literarischen Rezeption des Darwinismus* (Berlin, 1974).

Schmidt, J., 'Jakob von Uexküll und Houston Stewart Chamberlain. Ein Briefwechsel in Auszügen', *Medizinhistorisches Journal*, vol. 10 (1975), 121–9.

Schmincke, S., *Das Gesundheitswesen Neukölln* (Berlin, 1929).

Schmitz, S., *Adolf Neisser* (Düsseldorf, 1968).

Schmuhl, H.W., *Rassenhygiene, Nationalsozialismus, Euthanasie* (Göttingen, 1987).

Schneck, P., 'Die Entwicklung der Eugenik als soziale Bewegung in der Epoche des Imperialismus', Dietl (ed.), *Eugenik*, pp. 24–58.

'Wilhelm Liepmann (1878–1939) und die soziale Gynäkologie im Spiegel der Aktenbestände des Archivs der Humboldt-Universität zu Berlin', *NTM*, vol. 17 (1980), 102–20.

Schneider, W.H., 'Towards the Improvement of the Human Race: The History of Eugenics in France', *Journal of Modern History*, vol. 54 (1982), 268–91.

'Chance and Social Setting in the Application of the Discovery of Blood Groups', *Bulletin of the History of Medicine*, vol. 57 (1983), 545–62.

Schreiber, B., *The Men Behind Hitler* (London, nd).

Schreiber, G., *Deutsches Reich und Deutsche Medizin. Studien zur Medizinalpolitik des Reiches in der Nachkriegszeit (1918–1926)* (Leipzig, 1926).

Schriftenreihe zur Geschichte der Kinderheilkunde aus dem Archiv des Kaiserin Auguste Viktoria Hauses (KAVH) – Berlin, nos. 1–4 (1986–87).

Schroeder-Gudehus, B., 'The Argument for Self-Government and Public Support of

Science in Weimar Germany', *Minerva*, vol. 10 (1972), 537–70.

Schüler, W., *Der Bayreuther Kreis von seiner Entstehung bis zum Ausgang der wilhelminischen Ära* (Münster, 1971).

Schungel, W., *Alexander Tille. Leben und Ideen eines Sozialdarwinisten* (Husum, 1980).

Searle, G., *The Quest for National Efficiency* (Oxford, 1971).

Eugenics in Britain, 1900–1914 (Leyden, 1976).

Seeberg, R., *Der Geburtenrückgang in Deutschland: eine sozialethische Studie* (Leipzig, 1913).

Seidler, H. and A. Rett, *Das Reichssippenamt entscheidet. Rassenbiologie in Nationalsozialismus* (Vienna and Munich, 1982).

Sheehan, J.J. (ed.), *Imperial Germany* (New York, 1976).

German Liberalism in the Nineteenth Century (1978; London, 1982).

Shoen, E., *Emil Abderhalden* (Halle, 1952).

Shorter, E., 'Medizinische Theorien spezifisch weiblicher Nervenkrankheiten im Wandel' in A. Labisch and R. Spree (eds.), *Medizinische Deutungsmacht im Wandel* (Bonn, 1989).

Sohnrey, H., *Wegweiser für ländliche Wohlfahrts- und Heimatpflege* (Berlin, 1900).

Sommer, R., *Familienforschung und Vererbungslehre* (Leipzig, 1911).

Sontheimer, E., *Antidemokratisches Denken in der Weimarer Republik* (München, 1962, reprinted 1978).

Spree, R., 'Sozialisationsnormen in ärztlichen Ratgebern zur Säuglings- und Kleinkinderpflege. Von der Aufklärungs- zur naturwissenschaftlichen Pädiatrie', in J. Martin and A. Nitschke (eds.), *Zur Sozialgeschichte der Kindheit* (Freiburg and Munich, 1986), pp. 609–59.

Soziale Ungleichheit vor Krankheit und Tod (Göttingen, 1981). English edn translated by S. McKinnon-Evans and J. Halliday as: *Health and Social Class in Imperial Germany* (Oxford, 1988).

Stachura, P.D. (ed.), *Unemployment and the Great Depression in Weimar Germany* (Basingstoke, 1986).

The German Youth Movement (London, 1981).

Steakley, J.D., *The Homosexual Emancipation Movement in Germany* (New York, 1975).

Steinmetz, M., *Geschichte der Universität Jena*, 2 vols. (Jena, 1958).

Stenson, G.P., *Karl Kautsky 1854–1938* (Pittsburgh, 1978).

Stephenson, J., '"Reichsbund der Kinderreichen": the League of Large Families in the Population Policy of Nazi Germany', *European Studies Review*, vol. 9 (1979), 350–75.

The Nazi Organisation of Women (London, 1981).

Still, G.F., *Common Disorders and Diseases of Childhood* (London, 1912).

Stöcker, H., *Die Liebe und die Frauen* (Minden, 1906).

Stoeckel, W., *Erinnerungen eines Frauenarztes* (Leipzig, 1980).

Stollberg, G., 'Die Naturheilvereine im Deutschen Kaiserreich', *Archiv für Sozialgeschichte*, vol. 28 (1988), 287–305.

Stroka, A., *Carl Hauptmann's Werdegang als Denker und Dichter* (Wroclaw, 1965).

Strubel, K., W. Tetzner and W. Piechocki, *Zur Geschichte der Gründung des Zweigvereins zur Bekämpfung der Schwindsucht in der Stadt Halle am 15. Juni 1899* (Halle, 1974).

Stubbe, H., *Geschichte des Instituts für Kulturpflanzenforschung Gatersleben* (Berlin, 1982).

Stümke, H.-G. and R. Finkler, *Rosa Winkel, Rosa Listen* (Reinbek bei Hamburg, 1981).

Stürzbecher, M., 'Adolf Gottstein als Gesundheitspolitiker', *Medizinische Monatsschrift* (1959), 374–9.

'Zur Geschichte von Mutterschutz und Frühsterblichkeit', *Gesundheitspolitik*, vol. 8 (1966), 227–40.

100 Jahre Berliner Krippenverein (Berlin, 1977).

'Aus der Geschichte des Charlottenburger Gesundheitswesens', *Bär von Berlin* (1980), 43–113.

'Von den Berliner Stadtmedizinalräten, Stadtmedizinaldirektoren und Senatsdirektoren für das Gesundheitswesen', *Berliner-Aerzteblatt*, vol. 94 (1981), 789–90.

Teitelbaum, M.S. and J.M. Winter, *The Fear of Population Decline* (New York, 1985).

Teleky, L., 'Geschichtliches, Biographisches, Autobiographisches', Lesky (ed.), *Sozialmedizin*, pp. 355–70.

Tennstedt, F., 'Sozialismus, Lebensreform und Krankenkassenbewegung. Friedrich Landmann und Raphael Friedeberg als Ratgeber der Krankenkassen', *Soziale Sicherheit*, vol. 26 (1977), 210–14, 306–10, 332–6.

'Alfred Blaschko – das wissenschaftliche und sozialpolitische Wirken eines menschenfreundlichen Sozialhygienikers im Deutschen Reich', *Zeitschrift für Sozialreform*, vol. 25 (1979), 513–23, 600–14, 646–67.

'Arbeiterbewegung und Familiengeschichte bei Eduard Bernstein und Ignaz Zadek', *IWK*, vol. 18 (1982), 451–81.

Vom Proleten zum Industriearbeiter (Cologne, 1985).

Theilhaber, F.A., *Der Untergang der deutschen Juden: eine volkswirtschaftliche Studie* (Munich, 1911).

Das sterile Berlin. Eine volkswirtschaftliche Studie (Berlin, 1913).

Theweleit, K. *Männerphantasien* (Reinbek bei Hamburg, 1980).

Thom, A. and H. Spaar (eds.), *Medizin im Faschismus* (Berlin, 1983), new edn (Berlin, 1985).

Thomann, K.-D., *Alfons Fischer (1873–1936) und die Badische Gesellschaft für Sozialhygiene* (Cologne, 1980).

'Das Reichsgesundheitsamt und die Rassenhygiene', *Bundesgesundheitsblatt*, vol. 26 (1983), 206–13.

'Otmar Freiherr von Verschuer – ein Hauptvertreter der faschistischen Rassenhygiene', in Thom and Spaar (eds.), *Medizin im Faschismus*, pp. 38–41.

'Rassenhygiene und Anthropologie: Die zwei Karrieren des Prof. Verschuer', *Frankfurter Rundschau*, no. 116 (21 May 1985).

Thomas, R.H., *Nietzsche in German Politics and Society 1890–1918* (Manchester, 1985).

Tille, A., *Volksdienst – Von einem Sozialaristokraten* (Berlin and Leipzig, 1893).

Tönnies, A., 'Eugenik', *Schmollers Jahrbuch*, vol. 29 (1905), 1089–106.

'Zur naturwissenschaftichen Gesellschaftslehre', *Schmollers Jahrbuch*, vol. 29 (1905), 27–101, 1283–321; vol. 30 (1906), 121–46.

'Zur naturwissenschaftlichen Gesellschaftslehre. Eine Replik', *Schmollers Jahrbuch*, vol. 33 (1907), 487–552.

Töpner, K., *Gelehrte Politiker und politisierende Gelehrte. Die Revolution von 1918 im Urteil deutscher Hochschullehrer* (Göttingen, 1970).

Tröhler, U. and Maehle, A.-H., 'Anti-vivisection in Nineteenth-Century Germany and Switzerland: Motives and Methods', in N. Rupke (ed.), *Vivisection in Historical Perspective* (London, 1987), pp. 149–87.

Trüb, C.L.P., *Die Terminologie und Definition Sozialmedizin und Sozialhygiene in den literarischen Sekundärquellen der Jahre 1900 bis 1960* (Opladen, 1964).

Tutzke, D., 'Alfred Grotjahns Verhältnis zur Sozialdemokratie', *Zeitschrift für ärztliche Fortbildung*, vol. 54 (1960), 1183–7.

Alfred Grotjahn (Leipzig, 1979).

Uexküll, J. v., *H.S. Chamberlain. Natur und Leben* (Munich, 1928).

Unger, H., *Sendung und Gewissen* (Berlin, 1936).

Usborne, C., 'The Christian Churches and the Regulation of Sexuality in Weimar Germany', in J. Obelkevitch, L. Roper and K. Samuel (eds.), *Disciplines of Faith* (London, 1987), pp. 99–112.

'Abortion in Weimar Germany – the Discourse among the Medical Profession', unpublished MS.

Uschmann, G., *Geschichte der Zoologie und der zoologischen Anstalten in Jena 1779–1919* (Jena, 1959).

Ernst Haeckel. Eine Biographie in Briefen (Leipzig, 1983).

Vader, J.P., 'August Forel Defends the Persecuted Persian Baha' in 1925–27', *Gesnerus*, vol. 41 (1984), 53–60.

Verschuer, O. v., 'Rasse' in *Deutsche Politik, ein völkisches Handbuch* (Frankfurt-on-Main, 1925).

Sozialpolitik und Rassenhygiene (Langensalza, 1928).

Erbpathologie. Ein Lehrbuch für Ärzte (Dresden and Leipzig, 1934).

Erbananlage als Schicksal und Aufgabe (Berlin, 1944).

'Eugen Fischer', *Der Erbarzt*, vol. 12 (1944), 57–9.

Verworn, M., *Biologische Richtlinien der staatlichen Organisation* (Bonn, 1917).

Aphorismen (Jena, 1922).

Virchow, R., 'Ueber gewisse, die Gesundheit benachteiligende Einflüsse der Schulen', *Archiv für pathologische Anatomie und Physiologie und für klinische Medicin*, vol. 46 (1869), 447–70.

'Ueber die Methode der wissenschaftlichen Anthropologie', *Zeitschrift für Ethnologie*, vol. 4 (1872), 300–20.

'Die Freiheit der Wissenschaft in modernen Staat', *Amtlicher Bericht der 50. Versammlung deutscher Naturforscher und Aerzte in München* (1877), 65–77.

'The Founding of the Berlin University and the Transition from the Philosophic to the Scientific Age', *Annual Report of the Board of Regents of the Smithsonian Institution to July 1894* (Washington, 1896), pp. 681–95.

Vogel, M. (ed.), *Der Mensch* (Leipzig, 1930).

Volk & Gesundheit. Heilen & Vernichten im Nationalsozialismus (Tübingen, 1982).

Wall, R. and J. Winter (eds.), *The Upheaval of War. Family, Work and Welfare in Europe 1914–1918* (Cambridge, 1988).

Wallace, A.R., 'Menschliche Auslese', *Hardens Zukunft*, vol. 8 no. 93 (7 July 1894), 10–24.

Walser, H.H., *August Forel – Briefe, Correspondance 1864–1927* (Bern, 1968).

Ward Richardson, B., *Hygeia – a City of Health* (London, 1876).

Weber, E. v., *Die Folterkammern der Wissenschaft* (Berlin and Leipzig, 1879).

Wehler, H.-U., 'Sozialdarwinismus im expandierenden Industriestaat', in I. Geiss and B.J. Wendt (eds.), *Deutschland in der Weltpolitik des 19. and 20. Jahrhunderts* (Düsseldorf, 1974), pp. 138–42.

Weinberg, G.L. (ed.), *Hitlers Zweites Buch. Ein Dokument aus dem Jahr 1928* (Stuttgart, 1961).

Weinberg, W., *Die Kinder der Tuberkulösen, mit einem Begleitwort von Obermedizinalrat Professor Max von Gruber* (Leipzig, 1913).

Weindling, P.J., 'Theories of the Cell State in Imperial Germany', in C. Webster (ed.), *Biology, Medicine and Society 1840–1940* (Cambridge, 1981), pp. 99–155.

'Shattered Alternatives in Medicine. [Essay Review of the Verschütteten Alternativen Project]', *History Workshop Journal*, issue 16 (1983), 152–7.

'Die Preussische Medizinalverwaltung und die "Rassenhygiene"', in Thom and Spaar (eds.), *Medizin und Faschismus*, pp. 23–35, new edn (Berlin, 1985), pp. 48–56; extended version as 'Die Preussische Medizinalverwaltung und die Rassenhygiene. Anmerkun-

gen zur Gesundheitspolitik der Jahre 1905–1933', *Zeitschrift für Sozialreform*, vol. 30 (1984), 675–87.
'Was Social Medicine Revolutionary? Virchow on Famine and Typhus in 1848', *Bulletin of the Society for the Social History of Medicine*, no. 34 (1984), 13–18.
'Soziale Hygiene, Eugenik und medizinische Praxis: Der Fall Alfred Grotjahn', *Das Argument. Jahrbuch für kritische Medizin*, no. 119 (1984), 6–20.
'Blood, Race and Politics', *Times Higher Educational Supplement* (19 July 1985).
From Bacteriology to Social Hygiene. Handlist of the Papers of Martin Hahn (Oxford, 1985).
'Weimar Eugenics: The Kaiser Wilhelm Institute for Anthropology, Human Heredity and Eugenics in Social Context', *Annals of Science*, vol. 42 (1985), 303–18.
'Medicine and Modernization: the Social History of German Health and Medicine', *History of Science*, vol. 24 (1986), 277–301.
'German–Soviet Co-operation in Science. The Case of the Laboratory for Racial Research 1931–1938', *Nuncius*, vol. 1 (1987), 103–9.
'Compulsory Sterilization in National Socialist Germany', *German History*, no. 5 (1987), 10–24.
'Medical Practice in Imperial Berlin: The Casebook of Alfred Grotjahn', *Bulletin of the History of Medicine*, vol. 61 (1987), 391–440.
'From Philanthropy to International Science Policy. Rockefeller Funding of Biomedical Sciences in Germany 1920–1940', in N. Rupke (ed.), *Science, Politics and the Public Good. Essays in Honour of Margaret Gowing* (Basingstoke, 1988).
Darwinism and Social Darwinism in Imperial Germany: the Contribution of the Cell Biologist Oscar Hertwig (1849–1922) (Stuttgart, 1989).
'The Medical Profession, Social Hygiene and the Birth Rate in Germany 1914–1918', in Wall and Winter (eds.), *Upheaval of War*, 417–38.
Ernst Haeckel and the Secularization of Nature', in J. Moore (ed.), *History, Humanity and Evolution*, (Cambridge, 1989), 311–27.
'Fascism and Population Policies in Comparative European Perspective', in M. Teitelbaum and J. Winter (eds.), *Population, Resources and the Environment: the Interplay of Science, Ideology and Intellectual Traditions* (Cambridge, in press). Also in *Population and Development Review*, vol. 14 supplement (1989), 102–21.
'Hygienepolitik als sozialintegrative Strategie im späten Deutschen Kaiserreich', in A. Labisch and R. Spree (eds.), *Medizinische Deutungsmacht im Sozialen Wandel* (Bonn, in press).
Weindling, P.J., (ed.), *The Social History of Occupational Health* (London, 1985).
Weingart, P., 'Eugenic Utopias – Blueprints for the Rationalization of Human Evolution', *Sociology of the Sciences*, (1984), 173–87.
Weingart, P., J. Kroll and K. Bayertz, *Rasse, Blut und Gene. Geschichte der Eugenik und Rassenhygiene in Deutschland* (Frankfurt-on-Main, 1988).
Weinhandl, F. (ed.), *Gestalthaftes Sehen* (Darmstadt, 1974).
Weinreich, M., *Hitler's Professors. The Part of Scholarship in Germany's Crimes Against the Jewish People* (New York, 1946).
Weiser, J., 'Quellen zur Geschichte der Medizin und der Medizinalverwaltung in der Historischen Abteilung II des Deutschen Zentralarchivs', *NTM*, vol. 8 (1971), 82–91.
Weismann, A., *The Evolution Theory* (London, 1904).
Vorträge über Deszendenztheorie, 3rd edn (Jena, 1913).
Weiss, S., 'The Race Hygiene Movement in Germany', *Osiris*, 2nd series vol. 3 (1987), 193–236.
Race, Hygiene and National Efficiency (Berkeley and London, 1988).

Weizsäcker, V. v., *Soziale Krankheit und soziale Gesundung* (Berlin, 1930).

Wendel, G., *Die Kaiser-Wilhelm-Gesellschaft 1911–1914* (Berlin, 1975).

Westenhöfer, M., *Die Aufgaben der Rassenhygiene (des Nachkommenschutzes) im neuen Deutschland. Vortrag gehalten am 27. Februar 1919 in der Berliner Gesellschaft für Rassenhygiene* (Berlin, 1920), (= Veröffentlichungen aus dem Gebiete der Medizinal-verwaltung vol. 10 no. 2).

Weyl, T., *Soziale Hygiene* (Jena, 1904).

Whalen, R., *Bitter Wounds. German Victims of the Great War 1914–1939* (Ithaca and London, 1984).

Whyte, I.B., *Bruno Taut and the Architecture of Activism* (Cambridge, 1982).

Willett, S., *The New Society* (London, 1982).

Windorfer, A., and R. Schlenk, *Die Deutsche Gesellschaft für Kinderheilkunde* (Berlin, 1978).

Winter, I., 'Geschichte der Gesundheitspolitik der KPD in der Weimarer Republik', *Zeitschrift für ärztliche Fortbildung*, vol. 67 (1973), 455–72, 498–526.

Wolf, E., '"... nichts weiter als eben einen unmittelbaren persönlichen Nutzen ...". Zur Entstehung und Ausbreitung der homöopatischen Laienbewegung', *Jahrbuch des Instituts für Geschichte der Medizin der Robert Bosch Stiftung*, vol. 4 (1985), 61–97.

Wolf, F., *Aufsätze 1919–1944* (Berlin, 1967).

Wolf, J., *Der Geburtenrückgang* (Jena, 1912).

'Der Geburtenrückgang und seine Bekämpfung', *Berliner Klinische Wochenschrift*, vol. 49 (1912), 2297–301, 2351–4.

Wolff, C., *Magnus Hirschfeld* (London, 1986).

Woltmann, L. and H.K.E. Buhmann, 'Naturwissenschaft und Politik. Zur Einführung', *Politisch-anthropologische Revue*, vol. 1 (1902), 1–2.

Wunderlich, P., 'Arthur Schlossmann und seine Bemühungen um die Anerkennung der Kinderheilkunde in Dresden, 1893 bis 1906', *Beiträge zur Geschichte der Universität Erfurt*, vol. 12 (1965–66), 167–80.

Wuttke-Groneberg, W., *Medizin im Nationalsozialismus. Ein Arbeitsbuch* (Tübingen, 1980).

Young, E.J., *Gobineau und der Rassismus* (Meisenheim, 1968).

Zadek, I., *Die Arbeiterversicherung. Eine social-hygienische Kritik* (Jena, 1895).

Ziegler, H.E., *Die Naturwissenschaft und die Socialdemokratische Theorie. Die Verhältnisse dargelegt auf Grund der Werke von Darwin und Bebel* (Stuttgart, 1893).

'Ueber die Beziehungen der Zoologie zur Sociologie', *Verhandlungen der Deutschen Zoologischen Gesellschaft* (1893), vol. 3, 51–5.

Der Begriff des Instinktes einst und jetzt (Jena, 1920).

Ziegler, H.E., and E. Bresslau, *Zoologisches Wörterbuch*, 2nd edn (Jena, 1912).

Zirnstein, G., 'Zur gesellschaftlichen Stellung der wissenschaftlichen Pflanzenzüchtung in Deutschland während der zwanziger und dreissiger Jahre des 20. Jahrhundert', *NTM*, vol. 9 (1972), 60–9.

Zmarzlik, H.-G., 'Der Sozialdarwinismus als geschichtliches Problem', *Vierteljahreshefte für Zeitgeschichte*, vol. 11 (1963), 246–73.

Zuelzer, W., *The Nicolai Case* (Detroit, 1982).

INDEX

I wish to thank Ingrid Canning, Jean Loudon, Jill Paterson, Elizabeth Peretz and Ursula Slevogt for help in preparation of the index and text.

Index